A Guide to Success
Review for Licensure in Physical Therapy

Scott M. Giles M.S., P.T.

Clinical Assistant Professor
Department of Physical Therapy
University of New England
Biddeford, Maine

Copyright © 2002
ISBN 1890989-12-6

The enclosed material is the exclusive property of Mainely Physical Therapy. No part of this publication may be reproduced or transmitted, in any form, without the express written consent of Mainely Physical Therapy.

For additional information on our review texts and software for physical therapists and physical therapist assistants, please contact Mainely Physical Therapy.

Mainely Physical Therapy
P.O. Box 7242
Scarborough, Maine 04070-7242

Phone: (207) 885-0304
Toll Free: (866) PTEXAMS
Fax: (207) 883-8377
Web site: www.ptexams.com
email: ptexams@cybertours.com

Acknowledgments

Contributors

I would like to thank my wife Therese from the bottom of my heart for her many valuable contributions during the entire project. Her clinical expertise and willingness to create, edit, and revise various facets of the new edition were invaluable. Thank you for being my teammate and best friend. I love you.

Special Thanks

To my children Meghan, Erin, and Alexander. Thanks for tolerating the many long nights when Dad had to do "work." You are all an ongoing source of inspiration for me. Love always.

Special thanks to Gwenn Hoyt for her dedication to this project, attention to detail, and creative flair. It was a pleasure working with you!

I would like to offer my sincere thanks to Jerry Amash, Laura Anderson, Pauline Boyce, Shauna DeTurk, and Kathy Lavigne for their dedication and numerous contributions to this project.

Table of Contents

Academic Review

Introduction 1

Unit 1: Foundational Science 3

Anatomy and Physiology 3
    Joint Classification 3
    Specific Joints 3
    Joint Receptors 4
    Muscle Action 5
    Nerve Root Dermatomes, Myotomes, Reflexes, and Paresthetic Areas 7
    Nerves of the Brachial Plexus 9
    Lower Extremity Innervation 9

Neuroanatomy 10
    Cranial Nerves and Methods of Testing 10

Kinesiology 11
    Planes of the Body 11
    Classes of Levers 11

Exercise Physiology 11
    Energy Systems 11
        Anaerobic Metabolism 11
        Aerobic Metabolism 12
    Muscle Physiology 12
        Classification of Muscle Fibers 12
        Functional Characteristics of Muscle Fibers 12
        Muscle Receptors 12
    Resistive Training 12
        Types of Muscular Contraction 12
        Open-Chain versus Closed-Chain Activities 12
        Resistive and Overload Training 12
        Exercise Programs 13

Psychological Disorders 13
    Affective Disorders 13
    Neuroses Disorders 13
    Dissociative Disorders 14
    Somatoform Disorders 14
    Schizophrenia Disorders 14
    Personality Disorders 14

Psychiatric Medications 15
    Antianxiety 15
    Antidepressants 15
    Antipsychotics 15
    Sedatives-Hypnotics 15

Unit 2: Musculoskeletal 17

Orthopedics 17
    Examination 17
        Screening 17
            Upper Quarter Screening 17
            Lower Quarter Screening 17
            Scanning Examination to Rule Out Referral of Other Symptoms from Other Tissues 18
        Posture 19
            Good and Faulty Posture: Summary Chart 19

- Positioning of a Joint 21
  - Descriptions of Specific Positions 21
  - Resting (Loose Packed) Position of Joints 21
  - Close Packed Position of Joints 21
  - Common Capsular Patterns of Joints 21
  - End-Feel 22
- Muscle Testing 22
  - Manual Muscle Testing Grades 22
  - Recommended Positioning for Muscle Testing 23
- Gait 23
  - Standard versus Rancho Los Amigos Terminology 23
  - Standard Terminology 23
  - Rancho Los Amigos Terminology 24
  - Normal Gait 24
  - Range of Motion Requirements for Normal Gait 25
  - Peak Muscle Activity during the Gait Cycle 25
  - Gait Terminology 25
  - Abnormal Gait Patterns 25
  - Gait Deviations 26
- Range of Motion 27
  - Average Adult Range of Motion for the Upper and Lower Extremities 27
  - Process for Conducting Goniometric Measurements 27
  - Goniometric Technique 28
  - Muscle Insufficiency 30
- Special Tests 31
  - Special Tests Outline 31
  - Descriptions of Special Tests 32

Intervention
- Orthotics 38
  - Types of Orthoses 38
    - Lower Extremity 38
    - Spine 39
  - Functions of Orthotics 39
  - Orthotic Considerations 39
- Orthotic Profile 39
  - Examination 39
  - Intervention 39
  - Goals 40
- Mobilization 40
  - Grades of Movement 40
  - Mobilization Technique 40
  - Convex-Concave Rule 40

Orthopedic Profile 40
- Examination 40
- Intervention 41
- Goals 41

Orthopedic Surgical Procedures 41
- Total Hip Replacement 41
- Total Knee Replacement 41

Orthopedic Pathology 42
- Rheumatism 42
  - Osteoarthritis 42
  - Rheumatoid Arthritis 43
- Types of Fractures 43

Orthopedic Terminology 44
Orthopedic Medications 45

Amputations and Prosthetics 45
    Examination 45
        Factors that Influence Vascular Disease 45
        Risk Factors for Amputation 45
        Types of Lower Extremity Amputations 45
        Types of Amputation and Considerations for Prosthetic Training 46
        Potential Complications 46
        Components of a Prosthesis 46
    Intervention 47
        Types of Postoperative Dressings 47
        Wrapping Guidelines 47
        Gait Deviations 47
    Amputation and Prosthetic Profile 48
        Examination 48
        Preprosthetic Intervention 48
        Prosthetic Intervention 49
        Preprosthetic Goals 49
        Prosthetic Goals 49

Unit 3: Neuromuscular 51
Neurology 51
    Examination 51
        Cranial Nerve Testing 51
        Upper versus Lower Motor Neuron Disease 52
        Cerebral Hemisphere Function 52
        Hemisphere Specialization/Dominance 52
        Risk Factors for Cerebrovascular Accident 53
        Types of Cerebrovascular Accidents 53
        Expected Impairment Based on Vascular Involvement 53
        Characteristics of a Cerebrovascular Accident 54
        Synergy Patterns 54
        Types of Nerve Injury 55
    Intervention 55
        Theories of Neurological Intervention 55
            Bobath – Neuromuscular Developmental Treatment 55
            Brunnstrom – Movement Therapy in Hemiplegia 55
            Kabat, Knott, and Voss – Proprioceptive Neuromuscular Facilitation 56
            Motor Control: A Task Oriented Approach 59
            Rood 60
    Neurological Profile 60
        Examination 60
        Intervention 60
        Goals 60
    Neurological Terminology 61
Spinal Cord Injury 62
    Examination 62
        Types of Spinal Cord Injury 62
        Specific Incomplete Lesions 62
    Intervention 62
        Potential Complications of Spinal Cord Injury 62
        Functional Outcomes for Complete Lesions 64
    Spinal Cord Injury Profile 67
        Examination 67
        Intervention 67
        Goals 67
    Spinal Cord Injury Terminology 67
    Spinal Cord Injury Medications 68

Traumatic Brain Injury 68
    Examination 68
        Types of Injury 68
        Acute Diagnostic Management 68
        Levels of Consciousness 68
        Glasgow Coma Scale 69
        Memory Impairments 69
        Rancho Los Amigos Levels of Cognitive Functioning 69
    Intervention 70
        Guidelines for Treatment of Brain Injury 70
    Traumatic Brain Injury Profile 70
        Examination 70
        Intervention 70
        Goals 70
    Traumatic Brain Injury Medications 71

Unit 4: Cardiopulmonary 73

Cardiac 73
    Examination 73
        Anatomy of the Heart 73
        Cardiac Conduction System 73
        Korotkoff's Sounds 73
        Cardiac Facts 73
        Common Circulatory Pulse Locations 73
        Diagnostic Tests for Cardiac Dysfunction 74
        Electrocardiogram 75
        Pathological Changes in an ECG Denoting Disease 75
        Comparisons of Right and Left-Sided Heart Failure 75
        Vital Signs 76
            Blood Pressure 76
            Heart Rate 76
            Respiratory Rate 76
        Borg's Rate of Perceived Exertion Scale 76
        Metabolic Equivalents 76
        Risk Factors for Cardiac Pathology 77
        Symptoms of Cardiac Pathology 77
        Symptoms of Myocardial Infarction 77
        Diagnosis of Myocardial Infarction 77
    Intervention 77
        Methods to Determine Exercise Intensity 77
        Cardiac Rehabilitation 77
            Indications for Cardiac Rehabilitation 77
            Description of a Cardiac Rehabilitation Program 77
            Therapist Role During Inpatient Cardiac Rehabilitation 78
            Therapist Role During Outpatient Cardiac Rehabilitation 78
        Cardiopulmonary Resuscitation Standards 78
    Cardiac Profile 79
        Examination 79
        Intervention 79
        Inpatient Goals 79
        Outpatient Goals 79
    Cardiac Pathology 79
    Cardiac Medications 80

Pulmonary 81
    Examination 81
        Pulmonary Function Testing 81
        Pulmonary Function Reference Values 81
        Gas Pressure 81
        Arterial Blood Gases 81
        Physical Signs Observed in Various Disorders 82

   Interpretation of Abnormal Acid-Base Balance 83
  Intervention 83
   Indications for Chest Physical Therapy 83
   Contraindications for Chest Physical Therapy 83
   Guidelines for Chest Physical Therapy...83
   Goals for Chest Physical Therapy...83
   Bronchial Drainage 83
   Breathing Exercises 84
  Pulmonary Profile 85
   Examination 85
   Intervention 85
   Goals 85
  Pulmonary Pathology...85
  Pulmonary Medications 86

Unit 5: Integumentary 87
 Integumentary System 87
  Key Functions of the Integumentary System 87
 Burns 87
  Examination 87
   Types of Burns..87
   Burn Classification 87
   Rule of Nines 87
    Adult Values 87
    Children Values 87
  Intervention 88
   Positioning and Splinting 88
   Topical Agents Used in Burn Care 88
   Skin Graft Procedures 88
  Burn Profile..89
   Examination 89
   Intervention 89
   Goals 89
  Burn Terminology..89

Unit 6: Patient Care Skills 91
 Patient Management 91
  Body Mechanics...91
  Patient Communication 91
  Infection Control 91
  Category-Specific Isolation Precautions 92
  Transfers 92
   Communication during Transfers 92
   Levels of Physical Assistance 92
   Types of Transfers 93
  Wheelchairs..94
   Wheelchair Facts..94
   Components of a Wheelchair 94
   Standard Wheelchair Measurements for Proper Fit 94
  Ambulation 95
   Assistive Devices..95
   Assistive Device Selection..95
   Levels of Weight Bearing 95
   Gait Patterns..96
  Accessibility...96
   Americans with Disabilities Act 96
   Accessibility Requirements 97

Laboratory/Diagnostic Testing..97
    Laboratory Testing..97
    Reference Values in Hematology 98
    Reference Values for Clinical Chemistry (Blood, Serum, Plasma) 99
    Diagnostic Tests..99
Medical Equipment 100
    Tubes, Lines, and Equipment..100

Unit 7: Physical Agents 101
Therapeutic Modalities 101
Indications for Therapeutic Modalities 101
Principles of Heat Transfer 101
Cryotherapy..101
    Ice Massage...101
    Cold Pack...101
    Cold Bath 102
    Vapocoolant Spray..102
Superficial Heating Agents 102
    Fluidotherapy..102
    Hot Pack..102
    Infrared Lamp 103
    Paraffin 103
Deep Heating Agents 103
    Diathermy 103
    Ultrasound...104
Hydrotherapy 104
    Types of Hydrotherapy 105
    Contrast Bath 105
Mechanical Agents...106
    Traction...106
    Compression...106
Additional Physical Agents..107
    Ultraviolet...107
    Biofeedback..107
    Massage 108
Electrotherapy..109
    Treatment Parameters 109
        Types of Current...109
        Electrode Configuration...109
        Electrode Size...109
    Neuromuscular Electrical Stimulation 110
    Transcutaneous Electrical Nerve Stimulation 110
    Iontophoresis..110
    Electrical Equipment Care and Maintenance 110
    Electrotherapy Terminology 110

Unit 8: Research 113
Research Basics 113
Types of Research..113
Ethical Considerations 113
Reliability...113
Validity 113
Variables 113
Levels of Measurement..114
Research Design...114
Sampling 114
Research Terminology 115

Statistics 115
    Types of Statistics 115
    Measures of Central Tendency..115
    Measures of Variation 115
    Normal Distribution 116
    Steps in Testing a Statistical Hypothesis...116
    Parametric Statistics 116
    Nonparametric Statistics 116
    Correlation 117
    Graphs..117

Unit 9: Administration 119
Documentation..119
    Purpose of Documentation 119
    Records 119
    Referrals 119
    Progress Notes 119
    Discharge Summary...119
    S.O.A.P. Notes 119
    Guidelines for Physical Therapy Documentation 120
    Symbols Commonly Used in Clinical Practice 123
    Military Time 123
    Measurement..123
Ethics...123
    Ethical Principles 123
Management..124
    Quality Management Process..124
    Quality Assurance 124
Legal 124
    Elements of a Risk Management Program..124
    Recommendations to Avoid Litigation 124
    Legal Terminology...124
Delegation and Supervision 125
    American Physical Therapy Association Direction, Delegation, and Supervision
        in Physical Therapy Services 125
    Support Personnel Supervised by Physical Therapists..125
    Health Care Professions 126
Physical Therapy Practice 128
    The Elements of Patient/Client Management Leading to Optimal Outcomes 128
    Standards of Practice for Physical Therapy and the Criteria..128
    Code of Ethics...132
    Guide for Professional Conduct 133
Health Insurance...137
    Private Health Insurance Companies 137
    Independent Health Plans..137
    Government Health Insurance...137
    Fee for Service versus Managed Care 138

Unit 10: Special Topics..139
Obstetrics 139
    Exercise and Pregnancy 139
    American College of Obstetricians and Gynecologists Recommendations for Exercise
        in Pregnancy and Postpartum..140
    Contraindications for Exercise during Pregnancy 140
Pediatrics 140
    Developmental Gross and Fine Motor Skills 140
    Concepts of Development 142
    Pediatric Therapeutic Positioning 142
    Ideal Positioning 143
    Infant Reflexes and Possible Effects if Reflex Persists Abnormally..144

Federal Legislation Affecting Health and Education for Children
  with Disabilities 145
Pediatric Assessment Tools..146
Pediatric Profile 147
  Examination 147
  Intervention 147
  Goals 147
Pediatric Pathology 147
  Cardiopulmonary 147
  Musculoskeletal 148
  Neurological..149
  Oncology..151
  Rheumatory 152
Models of Disability 152
The Nagi Model 152
The International Classification of Impairment, Disabilities,
  and Handicaps Model 153
Disablement Model 153
Outcome Measurement Tools 153
Balance...153
Cognitive Assessment 154
Coordination and Manual Dexterity..154
Endurance 154
Motor Recovery 155
Pain 155
Self-Care and ADL 155
Pharmacology 156
Pharmacological Categories..156
Review of Systems: Side Effects/Subjective Complaints 157
Vitamins 158
Fat-Soluble Vitamins 158
Water-Soluble Vitamins 159
Minerals 160
Major Minerals 160
Trace Minerals 160

Unit 11: Education 163
Psychology 163
Maslow's Hierarchy of Needs..163
Classical Conditioning 163
Operant Conditioning..163
Social Learning Theory..163
Patient Education 163
Adult Learning 163
Guidelines to Promote Adult Learning 164
Domains of Learning 164
Learning Style 164
Teaching Methods 164
Guidelines for Effective Patient Education 164
Principles of Motivation..165
Cultural Influences 165
Designing Effective Patient Education Materials 165
Teaching Guidelines for Specific Patient Categories...165
Stages of Dying 166
Education Concepts 166
Practice...166
Feedback 166
Team Models 167

Clinical Application Templates

Introduction **169**
    Template 1: Achilles Tendon Rupture 171
    Template 2: Alzheimer's Disease..173
    Template 3: Amputation due to Arteriosclerosis Obliterans 175
    Template 4: Amyotrophic Lateral Sclerosis...177
    Template 5: Ankylosing Spondylitis...179
    Template 6: Anterior Cruciate Ligament Sprain – Grade III 181
    Template 7: Breast Cancer 183
    Template 8: Carpal Tunnel Syndrome 185
    Template 9: Cerebrovascular Accident 187
    Template 10: Cystic Fibrosis...189
    Template 11: Duchenne Muscular Dystrophy..191
    Template 12: Emphysema 193
    Template 13: Huntington's Disease..195
    Template 14: Medial Collateral Ligament Sprain – Grade II..197
    Template 15: Multiple Sclerosis...199
    Template 16: Myocardial Infarction...201
    Template 17: Parkinson's Disease 203
    Template 18: Patellofemoral Syndrome 205
    Template 19: Plantar Fasciitis 207
    Template 20: Restrictive Lung Disease..209
    Template 21: Rheumatoid Arthritis..211
    Template 22: Rotator Cuff Tendonitis 213
    Template 23: Scoliosis 215
    Template 24: Spina Bifida - Myelomeningocele..217
    Template 25: Spinal Cord Injury – C7 Tetraplegia 219
    Template 26: Systemic Lupus Erythematosus 221
    Template 27: Thoracic Outlet Syndrome 223
    Template 28: Total Hip Replacement 225
    Template 29: Total Knee Replacement 227
    Template 30: Urinary Stress Incontinence 229

Sample Examinations

Introduction..**231**
Exam One..**233**
    Questions..233
    Answer Sheets..257
    Explanations...259

Exam Two **271**
    Questions 271
    Answer Sheets..295
    Explanations...297

Exam Three **309**
    Questions 309
    Answer Sheets..333
    Explanations...335

Exam Four **347**
    Questions 347
    Answer Sheets..371
    Explanations...373

Bibliography..

Order Form..

Introduction

Introduction

Preparing for a comprehensive licensing examination that potentially encompasses all elements of a physical therapy academic program can be an overwhelming task. Students are often exhausted after completing a rigorous academic program and suddenly are faced with the daunting task of taking a 225 question examination that incorporates all elements of patient/client management. Anxiety, economics, and a strong desire to practice as a physical therapist only increase a candidate's sense of urgency. Often when faced with such an overwhelming task the reaction is to either procrastinate or to wander aimlessly through study sessions without real direction or focus.

A Guide to Success: Review for Licensure in Physical Therapy was designed to assist candidates with their preparation for the Physical Therapist Examination. The text consists of three distinct sections:

Section One: Academic Review
The academic review is divided into eleven specific units and is designed to highlight essential elements of a physical therapist academic curriculum. Candidates should make sure they are familiar with this foundational information prior to exploring specific content in greater breadth and depth.

Since the examination is designed to assess entry-level practice it is likely that candidates will encounter the information presented in the academic review frequently on the actual examination. Academic resources such as textbooks and class notes should be used to augment the academic review as necessary.

Section Two: Clinical Application Templates
Clinical application templates provide candidates with a unique study tool designed to broaden their exposure to a variety of medical conditions. The section presents 30 different clinical application templates commonly encountered in clinical practice. Candidates are encouraged to review the templates and carefully reflect on each of the elements of patient/client management.

Section Three: Sample Examinations
Sample examinations provide candidates with the opportunity to assess their current level of preparedness and at the same time gain valuable experience taking multiple-choice examinations. The section provides four complete sample examinations with explanation of answers and cited resources. Candidates should analyze questions that were answered correctly and incorrectly and attempt to identify content areas that may need additional review or formal remediation.

Each of the sections in *A Guide to Success* presents candidates with a unique opportunity to improve their performance on the examination. Subject matter encountered that candidates have limited familiarity with in the academic review, clinical application templates, and sample examinations sections should be explored in detail, while other more familiar subject matter should be reviewed more quickly.

Since there are an infinite number of possible questions on the examination, candidates should avoid familiarizing themselves with only the stated answers and instead use the presented information as a platform to explore a myriad of related topics. Candidates that have broad exposure to a diverse patient population during their didactic training combined with a meaningful study plan emphasizing applied knowledge can be richly rewarded on this challenging examination.

Congratulations on your decision to purchase *A Guide to Success*. We encourage you to leave no stone unturned in your preparation for this important examination and urge you to strive to make your examination score reflect your academic knowledge. We are confident that *A Guide to Success* will be a valuable component of your comprehensive study program. Although undoubtedly there will be many magical moments in your life, I am sure you will never forget the moment when you become licensed as a physical therapist. Best of luck on the examination and in your future career endeavors!

*Additional resources to assist candidates with their preparation for the Physical Therapist Examination are located at the conclusion of the text.

Academic Review

Unit One	Foundational Science	3
Unit Two	Musculoskeletal	17
Unit Three	Neuromuscular	51
Unit Four	Cardiopulmonary	73
Unit Five	Integumentary	87
Unit Six	Patient Care Skills	91
Unit Seven	Physical Agents	101
Unit Eight	Research	113
Unit Nine	Administration	119
Unit Ten	Special Topics	139
Unit Eleven	Education	163

Academic Review

Introduction

The Physical Therapist Examination is a generalist examination that attempts to determine if candidates possess the minimal qualifications necessary to practice as an entry-level physical therapist. The examination requires candidates to exhibit familiarity with each of the elements of patient/client management and apply that knowledge in a safe and effective manner. In order to successfully meet this requirement it is incumbent upon therapists to familiarize themselves with essential didactic information.

The academic review section of *A Guide to Success* presents information arranged in eleven distinct units. A detailed listing of the content of each unit is located in the table of contents. The academic review was designed to serve as a summary of the most essential elements of patient/client management. The majority of information presented in the academic review should be familiar to candidates, however due to the sheer volume of information included in a physical therapy academic program it is likely that candidates need to review much of the information. In addition the problem is magnified since invariably students do not have the opportunity to apply all of the didactic information during their clinical experiences.

Candidates should remember that the examination is designed to reflect current clinical practice and as a result topics that are commonly encountered in clinical practice will represent a vast majority of the actual questions on any version of the examination. Candidates should make sure that they are thoroughly familiar with this foundational information prior to expanding the breadth and depth of their academic review. This pragmatic approach allows candidates to significantly increase the utility of their study sessions and increase their examination score.

A prime example of this basic premise is as follows. Assume that a candidate is reviewing orthopedic special tests by utilizing the textbook Orthopedic Assessment by David Magee. The textbook offers a complete description of hundreds of special tests organized by area of the body. Although the textbook is a wonderful resource for students and faculty the sheer volume of special tests makes it impractical to attempt to review all of the presented information. In contrast the academic review section of *A Guide to Success* offers a summary of the most commonly encountered special tests organized by body part and by specific condition that the test is designed to identify.

Candidates have numerous resources that they can rely on for additional information such as the textbook by Magee, however as this example illustrates candidates must have a firm grasp on the basics before expanding the scope of their academic review.

Foundational Science

Anatomy and Physiology

Joint Classification

Fibrous Joints (synarthroses)
Fibrous joints are composed of bones that are united by fibrous tissue and are nonsynovial. Movement is minimal to none with the amount of movement permitted at the joint dependent on the length of the fibers uniting the bones.

Suture – (e.g. sagittal suture of the skull)
- Union of two bones by a ligament or membrane
- Immovable joint
- Eventual fusion is termed a synostosis

Syndesmosis – (e.g. the tibia and fibula with interosseous membrane)
- Bone connected to bone by a dense fibrous membrane or cord
- Very little motion

Gomphosis – (e.g. a tooth in its socket)
- Two bony surfaces connect as a peg in a hole
- The teeth and corresponding sockets in the mandible/maxilla are the only gomphosis joints in the body
- The periodontal membrane is the fibrous component of the joint

Cartilaginous Joints (amphiarthroses)
Cartilaginous joints have a hyaline cartilage or fibrocartilage that connects one bone to another. These are slightly moveable joints.

Synchondrosis – (e.g. sternum and true rib articulation)
- Hyaline cartilage
- Cartilage adjoins two ossifying centers of bone
- Provides stability during growth
- May ossify to a synostosis once growth is completed
- Slight motion

Symphysis – (e.g. pubic symphysis)
- Generally located at the midline of the body
- Two bones covered with hyaline cartilage
- Two bones connected by fibrocartilage
- Slight motion

Synovial Joints (diarthroses)
Synovial joints provide free movement between the bones they join. They have five distinguishing characteristics: joint cavity, articular cartilage, synovial membrane, synovial fluid, and fibrous capsule. The joints are the most complex and vulnerable to injury and are further classified by the type of movement and by the shape of articulating bones.

Uniaxial joint – one motion around a single axis in one plane of the body
- Hinge (ginglymus) – elbow joint
- Pivot (trochoid) – atlantoaxial joint

Biaxial joint – movement occurs in two planes and around two axes through the convex/concave surfaces
- Condyloid – metacarpophalangeal joint of a finger
- Saddle – carpometacarpal joint of the thumb

Multiaxial joint – movement occurs in three planes and around three axes
- Plane (gliding) – carpal joints
- Ball and socket – hip joint

Specific Joints

Shoulder
The shoulder complex consists of four separate articulations.

- **Sternoclavicular Joint:** Composed of the clavicle articulating with the manubrium of the sternum.

- **Acromioclavicular Joint:** Composed of the lateral end of the clavicle articulating with the acromion of the scapula.

- **Glenohumeral Joint:** Classified as a ball and socket joint, in which the round head of the humerus articulates with the shallow glenoid cavity of the scapula. The capsule of the glenohumeral joint is reinforced by the superior glenohumeral ligament, middle glenohumeral ligament, inferior glenohumeral ligament, and the coracohumeral ligament.

- **Scapulothoracic Articulation:** Composed of the articulation between the scapula and the posterior rib cage. The articulation is not considered to be a joint since it lacks connection by fibrous, cartilaginous or synovial tissue.

Elbow
The elbow is classified as a hinge joint. It is composed of the humerus, ulna, and radius. Flexion and extension occur at the articulation of the trochlea with the semilunar notch of the ulna.

The joint capsule is reinforced by the ulnar collateral ligament and the radial collateral ligament.

Wrist and Hand
The wrist complex consists of the radiocarpal and midcarpal joints. Motions at the wrist include flexion, extension, radial and ulnar deviation. The hand consists of the metacarpophalangeal joints, the proximal and distal interphalangeal joints, and the carpometacarpal joints.

Hip
The hip is classified as a ball and socket joint. It is formed by the articulation of the femur with the innominate bone. The head of the femur inserts into a deep socket called the acetabulum.

Stability is provided to the hip joint by the following:
- Acetabulum
- Iliofemoral ligament
- Pubofemoral ligament
- Ischiofemoral ligament

Knee
The knee is classified as a hinge joint. It is formed by the articulation of the tibia with the femur. The knee is extremely weak in terms of its bony arrangement.

Stability is provided to the knee joint by the following ligaments:
- Anterior cruciate ligament
- Posterior cruciate ligament
- Medial collateral ligament
- Lateral collateral ligament
- Deep medial capsular ligament

Ankle
The ankle is classified as a hinge joint which is formed by the articulation of the tibia and fibula with the talus. The distal ends of the tibia and fibula form a mortise that borders the talus. The bony arrangement provides the ankle with good lateral stability.

The ankle is structurally strong secondary to the bony and ligamentous arrangement.
- **Medial Ligaments:** Deltoid
- **Lateral Ligaments:** Anterior tibiofibular
  Anterior talofibular
  Calcaneofibular
  Lateral talocalcaneal
  Posterior talofibular

Joint Receptors

Free Nerve Endings
- **Location:** Joint capsule, ligaments, synovium, fat pads
- **Sensitivity:** One type sensitive to nonnoxious mechanical stress; other type sensitive to noxious mechanical or biochemical stimuli
- **Primary Distribution:** All joints

Golgi Ligament Endings
- **Location:** Ligaments, adjacent to ligaments' bony attachment
- **Sensitivity:** Tension or stretch on ligaments
- **Primary Distribution:** Majority of joints

Golgi-Mazzoni Corpuscles
- **Location:** Joint capsule
- **Sensitivity:** Compression of joint capsule
- **Primary Distribution:** Knee joint, joint capsule

Pacinian Corpuscles
- **Location:** Fibrous layer of joint capsule
- **Sensitivity:** High frequency vibration, acceleration, and high velocity changes in joint position
- **Primary Distribution:** All joints

Ruffini Endings
- **Location:** Fibrous layer of joint capsule
- **Sensitivity:** Stretching of joint capsule, amplitude, and velocity of joint position
- **Primary Distribution:** Greater density in proximal joints particularly in capsular regions

Muscle Action

Head

Temporomandibular Joint

Depress:
Lateral pterygoid
Suprahyoid
Infrahyoid

Protrusion:
Masseter
Lateral pterygoid
Medial pterygoid

Retrusion:
Temporalis
Masseter
Digastric

Elevate:
Temporalis
Masseter
Medial pterygoid

Side to Side:
Medial pterygoid
Lateral pterygoid
Masseter
Temporalis

Spine

Cervical Intervertebral Joints

Flexion Bending:
Sternocleidomastoid
Longus coli
Scalenus muscles

Rotation and Lateral Bending:
Sternocleidomastoid
Scalenus muscles
Splenius cervicis
Longissimus cervicis
Iliocostalis cervicis
Levator scapulae
Multifidus

Extension:
Splenius cervicis
Semispinalis cervicis
Iliocostalis cervicis
Longissimus cervicis
Multifidus
Trapezius

Thoracic and Lumbar Intervertebral Joints

Flexion Bending:
Rectus abdominis
Internal oblique
External oblique

Extension:
Erector spinae
Quadratus lumborum
Multifidus

Rotation and Lateral Bending:
Psoas major
Quadratus lumborum
External oblique
Internal oblique
Multifidus
Longissimus thoracis
Iliocostalis thoracis
Rotatores

Upper Extremity

Scapula

Elevation:
Trapezius
Levator scapulae

Protraction:
Serratus anterior
Pectoralis major
Pectoralis minor

Upward Rotation:
Trapezius
Serratus anterior

Depression:
Latissimus dorsi
Pectoralis major
Pectoralis minor

Retraction:
Trapezius
Rhomboids

Downward Rotation:
Lower trapezius
Rhomboids
Levator scapulae
Pectoralis minor

Shoulder Joint

Flexion:
Deltoid
Coracobrachialis
Pectoralis major
Biceps brachii

Abduction:
Deltoid
Supraspinatus
Infraspinatus

Lateral Rotation:
Teres minor
Infraspinatus
Deltoid

Extension:
Latissimus dorsi
Teres major and minor
Deltoid
Pectoralis major

Adduction:
Pectoralis major
Latissimus dorsi
Teres major

Medial Rotation:
Subscapularis
Teres major
Pectoralis major
Latissimus dorsi
Deltoid

Elbow Joint

Flexion:
Biceps brachii
Brachialis
Brachioradialis
Supinator

Extension:
Triceps brachii
Anconeus

Radioulnar Joint

Supination:
Biceps brachii
Supinator

Pronation:
Pronator teres
Pronator quadratus

UNIT ONE: FOUNDATIONAL SCIENCE

Wrist Joint

Flexion:
Flexor carpi radialis
Flexor carpi ulnaris
Palmaris longus

Radial Deviation
Flexor carpi radialis
Extensor carpi radialis
Extensor pollicis longus and brevis

Extension:
Extensor carpi radialis longus
Extensor carpi radialis brevis
Extensor carpi ulnaris

Ulnar Deviation
Flexor carpi ulnaris
Extensor carpi ulnaris

Ankle Joint

Plantar Flexion:
Gastrocnemius
Soleus
Peroneus longus
Peroneus brevis
Plantaris
Flexor hallucis

Inversion:
Tibialis anterior
Tibialis posterior
Flexor digitorum longus

Dorsiflexion:
Tibialis anterior
Extensor hallucis longus
Extensor digitorum longus
Peroneus tertius

Eversion:
Peroneus longus
Peroneus brevis
Peroneus tertius

Lower Extremity

Hip Joint

Flexion:
Iliopsoas
Sartorius
Rectus femoris
Pectineus

Abduction:
Gluteus medius
Gluteus minimus
Tensor fasciae latae
Piriformis

Medial Rotation:
Tensor fasciae latae
Gluteus medius
Gluteus minimus
Pectineus
Adductor longus

Extension:
Gluteus maximus and medius
Semitendinosus
Semimembranosus
Biceps femoris

Adduction:
Adductor magnus
Adductor longus
Adductor brevis
Gracilis

Lateral Rotation:
Gluteus maximus
Obturator externus
Obturator internus
Piriformis
Gemelli

Knee Joint

Flexion:
Biceps femoris
Semitendinosus
Semimembranosus
Sartorius

Medial Rotation of Flexed Leg:
Sartorius
Popliteus
Semitendinosus
Semimembranosus

Extension:
Rectus femoris
Vastus lateralis
Vastus intermedius
Vastus medialis

Lateral Rotation of Flexed Leg:
Biceps femoris

Nerve Root Dermatomes, Myotomes, Reflexes, and Paresthetic Areas

Nerve Root	Dermatome*	Muscle Weakness (Myotome)	Reflexes Affected	Paresthesias
C1	Vertex of skull	None	None	None
C2	Temple, forehead, occiput	Longus colli, sternocleidomastoid, rectus capitis	None	None
C3	Entire neck, posterior cheek, temporal area, prolongation forward under mandible	Trapezius, splenius capitis	None	Cheek, side of neck
C4	Shoulder area, clavicular area, upper scapular area	Trapezius, levator scapulae	None	Horizontal band along clavicle and upper scapula
C5	Deltoid area, anterior aspect of entire arm to base of thumb	Supraspinatus, infraspinatus, deltoid, biceps	Biceps, brachioradialis	None
C6	Anterior arm, radial side of hand to thumb and index finger	Biceps, supinator, wrist extensors	Biceps, brachioradialis	Thumb and index finger
C7	Lateral arm and forearm to index, long, and ring fingers	Triceps, wrist flexors (rarely, wrist extensors)	Triceps	Index, long, and ring fingers
C8	Medial arm and forearm to long, ring, and little fingers	Ulnar deviators, thumb extensors, thumb adductors (rarely, triceps)	Triceps	Little finger alone or with two adjacent fingers; not ring or long fingers, alone or together (C7)
T1	Medial side of forearm to base of little finger	Disc lesions at upper two thoracic levels do not appear to give rise to root weakness. Weakness of intrinsic muscles of the hand is due to other pathology (e.g., thoracic outlet pressure, neoplasm of lung, and ulnar nerve lesion). Dural and nerve root stress has T1 elbow flexion with arm horizontal. T1 and T2 scapulae forward and backward on chest wall. Neck flexion at any thoracic level.		
T2	Medial side of upper arm to medial elbow, pectoral and midscapular areas			
T3 – T12	T3-T6, upper thorax; T5-T7, costal margin; T8-T12, abdomen and lumbar region	Articular and dural signs and root pain are common. Root signs (cutaneous analgesia) are rare and have such indefinite area that they have little localizing value. Weakness is not detectable.		
L1	Back, over trochanter and groin	None	None	Groin; after holding posture, which causes pain
L2	Back, front of thigh to knee	Psoas, hip adductors	None	Occasionally anterior thigh
L3	Back, upper buttock, anterior thigh and knee, medial lower leg	Psoas, quadriceps, thigh atrophy	Knee jerk sluggish, PKB positive, pain on full SLR	Medial knee, anterior lower leg
L4	Medial buttock, lateral thigh, medial leg, dorsum of foot, big toe	Tibialis anterior, extensor hallucis	SLR limited neck flexion pain, weak or absent knee jerk, side flexion limited	Medial aspect of calf and ankle
L5	Buttock, posterior and lateral thigh, lateral aspect of leg, dorsum of foot, medial half of sole, first, second, and third toes	Extensor hallucis, peroneals, gluteus medius, dorsiflexors, hamstring and calf atrophy	SLR limited one side, neck flexion painful, ankle decreased, crossed-leg raising pain	Lateral aspect of leg, medial three toes

Nerve Root	Dermatome*	Muscle Weakness (Myotome)	Reflexes Affected	Paresthesias
S1	Buttock, thigh, and leg posterior	Calf and hamstring, wasting of gluteals, peroneals, plantar flexors	SLR limited, Achilles reflex weak or absent	Lateral two toes, lateral foot, lateral leg to knee, plantar aspect of foot
S2	Same as S1	Same as S1 except peroneals	Same as S1	Lateral leg, knee, and heel
S3	Groin, medial thigh to knee	None	None	None
S4	Perineum, genitals, lower sacrum	Bladder, rectum	None	Saddle area, genitals, anus, impotence, massive posterior herniation

*In any part of which pain may be felt.
PKB = prone knee bending; SLR = straight leg raising.

From Magee, DJ: Orthopedic Physical Assessment. W.B. Saunders Company, Philadelphia 1997, p.12, with permission.

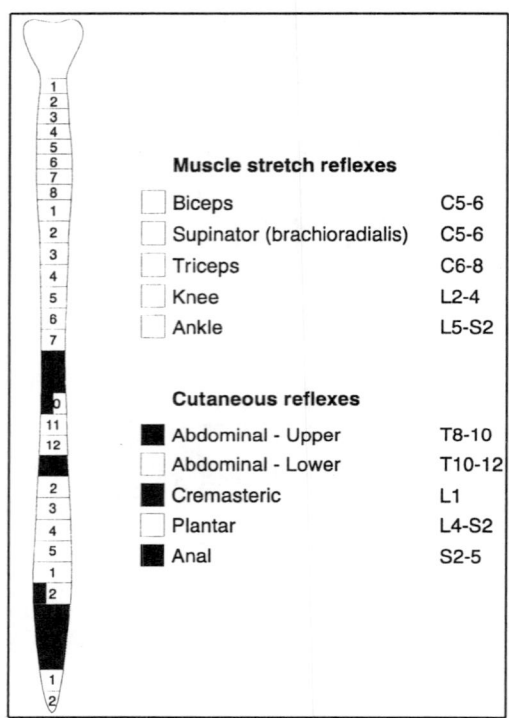

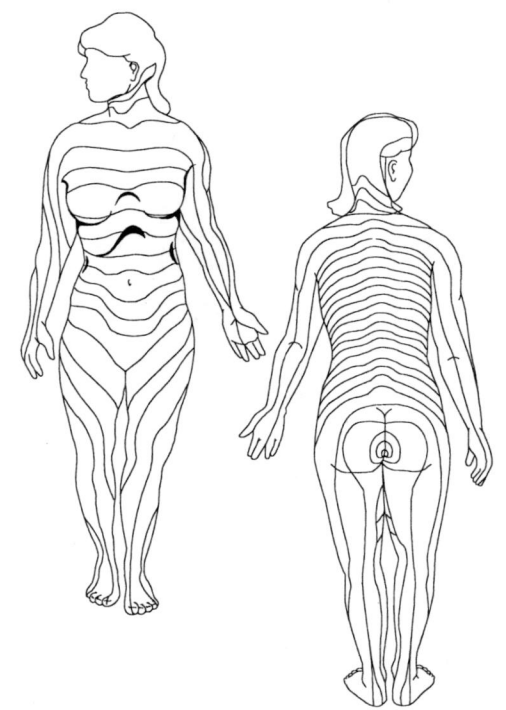

8 A GUIDE TO SUCCESS

Nerves of the Brachial Plexus

Origin	Nerves	Muscles
From the rami of the plexus:	Dorsal scapular	Rhomboids
		Levator scapulae
	Long thoracic	Serratus anterior
From the trunks of the plexus:	Nerve to subclavius	Subclavius
	Suprascapular	Infraspinatus
		Supraspinatus
From the lateral cord of the plexus:	Lateral pectoral	Pectoralis major
		Pectoralis minor
	Musculocutaneous	Coracobrachialis
		Biceps brachii
		Brachialis
	Lateral root of the median	Flexor muscles in the forearm, except flexor carpi ulnaris, and 5 muscles in the hand
From the medial cord of the plexus:	Medial pectoral	Pectoralis major
		Pectoralis minor
	Ulnar	1 ½ muscles of the forearm and most small muscles of the hand
	Medial root of the median	Flexor muscles in the forearm, except flexor carpi ulnaris, and 5 muscles of the hand
From the posterior cord of the plexus:	Upper subscapular	Subscapularis
	Thoracodorsal	Latissimus dorsi
	Lower subscapular	Subscapularis
		Teres major
	Axillary	Deltoid
		Teres minor
	Radial	Brachioradialis and the extensor muscles of the forearm

Lower Extremity Innervation

Lumbar Plexus:
- Psoas major
- Psoas minor

Sacral Plexus:
- Piriformis
- Obturator internus
- Quadratus femoris
- Superior gemelli
- Inferior gemelli

Superior Gluteal Nerve:
- Gluteus medius
- Gluteus minimus
- Tensor fasciae latae

Inferior Gluteal Nerve:
- Gluteus maximus

Femoral Nerve:
- Iliacus
- Rectus femoris
- Sartorius
- Pectineus
- Vastus lateralis
- Vastus medialis
- Vastus intermedius

Obturator Nerve:
- Adductor longus
- Adductor brevis
- Adductor magnus
- Gracilis
- Obturator externus

Sciatic Nerve (Tibial Division):
- Semitendinosus
- Soleus
- Popliteus
- Gastrocnemius
- Biceps femoris (long head)
- Semimembranosus
- Plantaris
- Tibialis posterior
- Flexor hallucis longus
- Flexor digitorum longus

Sciatic Nerve (Common Peroneal Division):
- Biceps femoris (short head)

Superficial Peroneal Nerve:
- Peroneus longus
- Peroneus brevis

Deep Peroneal Nerve:
- Extensor digitorum longus
- Tibialis anterior

Medial Plantar Nerve:
- Abductor hallucis
- Lumbricale I
- Flexor digitorum brevis
- Flexor hallucis longus

Lateral Plantar Nerve:
- Abductor digiti minimi
- Dorsal interossei
- Quadratus plantae
- Adductor hallucis
- Lumbricale II, III, IV
- Plantar interossei
- Flexor digiti minimi brevis

Neuroanatomy

Cranial Nerves and Methods of Testing

Nerve	Afferent (Sensory)	Efferent (Motor)	Test
Olfactory	Smell: Nose		Identify familiar odors (e.g., chocolate, coffee)
Optic	Sight: Eye		Test visual fields
Oculomotor		Voluntary motor: Levator of eyelid; superior, medial, and inferior recti; inferior oblique muscle of eyeball Autonomic: Smooth muscle of eyeball	Upward, downward, and medial gaze Reaction to light
Trochlear		Voluntary motor: Superior oblique muscle of eyeball	Downward and lateral gaze
Trigeminal	Touch, pain: Skin of face, mucous membranes of nose, sinuses, mouth, anterior tongue	Voluntary motor: Muscles of mastication	Corneal reflex Face sensation Clench teeth; push down on chin to separate jaws
Abducens		Voluntary motor: Lateral rectus muscle of eyeball	Lateral gaze
Facial	Taste: Anterior tongue	Voluntary motor: Facial muscles Autonomic: Lacrimal, submandibular, and sublingual glands	Close eyes tight Smile and show teeth Whistle and puff cheeks Identify familiar tastes (e.g., sweet, sour)
Vestibulocochlear (acoustic nerve)	Hearing: Ear Balance: Ear		Hear watch ticking Hearing tests Balance and coordination test
Glossopharyngeal	Touch, pain: Posterior tongue, pharynx Taste: Posterior tongue	Voluntary motor: Unimportant muscle of pharynx Autonomic: Parotid gland	Gag reflex Ability to swallow
Vagus	Touch, pain: Pharynx, larynx, bronchi Taste: Tongue, epiglottis	Voluntary motor: Muscles of palate, pharynx, and larynx Autonomic: Thoracic and abdominal viscera	Gag reflex Ability to swallow Say "Ahhh"
Accessory		Voluntary motor: Sternocleidomastoid and trapezius muscle	Resisted shoulder shrug
Hypoglossal		Voluntary motor: Muscles of tongue	Tongue protrusion (if injured, tongue deviates toward injured side)

From Magee, DJ: Orthopedic Physical Assessment. W.B. Saunders Company, Philadelphia 1997, p.55, with permission.

Kinesiology

Planes of the Body

Motions are described as occurring around three cardinal planes of the body (frontal, sagittal, transverse). Movement in the cardinal planes occurs around three corresponding axes (anterior-posterior, medial-lateral, vertical).

Frontal plane
The frontal plane divides the body into anterior and posterior sections. Motions in the frontal plane such as abduction and adduction occur around an anterior-posterior axis.

Sagittal plane
The sagittal plane divides the body into right and left sections. Motions in the sagittal plane such as flexion and extension occur around a medial-lateral axis.

Transverse plane
The transverse plane divides the body into upper and lower sections. Motions in the transverse plane such as medial and lateral rotation occur around a vertical axis.

Classes of Levers

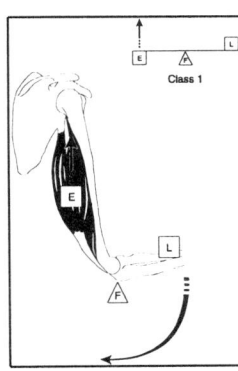

Class 1 lever
A class 1 lever has the axis of rotation (fulcrum) between the effort (force) and resistance (load). There are very few class 1 levers in the body. A class 1 lever is illustrated with the triceps brachii force on the olecranon with an external counter force pushing on the forearm. Another example of a class 1 lever is a see saw.

Class 2 lever
A class 2 lever has the resistance (load) between the axis of rotation (fulcrum) and the effort (force). The length of the effort arm is always longer than the resistance arm. In most instances, gravity is the effort and muscle activity is the resistance, however there are class 2 levers that the muscle is the effort when the distal attachment is on a weight bearing segment. An example of a class 2 lever is a wheelbarrow.

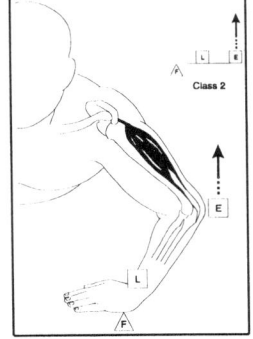

Class 3 lever
A class 3 lever has the effort (force) between the axis of rotation (fulcrum) and the resistance (load). The length of the effort arm is always shorter than the length of the resistance arm. Shoulder abduction with weight at the wrist is a class 3 lever. Class 3 levers usually permit large movements at rapid speeds and are the most common type of lever in the body. An example of a class 3 lever is elbow flexion.

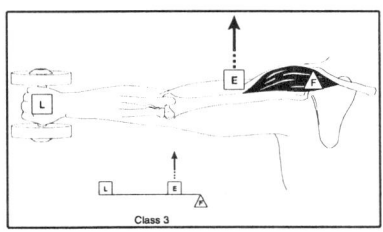

Exercise Physiology

Energy Systems

   ATP-PC or Phosphagen System
   Anaerobic Glycolysis or Lactic Acid System
   Aerobic or Oxygen System

Anaerobic Metabolism

ATP-PC System
This energy system is used for ATP production during high intensity, short duration exercise such as sprinting 100 meters. Phosphocreatine decomposes and releases a large amount of energy which is used to construct ATP. There is two to three times more phosphocreatine in cells of muscles than ATP. This process occurs almost instantaneously allowing for ready and available energy needed by the muscles. The system provides energy for muscle contraction for up to 15 seconds.

The phosphagen system represents the most rapidly available source of ATP for use by the muscle. Reasons for this rapid availability are as follows:
1. It does not depend on a long series of chemical reactions.
2. It does not depend on transporting the oxygen we breathe to the working muscles.
3. Both ATP and PC are stored directly within the contractile mechanisms of the muscle.

Anaerobic Glycolysis
This energy system is a major supplier of ATP during high intensity, short duration activities such as sprinting 400 or 800 meters. Stored glycogen is split into glucose, and through glycolysis, split again into pyruvic acid. The energy released during this process forms ATP. The process does not require oxygen. This system is approximately 50% slower than the

phosphocreatine system and can provide a person with 30 to 40 seconds of muscle contraction.
1. Anaerobic glycolysis results in the formation of lactic acid, which causes muscular fatigue.
2. It does not require the presence of oxygen.
3. It uses only carbohydrates (glycogen and glucose).
4. It releases enough energy for the resynthesis of only small amounts of ATP.

Aerobic Metabolism

The aerobic system is used predominantly during low intensity, long duration exercise such as running a marathon. The oxygen system yields by far the most ATP, but it requires several series of complex chemical reactions. This system provides energy through the oxidation of food. The combination of fatty acids, amino acids, and glucose with oxygen releases energy that forms ATP. This system will provide energy as long as there are nutrients to utilize.

Muscle Physiology

Classification of Muscle Fibers

Type I:
Aerobic
Red
Tonic
Slow twitch
Slow-oxidative

Type II:
Anaerobic
White
Phasic
Fast twitch
Fast-glycolytic

Functional Characteristics of Muscle Fibers

Type I:
Low fatigability
High capillary density
High myoglobin content
Smaller fibers
Extensive blood supply
Large amount of mitochondria

Example: marathon, swimming

Type II:
High fatigability
Low capillary density
Low myoglobin content
Larger fibers
Less blood supply
Fewer mitochondria

Example: high jump, sprinting

Muscle Receptors

Muscle Spindle
Muscle spindles are distributed throughout the belly of the muscle. They function to send information to the nervous system about muscle length and/or the rate of change of its length. The muscle spindle is important in the control of posture and with the help of the gamma system, involuntary movements.

Golgi Tendon Organ
Golgi tendon organs are encapsulated sensory receptors through which the muscle tendons pass immediately beyond their attachment to the muscle fibers. They are very sensitive to tension especially when produced from an active muscle contraction. They function to transmit information about tension or the rate of change of tension within the muscle.

An average of 10-15 muscle fibers are usually connected in series with each golgi tendon organ. The golgi tendon organ is stimulated through the tension produced by muscle fibers. Golgi tendon organs provide the nervous system with instantaneous information on the degree of tension in each small muscle segment.

Resistive Training

Types of Muscular Contraction

Isotonic: The muscle shortens or lengthens while resisting a constant load.

Isometric: Tension develops but there is no change in the length of the muscle.

Concentric: The muscle shortens while developing tension.

Eccentric: The muscle lengthens while developing tension.

Isokinetic: The tension developed by the muscle, while shortening or lengthening at a constant speed, is maximal over the full range of motion.

Open-Chain versus Closed-Chain Activities

Open-Chain: Open-chain activities involve the distal segment, usually the hand or foot, moving freely in space. An example of an open-chain activity is kicking a ball with the lower extremity.

Closed-Chain: Closed-chain activities involve the body moving over a fixed distal segment. An example of a closed-chain activity is a squat lift.

Resistive and Overload Training

Isometric Exercise
Muscular force is generated without a change in muscle length. Isometric exercises are often performed against an

immovable object. Submaximal isometric exercises are traditionally used in rehabilitation programs.

Isotonic Exercise
Muscular contraction in which the muscle exerts a constant tension. This can also be thought of as muscle movement with a constant load. Isotonic exercises are performed against resistance often employing equipment such as handheld weights.

Isokinetic Exercise
Exercise with a constant maximal speed and variable load. In isokinetic exercise the reaction force is identical to the force applied to the equipment. Cybex, Biodex, and Lido are a few of the companies making isokinetic exercise equipment.

Exercise Programs

DeLorme	Protocol
First Set	10 repetitions x 50% of 10 repetition maximum
Second Set	10 repetitions x 75% of 10 repetition maximum
Third Set	10 repetitions x 100% of 10 repetition maximum

Oxford Technique	Protocol
First Set	10 repetitions x 100% of 10 repetition maximum
Second Set	10 repetitions x 75% of 10 repetition maximum
Third Set	10 repetitions x 50% of 10 repetition maximum

Psychological Disorders

Affective Disorders

Affective disorders are classified by disturbances in mood or emotion. States of extreme happiness or sadness occur and mood can alternate without cause. These extreme emotions can become intense and unrealistic.

Depression
- Slower mental and physical activity
- Poor self-esteem
- Immobilized from everyday activities
- Sadness, hopelessness, and helplessness
- Desire to withdraw
- Delusions in severe cases

Mania
- Constantly active
- Impulses immediately expressed
- Unrealistic activity
- Elation and self-confidence
- Disagreement with a patient may produce patient aggression
- Disorganized thoughts and speech
- Very few patients are diagnosed with only a manic disorder

Bipolar
- Alternating periods of depression and mania
- Females are at greater risk
- Usually begins in a patient's twenties

Neuroses Disorders

Neuroses refer to a group of disorders that are characterized by individuals exhibiting fear and maladaptive strategies in dealing with stressful or everyday stimuli. Patients with neuroses are not dealing with psychosis, do not have delusions, and usually realize that they have a problem.

Obsessive-compulsive disorder
- Obsessions – persistent thoughts that will not leave
- Compulsions – repetitive ritual behaviors the patient cannot stop performing
- Thoughts or ritual behaviors that interfere with daily living
- Unable to control irrational behavior
- Most commonly begins in young adulthood

Anxiety disorder
- Constant high tension
- Overreacts in certain instances
- Presents with apprehension
- Chronic worry
- Acute anxiety attacks
  - --Lasts a few minutes in duration
  - --Excitation of the sympathetic autonomic nervous system
  - --Fear of impending doom or death
  - --Shortness of breath, heart palpitations, dizziness, nausea
  - --Initiated by unconscious and internal mechanisms

Phobia disorder
- Excessive fear of objects, occurrences, or situations
- Fear is considerably out of proportion and irrational
- Fear creates difficulty in everyday life
- Subclassifications are agorophobia, social phobia, and simple phobia
- May develop from traumatic experiences, observation, classical conditioning

- Simple phobias are the easiest to treat
  - --Acrophobia – fear of heights
  - --Agorophobia – fear of open spaces
  - --Astraphobia – fear of thunderstorms
  - --Belonephobia – fear of needles
  - --Claustrophobia – fear of being in closed-in places
  - --Pathophobia – fear of disease
  - --Pyrophobia – fear of fire
  - --Zoophobia – fear of animal(s)

Dissociative Disorders

Dissociative disorders develop when a person unconsciously dissociates (separates) one part of the mind from the rest.

Psychogenic amnesia
- Produced by the mind
- No physical cause
- Forgets all aspects of the past

Multiple personality
- A rare dissociative disorder
- Two or more independent personalities
- Each personality may or may not know about the other
- Causative factors are not understood
- Believed to allow a person to engage in behaviors that are against the patient's morality and normally produce guilt

Somatoform Disorders

Somatoform disorders are classified based on the physical symptoms present in each disorder.

Somatization disorder
- Primarily in women
- Often chronic and long lasting
- Complaints of symptoms with no physiological basis
- Symptoms usually lead to medications and medical visits
- Symptoms alter the patient's life
- Resembles hypochondriasis disorder
- Has familial association

Conversion disorder
- Physical complaint of neurological basis with no underlying cause
- Paralysis is the most common finding
- Other findings include deafness, blindness, paresthesia
- Freud believes this is mental anxiety transformed into physical symptoms
- Diagnosis can be made once testing is negative for physical ailments
- Both men and women can experience a conversion disorder

Hypochondriasis disorder
- Excessive fear of illness
- Believes that minor illnesses or medical problems indicate a serious or life threatening disease

Schizophrenia Disorders

Schizophrenia disorders are psychotic in nature and present with disorganization of thought, hallucinations, emotional dysfunction, anxiety, and perceptual impairments. Causative factors include traumatic events, genetic inheritance, biochemical imbalances, and environmental influence.

Catatonic schizophrenia
- Motor disturbances with rigid posturing
- Patients remain aware during episodes
- Episodes consist of uncontrolled movements
- Medications are required to regulate episodes

Paranoid schizophrenia
- Delusions of grandeur
- Delusions of persecution
- May believe they possess special powers

Disorganized schizophrenia
- Usually progressive and irreversible
- Inappropriate emotional responses
- Mumbled talking

Undifferentiated schizophrenia
- May possess a mix of symptoms
- Does not classify into one category

Personality Disorders

Personality disorders are classified by patterns of behavior, dysfunctional view of society, and level of sadness. Personality disorders are usually ongoing patterns of dysfunctional behavior.

Psychopathic personality
- Low morality
- Poor sense of responsibility
- No respect for others
- Impulsive behavior for immediate gratification
- High frustration
- Little guilt or remorse for all actions
- Inability to alter behavior even with punishment
- Expert liar

Antisocial behavior
- Results from particular causes (e.g. need for attention or involvement in a gang)
- Usually have some concern for others (e.g. their gang)
- Blames other institutions (e.g. family, school) for their actions

- Usually begins before 16 years of age
- Violates the rights of others
- Lacks responsibility and emotional stability

Narcissistic behavior
- Incapable of loving others
- Self-absorbed
- Obsessed with success and power
- Unrealistic perception of self-importance

Borderline behavior
- Instability in all aspects of life
- Can identify self from others as well as reality
- Uses projection, denial, defensiveness
- Intense and uncontrolled anger
- Chronic feelings of emptiness
- Unpredictable mood or behavior

Psychiatric Medications

Antianxiety Drugs

Antianxiety drugs are usually benzodiazepines that function to assist with alleviating anxiety without significant sedation. There is still the possibility of addiction with prolonged use and also the risk of increased anxiety once the medication is stopped.

Common drugs include:
- Librium
- Ativan
- Valium
- Serax

Anti depressants

Multiple classifications of drugs are used in treating depression. The latest theory as to depression's etiology is that there is some form of increased sensitivity within receptors of the central nervous system. Most antidepressants are believed to create a decrease in sensitivity at these synapses, thus alleviating clinical depression. Side effects range from sedation, confusion, and cardiovascular problems to irritability, agitation, and insomnia.

First Generation:
- **Tricyclics:** Elavil, Norpramin, Pamelor
- **Monoamine Oxidase Inhibitors:** Marplan, Nardil
- **Sympathomimetic Stimulants:** Dexedrine

Second Generation:
- **Newer Drugs:** Xanax, Merital, Desyrel

Antipsychotics

Drugs used in the treatment of schizophrenia. The latest theory indicates that schizophrenia occurs from increased dopamine transmission into areas of the brain such as the limbic area. This creates a very complex chain of interactions. Antipsychotic drugs block dopamine receptors. Side effects can be very serious and include abnormal movements, sedation, blurred vision, and hypotension.

Common drugs include:
- Thorazine
- Mellaril
- Navane
- Compazine
- Vesprin
- Haldol

Sedatives-Hypnotics

Barbituates are primarily used for their sedative effects. They are central nervous system depressants, however, can be fatal with overdose and are addictive. Benzodiazepines are presently the drug of choice to attain sedative-hypnotic effects.

Common drugs include:
- **Benzodiazepines:** Dalmane, Halcion, Restoril
- **Barbituates:** Seconal, Butisol, Amytal

Musculoskeletal

Orthopedics

Examination

Upper Quarter Screening

The upper quarter screen provides a rapid assessment of mobility and neurologic function of the cervical spine and upper extremities. The screen is traditionally performed with the patient in sitting.

The following is an example of the components of an upper extremity screening.

Posture
- Postural assessment

Range of Motion
- Active range of motion of the cervical spine
- Active range of motion of the upper extremities
- Passive overpressure of the cervical spine and upper extremities, if the patient does not exhibit signs and symptoms of pathology

Resistive Testing (C1-T1)

Resistive Test	Innervation Level
Cervical rotation	C1
Shoulder elevation	C2-C4
Shoulder abduction	C5
Elbow flexion	C5-C6
Wrist extension	C6
Elbow extension	C7
Wrist flexion	C7
Thumb extension	C8
Finger adduction	T1

Dermatome Testing (C2-T1)

Area of Skin	Innervation Level
Posterior head	C2
Posterior-lateral neck	C3
Acromioclavicular joint	C4
Lateral Arm	C5
Lateral forearm and thumb	C6
Palmar distal phalanx – middle finger	C7
Little finger and ulnar border of the hand	C8
Medial forearm	T1

Reflex Testing (C5-C7)

Reflex	Innervation Level
Biceps	C5
Brachioradialis	C6
Triceps	C7

Lower Quarter Screening

The lower quarter screen provides a rapid assessment of mobility and neurologic function of the lumbosacral spine and lower extremities. The screen is traditionally performed with the patient in standing or sitting.

The following is an example of the components of a lower extremity screening.

Posture
- Postural assessment

Range of Motion
- Active range of motion of the lumbosacral spine
- Active range of motion of the lower extremities
- Passive overpressure of the lumbosacral spine and lower extremities, if the patient does not exhibit signs and symptoms of pathology

Functional Testing (L4-S1)

Functional Test	Innervation Level
Heel walking	L4-L5
Toe walking	S1
Straight leg raise	L4-S1

Resistive Testing (L1-S1)

Resistive Test	Innervation Level
Hip flexion	L1-L2
Knee extension	L3-L4
Ankle dorsiflexion	L4-L5
Great toe extension	L5
Ankle plantar flexion	S1

Dermatome Testing (L2-S5)

Area of Skin	Innervation Level
Anterior thigh	L2
Middle third of anterior thigh	L3
Patella and medial malleolus	L4
Fibular head and dorsum of foot	L5
Lateral and plantar aspect of foot	S1
Medial aspect of posterior thigh	S2
Perianal area	S3-S5

Reflex Testing (L4-S1)

Reflex	Innervation Level
Patella	L4
Achilles	S1

Scanning Examination to Rule Out Referral of Symptoms from Other Tissues

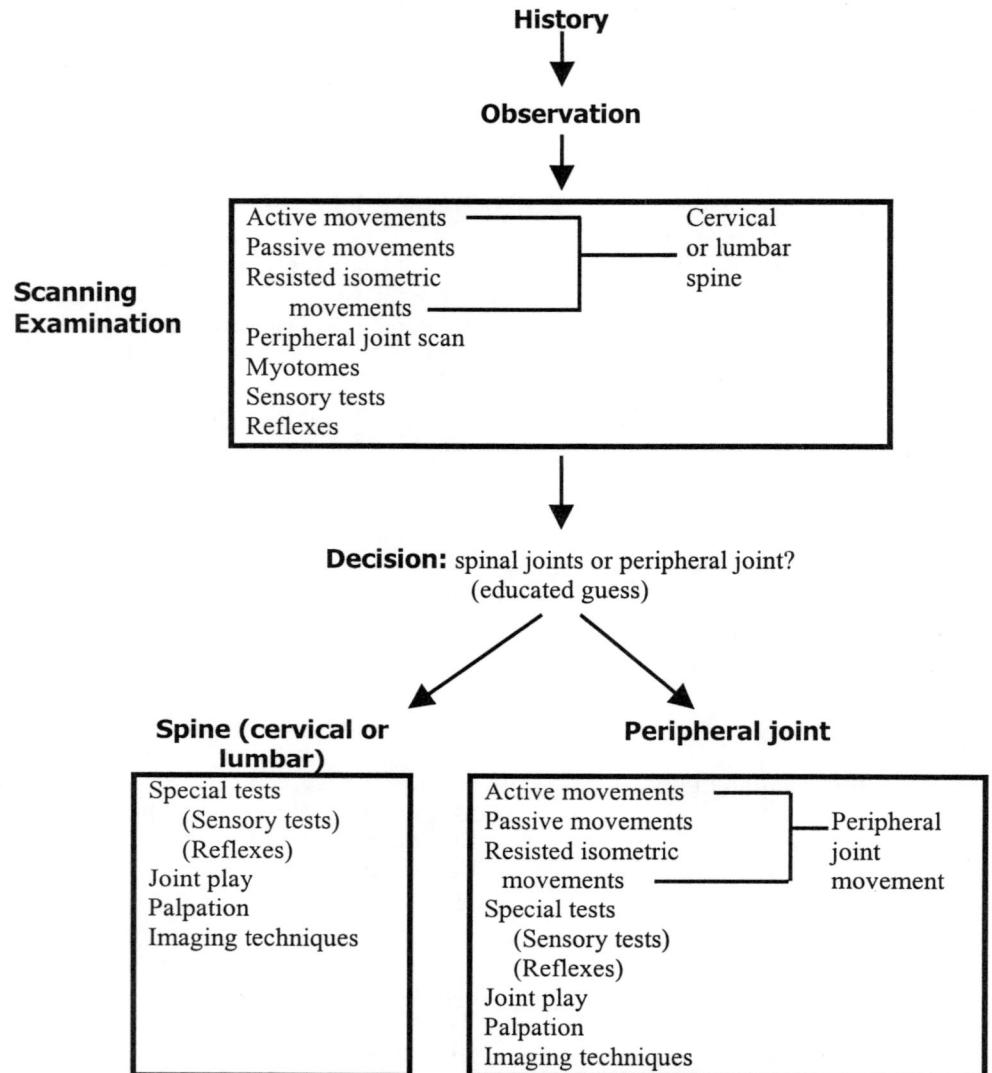

From Magee, DJ: Orthopedic Physical Assessment. W.B. Saunders Company, Philadelphia 1997, p.10, with permission.

18 A GUIDE TO SUCCESS

Posture

Good and Faulty Posture: Summary Chart

Good Posture	Part	Faulty Posture
In standing, the longitudinal arch has the shape of a half dome. Barefoot or in shoes without heels, the feet toe out slightly. In shoes with heels the feet are parallel. In walking with or without shoes, the feet are parallel and the weight is transferred from the heel along the outer border to the ball of the foot. In sprinting the feet are parallel or toe in slightly. The weight is on the balls of the feet and toes because the heels do not come in contact with the ground.	**Foot**	Low longitudinal arch or flat foot. Low metatarsal arch, usually indicated by calluses under the ball of the foot. Weight borne on the inner side of the foot (pronation). "Ankle rolls in." Weight borne on the outer border of the foot (supination). "Ankle rolls out." Toeing-out while walking, or while standing in shoes with heels ("slue-footed"). Toeing-in while walking or standing ("pigeon-toed").
Toes should be straight, that is, neither curled downward nor bent upward. They should extend forward in line with the foot and not be squeezed together or overlap.	**Toes**	Toes bend up at the first joint and down at middle joints so that the weight rests on the tips of the toes (hammer toes). This fault is often associated with wearing shoes that are too short. Big toe slants inward toward the midline of the foot (hallux valgus). "Bunion." This fault is often associated with wearing shoes that are too narrow and pointed at the toes.
Legs are straight up and down. Kneecaps face straight ahead when feet are in good position. Looking at the knees from the side, the knees are straight, i.e., neither bent forward nor locked backward.	**Knees and Legs**	Knees touch when feet are apart (knock-knees). Knees are apart when feet touch (bowlegs). Knee curves slightly backward (hyperextended knee). "Back-knee." Knee bends slightly forward, that is, it is not as straight as it should be (flexed knee). Kneecaps face slightly toward each other (medially rotated femurs). Kneecaps face slightly outward (laterally rotated femurs).
Ideally, the body weight is borne evenly on both feet, and the hips are level. One side is not more prominent than the other as seen from front or back, nor is one hip more forward or backward than the other as seen from the side. The spine does not curve to the left or the right side. (A *slight* deviation to the left in right-handed individuals and to the right in left-handed individuals is not uncommon. Also, a tendency toward a *slightly* low right shoulder and *slightly* high right hip is frequently found in right-handed people, and vice versa for left-handed people).	**Hips, Pelvis, and Spine Back View**	One hip is higher than the other (lateral pelvic tilt). Sometimes it is not really much higher but appears so because a sideways sway of the body has made it more prominent. (Tailors and dressmakers often notice a lateral tilt because the hemline of skirts or length of trousers must be adjusted to the difference.) The hips are rotated so that one is farther forward than the other (clockwise or counter clockwise rotation).

UNIT TWO: MUSCULOSKELETAL

Good Posture	Part	Faulty Posture
The front of the pelvis and the thighs are in a straight line. The buttocks are not prominent in back but slope slightly downward. The spine has four natural curves. In the neck and lower back the curve is forward, in the upper back and lowest part of the spine (sacral region) it is backward. The sacral curve is a fixed curve while the other three are flexible.	**Spine and Pelvis Side View**	The low back arches forward too much (lordosis). The pelvis tilts forward too much. The front of the thigh forms an angle with the pelvis when this tilt is present. The normal forward curve in the low back has straightened. The pelvis tips backward as in sway-back and flat-back postures. Increased backward curve in the upper back (kyphosis or round upper back). Increased forward curve in the neck. Almost always accompanied by round upper back and seen as a forward head. Lateral curve of the spine (scoliosis); toward one side (C-curve), toward both sides (S-curve).
In young children up to about the age of 10, the abdomen normally protrudes somewhat. In older children and adults it should be flat.	**Abdomen**	Entire abdomen protrudes. Lower part of the abdomen protrudes while the upper part is pulled in.
A good position of the chest is one in which it is slightly up and slightly forward (while the back remains in good alignment). The chest appears to be in a position about halfway between that of a full inspiration and a forced expiration.	**Chest**	Depressed, or "hollow-chest" position. Lifted and held up too high, brought about by arching the back. Ribs more prominent on one side than on the other. Lower ribs flaring out or protruding.
Arms hang relaxed at the sides with palms of the hands facing toward the body. Elbows are slightly bent, so forearms hang slightly forward. Shoulders are level and neither one is more forward or backward than the other when seen from the side. Shoulder blades lie flat against the rib cage. They are neither too close together or too wide apart. In adults, a separation of about 4 inches is average.	**Arms and Shoulders**	Arms held stiffly in any position forward, backward, or out from the body. Arms turned so that palms of hands face backward. One shoulder higher than the other. Both shoulders hiked-up. One or both shoulders drooping forward or sloping. Shoulders rotated either clockwise or counterclockwise. Shoulder blades pulled back too hard. Shoulder blades too far apart. Shoulder blades too prominent, standing out from the rib cage (winged scapulae).
Head is held erect in a position of good balance.	**Head**	Chin up too high. Head protruding forward. Head tilted or rotated to one side.

From Kendall F, McCreary E, Provance P: Muscle Testing and Function. Lippencott, William & Wilkens, Baltimore 1993, p.115-116, with permission

Positioning of a Joint

Descriptions of Specific Positions

	Loose Packed	Close Packed
Stress on joint:	Minimal	Maximal
Congruency of joint:	Minimal	Full
Ligament position:	Great laxity	Full tightness
Joint surface:	No volitional separation	Compressed

Resting (Loose Packed) Position of Joints

Joint:	Position:
Facet (spine)	Midway between flexion and extension
Temporomandibular	Mouth slightly open (freeway space)
Glenohumeral	55° abduction, 30° horizontal adduction
Acromioclavicular	Arm resting by side in normal physiological position
Ulnohumeral (elbow)	70° flexion, 10° supination
Radiohumeral	Full extension, full supination
Proximal radioulnar	70° flexion, 35° supination
Distal radioulnar	10° supination
Radiocarpal (wrist)	Neutral with slight ulnar deviation
Carpometacarpal	Midway between abduction - adduction and flexion - extension
Metacarpophalangeal	Slight flexion
Interphalangeal	Slight flexion
Hip	30° flexion, 30° abduction, slight lateral rotation
Knee	25° flexion
Talocrural (ankle)	10° plantar flexion, midway between maximum inversion and eversion
Subtalar	Midway between extremes of range of movement
Midtarsal	Midway between extremes of range of movement
Tarsometatarsal	Midway between extremes of range of movement
Metatarsophalangeal	Neutral
Interphalangeal	Slight flexion

From Magee, DJ: Orthopedic Physical Assessment. W.B. Saunders Company, Philadelphia 1997, p.38, with permission.

Close Packed Position of Joints

Joint:	Position:
Facet (spine)	Extension
Temporomandibular	Clenched teeth
Glenohumeral	Abduction and lateral rotation
Acromioclavicular	Arm abducted to 90°
Sternoclavicular	Maximum shoulder elevation
Ulnohumeral (elbow)	Extension
Radiohumeral	Elbow flexed 90°, forearm supinated 5°
Proximal radioulnar	5° supination
Distal radioulnar	5° supination
Radiocarpal (wrist)	Extension with radial deviation
Metacarpophalangeal (fingers)	Full flexion
Metacarpophalangeal (thumb)	Full opposition
Interphalangeal	Full extension
Hip	Full extension, medial rotation
Knee	Full extension, lateral rotation of tibia
Talocrural (ankle)	Maximum dorsiflexion
Subtalar	Supination
Midtarsal	Supination
Tarsometatarsal	Supination
Metatarsophalangeal	Full extension
Interphalangeal	Full extension

From Magee, DJ: Orthopedic Physical Assessment. W.B. Saunders Company, Philadelphia 1997, p.38, with permission.

Common Capsular Patterns of Joints

Joint:	Restriction:*
Temporomandibular	Limitation of mouth opening
Atlanto-occipital	Extension, side flexion equally limited
Cervical spine	Side flexion and rotation equally limited, extension
Glenohumeral	Lateral rotation, abduction, medial rotation
Sternoclavicular	Pain at extreme of range of movement
Acromioclavicular	Pain at extreme of range of movement
Humeroulnar	Flexion, extension
Radiohumeral	Flexion, extension, supination, pronation
Proximal radioulnar	Supination, pronation

UNIT TWO: MUSCULOSKELETAL

Joint:	Restriction:*
Distal radioulnar	Full range of movement, pain at extremes of rotation
Wrist	Flexion and extension equally limited
Trapeziometacarpal	Abduction, extension
Metacarpophalangeal and interphalangeal	Flexion, extension
Thoracic spine	Side flexion and rotation equally limited, extension
Lumbar spine	Side flexion and rotation equally limited, extension
Sacroiliac, symphysis pubis, and sacrococcygeal	Pain when joints are stressed
Hip**	Flexion, abduction, medial rotation (but in some cases medial rotation is most limited)
Knee	Flexion, extension
Tibiofibular	Pain when joint stressed
Talocrural	Plantar flexion, dorsiflexion
Talocalcaneal (subtalar)	Limitation of varus range of movement
Midtarsal	Dorsiflexion, plantar flexion, adduction, medial rotation
First metatarsophalangeal	Extension, flexion
Second to fifth metatarsophalangeal	Variable
Interphalangeal	Flexion, extension

* Movements are listed in order of restriction.
**For the hip, flexion, abduction, and medial rotation are always the movements most limited in a capsular pattern. However, the order of restriction may vary.

From Magee, DJ: Orthopedic Physical Assessment. W.B. Saunders Company, Philadelphia 1997, p.22, with permission.

End-Feel

End-feel is the type of resistance that is felt when passively moving a joint through the end range of motion. Certain tissues and joints have a consistent end-feel and are described as firm, hard, or soft. Pathology can be identified through noting the type of abnormal end-feel within a particular joint.

Normal end-feel
- **Firm (stretch)**
  Examples: Ankle dorsiflexion
  Finger extension
  Hip medial rotation
  Forearm supination
- **Hard (bone to bone)**
  Example: Elbow extension
- **Soft (soft tissue approximation)**
  Examples: Elbow flexion
  Knee flexion

Abnormal end-feel
Abnormal end-feel would consist of any end-feel that is felt at an abnormal or inconsistent point in the range of motion or in a joint that normally presents with a different end-feel.

- **Empty (cannot reach end-feel, usually due to pain)**
  Examples: Joint inflammation
  Fracture
  Bursitis
- **Firm**
  Examples: Increased tone
  Tightening of the capsule
  Ligament shortening
- **Hard**
  Examples: Fracture
  Osteoarthritis
  Osteophyte formation
- **Soft**
  Examples: Edema
  Synovitis
  Ligament instability/tear

Muscle Testing

Manual Muscle Testing Grades

Zero (0/5)	The subject demonstrates no palpable muscle contraction.
Trace (1/5)	The subject's muscle contraction can be palpated, but there is no joint movement.
Poor Minus (2-/5)	The subject does not complete range of motion in a gravity eliminated position.
Poor (2/5)	The subject completes range of motion with gravity eliminated.
Poor Plus (2+/5)	The subject is able to initiate movement against gravity.
Fair Minus (3-/5)	The subject does not complete the range of motion against gravity, but does complete more than half of the range.
Fair (3/5)	The subject completes range of motion against gravity without manual resistance.

Fair Plus (3+/5) — The subject completes range of motion against gravity with only minimal resistance.

Good Minus (4-/5) — The subject completes range of motion against gravity with minimal-moderate resistance.

Good (4/5) — The subject completes range of motion against gravity with moderate resistance.

Good Plus (4+/5) — The subject completes range of motion against gravity with moderate-maximal resistance.

Normal (5/5) — The subject completes range of motion against gravity with maximal resistance.

Recommended Positioning for Muscle Testing

Supine:
Abdominals
Biceps
Finger flexors
Iliopsoas
Lateral rotators of shoulder*
Neck flexors
Pectoralis minor
Pronators
Serratus anterior
Tensor fasciae latae
Thumb muscles
Tibialis posterior
Toe flexors
Wrist extensors
Anterior deltoid*
Brachioradialis
Finger extensors
Infraspinatus
Medial rotators of shoulder*
Pectoralis major
Peroneals
Sartorius
Supinators
Teres minor
Tibialis anterior
Toe extensors
Triceps*
Wrist flexors

Sidelying:
Gluteus medius
Hip adductors
Gluteus minimus
Lateral abdominals

Prone:
Back extensors
Gluteus maximus
Lateral rotators of the shoulder*
Lower trapezius
Middle trapezius
Posterior deltoid*
Rhomboids
Teres major
Gastrocnemius
Hamstrings*
Latissimus dorsi
Medial rotators of the shoulder*
Neck extensors
Quadratus lumborum
Soleus
Triceps*

Sitting:
Coracobrachialis
Hip flexors*
Medial rotators of hip
Upper trapezius
Deltoid*
Lateral rotators of hip
Quadriceps
Serratus anterior*

Standing:
Ankle plantar flexors
Serratus anterior*

*Indicates multiple acceptable positions for muscle testing

Gait

Standard versus Rancho Los Amigos Terminology

	Standard Terminology	Rancho Los Amigos Terminology
Stance Phase (60% of gait cycle)	Heel strike	Initial contact
	Foot flat	Loading response
	Mid-stance	Mid-stance
	Heel off	Terminal stance
	Toe off	Pre-swing
Swing Phase (40% of gait cycle)	Acceleration	Initial swing
	Mid-swing	Mid-swing
	Deceleration	Terminal swing

Standard Terminology

Stance phase:
Heel strike: Heel strike is the instant that the heel touches the ground to begin stance phase.

Foot flat: Foot flat is the point in which the entire foot makes contact with the ground and should occur directly after heel strike.

Mid-stance: Mid-stance is the point during the stance phase when the entire body weight is directly over the stance limb.

Heel off: Heel off is the point in which the heel of the stance limb leaves the ground.

Toe off: Toe off is the point in which only the toe of the stance limb remains on the ground.

Swing phase:
Acceleration: Acceleration begins when toe off is complete and the reference limb swings until positioned directly under the body.

Mid-swing: Mid-swing is the point when the swing limb is directly under the body.

UNIT TWO: MUSCULOSKELETAL

Deceleration: Deceleration begins directly after mid-swing as the swing limb begins to extend and ends just prior to heel strike.

Rancho Los Amigos Terminology

Stance Phase:

Initial contact: Initial contact is the beginning of the stance phase that occurs when the foot touches the ground.

Loading response: Loading response corresponds to the amount of time between initial contact and the beginning of the swing phase for the other leg.

Mid-stance: Mid-stance corresponds to the point in stance phase when the other foot is off the floor until the body is directly over the stance limb.

Terminal stance: Terminal stance begins when the stance limb's heel rises and ends when the other foot touches the ground.

Pre-swing: Pre-swing phase begins when the other foot touches the ground and ends when the stance foot reaches toe off.

Swing Phase:

Initial swing: Initial swing phase begins when the stance foot lifts from the floor and ends with maximal knee flexion during swing.

Mid-swing: Mid-swing phase begins with maximal knee flexion during swing and ends when the tibia is perpendicular with the ground.

Terminal swing: Terminal swing phase begins when the tibia is perpendicular to the floor and ends when the foot touches the ground.

Normal Gait

	SWING 40 %			**STANCE 60 %**				
	Initial Swing	Mid-Swing	Terminal Swing	Initial Contact	Loading Response	Mid-Stance	Terminal Stance	Pre-Swing
Trunk	Erect Neutral	Erect Neutral	Erect Neutral	Erect Neutral	Erect Neutral	Erect Neutral	Erect Neutral	Erect Neutral
Pelvis	Level; Backward Rotation 5°	Level; Neutral Rotation	Level; Forward Rotation 5°	Level; Maintains Forward Rotation	Level; Less Forward Rotation	Level; Neutral Rotation	Level; Backward Rotation 5°	Level; Backward Rotation 5°
Hip	Flexion 20° Neutral -Rotation -Abduction -Adduction	Flexion 20°-30° Neutral -Rotation -Abduction -Adduction	Flexion 30° Neutral -Rotation -Abduction -Adduction	Flexion 30° Neutral -Rotation -Abduction -Adduction	Flexion 30° Neutral -Rotation -Abduction -Adduction	Extending to Neutral Neutral -Rotation -Abduction -Adduction	Apparent Hyperext 10° Neutral -Rotation -Abduction -Adduction	Neutral Extension Neutral -Rotation -Abduction -Adduction
Knee	Flexion 60°	From 60° to 30° Flexion	Extension to 0°	Full Extension	Flexion 15°	Extending to Neutral	Full Extension	Flexion 35°
Ankle	Plantar Flexion 10°	Neutral	Neutral	Neutral Heel First	Plantar Flexion 15°	From Plantar Flexion to 10° Dorsiflexion	Neutral with Tibia Stable and Heel Off Prior to Initial Contact Opposite Foot	Plantar Flexion 20°
Toes	Neutral	Neutral	Neutral	Neutral	Neutral	Neutral	Neutral IP Extended MP	Neutral IP Extended MP

From Rancho Los Amigos National Rehabilitation Center: Normal and Pathological Gait Syllabus, p.11. Downey, California, with permission.

Range of Motion Requirements for Normal Gait

Hip flexion:	0 – 30 degrees
Hip extension:	0 – 15 degrees
Knee flexion:	0 – 60 degrees
Knee extension:	0 degrees
Ankle dorsiflexion:	0 – 10 degrees
Ankle plantar flexion:	0 – 20 degrees

Peak Muscle Activity During the Gait Cycle

Tibialis anterior: Peak activity is just after heel strike. Responsible for eccentric lowering of the foot into plantar flexion.

Gastroc-soleus: Peak activity is during late stance phase. Responsible for concentric raising of the heel during toe off.

Quadriceps group: Two periods of peak activity. In periods of single support during early stance phase and just before toe off to initiate swing phase.

Hamstrings group: Peak activity is during late swing phase. Responsible for decelerating the unsupported limb.

Gait Terminology

Base of support: The distance measured between the left and right foot during progression of gait. The distance decreases as cadence increases. The average base of support for an adult is two to four inches.

Cadence: The number of steps an individual will walk over a period of time. The average value for an adult is 110 – 120 steps per minute.

Degree of toe out: The angle formed by each foot's line of progression and a line intersecting the center of the heel and second toe. The average degree of toe out for an adult is seven degrees.

Double support phase: The double support phase refers to the two times during a gait cycle where both feet are on the ground. The time of double support increases as the speed of gait decreases. This phase does not exist with running.

Gait cycle: The gait cycle refers to the sequence of motions that occur from one initial contact of the heel to the next consecutive initial contact of the same heel.

Pelvic rotation: Rotation of the pelvis opposite the thorax in order to maintain balance and regulate speed. The pelvic rotation during gait for an adult is a total of 8 degrees (4 degrees forward with the swing leg and 4 degrees backward with the stance leg).

Single support phase: The single support phase occurs when only one foot is on the ground and occurs twice during a single gait cycle.

Step length: The distance measured between right heel strike and left heel strike. The average step length for an adult is 13 to 16 inches.

Stride: The distance measured between right heel strike and the following right heel strike. The average stride length for an adult is 26 to 32 inches.

Abnormal Gait Patterns

Antalgic: A protective gait pattern where the involved step length is decreased in order to avoid weight bearing on the involved side usually secondary to pain.

Ataxic: Characterized by staggering and unsteadiness. There is usually a wide base of support and movements are exaggerated.

Cerebellar: A staggering gait pattern seen in cerebellar disease.

Circumduction: Characterized by a circular motion to advance the leg during swing phase; this may be used to compensate for insufficient hip or knee flexion or dorsiflexion.

Double step: Gait in which alternate steps are of a different length or at a different rate.

Equine: Characterized by high steps; usually involves excessive activity of the gastrocnemius.

Festinating: Patient walks on toes as though pushed. Starts slowly, increases, and may continue until the patient grasps an object in order to stop.

Hemiplegic: Gait in which patients abduct the paralyzed limb, swing it around, and bring it forward so the foot comes to the ground in front of them.

Parkinsonian: Increased forward flexion of the trunk and knees; gait is shuffling with quick and small steps; festinating may occur.

Scissor: Gait in which the legs cross midline upon advancement.

Spastic: A stiff movement, toes seeming to catch and drag, legs held together, hip and knee joints slightly flexed. Commonly seen in spastic paraplegia.

Steppage: Gait in which the feet and toes are lifted through hip and knee flexion to excessive heights; usually secondary to dorsiflexor weakness. The foot will slap at initial contact with the ground secondary to the decreased control.

Tabetic: High stepping ataxic gait in which the feet slap the ground.

Trendelenburg: Denotes gluteus medius weakness; excessive lateral trunk flexion and weight shifting over the stance leg.

Vaulting: The swing leg advances by compensating through the combination of elevation of the pelvis and plantar flexion of the stance leg.

Gait Deviations

Ankle and Foot	*Foot slap* -- Weak dorsiflexors -- Dorsiflexor paralysis	*Toe down instead of heel strike* -- Plantar flexor spasticity -- Plantar flexor contracture -- Weak dorsiflexors -- Dorsiflexor paralysis -- Leg length discrepancy -- Hindfoot pain	*Clawing of toes* -- Toe flexor spasticity -- Positive support reflex	*Heel lift during mid-stance* -- Insufficient dorsiflexion range -- Plantar flexor spasticity	*No toe off* -- Forefoot/toe pain -- Weak plantar flexors -- Weak toe flexors -- Insufficient plantar flexion range of motion
Knee	*Exaggerated knee flexion at contact* -- Weak quadriceps -- Quadriceps paralysis -- Hamstrings spasticity -- Insufficient extension range of motion	*Hyperextension in stance* -- Compensation for weak quadriceps -- Plantar flexor contracture	*Exaggerated knee flexion at terminal stance* -- Knee flexion contracture -- Hip flexion contracture	*Insufficient flexion with swing* -- Knee effusion -- Quadriceps extension spasticity -- Plantar flexor spasticity -- Insufficient flexion range of motion	*Excessive flexion with swing* -- Flexor withdrawal reflex -- Lower extremity flexor synergy
Hip	*Insufficient hip flexion at initial contact* -- Weak hip flexors -- Hip flexor paralysis -- Hip extensor spasticity -- Insufficient hip flexion range of motion	*Insufficient hip extension at stance* -- Insufficient hip extension range of motion -- Hip flexion contracture -- Lower extremity flexor synergy	*Circumduction during swing* -- Compensation for weak hip flexors -- Compensation for weak dorsiflexors -- Compensation for weak hamstrings	*Hip hiking during swing* -- Compensation for weak dorsiflexors -- Compensation for weak knee flexors -- Compensation for extensor synergy pattern	*Exaggerated hip flexion during swing* -- Lower extremity flexor synergy -- Compensation for insufficient hip flexion or dorsiflexion

26 A GUIDE TO SUCCESS

Range of Motion

Average Adult Range of Motion for the Upper and Lower Extremities

Upper Extremity

- **Shoulder:**

Flexion	0-180
Extension	0-60
Abduction	0-180
Medial rotation	0-70
Lateral rotation	0-90

- **Elbow:**

Flexion	0-150

- **Forearm:**

Pronation	0-80
Supination	0-80

- **Wrist:**

Flexion	0-80
Extension	0-70
Radial deviation	0-20
Ulnar deviation	0-30

- **Thumb:**
  - **Carpometacarpal**

Abduction	0-70
Flexion	0-15
Extension	0-20
Opposition	Tip of thumb to base of fifth digit

  - **Metacarpophalangeal**

Flexion	0-50

  - **Interphalangeal**

Flexion	0-80

- **Digits – Second to Fifth:**
  - **Metacarpophalangeal**

Flexion	0-90
Hyperextension	0-45

  - **Proximal interphalangeal**

Flexion	0-100

  - **Distal interphalangeal**

Flexion	0-90
Hyperextension	0-10

Lower Extremity

- **Hip:**

Flexion	0-120
Extension	0-30
Abduction	0-45
Adduction	0-30
Medial rotation	0-45
Lateral rotation	0-45

- **Knee:**

Flexion	0-135

- **Ankle:**

Dorsiflexion	0-20
Plantar flexion	0-50
Inversion	0-35
Eversion	0-15

- **Subtalar:**

Inversion	0-5
Eversion	0-5

From Norkin and White: Measurement of Joint Motion: A Guide to Goniometry. F.A. Davis Company, Philadelphia, 1995, p.221-222, with permission.

Process for Conducting Goniometric Measurements

1. Place the subject in the recommended testing position.
2. Stabilize the proximal joint segment.
3. Move the distal joint segment through the available range of motion. Make sure that the passive range of motion is performed slowly, the end of the range is attained, and the end-feel determined.
4. Make a clinical estimate of the range of motion.
5. Return the distal joint segment to the starting position.
6. Palpate bony anatomical landmarks.
7. Align the goniometer.
8. Read and record the starting position. Remove the goniometer.
9. Stabilize the proximal joint segment.
10. Move the distal segment through the full range of motion.
11. Replace and realign the goniometer. Palpate the anatomical landmarks again if necessary.
12. Read and record the range of motion.

Adapted from Norkin and White: Measurement of Joint Motion: A Guide to Goniometry. F.A. Davis Company, Philadelphia, 1995, p.32, with permission.

UNIT TWO: MUSCULOSKELETAL

Goniometric Technique

Upper Extremity

- **Shoulder:**
  Flexion
  Axis: acromial process
  Stationary arm: midaxillary line of the thorax
  Moveable arm: lateral midline of the humerus using the lateral epicondyle of the humerus for reference

  Extension
  Axis: acromial process
  Stationary arm: midaxillary line of the thorax
  Moveable arm: lateral midline of the humerus using the lateral epicondyle of the humerus for reference

  Abduction
  Axis: anterior aspect of the acromial process
  Stationary arm: parallel to the midline of the anterior aspect of the sternum
  Moveable arm: medial midline of the humerus

  Adduction
  Axis: anterior aspect of the acromial process
  Stationary arm: parallel to the midline of the anterior aspect of the sternum
  Moveable arm: medial midline of the humerus

  Medial rotation
  Axis: olecranon process
  Stationary arm: parallel or perpendicular to the floor
  Moveable arm: ulna using the olecranon process and ulnar styloid for reference

  Lateral rotation
  Axis: olecranon process
  Stationary arm: parallel or perpendicular to the floor
  Moveable arm: ulna using the olecranon process and ulnar styloid process for reference

- **Elbow:**
  Flexion
  Axis: lateral epicondyle of the humerus
  Stationary arm: lateral midline of the humerus using the center of the acromial process for reference
  Moveable arm: lateral midline of the radius using the radial head and radial styloid process for reference

  Extension
  Axis: lateral epicondyle of the humerus
  Stationary arm: lateral midline of the humerus using the center of the acromial process for reference
  Moveable arm: lateral midline of the radius using the radial head and radial styloid process for reference

- **Forearm:**
  Pronation
  Axis: lateral to the ulnar styloid process
  Stationary arm: parallel to the anterior midline of the humerus
  Moveable arm: dorsal aspect of the forearm, just proximal to the styloid process of the radius and ulna

  Supination
  Axis: medial to the ulnar styloid process
  Stationary arm: parallel to the anterior midline of the humerus
  Moveable arm: ventral aspect of the forearm, just proximal to the styloid process of the radius and ulna

- **Wrist:**
  Flexion
  Axis: lateral aspect of the wrist over the triquetrum
  Stationary arm: lateral midline of the ulna using the olecranon and ulnar styloid process for reference
  Moveable arm: lateral midline of the fifth metacarpal

  Extension
  Axis: lateral aspect of the wrist over the triquetrum
  Stationary arm: lateral midline of the ulna using the olecranon and ulnar styloid process for reference
  Moveable arm: lateral midline of the fifth metacarpal

  Radial deviation
  Axis: over the middle of the dorsal aspect of the wrist over the capitate
  Stationary arm: dorsal midline of the forearm using the lateral epicondyle of the humerus for reference
  Moveable arm: dorsal midline of the third metacarpal

  Ulnar deviation
  Axis: over the middle of the dorsal aspect of the wrist over the capitate
  Stationary arm: dorsal midline of the forearm using the lateral epicondyle of the humerus for reference
  Moveable arm: dorsal midline of the third metacarpal

- **Thumb:**
  --Carpometacarpal
  Flexion
  Axis: over the palmar aspect of the first carpometacarpal joint
  Stationary arm: ventral midline of the radius using the ventral surface of the radial head and radial styloid process for reference
  Moveable arm: ventral midline of the first metacarpal

Extension
  Axis: over the palmar aspect of the first carpometacarpal joint
  Stationary arm: ventral midline of the radius using the ventral surface of the radial head and radial styloid process for reference
  Moveable arm: ventral midline of the first metacarpal

Abduction
  Axis: over the lateral aspect of the radial styloid process
  Stationary arm: lateral midline of the second metacarpal using the center of the second metacarpophalangeal joint for reference
  Moveable arm: lateral midline of the first metacarpal using the center of the first metacarpophalangeal joint for reference

Adduction
  Axis: over the lateral aspect of the radial styloid process
  Stationary arm: lateral midline of the second metacarpal using the center of the second metacarpophalangeal joint for reference
  Moveable arm: lateral midline of the first metacarpal using the center of the first metacarpophalangeal joint for reference

- **Fingers:**
  --**Metacarpophalangeal**
  Flexion
    Axis: over the dorsal aspect of the metacarpophalangeal joint
    Stationary arm: over the dorsal midline of the metacarpal
    Moveable arm: over the dorsal midline of the proximal phalanx

  Extension
    Axis: over the dorsal aspect of the metacarpophalangeal joint
    Stationary arm: over the dorsal midline of the metacarpal
    Moveable arm: over the dorsal midline of the proximal phalanx

  Abduction
    Axis: over the dorsal aspect of the metacarpophalangeal joint
    Stationary arm: over the dorsal midline of the metacarpal
    Moveable arm: dorsal midline of the proximal phalanx

  Adduction
    Axis: over the dorsal aspect of the metacarpophalangeal joint
    Stationary arm: over the dorsal midline of the metacarpal
    Moveable arm: dorsal midline of the proximal phalanx

  --**Proximal Interphalangeal**
  Flexion
    Axis: over the dorsal aspect of the proximal interphalangeal joint
    Stationary arm: over the dorsal midline of the proximal phalanx
    Moveable arm: over the dorsal midline of the middle phalanx

  Extension
    Axis: over the dorsal aspect of the proximal interphalangeal joint
    Stationary arm: over the dorsal midline of the proximal phalanx
    Moveable arm: over the dorsal midline of the middle phalanx

  --**Distal Interphalangeal**
  Flexion
    Axis: over the dorsal aspect of the distal interphalangeal joint
    Stationary arm: over the dorsal midline of the middle phalanx
    Moveable arm: over the dorsal midline of the distal phalanx

  Extension
    Axis: over the dorsal aspect of the distal interphalangeal joint
    Stationary arm: over the dorsal midline of the middle phalanx
    Moveable arm: over the dorsal midline of the distal phalanx

Lower Extremity

- **Hip:**
  Flexion
    Axis: over the lateral aspect of the hip joint using the greater trochanter of the femur for reference
    Stationary arm: lateral midline of the pelvis
    Moveable arm: lateral midline of the femur using the lateral epicondyle for reference

  Extension
    Axis: over the lateral aspect of the hip joint using the greater trochanter of the femur for reference
    Stationary arm: lateral midline of the pelvis
    Moveable arm: lateral midline of the femur using the lateral epicondyle for reference

Abduction
- **Axis:** over the anterior superior iliac spine (ASIS) of the extremity being measured
- **Stationary arm:** align with imaginary horizontal line extending from one ASIS to the other ASIS
- **Moveable arm:** anterior midline of the femur using the midline of the patella for reference

Adduction
- **Axis:** over the anterior superior iliac spine (ASIS) of the extremity being measured
- **Stationary arm:** align with imaginary horizontal line extending from one ASIS to the other ASIS
- **Moveable arm:** anterior midline of the femur using the midline of the patella for reference

Medial rotation
- **Axis:** anterior aspect of the patella
- **Stationary arm:** perpendicular to the floor or parallel to the supporting surface
- **Moveable arm:** anterior midline of the lower leg using the crest of the tibia and a point midway between the two malleoli for reference

Lateral rotation
- **Axis:** anterior aspect of the patella
- **Stationary arm:** perpendicular to the floor or parallel to the supporting surface
- **Moveable arm:** anterior midline of the lower leg using the crest of the tibia and a point midway between the two malleoli for reference

- **Knee:**
  Flexion
  - **Axis:** lateral epicondyle of the femur
  - **Stationary arm:** lateral midline of the femur using the greater trochanter for reference
  - **Moveable arm:** lateral midline of the fibula using the lateral malleolus and fibular head for reference

  Extension
  - **Axis:** lateral epicondyle of the femur
  - **Stationary arm:** lateral midline of the femur using the greater trochanter for reference
  - **Moveable arm:** lateral midline of the fibula using the lateral malleolus and fibular head for reference

- **Ankle:**
  Dorsiflexion
  - **Axis:** lateral aspect of the lateral malleolus
  - **Stationary arm:** lateral midline of the fibula using the head of the fibula for reference
  - **Moveable arm:** parallel to the lateral aspect of the fifth metatarsal

  Plantar flexion
  - **Axis:** lateral aspect of the lateral malleolus
  - **Stationary arm:** lateral midline of the fibula using the head of the fibula for reference
  - **Moveable arm:** parallel to the lateral aspect of the fifth metatarsal

  Inversion
  - **Axis:** anterior aspect of the ankle midway between the malleoli
  - **Stationary arm:** anterior midline of the lower leg using the tibial tuberosity for reference
  - **Moveable arm:** anterior midline of the second metatarsal

  Eversion
  - **Axis:** anterior aspect of the ankle midway between the malleoli
  - **Stationary arm:** anterior midline of the lower leg using the tibial tuberosity for reference
  - **Moveable arm:** anterior midline of the second metatarsal

- **Subtalar:**
  Inversion
  - **Axis:** posterior aspect of the ankle midway between the malleoli
  - **Stationary arm:** posterior midline of the lower leg
  - **Moveable arm:** posterior midline of the calcaneus

  Eversion
  - **Axis:** posterior aspect of the ankle midway between the malleoli
  - **Stationary arm:** posterior midline of the lower leg
  - **Moveable arm:** posterior midline of the calcaneus

Muscle Insufficiency

A muscle contraction that is less than optimal due to an extremely lengthened or shortened position of the muscle. There are two types of insufficiency:

Active: when a two joint muscle contracts across both joints simultaneously

Passive: when a two joint muscle is lengthened over both joints simultaneously

Special Tests

Special Tests Outline

Upper Extremity

- **Shoulder**
  --**Dislocation**
   Apprehension test for anterior shoulder dislocation
   Apprehension test for posterior shoulder dislocation

  --**Biceps Tendon Pathology**
   Ludington's test
   Speed's test
   Yergason's test

  --**Rotator Cuff Pathology/Impingement**
   Drop arm test
   Hawkins-Kennedy impingement test
   Neer impingement test
   Supraspinatus test

  --**Thoracic Outlet Syndrome**
   Adson maneuver
   Allen test
   Costoclavicular syndrome test
   Roos test
   Wright test (hyperabduction test)

  --**Miscellaneous**
   Glenoid labrum tear test

- **Elbow**
  --**Ligamentous Instability**
   Varus stress test
   Valgus stress test

  --**Epicondylitis**
   Cozen's test
   Lateral epicondylitis test
   Medial epicondylitis test
   Mill's test

  --**Neurological Dysfunction**
   Tinel's sign

- **Wrist/Hand**
  --**Ligamentous Instability**
   Ulnar collateral ligament instability test

  --**Vascular Insufficiency**
   Allen test
   Capillary refill test

  --**Contracture/Tightness**
   Bunnel-Littler test
   Tight retinacular ligament test

  --**Neurological Dysfunction**
   Froment's sign
   Phalen's test
   Tinel's sign

  --**Miscellaneous**
   Finkelstein test
   Grind test
   Murphy sign

Lower Extremity

- **Hip**
  --**Contracture/Tightness**
   Ely's test
   Ober's test
   Piriformis test
   Thomas test
   Tripod sign
   90-90 straight leg raise test

  --**Pediatric Tests**
   Barlow's test
   Ortolani's test

  --**Miscellaneous**
   Craig's test
   Patrick's test (Faber test)
   Quadrant scouring test
   Trendelenburg test

- **Knee**
  --**Ligamentous Instability**
   Anterior drawer test
   Lachman test
   Lateral pivot shift test
   Posterior drawer test
   Posterior sag sign
   Slocum test
   Valgus stress test
   Varus stress test

  --**Meniscal Pathology**
   Apley's compression test
   Bounce home test
   McMurray test

  --**Swelling**
   Brush test
   Patellar tap test

  --**Miscellaneous**
   Clarke's sign
   Hughston's plica test
   Noble compression test
   Patellar apprehension test

- **Ankle**
  - --**Ligamentous Instability**
    - Anterior drawer test
    - Talar tilt

  - --**Miscellaneous**
    - Homans' sign
    - Thompson test
    - Tibial torsion test
    - True leg length discrepancy test

Spine

- --**Cervical Region**
  - Foraminal compression test
  - Vertebral artery test

- --**Lumbar/Sacroiliac Region**
  - Sacroiliac joint stress test
  - Sitting flexion test
  - Standing flexion test

Descriptions of Special Tests

Upper Extremity

- **Shoulder**
  - --**Dislocation**

    Apprehension test for anterior shoulder dislocation
    The patient is positioned in supine with the arm in 90 degrees of abduction. The therapist laterally rotates the patient's shoulder. A positive test is indicated by a look of apprehension or a facial grimace prior to reaching an end point.

    Apprehension test for posterior shoulder dislocation
    The patient is positioned in supine with the arm in 90 degrees of flexion and medial rotation. The therapist applies a posterior force through the long axis of the humerus. A positive test is indicated by a look of apprehension or a facial grimace prior to reaching an end point.

  - --**Biceps Tendon Pathology**

    Ludington's test
    The patient is positioned in sitting and is asked to clasp both hands behind the head with the fingers interlocked. The patient is then asked to alternately contract and relax the biceps muscles. A positive test is indicated by absence of movement in the biceps tendon and may be indicative of a rupture of the long head of the biceps.

    Speed's test
    The patient is positioned in sitting or standing with the elbow extended and the forearm supinated. The therapist places one hand over the bicipital groove and the other hand on the volar surface of the forearm. The therapist resists active shoulder flexion. A positive test is indicated by pain or tenderness in the bicipital groove region and may be indicative of bicipital tendonitis.

    Yergason's test
    The patient is positioned in sitting with 90 degrees of elbow flexion and the forearm pronated. The humerus is stabilized against the patient's thorax. The therapist places one hand on the patient's forearm and the other hand over the bicipital groove. The patient is directed to actively supinate and laterally rotate against resistance. A positive test is indicated by pain or tenderness in the bicipital groove and may be indicative of bicipital tendonitis.

  - --**Rotator Cuff Pathology/Impingement**

    Drop arm test
    The patient is positioned in sitting or standing with the arm in 90 degrees of abduction. The patient is asked to slowly lower the arm to his/her side. A positive test is indicated by the patient failing to slowly lower the arm to his/her side or by the presence of severe pain and may be indicative of a tear in the rotator cuff.

    Hawkins-Kennedy impingement test
    The patient is positioned in sitting or standing. The therapist flexes the patient's shoulder to 90 degrees and then medially rotates the arm. A positive test is indicated by pain and may be indicative of shoulder impingement involving the supraspinatus tendon.

    Neer impingement test
    The patient is positioned in sitting or standing. The therapist positions one hand on the posterior aspect of the patient's scapula and the other hand stabilizing the elbow. The therapist elevates the patient's arm through flexion. A positive test is indicated by a facial grimace or pain and may be indicative of shoulder impingement involving the supraspinatus tendon.

    Supraspinatus test
    The patient is positioned with the arm in 90 degrees of abduction followed by 30 degrees of horizontal adduction with the thumb pointing downward. The therapist resists the patient's attempt to abduct the arm. A positive test is indicated by weakness or pain and may be indicative of a tear of the supraspinatus tendon, impingement, or suprascapular nerve involvement.

  - --**Thoracic Outlet Syndrome**

    Adson maneuver
    The patient is positioned in sitting or standing. The therapist monitors the radial pulse and asks the patient to rotate his/her head to face the test shoulder. The patient is then asked to extend his/her head while the therapist laterally rotates and extends the patient's shoulder. A positive test is indicated by an absent or diminished radial pulse and may be indicative of thoracic outlet syndrome.

32   A GUIDE TO SUCCESS

Allen test
The patient is positioned in sitting or standing with the test arm in 90 degrees of abduction, lateral rotation, and elbow flexion. The patient is asked to rotate the head away from the test shoulder while the therapist monitors the radial pulse. A positive test is indicated by an absent or diminished pulse when the head is rotated away from the test shoulder. A positive test may be indicative of thoracic outlet syndrome.

Costoclavicular syndrome test
The patient is positioned in sitting. The therapist monitors the patient's radial pulse and assists the patient to assume a military posture. A positive test is indicated by an absent or diminished radial pulse and may be indicative of thoracic outlet syndrome caused by compression of the subclavian artery between the first rib and the clavicle.

Roos test
The patient is positioned in sitting or standing with the arms positioned in 90 degrees of abduction, lateral rotation, and elbow flexion. The patient is asked to open and close his/her hands for three minutes. A positive test is indicated by an inability to maintain the test position, weakness of the arms, sensory loss, or ischemic pain. A positive test may be indicative of thoracic outlet syndrome.

Wright test (hyperabduction test)
The patient is positioned in sitting or supine. The therapist moves the patient's arm overhead in the frontal plane while monitoring the patient's radial pulse. A positive test is indicted by an absent or diminished radial pulse and may be indicative of compression in the costoclavicular space.

--**Miscellaneous**
Glenoid labrum tear test
The patient is positioned in supine. The therapist places one hand on the posterior aspect of the patient's humeral head while the other hand stabilizes the humerus proximal to the elbow. The therapist passively abducts and laterally rotates the arm over the patient's head and then proceeds to apply an anterior directed force to the humerus. A positive test is indicated by a clunk or grinding sound and may be indicative of a glenoid labrum tear.

- **Elbow**
  --**Ligamentous Instability**
  Varus stress test
  The patient is positioned in sitting with the elbow in 20 to 30 degrees of flexion. The therapist places one hand on the elbow and the other hand proximal to the patient's wrist. The therapist applies a varus force to test the lateral collateral ligament while palpating the lateral joint line. A positive test is indicated by increased laxity in the lateral collateral ligament when compared to the contralateral limb, apprehension or pain. A positive test may be indicative of a lateral collateral ligament sprain.

Valgus stress test
The patient is positioned in sitting with the elbow in 20 to 30 degrees of flexion. The therapist places one hand on the elbow and the other hand proximal to the patient's wrist. The therapist applies a valgus force to test the medial collateral ligament while palpating the medial joint line. A positive test is indicated by increased laxity in the medial collateral ligament when compared to the contralateral limb, apprehension or pain. A positive test may be indicative of a medial collateral ligament sprain.

--**Epicondylitis**
Cozen's test
The patient is positioned in sitting with the elbow in slight flexion. The therapist places his/her thumb on the patient's lateral epicondyle while stabilizing the elbow joint. The patient is asked to make a fist, pronate the forearm, radially deviate, and extend the wrist against resistance. A positive test is indicated by pain in the lateral epicondyle region or muscle weakness and may be indicative of lateral epicondylitis.

Lateral epicondylitis test
The patient is positioned in sitting. The therapist stabilizes the elbow with one hand and places the other hand on the dorsal aspect of the patient's hand distal to the proximal interphalangeal joint. The patient is asked to extend the third digit against resistance. A positive test is indicated by pain in the lateral epicondyle region or muscle weakness and may be indicative of lateral epicondylitis.

Medial epicondylitis test
The patient is positioned in sitting. The therapist palpates the medial epicondyle and supinates the patient's forearm, extends the wrist, and extends the elbow. A positive test is indicated by pain in the medial epicondyle region and may be indicative of medial epicondylitis.

Mill's test
The patient is positioned in sitting. The therapist palpates the lateral epicondyle and pronates the patient's forearm, flexes the wrist, and extends the elbow. A positive test is indicated by pain in the lateral epicondyle region and may be indicative of lateral epicondylitis.

--**Neurological Dysfunction**
Tinel's sign
The patient is positioned in sitting with the elbow in slight flexion. The therapist taps with the index finger between the olecranon process and the medial epicondyle. A positive test is indicated by a tingling sensation in the ulnar nerve distribution of the forearm,

hand, and fingers. A positive test may be indicative of ulnar nerve compression or compromise.

- **Wrist/Hand**
  --Ligamentous Instability
  Ulnar collateral ligament instability test
  The patient is positioned in sitting. The therapist holds the patient's thumb in extension and applies a valgus force to the metacarpophalangeal joint of the thumb. A positive test is indicated by excessive valgus movement and may be indicative of a tear of the ulnar collateral and accessory collateral ligaments. This type of injury is referred to as gamekeeper's or skier's thumb.

  --Vascular Insufficiency
  Allen test
  The patient is positioned in sitting or standing. The patient is asked to open and close the hand several times in succession and then maintain the hand in a closed position. The therapist compresses the radial and ulnar arteries. The patient is then asked to relax the hand and the therapist releases the pressure on one of the arteries while observing the color of the hand and fingers. A positive test is indicated by delayed or absent flushing of the radial or ulnar half of the hand and may be indicative of an occlusion in the radial or ulnar artery.

  Capillary refill test
  The patient is positioned in sitting or standing. The therapist compresses the patient's nailbed and after releasing the pressure notes the amount of time taken for the color to return to the nail. A positive test is indicated by a delayed or muted response (greater than two seconds) and may be indicative of arterial insufficiency.

  --Contracture/Tightness
  Bunnel-Littler test
  The patient is positioned in sitting with the metacarpophalangeal joint held in slight extension. The therapist attempts to move the proximal interphalangeal joint into flexion. If the proximal interphalangeal joint does not flex with the metacarpophalangeal joint extended, there may be a tight intrinsic muscle or capsular tightness. If the proximal interphalangeal joint fully flexes with the metacarpophalangeal joint in slight flexion, there may be intrinsic muscle tightness without capsular tightness.

  Tight retinacular ligament test
  The patient is positioned in sitting with the proximal interphalangeal joint in neutral and the distal interphalangeal joint flexed. If the therapist is unable to flex the distal interphalangeal joint the retinacular ligaments or capsule may be tight. If the therapist is able to flex the distal interphalangeal joint with the proximal interphalangeal joint in flexion, the retinacular ligaments may be tight and the capsule may be normal.

  --Neurological Dysfunction
  Froment's sign
  The patient is positioned in sitting or standing and is asked to hold a piece of paper between the thumb and index finger. The therapist attempts to pull the paper away from the patient. A positive test is indicated by the patient flexing the distal phalanx of the thumb due to adductor pollicis muscle paralysis. If at the same time the patient hyperextends the metacarpophalangeal joint of the thumb it is termed Jeanne's sign. Both objective findings may be indicative of ulnar nerve compromise or paralysis.

  Phalen's test
  The patient is positioned in sitting or standing. The therapist flexes the patient's wrists maximally and asks the patient to hold the position for 60 seconds. A positive test is indicated by tingling in the thumb, index finger, middle finger, and lateral half of the ring finger and may be indicative of carpal tunnel syndrome due to median nerve compression.

  Tinel's sign
  The patient is positioned in sitting or standing. The therapist taps over the volar aspect of the patient's wrist. A positive test is indicated by tingling in the thumb, index finger, middle finger, and lateral half of the ring finger distal to the contact site at the wrist. A positive test may be indicative of carpal tunnel syndrome due to median nerve compression.

  --Miscellaneous
  Finkelstein test
  The patient is positioned in sitting or standing and is asked to make a fist with the thumb tucked inside the fingers. The therapist stabilizes the patient's forearm and ulnarly deviates the wrist. A positive test is indicated by pain over the abductor pollicis longus and extensor pollicis brevis tendons at the wrist and may be indicative of tenosynovitis in the thumb (de Quervain's disease).

  Grind test
  The patient is positioned in sitting or standing. The therapist stabilizes the patient's hand and grasps the patient's thumb on the metacarpal. The therapist applies compression and rotation through the metacarpal. A positive test is indicated by pain and may be indicative of degenerative joint disease in the carpometacarpal joint.

  Murphy sign
  The patient is positioned in sitting or standing and is asked to make a fist. A positive test is indicated by the patient's third metacarpal remaining level with the second and fourth metacarpals. A positive test may be indicative of a dislocated lunate.

Lower Extremity

- **Hip**
  - **Contracture/Tightness**

    Ely's test
    The patient is positioned in prone while the therapist passively flexes the patient's knee. A positive test is indicated by spontaneous hip flexion occurring simultaneously with knee flexion and may be indicative of a rectus femoris contracture.

    Ober's test
    The patient is positioned in sidelying with the lower leg flexed at the hip and the knee. The therapist moves the test leg into hip extension and abduction and then attempts to slowly lower the test leg. A positive test is indicated by an inability of the test leg to adduct and touch the table and may be indicative of a tensor fasciae latae contracture.

    Piriformis test
    The patient is positioned in sidelying with the test leg positioned toward the ceiling and the hip flexed to 60 degrees. The therapist places one hand on the patient's pelvis and the other hand on the patient's knee. While stabilizing the pelvis, the therapist applies a downward (adduction) force on the knee. A positive test is indicated by pain or tightness, and may be indicative of piriformis tightness or compression on the sciatic nerve caused by the piriformis.

    Thomas test
    The patient is positioned in supine with the legs fully extended. The patient is asked to bring one of his/her knees to the chest in order to flatten the lumbar spine. The therapist observes the position of the contralateral hip while the patient holds the flexed hip. A positive test is indicated by the straight leg rising from the table and may be indicative of a hip flexion contracture.

    Tripod sign
    The patient is positioned in sitting with the knees flexed to 90 degrees over the edge of a table. The therapist passively extends one knee. A positive test is indicated by tightness in the hamstrings or extension of the trunk in order to limit the effect of the tight hamstrings.

    90-90 straight leg raise test
    The patient is positioned in supine and is asked to stabilize the hips in 90 degrees of flexion with the knees relaxed. The therapist instructs the patient to alternately extend each knee as much as possible while maintaining the hips in 90 degrees of flexion. A positive test is indicated by the knee remaining in 20 degrees or more of flexion and is indicative of hamstrings tightness.

  - **Pediatric Tests**

    Barlow's test
    The patient is positioned in supine with the hips flexed to 90 degrees and the knees flexed. The therapist tests each hip individually by stabilizing the femur and pelvis with one hand while the other hand moves the test leg into abduction while applying forward pressure posterior to the greater trochanter. A positive test is indicated by a click or a clunk and may be indicative of a hip dislocation being reduced. The test is considered to be a variation of Ortolani's test.

    Ortolani's test
    The patient is positioned in supine with the hips flexed to 90 degrees and the knees flexed. The therapist grasps the legs so that his/her thumbs are placed along the patient's medial thighs and the fingers are placed on the lateral thighs toward the buttocks. The therapist abducts the infant's hips and gentle pressure is applied to the greater trochanters until resistance is felt at approximately 30 degrees. A positive test is indicated by a click or a clunk and may be indicative of a dislocation being reduced.

  - **Miscellaneous**

    Craig's test
    The patient is positioned in prone with the test knee flexed to 90 degrees. The therapist palpates the posterior aspect of the greater trochanter and medially and laterally rotates the hip until the greater trochanter is parallel with the table. The degree of anteversion corresponds to the angle formed by the lower leg with the perpendicular axis of the table. Normal anteversion for an adult is 8-15 degrees.

    Patrick's test (Faber test)
    The patient is positioned in supine with the test leg flexed, abducted, and laterally rotated on the opposite leg. The therapist slowly lowers the test leg in abduction toward the table. A positive test is indicated by a failure of the test leg to abduct below the level of the opposite leg and may be indicative of iliopsoas, sacroiliac, or hip joint abnormalities.

    Quadrant scouring test
    The patient is positioned in supine. The therapist passively flexes and adducts the hip with the knee in maximal flexion. The therapist applies a compressive force through the shaft of the femur while continuing to passively move the patient's hip. A positive test is indicated by grinding, catching, or crepitation in the hip and may be indicative of pathologies such as arthritis, avascular necrosis, or an osteochondral defect.

    Trendelenburg test
    The patient is positioned in standing and is asked to stand on one leg for approximately ten seconds. A positive test is indicated by a drop of the pelvis on the unsupported side and may be indicative of weakness of the gluteus medius muscle on the supported side.

- **Knee**
  - **--Ligamentous Instability**

    Anterior drawer test
    The patient is positioned in supine with the knee flexed to 90 degrees and the hip flexed to 45 degrees. The therapist stabilizes the lower leg by sitting on the forefoot. The therapist grasps the patient's proximal tibia with two hands and places his/her thumbs on the tibial plateau and administers an anterior directed force to the tibia on the femur. A positive test is indicated by excessive anterior translation of the tibia on the femur with a diminished or absent end-point and may be indicative of an anterior cruciate ligament injury.

    Lachman test
    The patient is positioned in supine with the knee flexed to 20-30 degrees. The therapist stabilizes the distal femur with one hand and places the other hand on the proximal tibia. The therapist applies an anterior directed force to the tibia on the femur. A positive test is indicated by excessive anterior translation of the tibia on the femur with a diminished or absent end-point and may be indicative of an anterior cruciate ligament injury.

    Lateral pivot shift test
    The patient is positioned in supine with the hip flexed and abducted to 30 degrees with slight medial rotation. The therapist grasps the leg with one hand and places the other hand over the lateral surface of the proximal tibia. The therapist medially rotates the tibia and applies a valgus force to the knee while the knee is slowly flexed. A positive test is indicated by a palpable shift or clunk occurring between 20 and 40 degrees of flexion and is indicative of anterolateral rotary instability. The shift or clunk results from the reduction of the tibia on the femur.

    Posterior drawer test
    The patient is positioned in supine with the knee flexed to 90 degrees and the hip flexed to 45 degrees. The therapist stabilizes the lower leg by sitting on the forefoot. The therapist grasps the patient's proximal tibia with two hands and places his/her thumbs on the tibial plateau and administers a posterior directed force to the tibia on the femur. A positive test is indicated by excessive posterior translation of the tibia on the femur with a diminished or absent end-point and may be indicative of a posterior cruciate ligament injury.

    Posterior sag sign
    The patient is positioned in supine with the knee flexed to 90 degrees and the hip flexed to 45 degrees. A positive test is indicated by the tibia sagging back on the femur and may be indicative of a posterior cruciate ligament injury.

    Slocum test
    The patient is positioned in supine with the knee flexed to 90 degrees and the hip flexed to 45 degrees. The therapist rotates the patient's foot 30 degrees medially to test anterolateral instability or 15 degrees laterally to test anteromedial instability. The therapist stabilizes the lower leg by sitting on the forefoot. The therapist grasps the patient's proximal tibia with two hands and places his/her thumbs on the tibial plateau and administers an anterior directed force to the tibia on the femur. A positive test is indicated movement of the tibia occurring primarily on the lateral side and may be indicative of anterolateral instability.

    Valgus stress test
    The patient is positioned in supine with the knee flexed to 20-30 degrees. The therapist positions one hand on the medial surface of the patient's ankle and the other hand on the lateral surface of the knee. The therapist applies a valgus force to the knee with the distal hand. A positive test is indicated by excessive valgus movement and may be indicative of a medial collateral ligament sprain. A positive test with the knee in full extension may be indicative of damage to the medial collateral ligament, posterior cruciate ligament, posterior oblique ligament, and posteromedial capsule.

    Varus stress test
    The patient is positioned in supine with the knee flexed to 20-30 degrees. The therapist positions one hand on the lateral surface of the patient's ankle and the other hand on the medial surface of the knee. The therapist applies a varus force to the knee with the distal hand. A positive test is indicated by excessive varus movement and may be indicative of a lateral collateral ligament sprain. A positive test with the knee in full extension may be indicative of damage to the lateral collateral ligament, posterior cruciate ligament, arcuate complex, and posterolateral capsule.

  - **--Meniscal Pathology**

    Apley's compression test
    The patient is positioned in prone with the knee flexed to 90 degrees. The therapist stabilizes the patient's femur using one hand and places the other hand on the patient's heel. The therapist medially and laterally rotates the tibia while applying a compressive force through the tibia. A positive test is indicated by pain or clicking and may be indicative of a meniscal lesion.

    Bounce home test
    The patient is positioned in supine. The therapist grasps the patient's heel and maximally flexes the knee. The patient's knee is extended passively. A positive test is indicated by incomplete extension or a rubbery end-feel and may be indicative of a meniscal lesion.

    McMurray test
    The patient is positioned in supine. The therapist grasps the distal leg with one hand and palpates the knee joint line with the other. With the knee fully flexed the therapist medially rotates the tibia and extends the knee. The therapist repeats the same

procedure while laterally rotating the tibia. A positive test is indicated by a click or pronounced crepitation felt over the joint line and may be indicative of a posterior meniscal lesion.

--Swelling
Brush test
The patient is positioned in supine. The therapist places one hand below the joint line on the medial surface of the patella and strokes proximally with the palm and fingers as far as the suprapatellar pouch. The other hand then strokes down the lateral surface of the patella. A positive test is indicated by a wave of fluid just below the medial distal border of the patella and is indicative of effusion in the knee.

Patellar tap test
The patient is positioned in supine with the knee flexed or extended to a point of discomfort. The therapist applies a slight tap over the patella. A positive test is indicated if the patella appears to be floating and may be indicative of joint effusion.

--Miscellaneous
Clarke's sign
The patient is positioned in supine with the knees extended. The therapist applies slight pressure with the web space of his/her hand over the superior pole of the patella. The therapist then asks the patient to contract the quadriceps muscle while maintaining pressure on the patella. A positive test is indicated by failure to complete the contraction without pain and may be indicative of patellofemoral dysfunction.

Hughston's plica test
The patient is positioned in supine. The therapist flexes the knee and medially rotates the tibia with one hand while the other hand attempts to move the patella medially and palpate the medial femoral condyle. A positive test is indicated by a popping sound over the medial plica while the knee is passively flexed and extended.

Noble compression test
The patient is positioned in supine with the hip slightly flexed and the knee in 90 degrees of flexion. The therapist places the thumb of one hand over the lateral epicondyle of the femur and the other hand around the patient's ankle. The therapist maintains pressure over the lateral epicondyle while the patient is asked to slowly extend the knee. A positive test is indicated by pain over the lateral femoral epicondyle at approximately 30 degrees of knee flexion and may be indicative of iliotibial band friction syndrome.

Patellar apprehension test
The patient is positioned in supine with the knees extended. The therapist places both thumbs on the medial border of the patella and applies a laterally directed force. A positive test is indicated by a look of apprehension or an attempt to contract the quadriceps in an effort to avoid subluxation and may be indicative of patella subluxation or dislocation.

• Ankle
--Ligamentous Instability
Anterior drawer test
The patient is positioned in supine. The therapist stabilizes the distal tibia and fibula with one hand, while the other hand holds the foot in 20 degrees of plantar flexion and draws the talus forward in the ankle mortise. A positive test is indicated by excessive anterior translation of the talus away from the ankle mortise and may be indicative of an anterior talofibular ligament sprain.

Talar tilt
The patient is positioned in sidelying with the knee flexed to 90 degrees. The therapist stabilizes the distal tibia with one hand while grasping the talus with the other hand. The foot is maintained in a neutral position. The therapist tilts the talus into abduction and adduction. A positive test is indicated by excessive adduction and may be indicative of a calcaneofibular ligament sprain.

--Miscellaneous
Homans' sign
The patient is positioned in supine. The therapist maintains the leg in extension and passively dorsiflexes the patient's foot. A positive test is indicated by pain in the calf and may be indicative of deep vein thrombophlebitis.

Thompson test
The patient is positioned in prone with the feet extended over the edge of a table. The therapist asks the patient to relax and proceeds to squeeze the muscle belly of the gastrocnemius and soleus muscles. A positive test is indicated by the absence of plantar flexion and may be indicative of a ruptured Achilles tendon.

Tibial torsion test
The patient is positioned in sitting with the knees over the edge of a table. The therapist places the thumb and index finger of one hand over the medial and lateral malleolus. The therapist then measures the acute angle formed by the axes of the knee and ankle. Normal lateral rotation of the tibia is considered to be 12-18 degrees in an adult.

True leg length discrepancy test
The patient is positioned in supine with the hips and knees extended and the legs 15 to 20 cm apart with the pelvis in balance with the legs. Using a tape measure the therapist measures from the distal point of the anterior superior iliac spines to the distal point of the medial malleoli. A positive test is indicated by a

bilateral variation of greater than one centimeter and may by indicative of a true leg length discrepancy.

Spine

--Cervical Region

Foraminal compression test
The patient is positioned in sitting with the head laterally flexed. The therapist places both hands on top of the subject's head and exerts a downward force. A positive test is indicated by pain radiating into the arm toward the flexed side and may be indicative of nerve root compression.

Vertebral artery test
The patient is positioned in supine. The therapist places the patient's head in extension, lateral flexion, and rotation to the ipsilateral side. A positive test is indicated by dizziness, nystagmus, slurred speech or loss of consciousness and may be indicative of compression of the vertebral artery.

--Lumbar/Sacroiliac Region

Sacroiliac joint stress test
The patient is positioned in supine. The therapist crosses his/her arms placing the palms of the hands on the patient's anterior superior iliac spines. The therapist applies a downward and lateral force to the pelvis. A positive test is indicated by unilateral pain in the sacroiliac joint or gluteal area and may be indicative of sacroiliac joint dysfunction.

Sitting flexion test
The patient is positioned in sitting with the knees flexed to 90 degrees and the feet on the floor. The patient's hips should be abducted to allow the patient to bend forward. The therapist places his/her thumbs on the inferior margin of the posterior superior iliac spines and monitors the movement of the bony structures as the patient bends forward and reaches toward the floor. A positive test is indicated by one posterior superior iliac spine moving further in a cranial direction and may be indicative of an articular restriction.

Standing flexion test
The patient is positioned in standing with the feet 12 inches apart. The therapist places his/her thumbs on the inferior margin of the posterior superior iliac spines and monitors the movement of the bony structures as the patient bends forward with the knees extended. A positive test is indicated by one posterior superior iliac spine moving further in a cranial direction and may be indicative of an articular restriction.

Intervention

Orthotics

Types of Orthoses

Lower Extremity

- **Foot orthotics**
A semirigid or rigid insert worn inside a shoe that corrects foot alignment and improves function. May also be used to relieve pain. Foot orthotics are custom molded and are often designed for a specific level of functioning.

- **Ankle-foot orthosis (AFOs)**
A metal ankle-foot orthosis consists of two metal uprights connected proximally to a calf band and distally to a mechanical ankle joint and shoe. The ankle joint may have the ability to be locked and not allow any motion, or set to have limited anterior/posterior capability depending on the patient's need. A plastic ankle-foot orthosis is fabricated by a cast mold of the patient's lower extremity. The use of plastic is more cosmetic, lighter, and requires that if a patient presents with edema it does not significantly fluctuate. Proper fit of a plastic ankle-foot orthosis requires that a patient be casted in a subtalar neutral position. A foot plate can be incorporated into the ankle-foot orthosis to assist with tone reduction. Solid ankle-foot orthoses control dorsiflexion/plantar flexion and also inversion/eversion with a trimline anterior to the malleoli. They can be fabricated to keep an ankle positioned at 90 degrees or can be fabricated with an articulating ankle joint. This articulation allows the tibia to advance over the foot during the mid to late stance phase of gait. A posterior leaf spring is a plastic AFO with a trimline posterior to the malleoli. Its primary purpose is to assist with dorsiflexion and prevent footdrop. It requires adequate medial/lateral control by the patient. Ankle-foot orthoses can also influence knee control. A floor reaction AFO assists with knee extension during stance through positioning of a calf band and/or positioning at the ankle. Ankle-foot orthoses are commonly prescribed for patients with peripheral neuropathy, nerve lesions or hemiplegia.

- **Knee-ankle-foot orthosis (KAFOs)**
Knee-ankle-foot orthoses provide support and stability to the knee and ankle. The orthoses can be fabricated using two metal uprights extending from the foot/shoe to the thigh with calf and thigh bands. Plastic knee-ankle-foot orthoses are fabricated by a cast mold of the patient's lower extremity. A plastic thigh shell is connected to a plastic ankle-foot orthosis through metal uprights lateral and medial to the knee joint. Both types allow for a lock mechanism at the knee that provides stability. The ankle is also held in proper alignment.

- **Craig-Scott knee-ankle-foot orthosis**
  A knee-ankle-foot orthosis designed specifically for persons with paraplegia. This design allows a person to stand with a posterior lean of the trunk.

- **Hip-knee-ankle-foot orthosis (HKAFOs)**
  A hip-knee-ankle orthosis is indicated for patients with hip, foot, knee, and ankle weakness. It consists of bilateral knee-ankle-foot orthoses with an extension to the hip joints with use of a pelvic band. The orthosis can control rotation at the hip and abduction/adduction. The orthosis is heavy and restricts patients to a swing-to or swing-through gait pattern.

- **Reciprocating gait orthosis (RGOs)**
  Reciprocating gait orthoses are a derivative of the HKAFO and incorporate a cable system to assist with advancement of the lower extremities during gait. When the patient shifts weight onto a selected lower extremity, the cable system advances the opposite lower extremity. The orthoses are used primarily for patients with paraplegia.

- **Parapodiums**
  A standing frame designed to allow a patient to sit when necessary. It is a prefabricated frame and ambulation is achieved by shifting weight and rocking the base across the floor. It is primarily used by the pediatric population.

Spine
- **Corset**
  A corset is constructed of fabric and may have metal uprights within the material to provide abdominal compression and support. Corsets are utilized to provide pressure and relieve pain associated with mid and low back pathologies.

- **Halo vest orthosis**
  The halo vest is an invasive cervical thoracic orthosis that provides full restriction of all cervical motion. A metal ring with four posts that attach to a vest is placed on a patient and secured by inserting four pins through the ring into the skull. This orthosis is commonly used with cervical spinal cord injuries to prevent further damage or dislocation during the recovery period. A patients will wear a halo vest until the spine becomes stable.

- **Milwaukee orthosis**
  The Milwaukee orthosis is designed to promote realignment of the spine due to scoliotic curvature. The orthosis is custom made and extends from the pelvis to the upper chest. Corrective padding is applied based on the location and severity of the curve.

- **Taylor brace**
  The Taylor brace is a thoracolumbosacral orthosis that limits trunk flexion and extension through a three-point control design.

- **Thoracolumbosacral orthosis (TLSO)**
  A custom molded TLSO is utilized to prevent all trunk motions and is commonly utilized as a means of postsurgical stabilization. The rigid shell is fabricated from plastics in a bivalve style using straps/velcro to secure the orthosis.

Functions of Orthotics

- Prevent deformity
- Assist function of a weak limb
- Maintain proper alignment of joints
- Inhibit tone
- Protect against injury of a weak joint
- Allow for maximal functional independence
- Facilitate motion

Orthotic Considerations

- Do not overprescribe
- Cost
- Energy efficiency
- Cosmesis
- Temporary versus permanent
- Dynamic versus static
- Encourage normal movement

Orthotic Profile

Examination

- Past medical history
- History of current condition
- Social history (caregiver support)
- Medications
- Living environment
- Systems review
- Skin assessment
- Edema/girth measurements
- Postural tone assessment
- Pathological reflex assessment
- Sensation, proprioception, and kinesthesia
- Range of motion
- Motor assessment/strength
- Mobility skills

Intervention

- Ensure continued proper fit
- Donning/doffing orthosis
- Implement progressive wearing schedule

UNIT TWO: MUSCULOSKELETAL

- Patient/caregiver teaching:
  --Skin inspection
  --Care of orthosis
- Mobility training with orthosis

Goals

- Maximize functional mobility skills with orthosis
- Maximize independence with donning/doffing
- Maximize independence with wearing schedule
- Maximize independence with skin inspection
- Maximize competence with care of orthosis

Mobilization

Mobilization is a passive movement technique designed to improve joint function.

Grades of Movement

Grade I	Small amplitude movement performed at the beginning of range.
Grade II	Large amplitude movement performed within the range, but not reaching the limit of the range and not returning to the beginning of range.
Grade III	Large amplitude movement performed to the limit of range.
Grade IV	Small amplitude movement performed at the limit of range.

Mobilization Technique

- The patient should have a general understanding of the purpose of mobilization.
- The patient should be completely relaxed during treatment.
- The therapist should be in a comfortable position while performing mobilization activities.
- The therapist's position should allow for optimal control of movement.
- Explain specific mobilization techniques to the patient prior to beginning treatment.
- Complete a general examination of each patient prior to beginning mobilization activities.
- Use gravity to assist with mobilization whenever possible.
- Mobilization activities are usually performed initially with the joint in a loose packed position.
- Maintain contact with the mobilizing hand as close to the joint space as possible.
- Allow one digit to palpate the joint line when possible.
- Mobilize one joint in one direction at a time.
- Use a mobilization belt or wedge to assist with stabilization when necessary.
- Constantly modify mobilization techniques based on individual patient response.
- Compare the quality and quantity of joint play bilaterally.
- Reassess each patient prior to each treatment session.

Convex-Concave Rule

Determines the direction of decreased joint gliding and the appropriate direction for the mobilizing force.

Convex surface moving on a concave surface:
- Roll and slide occur in the opposite direction
- Mobilizing force should be applied in the opposite direction of the bone movement

Concave surface moving on a convex surface:
- Roll and slide occur in the same direction
- Mobilizing force should be applied in the same direction as the bone movement

Indications: restricted joint mobility, restricted accessory motion, desired neurophysiological effects

Contraindications: active disease, infection, advanced osteoporosis, articular hypermobility, fracture, acute inflammation, muscle guarding, joint replacement

Orthopedic Profile

Examination

- Past medical history
- History of current condition
  --Surgical procedures
  --Precautions/contraindications
- Social history
- Medications
- Living environment
- Systems review
  --Vital signs
- Observation/inspection
- Postural assessment
- Reflex assessment
- Special tests
- Pain
- Range of motion
- Gait
- Mobility skills
- Strength

Intervention

- Exercise training
- Edema control
- Pain management
- Electrotherapeutic modalities
- Physical agents
- Joint mobilization
- Mobility training
- Patient/caregiver teaching:
  - --Precautions/contraindications
  - --Exercise program
  - --Positioning
  - --Competence with an assistive device
  - --Proper body mechanics

Goals

- Maximize functional mobility skills
- Reduce edema to the affected areas
- Maximize strength and endurance
- Maximize range of motion
- Minimize pain
- Maximize proper posture
- Maximize tissue healing
- Maximize patient/caregiver competence with:
  - --Safe use of assistive device
  - --Body mechanics
  - --Home exercise program
- Safe positioning for mobility

Orthopedic Surgical Procedures

Total Hip Replacement (THR)

Surgical Indications:
Osteoarthritis
Avascular necrosis
Bone tumor
Failed internal fixation of a fracture
Rheumatoid arthritis
Developmental dysplasia
Osteomyelitis

Surgical Contraindications:
Inadequate bone mass
Active infection
Poor periarticular support
Sepsis

Types of Total Hip Replacement:
- *Cemented*
  - --Immediate weight bearing as tolerated
  - --May require more bone tissue removal
  - --May experience loosening of the prosthesis
- *Noncemented*
  - --Toe touch weight bearing for up to six weeks
  - --Longer life expectancy than cemented
  - --Allows a larger amount of bone tissue to remain intact
  - --Allows for continued tissue growth

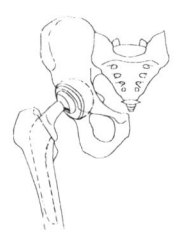

Potential Postsurgical Complications:
Deep vein thrombosis
Pulmonary embolus
Sciatic nerve injury
Dislocation or subluxation of the femoral head
Infection
Periprosthetic fracture
Heterotopic ossification

General Postoperative Precautions (Posterolateral approach):
- Use an abduction pillow
- Maintain appropriate weight bearing status
- Avoid hip adduction
- Avoid hip medial rotation
- Avoid hip flexion > 90 degrees
- Do not sit on low surfaces
- Do not bend over towards the ground
- Do not lean over to get up from a chair
- Do not bend over to tie shoes
- Do not pivot towards the surgical side
- Do not cross the legs when sitting or lying down
- Use a pillow between the legs when sidelying

Physical Therapy Intervention:
- Maintain appropriate weight bearing status
- Mobility training using hip precautions
- Early ambulation training
- Initiate strengthening with isometric exercises and progress as tolerated
- Implement gentle stretching using hip precautions

Total Knee Replacement (TKR)

Surgical Indications:
Disabling pain
Failed conservative treatment
Impaired mobility due to advanced arthritis

Surgical Contraindications:
Active infection
Advanced osteoporosis
Severe peripheral vascular disease
Sepsis
Morbid obesity

UNIT TWO: MUSCULOSKELETAL

Types of Total Knee Replacement:
- *Cemented*
  - --Immediate weight bearing as tolerated
  - --Used with older and sedentary patients

- *Hybrid*
  - --Toe touch weight bearing for up to six weeks
  - --Cemented tibial component and noncemented femoral and patellar components

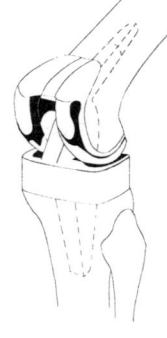

- *Noncemented*
  - --Toe touch weight bearing for up to six weeks
  - --Femoral, tibial, and patellar components are all noncemented
  - --Longer life expectancy than cemented
  - --Preferred for younger patients

Potential Postsurgical Complications:
Deep vein thrombosis
Pulmonary embolus
Peroneal nerve palsy
Restricted range of motion
Infection
Chronic joint effusion
Periprosthetic fracture

General Postoperative Precautions:
- Maintain appropriate weight bearing status
- Postsurgical use of knee immobilizer for stability

Physical Therapy Intervention:
- Maintain appropriate weight bearing status
- Mobility training
- Early ambulation training with knee immobilizer
- Use of a continuous passive motion machine (CPM)
- Initiate strengthening with isometric exercises
- Initiate passive range of motion to attain 90 degrees of knee flexion and 0 degrees of knee extension
- Use compression stockings for excess edema
- Wean from the knee immobilizer once the patient gains quadriceps control

Orthopedic Pathology

Rheumatism

A condition found in a number of disorders characterized by inflammation, degeneration or metabolic derangement of the connective tissue, soreness, joint pain, and stiffness of muscles. Some conditions that present with rheumatism include: osteoarthritis, rheumatoid arthritis, juvenile rheumatoid arthritis, gout, systemic lupus erythematosus, and ankylosing spondylitis.

Physical Therapy Examination:
- Measurement of independence with functional activities
- Measurement of joint inflammation
- Measurement of joint range of motion
- Determination of limiting factors including pain, weakness, and fatigue

Physical Therapy Goals:

Short-Term Goals (Acute or Exacerbation)	Alleviate pain
	Decrease inflammation
	Maintain strength and endurance to activity
	Provide splinting and/or assistive devices to increase safety
Long-Term Goals	Patient independence and competence with:
	• Proper body mechanics
	• Reduction of biomechanical stressors
	• Exercise program
	Maximize functional mobility
	Maximize endurance to tolerate activities of daily living
	Demonstrate safety with ambulation and all mobility
	Management of pain

Osteoarthritis

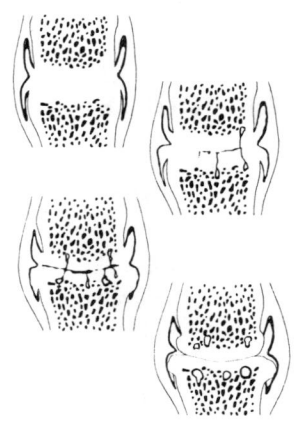

A chronic disease that primarily involves the weight bearing joints. Osteoarthritis causes a degeneration of articular cartilage. Subsequent deformity and thickening of subchondral bone occurs with an outcome of impaired functional status. Any joint may be involved, however the most commonly affected sites include: cervical spine (C5-C6), lumbar spine, hips, and knees.

It is common to be affected by osteoarthritis after age 40. The disease affects men more than women. Risk factors include trauma, repetitive microtrauma, and obesity.

Pathogenesis:
- Cartilage becomes soft and damaged
- Osteophytes form
- Subchondral bone thickens
- Synovitis is mild to moderate

42 A GUIDE TO SUCCESS

Clinical Presentation:
- Gradual onset
- Pain present at the affected joint
- Increased pain after exercise
- Joint crepitus
- Joints may become enlarged
- Bouchard's nodes
- Usually localized to a few joints
- Increased pain with weather changes
- Joint motion limitation
- Joint stiffness < 15 minutes
- Heberden's nodes

Medications:
Goal: To decrease inflammation and alleviate pain.
- **NSAIDs** — *See Orthopedic Medications page 45*

Physical Therapy Intervention:
1. Rest required for the affected joints
2. Patient education on disease process, energy conservation, body mechanics, and joint protection techniques
3. Splinting
4. Use of cold and/or heat
5. Ultrasound, hydrotherapy, paraffin
6. Use of assistive devices to reduce weight bearing on affected joints
7. Weight loss
8. Isometric exercise followed by gradual progression to isotonic exercise
9. Transcutaneous electrical nerve stimulation
10. NSAIDs
11. Orthopedic surgical intervention

Rheumatoid Arthritis

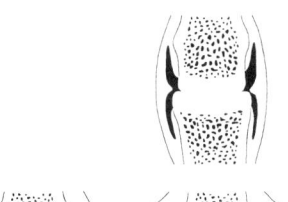

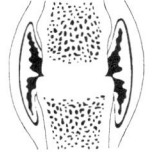

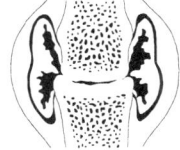

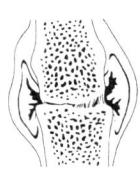

A systemic autoimmune disorder of unknown etiology. The disease presents with a chronic inflammatory reaction in the synovial tissues of a joint that results in erosion of cartilage and supporting structures within the capsule. One percent of the American population is affected. Women are affected three times more than men and the most common age of onset falls between thirty and fifty years of age. Onset of rheumatoid arthritis may occur first at any joint, but it is common to find it in the small joints of the hand, foot, wrist, and ankle. This disease has periods of exacerbation and remission.

Pathogenesis:
- Thickening of synovial membrane in affected joints
- Colonization of lymphocytes which synthesize the rheumatoid factor
- Subsequent erosion of cartilage and supporting structures

Clinical Presentation:
- Onset may be gradual or immediate
- Pain and tenderness of affected joints
- Warm joints
- Decrease in appetite
- Boutonniere deformity – DIP extension PIP flexion
- Symmetrical polyarthritis
- Morning stiffness > one hour
- Malaise and increased fatigue
- Redness at joints
- Swan neck deformity – DIP flexion PIP hyperextension

Medications:
Goal: To decrease inflammation and pain as well as to stop progression of the disease process.

NSAIDs	*See Orthopedic Medications page 45*
Corticosteroids	*Examples:* Decadron, Hydrocortone, Celestone
Disease Modifying Medications	*Gold compounds:* Solganal, Ridaura *Antimalarial:* Aralen, Plaquenil *Immunosuppressants:* Azathioprine *Antimetabolite:* Methotrexate

Physical Therapy Intervention:
1. Complete bedrest or regular rest periods my be indicated
2. NSAIDs or other medications
3. Patient education on disease process, energy conservation, body mechanics, and joint protection techniques
4. Modalities such as hydrotherapy, hot pack, paraffin, or use of cold - avoid deep heat
5. Splinting
6. Use of assistive devices
7. Passive range of motion during acute stage
8. Active range of motion once in the subacute stages
9. Hydrotherapy and isometrics once in the subacute stages
10. Exercise which may include swimming, stationary bicycle, or walking may be indicated
11. Orthopedic intervention

Types of Fractures

Avulsion fracture: A portion of a bone becomes fragmented at the site of tendon attachment from a traumatic and sudden stretch of the tendon.

Closed fracture: A break in a bone where the skin over the site remains intact.

Comminuted fracture: A bone breaks into fragments at the site of injury.

Compound fracture: A break in a bone that protrudes through the skin.

Greenstick fracture: A break on one side of a bone that does not damage the periosteum on the opposite side. This type of fracture is often seen in children.

Nonunion fracture: A break in a bone that has failed to unite and heal after nine to twelve months.

Stress fracture: A break in a bone due to repeated forces to a particular portion of the bone.

Spiral fracture: A break in a bone shaped as an "S" due to torsion and twisting.

Orthopedic Terminology

Bursitis: A condition caused by acute or chronic inflammation of the bursae. Symptoms may include a limitation in active range of motion secondary to pain and swelling.

Contusion: A sudden blow to a part of the body that can result in mild to severe damage to superficial and deep structures. Treatment includes active range of motion, ice, and compression.

Edema: An increased volume of fluid in the soft tissue outside of a joint capsule.

Effusion: An increased volume of fluid within a joint capsule.

Genu valgum: A condition where the knees touch while standing with the feet separated. Genu valgum will increase compression of the lateral condyle and increase stress to the medial structures. Genu valgum is also termed knock-knee.

Genu varum: A condition where there is bowing of the legs with added space between the knees while standing with the feet together. Genu varum will increase compression of the medial tibial condyle and increase stress to the lateral structures. Genu varum is also termed bowleg.

Kyphosis: An excessive curvature of the spine in a posterior direction usually identified in the thoracic spine. Common causes include osteoporosis, compression fractures, and poor posture secondary to paralysis.

Lordosis: An excessive curvature of the spine in an anterior direction usually identified in the cervical or lumbar spine. Common causes include weak abdominal muscles, pregnancy, excessive weight in the abdominal area, and hip flexion contractures.

Myositis ossificans: A condition of heterotopic bone formation that occurs three to four weeks after a contusion or trauma within the soft tissue.

Osteoporosis: The thinning of bone matrix with eventual bone loss and an increased risk for fracture. Osteoporosis is usually found in postmenopausal women. Causative factors for osteoporosis include decreased weight bearing, inactivity, family history, smoking, and drinking. Diagnosis of osteoporosis is made through bone density screening. Medications used to assist against the progression of osteoporosis include estrogen, calcium, vitamin D, calcitonin, and fluoride.

Q angle: The degree of angulation present when measuring from the midpatella to the anterosuperior iliac spine and to the tibial tubercle. A normal Q angle measured in supine with the knee straight is 13 degrees for a male and is 18 degrees for a female. An excessive Q angle can lead to pathology and abnormal tracking.

Scoliosis: A lateral curvature of the spine. Scoliosis can occur in the cervical, thoracic or lumbar curves. Classifications of scoliosis include idiopathic, nonstructural, and structural.

Shoulder dislocation: A true separation of the humerus from the glenoid fossa.

Shoulder separation: A disruption in the stability of the acromioclavicular joint.

Sprain: An acute injury involving a ligament.
- Grade I – mild pain and swelling, little to no tear of the ligament
- Grade II – moderate pain and swelling, minimal instability of the joint, minimal to moderate tearing of the ligament, decreased range of motion
- Grade III – severe pain and swelling, substantial joint instability, total tear of the ligament, substantial decrease in range of motion

Strain: An injury involving the musculotendinous unit that involves a muscle, tendon or their attachments to bone.
- Grade I – localized pain, minimal swelling, and tenderness
- Grade II – localized pain, moderate swelling, tenderness, and impaired motor function
- Grade III – a palpable defect of the muscle, severe pain, and poor motor function

Tendonitis: A condition caused by acute or chronic inflammation of a tendon. Symptoms may include gradual onset, tenderness, swelling, and pain.

Orthopedic Medications

Opioids:
- Narcotics
- Pain medications
- Can be addictive
- May develop physical dependence
- Used for moderate to severe pain
- May produce sedation
- May produce mood swings
- May produce gastrointestinal side effects
- May produce constipation
- May produce orthostatic hypotension

Specific Drugs:
Codeine	Hydrocodone (Hycodan)
Meperidine (Demerol)	Methadone (Dolophine)
Morphine	Oxycodone (Percodan)
Propoxyphene (Darvon)	

Nonopioids:
- Nonsteroidal anti-inflammatory drugs and acetaminophen
- Analgesia
- Anti-inflammatory (except acetaminophen)
- Reduces fever
- Reduces risk of clotting (except acetaminophen)
- For mild to moderate pain
- May produce gastrointestinal side effects
- May produce liver/kidney toxicity

Specific Drugs:
Aspirin	Voltaren
Dolobid	Lodine
Ibuprofen	Indocin
Toradol	Naproxen
Daypro	Feldene
Clinoril	Anaprox

Glucocorticoids:
- Decrease inflammation
- May produce drug induced Cushing's syndrome
- May produce muscle atrophy
- May produce gastrointestinal ulcers
- May produce glaucoma

Specific Drugs:
Cortisone	Prednisone
Hydrocortisone	Dexamethasone (Decadron)
Prednisolone	

Amputations and Prosthetics

Examination

Factors that Influence Vascular Disease

- Hypertension
- Aging
- Diabetes mellitus
- Infection
- Poor nutrition
- Cigarette smoking

Risk Factors for Amputation

- Vascular disease
  - --Atherosclerosis/arteriosclerosis
  - --Venous insufficiency
  - --Buerger's disease
  - --Diabetes mellitus
- Malignancy/tumor
  - --Osteosarcoma
- Congenital deformities
- Infection
- Trauma

Types of Lower Extremity Amputations

Hemicorporectomy: Surgical removal of the pelvis and both lower extremities

Hemipelvectomy: Surgical removal of one half of the pelvis and the lower extremity

Hip Disarticulation: Surgical removal of the lower extremity from the pelvis

Transfemoral: Surgical removal of the lower extremity above the knee joint

Knee Disarticulation: Surgical removal through the knee joint

Transtibial: Surgical removal of the lower extremity below the knee joint

Syme's: Surgical removal of the foot at the ankle joint with removal of the malleoli

Chopart's: Disarticulation at the midtarsal joint

Transmetatarsal: Surgical removal of the midsection of the metatarsals

Types of Amputation and Considerations for Prosthetic Training

Hemipelvectomy and Hip Disarticulation
- All functions of the hip, knee, ankle, and foot are absent
- Most common cause is malignancy
- Does not allow for activation of the prosthesis through a residual limb
- Prosthetic motion must be initiated through weight bearing

Transfemoral Amputation
- Length of the residual limb with regard to leverage and energy expenditure
- No ability to weight bear through the end of the residual limb
- Susceptible to hip flexion contracture
- Adaptation required for balance, weight of prosthesis, and energy expenditure

Knee Disarticulation
- Loss of all knee, ankle, and foot function
- The residual limb can weight bear through its end
- Susceptible to hip flexion contracture
- Knee axis of the prosthesis is below the natural axis of the knee
- Gait deviations can occur secondary to the malalignment of the knee axis

Transtibial Amputation
- Loss of ankle and foot functions
- Residual limb does not allow for weight bearing at its end
- Weight bearing in the prosthesis should be distributed over the total residual limb
- Patella tendon should be the area of primary weight bearing
- Adaptations required for balance
- Susceptible to knee flexion contracture

Syme's Amputation
- Loss of all foot functions
- Residual limb can weight bear through its end
- Residual limb is bulbous with a noncosmetic appearance
- Dog ears must be reduced for proper prosthetic fit
- Adaptation required for the increased weight of the prosthesis
- Adaptation required due to diminished toe off during gait

Transmetatarsal and Chopart's Amputation
- Loss of forefoot leverage
- Loss of balance
- Loss of weight bearing surface
- Loss of proprioception
- Tendency to develop equinus deformity

Potential Complications

Neuroma
A neuroma is a bundle of nerve endings that group together and can produce pain due to scar tissue, pressure from the prosthesis or tension on the residual limb.

Phantom Limb
Phantom limb refers to a painless sensation where the patient feels that the limb is still present. This is seen soon after the amputation and will usually subside with desensitization and prosthetic use, however may continue for extended periods of time for some patients.

Phantom Pain
Phantom pain refers to the patient's perception of some form of painful stimuli. The pain can be continuous or intermittent, local or general, and short-term or permanent. This type of pain can disable the patient and interfere with successful rehabilitation. Treatment options include TENS, ultrasound, icing, relaxation techniques, desensitization techniques, and prosthetic use.

Components of a Prosthesis

	Transfemoral	*Transtibial*
Socket:	• Quadrilateral socket • Ischial containment socket	• Patella tendon bearing socket (PTB) • Supracondylar patella tendon socket (PTS) • Supracondylar – suprapatellar socket (SC-SP)
Suspension:	• Complete suction • Partial suction --Silesian bandage --Pelvic belt/band	• Supracondylar cuff • Thigh corset • Supracondylar brim • Rubber sleeve suspension • Waistbelt with fork strap
Knee:	• Single axis knee • Polycentric knee **Friction mechanisms:** --Constant friction --Variable friction --Sliding friction --Hydraulic friction --Pneumatic friction	• Not needed

Shank:	• Exoskeleton – rigid exterior • Endoskeleton – pylon covered with foam	• Same as transfemoral shank
Foot:	• Solid ankle cushion heel (SACH) • Stationary attachment flexible endoskeleton (SAFE) • Single axis foot • Multi axis foot	• Same as transfemoral foot

Intervention

Types of Postoperative Dressings

Rigid (Plaster of Paris):

Advantages
Allows early ambulation with pylon
Promotes circulation and healing
Stimulates proprioception
Provides protection
Provides soft tissue support
Limits edema

Disadvantages
Immediate wound inspection is not possible
Does not allow for daily dressing change
Requires professional application

Semi-rigid (Una paste, air splint):

Advantages
Reduces postoperative edema
Provides soft tissue support
Allows for earlier ambulation
Provides protection
Easily changed

Disadvantages
Does not protect as well as the rigid dressing
Requires more changing than rigid dressing
May loosen and allow for development of edema

Soft (Ace wrap, shrinker):

Advantages
Reduces postoperative edema
Provides some protection
Relatively inexpensive

Disadvantages
Tissue healing is interrupted by frequent dressing changes
Joint range of motion may delay the healing of the incision
Increased risk of joint contractures

Advantages
Provides soft tissue support
Easily removed for wound inspection
Allows for active joint range of motion

Disadvantages
Less control of residual limb pain
Cannot control the amount of tension in the bandage
Risk of a tourniquet effect

Wrapping Guidelines

- Elastic wrap should not have any wrinkles
- Diagonal and angular patterns should be used
- Do not wrap in circular patterns
- Provide pressure distally to enhance shaping
- Anchor wrap above the knee for transtibial amputations
- Anchor wrap around pelvis for transfemoral amputations
- Promote full knee extension for transtibial amputations
- Promote full hip extension for transfemoral amputations
- Secure the wrap with tape; do not use clips as they are unsafe
- Use 3-4 inch wrap for transtibial amputations
- Use 6 inch wrap for transfemoral amputations
- Rewrap frequently to maintain adequate pressure

Gait Deviations

Lateral Bending:

Prosthetic Causes
Prosthesis may be too short
Improperly shaped lateral wall
High medial wall
Prosthesis aligned in abduction

Amputee Causes
Poor balance
Abduction contracture
Improper training
Short residual limb
Weak hip abductors on prosthetic side
Hypersensitive and painful residual limb

Abducted Gait:

Prosthetic Causes
Prosthesis may be too long
High medial wall
Improperly shaped lateral wall
Prosthesis positioned in abduction
Inadequate suspension
Excessive knee friction

Amputee Causes
Abduction contracture
Improper training
Adductor roll
Weak hip flexors and adductors
Pain over lateral residual limb

UNIT TWO: MUSCULOSKELETAL

Circumducted Gait:
Prosthetic Causes
Prosthesis may be too long
Too much friction in the knee
Socket is too small
Excessive plantar flexion of prosthetic foot

Amputee Causes
Abduction contracture
Improper training
Weak hip flexors
Lacks confidence to flex the knee
Painful anterior distal stump
Inability to initiate prosthetic knee flexion

Excessive Knee Flexion During Stance:
Prosthetic Causes
Socket set forward in relation to foot
Foot set in excessive dorsiflexion
Stiff heel
Prosthesis too long

Amputee Causes
Knee flexion contracture
Hip flexion contracture
Pain anteriorly in residual limb
Decrease in quadriceps strength
Poor balance

Vaulting:
Prosthetic Causes
Prosthesis may be too long
Inadequate socket suspension
Excessive alignment stability
Foot in excess plantar flexion

Amputee Causes
Residual limb discomfort
Improper training
Fear of stubbing toe
Short residual limb
Painful hip or residual limb

Rotation of Forefoot at Heel Strike:
Prosthetic Causes
Excessive toe out built in
Loose fitting socket
Inadequate suspension
Rigid SACH heel cushion

Amputee Causes
Poor muscle control
Improper training
Weak medial rotators
Short residual limb

Forward Trunk Flexion:
Prosthetic Causes
Socket too big
Poor suspension
Knee instability

Amputee Causes
Hip flexion contracture
Weak hip extensors
Pain with ischial weight bearing
Inability to initiate prosthetic knee flexion

Medial or Lateral Whip:
Prosthetic Causes
Excessive rotation of the knee
Tight socket fit
Valgus in the prosthetic knee
Improper alignment of toe break

Amputee Causes
Improper training
Weak hip rotators
Knee instability

Amputation and Prosthetic Profile

Examination

- Past medical history
- History of current condition
- Social history (caregiver support)
- Medications
- Living environment
- Systems review
- Residual limb assessment
  --Level of healing
  --Color
  --Shape
  --Pulses
  --Edema
  --Girth and length
- Sensation
- Skin assessment
- Range of motion
- Balance
- Endurance
- Pain
  --Phantom sensation
  --Phantom pain
  --Neuroma
- Mobility skills

Preprosthetic Intervention

- Positioning
  --Prone lying
- Residual limb care
- Patient/caregiver teaching:
  --Nutrition
  --Desensitization
  --Positioning
  --Wrapping technique
  --Skin inspection and care
- Range of motion
- Strengthening
- Edema control
- Physical agents
- Electrotherapeutic modalities

- Pain management
- Endurance activities
- Balance activities
- Mobility training
- Gait training
- Wheelchair prescription
- Assistive device training

Prosthetic Intervention

- Proper adjustment/alignment of prosthesis
- Development of wearing schedule
- Skin inspection with prosthetic use
- Donning/doffing prosthesis
- Mobility training with prosthesis

Preprosthetic Goals

- Maximize functional mobility
- Maximize range of motion
- Maximize strength and endurance
- Reduce edema and promote proper shaping
- Maximize independence with wheelchair management and assistive devices
- Maximize balance
- Maximize patient/caregiver competence with:
  --Skin care and inspection
  --Wrapping
  --Desensitization techniques
  --Positioning

Prosthetic Goals

- Maximize functional mobility using prosthesis
- Maximize independence with donning/doffing prosthesis
- Maximize wearing tolerance of prosthesis
- Maximize competence with prosthetic care and use

Neuromuscular

Neurology

Examination

Cranial Nerve Testing

The cranial nerves refer to twelve pairs of nerves that have their origin in the brain. The majority of cranial nerves contain both sensory and motor fibers, however there are several exceptions. Since lesions affecting the cranial nerves produce specific and predictable alterations, it is often prudent to perform cranial nerve testing as part of a neurological examination. The following information is a summary of some of the more common methods of testing selected cranial nerves.

Cranial Nerve I - Olfactory
The patient is positioned in sitting with the eyes closed or blindfolded. The therapist places an item with a familiar odor under the patient's nostril and the patient is asked to identify the odor. A positive test may be indicated by an inability to identify familiar odors.

Cranial Nerve II - Optic
The patient is positioned in standing a selected distance from a chart or diagram. The therapist asks the patient to identify objects or read selected items from the chart or diagram. A positive test may be indicated by an inability to identify objects at a reasonable distance.

Cranial Nerve III - Oculomotor
The patient is positioned in sitting and is asked to follow an object such as a writing utensil with his/her eyes as it is moved vertically, horizontally, and diagonally. The therapist should make sure the patient does not rotate his/her head during the testing and should inspect the patient's eyes for asymmetry or ptosis. A positive test may be indicated by a tracking deficit, asymmetry, or ptosis.

Cranial Nerve IV - Trochlear
The patient is positioned in sitting and asked to follow an object such as a writing utensil with his/her eyes as it is moved in a superior direction. The therapist should make sure the patient does not move his head upward. A positive test may be indicated by an inability to elevate the eyes.

Cranial Nerve V - Trigeminal
The patient is positioned in sitting and is asked to close his/her eyes. The therapist uses a piece of cotton and a safety pin to alternately touch the patient's face. The patient is asked to classify each contact with the face as 'sharp' or 'dull.' A positive test for the sensory component may be identified by impaired or absent sensation or the inability to differentiate between 'sharp' or 'dull'. The motor component is tested by asking the patient to perform mandibular protrusion, retrusion, and lateral deviation. A positive test may be indicated by an impaired ability to move the mandible through the specified motions.

Cranial Nerve VI - Abducens
The patient is positioned in sitting. The therapist asks the patient to abduct his/her eyes without rotating the head. A positive test may be indicated by an inability to abduct the eyes.

Cranial Nerve VII - Facial
The patient is positioned in sitting and is asked to distinguish between sweet and salty substances placed on the anterior portion of the tongue. A positive test for the sensory component may be identified by an inability to accurately identify sweet and salty substances. The motor component is tested by performing a manual muscle test of selected muscles involved in facial expression. A positive test for the motor component may be indicated by an inability to mimic selected facial expressions due to muscle impairment.

Cranial Nerve VIII - Vestibulocochlear
The patient is positioned in sitting in a quiet location. The therapist, positioned behind the patient and to one side, slowly brings a ticking watch toward the patient's ear. The therapist records the distance from the ear when the patient is able to identify the ticking sound. The therapist repeats the procedure on the contralateral ear and compares the measurements. A positive test is indicated by an inability to hear the ticking sound at 18-24 inches or a significant bilateral difference. Alternate tests include the Weber and Rinne tests which require a 512 Hz tuning fork.

Cranial Nerve IX - Glossopharyngeal
The patient is positioned in sitting. The therapist touches the pharynx with a tongue depressor. A positive test may be indicated by lack of gagging or an inability to feel the tongue depressor touch the back of the throat. The sensory component is tested by assessing the patient's ability to distinguish objects by taste after they are placed on the posterior portion of the tongue. A positive test for the sensory component may be identified by an inability to accurately identify tasted substances, especially sour and bitter substances, placed on the posterior third of the tongue.

Cranial Nerve X - Vagus
The patient is positioned in sitting. The therapist touches the pharynx with a tongue depressor. A positive test may be indicated by a lack of gagging or an inability to feel the tongue

depressor touch the back of the throat. (Same description for Cranial Nerve IX - Glossopharyngeal). If the gag reflex is absent the therapist should carefully assess the movement of the soft palate and uvula.

Cranial Nerve XI - Accessory
The patient is positioned in sitting with the arms at the side. The therapist asks the patient to shrug his/her shoulders and maintain the position while the therapist applies resistance through the shoulders in the direction of shoulder depression. A positive test may be indicated by an inability to maintain the test position against resistance.

Cranial Nerve XII - Hypoglossal
The patient is positioned in sitting. The therapist asks the patient to protrude the tongue. A positive test may be indicated by an inability to fully protrude the tongue or the tongue deviating to one side during protrusion.

Upper versus Lower Motor Neuron Disease

	UMND	LMND
Reflexes	Hyperactive	Diminished or absent
Atrophy	Mild from disuse	Present
Fasciculations	Absent	Present
Tone	Hypertonic	Hypotonic to flaccid

Upper Motor Neuron Disease
Upper motor neuron diseases are characterized by lesions found in descending motor tracts within the cerebral motor cortex, internal capsule, brainstem, or spinal cord. Symptoms include weakness of involved muscles, hypertonicity, hyperreflexia, mild disuse atrophy, and abnormal reflexes. Damaged tracts are in the lateral white column of the spinal cord.

Examples of upper motor neuron lesions include cerebral palsy, hydrocephalus, CVA, birth injuries, multiple sclerosis, and brain tumors.

Lower Motor Neuron Disease
Lower motor neuron diseases are characterized by lesions which affect nerves or their axons at or below the level of the brainstem, usually within the "final common pathway." The ventral gray column of the spinal cord may also be affected. Symptoms include flaccidity or weakness of the involved muscles, decreased tone, fasciculations, muscle atrophy, and decreased or absent reflexes.

Examples of lower motor neuron lesions include poliomyelitis, tumors involving the spinal cord, trauma, infection, and muscular dystrophy.

Cerebral Hemisphere Function

Frontal lobes:
- Primary motor areas
- Voluntary control of motor activities
- Strong influence over mood, judgment, abstract thinking, and attention
- Prefrontal cortex integrates information received from other systems (e.g. limbic system)
- Broca's area
  Left – movement of mouth for speech
  Right – nonverbal communication

Parietal lobes:
- Primary sensory areas
- Perception of sensory information
- Role in short-term memory
- Sensory homunculus

Temporal lobes:
- Primary auditory areas
- Wernicke's area hears and understands spoken language
- Visual perception
- Musical discrimination
- Role in long-term memory

Occipital lobes:
- Primary visual cortex
- Organization and interpretation for visual information

Hemisphere Specialization/Dominance

Left:
- Language
- Process verbally coded information in an organized, logical, and sequential manner
- Understand language
- Produce written and spoken language
- Analytical
- Controlled
- Logical
- Rational
- Sequence and perform movements
- Mathematical calculations
- Express positive emotions such as love and happiness

Right:
- Nonverbal processing
- Process information in a holistic manner
- Artistic abilities
- General concept comprehension
- Hand-eye coordination
- Spatial relationships
- Kinesthetic awareness
- Understanding music
- Understanding nonverbal communication
- Body image awareness
- Express negative emotions
- Mathematical reasoning

Cerebellum:
- Balance
- Higher level muscular movements
- Integration and coordination of multijoint movements
- Initiation, timing, and sequencing of muscle contraction
- Creative
- Pictorial
- Intuitive

Risk Factors for Cerebrovascular Accident

Primary:
- Hypertension
- Heart disease
- Diabetes mellitus
- Cigarette smoking
- Transient ischemic attacks

Secondary:
- Obesity
- High cholesterol
- Behaviors related to hypertension
- Physical inactivity
- Increased alcohol consumption

Types of Cerebrovascular Accidents

Completed Stroke
A CVA that presents with total neurological deficits at the onset.

Stroke in Evolution
A CVA, usually caused by a thrombus, that gradually progresses. Total neurological deficits are not seen for one to two days after onset.

Embolus
Associated with cardiovascular disease, an embolus may be a solid, liquid or gas, and can originate in any part of the body. The embolus travels through the bloodstream to the cerebral arteries causing occlusion of a blood vessel and a resultant infarct. The middle cerebral artery is most commonly affected by an embolus from the internal carotid arteries. Due to the sudden onset of occlusion, tissues distal to the infarct can sustain higher permanent damage than those of thrombotic infarcts. An embolic CVA occurs rapidly with no warning, often presents with a headache, and can be associated with heart disease.

Hemorrhage
An abnormal bleeding in the brain due to a rupture in blood supply. The infarct is due to disruption of oxygen to an area of the brain and compression from the accumulation of blood. Hypertension is usually a precipitating factor causing rupture of an aneurysm or arteriovenous malformation. Trauma can also precipitate hemorrhage and subsequent CVA. Characteristics include severe headache, vomiting, high blood pressure, and abrupt onset of symptoms. Hemorrhage usually occurs during the day with symptoms evolving in relation to the speed of the bleed.

Thrombus
An atherosclerotic plaque develops in an artery and eventually occludes the artery or a branching artery causing an infarct. This type of CVA is extremely variable in onset where symptoms can appear in minutes or over several days. A thrombotic CVA usually occurs during sleep or upon awakening, after a myocardial infarction or postsurgical procedure.

Transient Ischemic Attack (TIA)
A transient ischemic attack is usually linked to an atherosclerotic thrombosis. There is a temporary interruption of blood supply to an area. The effects may be similar to a CVA, but symptoms resolve quickly. A TIA most often occurs in the carotid and vertebrobasilar arteries and may indicate future CVA.

Expected Impairment Based on Vascular Involvement

Anterior Cerebral Artery:
- Increased lower extremity involvement
- Loss of bowel and bladder control
- Loss of behavioral inhibition
- Significant mental changes
- May see neglect
- May see aphasia
- May see apraxia and agraphia
- Perseveration

Vertebral-Basilar Artery:
- Loss of consciousness
- Hemiplegia or quadriplegia
- Comatose or vegetative state
- Inability to speak
- Locked-in syndrome

Posterior Cerebral Artery:
- Thalamic pain syndrome
- Contralateral hemiplegia (central area)
- Pain and temperature sensory loss
- Ataxia, athetosis or choreiform movement
- Quality of movement is impaired
- Anomia
- Mild hemiparesis
- Hemiballismus
- Visual agnosia
- Prosopagnosia with occipital infarct
- Homonymous hemianopsia
- Memory impairment

Middle Cerebral Artery:
- Most common site of a CVA
- Aphasia in left hemisphere
- Homonymous hemianopsia
- Apraxia
- Flat affect in right hemisphere
- Impaired body schema
- Impaired spatial relations
- Superficial MCA – greater face and arm involvement
- Deep MCA – pure motor hemiplegia without sensory impairment

Lacunar Infarct:
- Cystic cavity after infarct
- Contralateral weakness
- Sensory loss
- Ataxia
- Dysarthria
- Deep regions of the brain:
  --internal capsule
  --thalamus
  --basal ganglia
  --pons

Cerebellum:
- Decreased balance
- Ataxia
- Decreased coordination
- Nausea
- Decreased ability for postural adjustment
- Nystagmus

Characteristics of a Cerebrovascular Accident

Right Hemisphere:
- Weakness, paralysis of the left side
- Decreased attention span
- Left hemianopsia
- Decreased awareness and judgment
- Memory deficits
- Left inattention
- Decreased abstract reasoning
- Emotional lability
- Impulsive behaviors
- Decreased spatial orientation

Left Hemisphere:
- Weakness, paralysis of the right side
- Increased frustration
- Decreased processing
- Possible aphasia (expressive, receptive, global)
- Possible dysphagia
- Possible motor apraxia (ideomotor and ideational)
- Decreased discrimination between left and right
- Right hemianopsia

Brainstem:
- Unstable vital signs
- Decreased consciousness
- Decreased ability to swallow
- Weakness on both sides of the body
- Paralysis on both sides of the body

Synergy Patterns

Upper Limb

	Flexor Synergy:	Extensor Synergy:
Scapula	Elevation and retraction	Depression and protraction
Shoulder	Abduction and lateral rotation	Medial rotation and adduction
Elbow	Flexion	Extension
Forearm	Supination	Pronation
Wrist	Flexion	Extension
Fingers	Flexion with adduction	Flexion with adduction
Thumb	Flexion and adduction	Adduction and flexion

- The flexor synergy is seen when the patient attempts to lift up their arm or reach for an object.

Lower Limb

	Flexor Synergy:	Extensor Synergy:
Hip	Abduction and lateral rotation	Extension, medial rotation and adduction
Knee	Flexion	Extension
Ankle	Dorsiflexion with supination	Plantar flexion with inversion
Toes	Extension	Flexion and adduction

- The flexor synergy is characterized by great toe extension and flexion of the remaining toes secondary to spasticity.

When the central nervous system is damaged as with a CVA, the higher centers of the brain are also damaged. The higher centers are responsible for both complex motor patterns and the inhibition of massive gross motor patterns. Synergy patterns result when the higher centers of the brain lose control and the uncontrolled or partially controlled stereotyped patterns of the middle and lower centers emerge.

Types of Nerve Injury

Neurapraxia: A nerve injury classified as a conduction block usually due to myelin dysfunction. The nerve fibers are not damaged and recovery usually occurs within six weeks.

Axonotmesis: A nerve injury classified as a reversible injury to damaged nerve fibers. Injury occurs distal to the site of damage and can regenerate at a rate of one millimeter per day.

Neurotmesis: A nerve injury classified as an irreversible injury. The nerve has severe damage and is unable to regenerate. All motor and sensory loss distal to the site of injury becomes a permanent condition.

Intervention

Theories of Neurological Rehabilitation

Bobath

Neuromuscular Developmental Treatment (NDT)
An approach developed by Karl and Berta Bobath based on the hierarchical model of neurophysiologic function. Abnormal postural reflex activity and abnormal muscle tone is caused by the loss of central nervous system control at the brainstem and spinal cord levels. The concept recognizes that interference of normal function of the brain caused by central nervous system dysfunction leads to a slowing down or cessation of motor development and the inhibition of righting reactions, equilibrium reactions, and automatic movements.

Key Terminology
Facilitation: A technique utilized to elicit voluntary muscular contraction.

Inhibition: A technique utilized to decrease excessive tone or movement.

Key points of control: Specific handling of designated areas of the body (shoulder, pelvis, hand, and foot) will influence and facilitate posture, alignment, and control.

Placing: The act of moving an extremity into a position that the patient must hold against gravity.

Reflex inhibiting posture: Designated static positions that Bobath found to inhibit abnormal tonal influences and reflexes.

Intervention
- Inhibition of abnormal patterns with facilitation of normal patterns
- Alteration of abnormal tone and influencing isolated active movement
- Avoid utilization of abnormal reflexes
- Manual contact and handling through key points of control for facilitation and inhibition
- Achieve a balance between muscle groups
- Use of developmental sequence
- Provide the patient with the sensation of normal movement by inhibiting abnormal postural reflex activity
- Use of dynamic reflex inhibiting patterns
- Use of functional activities with varying levels of difficulty
- Treatment should be active and dynamic
- Avoid associated reactions
- Emphasize the component of rotation during treatment activities
- Orientation to midline control by moving in and out of midline with dynamic activity

Brunnstrom

Movement Therapy in Hemiplegia
Movement therapy in hemiplegia developed by Signe Brunnstrom is based on the hierarchical model by Hughlings Jackson. This approach created and defined the term synergy and initially encouraged the use of synergy patterns during rehabilitation. The belief was to immediately practice synergy patterns and subsequently develop combinations of movement patterns outside of the synergy. Synergies are considered primitive patterns that occur at the spinal cord level as a result of the hierarchical organization of the central nervous system. Reinforcing synergy patterns is rarely utilized now as research has indicated that reinforced synergy patterns are very difficult to change. Brunnstrom developed the *seven stages of recovery*, which are used for evaluation and documentation of patient progress.

Key Terminology
Associated reactions: An involuntary and automatic movement of a body part as a result of an intentional active or resistive movement in another body part.

Homolateral synkinesis: A flexion pattern of the involved upper extremity facilitates flexion of the involved lower extremity.

Limb synergies: A group of muscles that produce a predictable pattern of movement in flexion or extension patterns.

Raimiste's phenomenon: The involved lower extremity will abduct/adduct with applied resistance to the uninvolved lower extremity in the same direction.

Souque's phenomenon: Raising the involved upper extremity above 100 degrees with elbow extension will produce extension and abduction of the fingers.

Stages of recovery: Brunnstrom separates neurological recovery into seven separate stages based on progression through abnormal tone and spasticity. These seven stages of recovery describe tone, reflex activity, and volitional movement.

Seven Stages of Recovery

Stage 1: No volitional movement initiated.

Stage 2: The appearance of basic limb synergies. The beginning of spasticity.

Stage 3: The synergies are performed voluntarily; spasticity increases.

Stage 4: Spasticity begins to decrease. Movement patterns are not dictated solely by limb synergies.

Stage 5: A further decrease in spasticity is noted with independence from limb synergy patterns.

Stage 6: Isolated joint movements are performed with coordination.

Stage 7: Normal motor function is restored.

Intervention
- Evaluation of strength focuses on patterns of movement rather than straight plane motion at a joint
- Sensory examination is required to assist with treating motor deficits
- Initially limb synergies were encouraged as a necessary milestone for recovery
- Encourage overflow to recruit active movement of the weak side
- Use of repetition of task and positive reinforcement
- A patient will follow the stages of recovery, but may experience a plateau at any point so that full recovery is not achieved

Kabat, Knott, and Voss

Proprioceptive Neuromuscular Facilitation (PNF)
PNF was introduced in the early 1950's using the hierarchical model as its framework. The original goal of treatment was to lay down gross motor patterns within the central nervous system. This approach is based on the premise that stronger parts of the body are utilized to stimulate and strengthen the weaker parts. Normal movement and posture is based on a balance between control of antagonist and agonist muscle groups. Development will follow the normal sequence through a component of motor learning. This theory places great emphasis on manual contacts and correct handling. Short and concise verbal commands are used along with resistance throughout the full movement pattern. The PNF approach utilizes methods that promote or hasten the response of the neuromuscular mechanism through stimulation of the proprioceptors. Movement patterns follow diagonals or spirals that each possess a flexion, extension, and rotatory component and are directed toward or away from midline.

Key Terminology
Chopping: A combination of bilateral upper extremity asymmetrical extensor patterns performed as a closed chain activity.

Developmental sequence: A progression of motor skill acquisition. The stages of motor control include mobility, stability, controlled mobility, and skill.

Mass movement patterns: The hip, knee, and ankle move into flexion or extension simultaneously.

Overflow: Muscle activation of an involved extremity due to intense action of an uninvolved muscle or group of muscles.

Intervention
- A patient learns diagonal patterns of movement
- Techniques must have accurate timing, specific commands, and correct hand placement
- Verbal commands must be short and concise
- Repetition is important in motor learning
- Resistance given during the movement pattern is greater if the objective is stability, less if the objective is mobility
- Techniques utilize isometric and isotonic muscle contractions
- Treatment objectives will dictate the use of techniques through either full movement or at points within the range
- Developmental sequence is used in conjunction with PNF techniques in order to increase the balance between agonists and antagonists
- PNF techniques are implemented to progress a patient through the stages of motor control
- Functional patterns of movement are used to increase control
- Techniques should be utilized that increase strength or improve relaxation by enhancing irradiation from the stronger to the weaker muscles

Levels of Motor Control

Mobility
The ability to initiate movement through a functional range of motion.

Stability
The ability to maintain a position or posture through cocontraction and tonic holding around a joint. Unsupported sitting with midline control is an example of stability.

Controlled Mobility
The ability to move within a weight bearing position or rotate around a long axis. Activities in prone on elbows or weight shifting in quadruped are examples of controlled mobility.

Skill
The ability to consistently perform functional tasks and manipulate the environment with normal postural reflex mechanisms and balance reactions. Skill activities include ADLs and community locomotion.

PNF Diagonal Patterns – Upper Extremity Responses

	D1 Flexion Pattern	D1 Extension Pattern	D2 Flexion Pattern	D2 Extension Pattern
Scapula	Elevation Abduction Upward rotation	Depression Adduction Downward rotation	Elevation Adduction Upward rotation	Depression Abduction Downward rotation
Shoulder	Flexion Adduction Lateral rotation	Extension Abduction Medial rotation	Flexion Abduction Lateral rotation	Extension Adduction Medial rotation
Elbow	Flexion or extension	Flexion or extension	Flexion or extension	Flexion or extension
Radioulnar	Supination	Pronation	Supination	Pronation
Wrist	Flexion Radial deviation	Extension Ulnar deviation	Extension Radial deviation	Flexion Ulnar deviation
Thumb	Adduction	Abduction	Extension	Opposition

PNF Diagonal Patterns – Lower Extremity Responses

	D1 Flexion Pattern	D1 Extension Pattern	D2 Flexion Pattern	D2 Extension Pattern
Pelvis	Protraction	Retraction	Elevation	Depression
Hip	Flexion Adduction Lateral rotation	Extension Abduction Medial rotation	Flexion Abduction Medial rotation	Extension Adduction Lateral rotation
Knee	Flexion or extension	Flexion or extension	Flexion or extension	Flexion or extension
Ankle and Toes	Dorsiflexion Inversion	Plantar flexion Eversion	Dorsiflexion Eversion	Plantar flexion Inversion

PNF Therapeutic Exercises

Technique	Mobility		Stability	Controlled Mobility	Skill		Strength
	Increased ROM	Initiate Movement			Distal Functional Movement	Proximal Dynamic Stability	
Agonistic Reversals				X		X	
Alternating Isometrics			X				
Contract-Relax	X						
Hold-Relax	X						
Hold-Relax Active Movement		X					
Joint Distraction	X	X					
Normal Timing					X		
Repeated Contractions		X					X
Resisted Progression						X	
Rhythmic Initiation		X					
Rhythmical Rotation	X	X					
Rhythmic Stabilization	X		X				
Slow Reversal			X	X	X		
Slow Reversal Hold			X	X	X		
Timing for Emphasis							X

PNF Therapeutic Exercise Descriptions*

*Italicized terms indicate level of developmental sequence.

Agonistic Reversals (AR)
Controlled mobility, skill - An isotonic concentric contraction performed against resistance followed by alternating concentric and eccentric contractions with resistance. AR requires use in a slow and sequential manner, and may be used in increments throughout the range to attain maximum control.

Alternating Isometrics (AI)
Stability - Isometric contractions are performed alternating from muscles on one side of the joint to the other side without rest. AI emphasizes endurance or strengthening.

Contract-Relax (CR)
Mobility - A technique used to increase range of motion. As the extremity reaches the point of limitation the patient performs a maximal contraction of the antagonistic muscle group. The therapist resists movement for eight to ten seconds with relaxation to follow. The technique is repeated until no further gains in range of motion are noted during the session.

Hold-Relax (HR)
Mobility - An isometric contraction used to increase range of motion. The contraction is facilitated for all muscle groups at the limiting point in the range of motion. Relaxation occurs and the extremity moves through the newly acquired range to the next point of limitation until no further increases in range of motion occur. The technique is often used for patients that present with pain.

Hold-Relax Active Movement (HRAM)
Mobility - A technique to improve initiation of movement to muscle groups tested at 1/5 or less. An isometric contraction is performed once the extremity is passively placed into a shortened range within the pattern. Overflow and facilitation may be used to assist with the contraction. Upon relaxation the extremity is immediately moved into a lengthened position of the pattern with a quick stretch. The patient is asked to return the extremity to the shortened position through an isotonic contraction.

Joint Distraction
Mobility - A proprioceptive component used to increase range of motion around a joint. Consistent manual traction is provided slowly and usually in combination with mobilization techniques. It can also be used in combination with quick stretch to initiate movement.

Normal Timing (NT)
Skill - A technique used to improve coordination of all components of a task. NT is performed in a distal to proximal sequence. Proximal components are restricted until the distal components are activated and initiate movement. Repetition of the pattern produces a coordinated movement of all components.

Repeated Contractions (RC)
Mobility – A technique used to initiate movement and sustain a contraction through the range of motion. Repeated contractions is used to initiate a movement pattern, throughout a weak movement pattern or at a point of weakness within a

58   A GUIDE TO SUCCESS

movement pattern. The therapist provides a quick stretch followed by isometric or isotonic contractions.

Resisted Progression (RP)
Skill - A technique used to emphasize coordination of proximal components during gait. Resistance is applied to an area such as the pelvis, hips, or extremity during the gait cycle in order to enhance coordination, strength or endurance.

Rhythmic Initiation (RI)
Mobility - A technique used to assist initiating movement when hypertonia exists. Movement progresses from passive ("let me move you"), to active assistive ("help me move you"), to slightly resistive ("move against the resistance"). Movements must be slow and rhythmical to reduce the hypertonia and allow for full range of motion.

Rhythmical Rotation (RR)
Mobility - A passive technique used to decrease hypertonia by slowly rotating an extremity around the longitudinal axis. Relaxation of the extremity will increase range of motion.

Rhythmic Stabilization (RS)
Mobility, stability - A technique used to increase range of motion and coordinate isometric contractions. The technique requires isometric contractions of all muscles around a joint against progressive resistance. The patient should relax and move into the newly acquired range and repeat the technique. If stability is the goal, RS should be applied as progression from AI in order to simultaneously stabilize all muscle groups around the specific body part.

Slow Reversal (SR)
Stability, controlled mobility, skill - A technique of slow and resisted concentric contractions of agonists and antagonists around a joint without rest between reversals. This technique is used to improve control of movement and posture.

Slow Reversal Hold (SRH)
Stability, controlled mobility, skill - Using slow reversal with the addition of an isometric contraction that is performed at the end of each movement in order to gain stability.

Timing for Emphasis (TE)
Skill - Used to strengthen the weak component of a motor pattern. Isotonic and isometric contractions produce overflow to weak muscles.

Motor Control: A Task Oriented Approach

Theories of motor control have been documented since the late nineteenth century when Sir Charles Sherrington postulated the reflex theory of motor control. Motor control refers to the ability to produce, regulate, and alter mechanisms that produce movement and control posture. The various theories are based on a specific interpretation of how the brain functions and interacts with other body systems. A task oriented approach to motor control utilizes a systems theory of motor control that views the entire body as a mechanical system with many interacting subsystems that all work cooperatively in managing internal and environmental influences. The task oriented approach utilizes an examination that consists of observation of functional performance, analysis of strategies used to accomplish tasks, and assessment of impairments. Treatment attempts to resolve impairments, design and implement effective recovery and compensatory strategies, and retrain using functional activities.

Key Terminology
Compensation: The ability to utilize alternate motor and sensory strategies due to an impairment that limits the normal completion of a task.

Motor learning: The ability to perform a movement as a result of internal processes that interact with the environment and produce a consistent strategy to generate the correct movement.

Plasticity: The ability to modify or change at the synapse level either temporarily or permanently in order to perform a particular function.

Postural control: The ability of the motor and sensory systems to stabilize position and control movement.

Recovery: The ability to utilize previous strategies to return to the same level of functioning.

Strategy: A plan used to produce a specific result or outcome that will influence the whole structure or system.

Intervention
- Models of motor control vary based on the interpretation of brain function
- Evaluation determines the degree of impairment
- Intervention is designed at the level of impairment
- Sensory, motor, and cognitive strategies are used to acquire postural control
- Focus is both on recovery and compensatory techniques
- Tasks are broken down into components of the task for practice
- Sensory, motor, and perceptual input contribute to motor control
- Movement is based around a behavioral goal
- Variable practice allows for training in a different and changing environment
- Type and amount of feedback (visual, verbal) should be evaluated for each individual patient
- Emphasis on postural control, alignment, and sequencing of movements is essential
- Intervention should create multiple ways to solve a movement disorder
- Environmental factors must be considered with intervention, planning, and implementation

Rood

This theory is based on Sherrington and the reflex stimulus model. Rood believed that all motor output was the result of both past and present sensory input. Treatment is based on sensorimotor learning. It takes into account the autonomic nervous system and emotional factors as well as motor ability. Rood used a developmental sequence, which was seen as "key patterns" in the enhancement of motor control. A goal of this approach is to obtain homeostasis in motor output and to activate muscles and perform a task independently of a stimulus. Exercise is seen as a treatment technique only if the response is correct and if it provides sensory feedback that enhances the motor learning of that response. Once a response is obtained during treatment the stimulus should be withdrawn. Rood introduced the use of sensory stimulation to facilitate or inhibit responses such as icing and brushing in order to elicit desired reflex motor responses.

Sensory Stimulation Techniques

Facilitation:
- Approximation
- Joint compression
- Icing
- Light tough
- Quick stretch
- Resistance
- Tapping
- Traction

Inhibition:
- Deep pressure
- Prolonged stretch
- Warmth
- Prolonged cold
- Carotid reflex

Key Terminology

Heavy work: A method used to develop stability by performing an activity (work) against gravity or resistance. Heavy work focuses on the strengthening of postural muscles.

Light work: A method used to develop controlled movement and skilled function by performing an activity (work) without resistance. Light work focuses on the extremities.

Key patterns: A developmental sequence designed by Rood that directs patients' mobility recovery from synergy patterns through controlled motion.

Intervention
- Use of sensory stimulation to achieve motor output
- Movement is considered autonomic and noncognitive
- Homeostasis of all systems is essential
- Use of techniques such as neutral warmth, maintained pressure, and slow rhythmical stroking to calm a patient
- Tactile stimulation is used to facilitate normal movement
- Exercise must provide proper sensory feedback in order to be therapeutic

Neurological Profile

Examination

- Past medical history
- History of current condition
- Social history (caregiver support)
- Medications
- Living environment
- Systems review
- Cognitive and language assessment
- Respiratory assessment
- Postural tone assessment
- Righting and equilibrium reaction assessment
- Pathological reflex assessment
- Pain
- Sensation, proprioception, and kinesthesia
- Range of motion
- Motor assessment
- Mobility skills

Intervention

- Postural control
- Positioning
- Therapeutic exercise
- Developmental activities training
- Facilitation/inhibition techniques
- Motor function retraining
- Sensory integration
- Wheelchair and orthotic prescription
- Mobility training

Goals

- Maximize functional mobility
- Normalize tonal abnormalities
- Maximize active isolated movement and strength
- Maximize range of motion and joint integrity
- Maximize independence with adaptive equipment
- Maximize static and dynamic balance
- Maximize patient/caregiver competence with:
    - --Diagnosis and prognosis
    - --Positioning
    - --Use of adaptive equipment and orthotic devices
    - --Home exercise programs

Neurological Terminology

Agnosia: The inability to interpret information.

Agraphesthesia: The inability to recognize symbols, letters or numbers traced on the skin.

Agraphia: The inability to write due to a lesion within the brain.

Akinesia: The inability to initiate movement; commonly seen in patients with Parkinson's disease.

Aphasia: The inability to communicate or comprehend due to damage to specific areas of the brain.

Apraxia: The inability to perform purposeful learned movements, although there is no sensory or motor impairment.

Astereognosis: The inability to recognize objects by sense of touch.

Ataxia: The inability to perform coordinated movements.

Athetosis: A condition that presents with involuntary movements combined with instability of posture. Peripheral movements occur without central stability.

Bradykinesia: Movement that is very slow.

Broca's aphasia: An infarct to a specific area of the frontal lobe that produces the inability to verbally communicate. Speech is difficult, but comprehension is usually functional or normal.

Chorea: Movements that are sudden, random, and involuntary.

Clonus: A characteristic of an upper motor neuron lesion; involuntary alternating spasmotic contraction of a muscle precipitated by a quick stretch reflex.

Constructional apraxia: The inability to reproduce geometric figures and designs. This person is visually unable to analyze how to perform a task.

Decerebrate rigidity: A characteristic of a corticospinal lesion at the level of the brainstem that results in extension of the trunk and all extremities.

Decorticate rigidity: A characteristic of a corticospinal lesion at the level of the diencephalon where the trunk and lower extremities are positioned in extension and the upper extremities are positioned in flexion.

Diplopia: Double vision

Dysarthria: Slurred and impaired speech due to a motor deficit of the tongue or other muscles essential for speech.

Dysdiadochokinesia: The inability to perform rapidly alternating movements.

Dysmetria: The inability to control the range of a movement and the force of muscular activity.

Dysphagia: The inability to properly swallow.

Dystonia: Closely related to athetosis, however there is larger axial muscle involvement rather than appendicular muscles.

Emotional lability: A characteristic of a right hemisphere infarct where there is an inability to control emotions and outbursts of laughing or crying that are inconsistent with the situation.

Expressive aphasia: A condition due to a lesion within the brain where language and communication skills such as reading, writing, and speaking are impaired.

Global aphasia: A type of aphasia that presents with both expressive and receptive deficits. Prognosis for recovery of speech is usually poor. The patient's speech is nonfluent and comprehension is significantly impaired.

Hemiballism: An involuntary and violent movement of a large body part.

Hemiparesis: A condition of weakness on one side of the body.

Hemiplegia: A condition of paralysis on one side of the body.

Homonymous hemianopsia: The loss of the right or left half of the field of vision in both eyes.

Ideational apraxia: The inability to formulate an initial motor plan and sequence tasks where the proprioceptive input necessary for movement is impaired.

Ideomotor apraxia: A condition where a person plans a movement or task but cannot volitionally perform it. Automatic movement may occur, however a person cannot impose additional movement on command.

Kinesthesia: The ability to perceive the direction and extent of movement of a joint or body part.

Neglect: The inability to interpret stimuli on the left side of the body due to a lesion of the right frontal lobe of the brain.

Perseveration: The state of repeatedly performing the same segment of a task or repeatedly saying the same word/phrase without purpose.

Proprioception: The ability to perceive the static position of a joint or body part.

Receptive aphasia: The inability to comprehend normal speech.

Rigidity: A state of severe hypertonicity where a sustained muscle contraction does not allow for any movement at a specified joint.

Synergy: A result of brain damage that presents with mass movement patterns that are primitive in nature and coupled with spasticity.

Wernicke's aphasia: An infarct to a specific area of the temporal lobe that severely affects the patient's level of comprehension. The person is usually able to verbalize, but is frequently nonfunctional.

Spinal Cord Injury

Examination

Types of Spinal Cord Injury

Complete lesion: A lesion to the spinal cord where there is no preserved motor or sensory function below the level of lesion.

Incomplete lesion: A lesion to the spinal cord with incomplete damage to the cord. There may be scattered motor function, sensory function or both below the level of lesion.

Specific Incomplete Lesions

Anterior cord syndrome
An incomplete lesion that results from compression and damage to the anterior part of the spinal cord or anterior spinal artery. The mechanism of injury is usually cervical flexion. There is loss of motor function and pain and temperature sense below the lesion due to damage of the corticospinal and spinothalamic tracts.

Brown-Sequard's syndrome
An incomplete lesion usually caused by a stab wound, which produces hemisection of the spinal cord. There is paralysis and loss of vibratory and position sense on the same side as the lesion due to the damage to the corticospinal tract and dorsal columns. There is a loss of pain and temperature sense on the opposite side of the lesion from damage to the lateral spinothalamic tract. Pure Brown-Sequard's syndrome is rare since most spinal cord lesions are atypical.

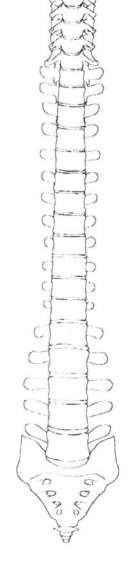

Cauda equina injuries
An injury that occurs below the L1 spinal level where the long nerve roots transcend. Cauda equina injuries can be complete, however are frequently incomplete due to the large number of nerve roots in the area. A cauda equina injury is considered a peripheral nerve injury. Characteristics include flaccidity, areflexia, and impairment of bowel and bladder function. Full recovery is not typical due to the distance needed for axonal regeneration.

Central cord syndrome
An incomplete lesion that results from compression and damage to the central portion of the spinal cord. The mechanism of injury is usually cervical hyperextension that damages the spinothalamic tract, corticospinal tract, and dorsal columns. The upper extremities present with greater involvement than the lower extremities and greater motor deficits exist as compared to sensory deficits.

Posterior cord syndrome
A relatively rare syndrome that is caused by compression of the posterior spinal artery and is characterized by loss of pain perception, proprioception, two-point discrimination, and stereognosis. Motor function is preserved.

Intervention

Potential Complications of Spinal Cord Injury

Autonomic Dysreflexia
Autonomic dysreflexia is perhaps the most dangerous complication of spinal cord injury and can occur in patients with lesions above T6. A noxious stimulus below the level of the lesion triggers the autonomic nervous system causing a sudden elevation in blood pressure. Common causes include distended or full bladder, kink or blockage in the catheter, bladder infections, pressure ulcers, extreme temperature changes, tight clothing, or even an ingrown toenail. If not treated, this condition can lead to convulsions, hemorrhage, and death.

Symptoms: High blood pressure, severe headache, blurred vision, stuffy nose, profuse sweating, goose bumps below the level of the lesion, and vasodilation (flushing) above the level of injury

Treatment: The first reaction to this medical crisis is to check the catheter for blockage. The bowel should also be checked for impaction. A patient should remain in a sitting position. Lying a patient down is contraindicated and will only assist to further elevate blood pressure. The patient should be examined for any other irritating stimuli. If the cause remains unknown, the patient should receive immediate medical intervention.

Deep Vein Thrombosis (DVT)

Deep vein thrombosis results from the formation of a blood clot that becomes dislodged and is termed an embolus. This is considered a serious medical condition since the embolus may obstruct a selected artery. A patient with a spinal cord injury has a greater risk of developing a DVT due to the absence or decrease in the normal pumping action by active contractions of muscles in the lower extremities. Homans' sign is a special test designed to confirm the presence of a DVT. Prevention of a DVT should include prophylactic anticoagulant therapy, maintaining a positioning schedule, range of motion, proper positioning to avoid excessive venous stasis, and use of elastic stockings.

Symptoms: Swelling of the lower extremity, pain, sensitivity over the area of the clot, and warmth in the area.

Treatment: Once a DVT is suspected there should be no active or passive movement performed to the involved lower extremity. Bed rest and anticoagulant drug therapy are usually indicated. Surgical procedures can be performed if necessary.

Ectopic Bone

Ectopic bone or heterotopic ossification refers to the spontaneous formation of bone in the soft tissue. It typically occurs adjacent to larger joints such as the knees or the hips. Theories regarding etiology range from tissue hypoxia to abnormal calcium metabolism.

Symptoms: Early symptoms include edema, decreased range of motion, and increased temperature of the involved joint

Treatment: Drug intervention usually involves diphosphates that inhibit ectopic bone formation. Physical therapy and surgery are often incorporated into treatment. Physical therapy must focus on maintaining functional range of motion and allowing the patient the most independent functional outcome possible.

Orthostatic Hypotension

Orthostatic hypotension or postural hypotension occurs due to a loss of sympathetic control of vasoconstriction in combination with absent or severely reduced muscle tone. Venous pooling is fairly common during the early stages of rehabilitation. A decrease in systolic blood pressure greater than 20 mm Hg after moving from a supine position to a sitting position is typically indicative of orthostatic hypotension.

Symptoms: Complaints of dizziness, light-headedness, nausea, and "blacking out" when going from a horizontal to a vertical position

Treatment: Monitoring vital signs assists with minimizing the effects of orthostatic hypotension. The use of elastic stockings, ace wraps to the lower extremities, and abdominal binders are common. Gradual progression to a vertical position using a tilt table is often indicated. Drug intervention may be indicated in order to increase blood pressure.

Pressure Ulcers

A pressure ulcer is caused by sustained pressure, friction, and/or shearing to a surface. The most common areas susceptible to pressure ulcers are the coccyx, sacrum, ischium, trochanters, elbows, buttocks, malleoli, scapulae, and prominent vertebrae. Pressure ulcers require immediate medical intervention and often can significantly delay the rehabilitation process.

Symptoms: A reddened area that persists; an open area

Treatment: Prevention is of greatest importance. A patient should change position frequently, maintain proper skin care, sit on an appropriate cushion, consistently weight shift, and maintain proper nutrition and hydration. Surgical intervention is often necessary with advanced pressure ulcers.

Spasticity

Spasticity can occasionally be useful to a patient with a spinal cord injury, however more often serves to interfere with functional activities. Spasticity can be enhanced by both internal and external sources such as stress, decubiti, urinary tract infections, bowel or bladder obstruction, temperature changes or touch.

Symptoms: Increased involuntary contraction of muscle groups, increased tonic stretch reflexes, excessive deep tendon reflexes

Treatment: Medications are usually administered in an attempt to reduce the degree of spasticity (Dantrium, Baclofen, Lioresal). Aggressive treatment includes phenol blocks, rhizotomies, myelotomies, and other surgical intervention. Physical therapy intervention includes positioning, aquatic therapy, weight bearing, functional electrical stimulation, range of motion, resting splints, and inhibitive casting.

Functional Outcomes for Complete Lesions

Functional Skills	Level of Assistance Required (by SCI level groups)			
	High Tetraplegia (C1-C5)	**Mid-Level Tetraplegia (C6)**	**Low Tetraplegia (C7-C8)**	**Paraplegia**
Bed Mobility • Rolling side to side • Rolling supine/prone • Supine/sitting • Scooting all directions	-Dependent (C1-C4) -Moderate to maximal assistance (C5) -Able to verbally direct	-Minimal assistance to modified independent with equipment -Able to verbally direct	-Independent with all	-Independent
Transfers • Bed • Car • Toilet • Bath equipment • Floor • Upright wheelchair	-Dependent (C1-C4) -Maximal assistance with level sliding board transfers (C5) -Able to verbally direct	-Minimal assistance to modified independent for sliding board transfers -Dependent with wheelchair loading in car -Dependent with floor transfers and uprighting wheelchair -Able to verbally direct	-Modified independent to independent with level surface transfer (sliding board or depression) -Moderate assistance to modified independent with car transfer -Maximal to moderate assistance with floor transfers and uprighting wheelchair -Able to verbally direct	-Independent with level surface and car transfers (depression) -Minimal assistance to independent with floor transfers and uprighting wheelchair -Able to verbally direct
Weight Shifts • Pressure relief • Repositioning in wheelchair	-Set-up to modified independent with power recline/tilt weight shift -Dependent with manual recline/tilt/lean weight shift -Able to verbally direct	-Modified independent with power recline/tilt weight shift -Minimal assistance to modified independent with side to side/forward lean weight shift -Able to verbally direct	-Modified independent with side to side/forward lean, or depression weight shift	-Modified independent with depression weight shift
Wheelchair Management • Wheel locks • Armrests • Foot rests/legrests • Safety strap(s) • Cushion adjustment • Anti-tip levers • Wheelchair maintenance	-Dependent with all -Able to verbally direct	-Some assistance required -Able to verbally direct	-May require assistance with cushion adjustment, anti-tip levers, and wheelchair maintenance -Able to verbally direct	-Independent with all

Level of Assistance Required (by SCI level groups)

Functional Skills	High Tetraplegia (C1-C5)	Mid-Level Tetraplegia (C6)	Low Tetraplegia (C7-C8)	Paraplegia
Wheelchair Mobility • Smooth surfaces • Up/down ramps • Up/down curbs • Rough terrain • Up/down steps (manual wheelchair only)	-Supervision/set-up to modified independent on smooth, ramp, and rough terrain with power wheelchair -Modified independent with manual wheelchair on smooth surface in forward direction (C5) -Maximal assistance to dependent with manual wheelchair in all other situations (C5) -Able to verbally direct	-Modified independent in smooth, ramp, and rough terrain with power wheelchair -Dependent to maximal assistance up/down curb with power wheelchair -Modified independent on smooth surfaces with manual wheelchair -Moderate to minimal assistance on ramps and rough terrain with manual wheelchair -Maximal to moderate assistance up/down curbs with manual wheelchair -Able to verbally direct	-Modified independent on smooth, ramp, and rough terrain with power wheelchair -Dependent to maximal assistance up/down curb with power wheelchair -Modified independent on smooth surfaces and up/down ramps with manual wheelchair -Minimal assistance to modified independent on rough terrain -Moderate to minimal assistance up/down curbs with manual wheelchair -Dependent to maximal assistance up/down steps with manual wheelchair -Able to verbally direct	-Minimal assistance to modified independent up/down 6" curbs with manual wheelchair -Modified independent with descending steps with manual wheelchair -Maximal to minimal assistance to ascend steps with manual wheelchair -Able to verbally direct
Gait • Don/doff orthoses • Sit/stand • Smooth surfaces • Up/down ramps • Up/down curbs • Up/down steps • Rough terrain • Safe falling	-Not applicable	-Not applicable	-Not applicable	Abilities range from: -exercise only with KAFOs* -household ambulation with KAFOs -limited community ambulation with KAFOs or AFOs* -functional community ambulation with or without orthoses
ROM/Positioning • PROM to trunk, legs, and arms • Pad/position in bed	-Dependent -Able to verbally direct	-Moderate assistance to modified independent with all -Able to verbally direct	-Minimal assistance to modified independent with all -Able to verbally direct	-Independent
Feeding • Drinking • Finger feeding • Utensil feeding	-Dependent (C1-C4) -Minimal assistance with adaptive equipment (C5) -Able to verbally direct	-Modified independent with adaptive equipment	-Modified independent with adaptive equipment (C7)	-Independent

UNIT THREE: NEUROMUSCULAR

Functional Skills	High Tetraplegia (C1-C5)	Mid-Level Tetraplegia (C6)	Low Tetraplegia (C7-C8)	Paraplegia
Grooming • Face • Teeth • Hair • Makeup • Shaving face	-Dependent (C1-C4) -Minimal assistance with adaptive equipment for face, teeth, makeup/shaving (C5) -Maximal to moderate assistance for hair grooming (C5) -Able to verbally direct	-Modified independent with adaptive equipment	-Modified independent	-Independent
Dressing • Dressing/undressing (in bed/wheelchair) • Upper body/lower body (in bed/wheelchair)	-Dependent -Able to verbally direct	-Modified independent for upper body in bed or wheelchair -Minimal assistance with lower body dressing in bed -Moderate assistance with lower body undressing in bed -Able to verbally direct	-Modified independent for upper/lower body dressing/undressing in bed -Minimal assistance with lower body dressing/undressing in wheelchair (C7) -Modified independent for upper/lower body dressing/undressing in wheelchair (C8) -Able to verbally direct	-Modified independent
Bathing • Bathing and drying off • Upper body and lower body	-Dependent -Able to verbally direct	-Minimal assistance for upper body bathing and drying -Moderate assistance for lower body bathing and drying -Use of shower or tub chair -Able to verbally direct	-Modified independent with all using shower or tub chair	-Modified independent with all on tub bench or tub bottom cushion
Bowel/Bladder Problems • Intermittent catheterization • Leg bag care • Condom application • Clean up • In bed/wheelchair (bladder) • Feminine hygiene • Bowel program	-Dependent -Able to verbally direct	**Bladder:** -minimal assistance for male in bed or wheelchair -moderate assistance for female in bed **Bowel:** -moderate assistance with use of equipment -Able to verbally direct	**Bladder:** -modified independent for male in bed or wheelchair -modified independent for female in bed; moderate assistance for female in wheelchair **Bowel:** -minimal assistance to modified independent with use of equipment -Able to verbally direct	**Bladder:** -modified independent for male and female **Bowel:** -modified independent for male and female

*KAFO, knee-ankle-foot orthosis; AFO = ankle-foot orthosis

From Umphred DA: Neurological Rehabilitation. Mosby-Year Book, Inc. 1995, p. 502-505, with permission.

Spinal Cord Injury Profile

Examination

- Past medical history
- History of current condition
- Social history (caregiver support)
- Medications
- Living environment
- Systems review
- Cognitive assessment
- Skin assessment
- American Spinal Cord Injury Association (ASIA) Standard Neurological Classification
    - --Sensory examination
    - --Motor examination
- American Spinal Cord Injury Association (ASIA) impairment scale
- Respiratory assessment
    - --Cough
    - --Chest expansion
    - --Accessory muscle use
    - --Vital capacity
- Range of motion
- Pain
- Mobility skills

Intervention

- Positioning
- Family/caregiver teaching
- Respiratory training
    - --Assisted cough and secretion clearance
    - --Breathing exercises
- Wheelchair, cushion, and orthotic prescription
- Pressure relief
- Range of motion
- Motor function retraining
- Mobility training
- Gait training (T9 or lower)

Goals

- Maximize functional mobility based on level of injury (please refer to "functional outcome" chart)
- Maximize respiratory function
- Attain functional range of motion for all joints
- Maximize strength of available muscle groups
- Maximize patient/caregiver competence with:
    - --Pressure relief
    - --Positioning
    - --Range of motion
    - --Strengthening
    - --Wheelchair management

Spinal Cord Injury Terminology

Cauda equina injury: A term used to describe injuries that occur below the L1 level of the spine. A cauda equina injury is considered to be a lower motor neuron lesion.

Dermatome: Designated sensory areas based on spinal segment innervation.

Myelotomy: A surgical procedure that severs certain tracts within the spinal cord in order to decrease spasticity and improve function.

Myotome: Designated motor areas based on spinal segment innervation.

Neurectomy: A surgical removal of a segment of a nerve in order to decrease spasticity and improve function.

Neurogenic bladder: The bladder empties reflexively for a patient with an injury above the level of S2. The sacral reflex arc remains intact.

Neurologic level: The lowest segment (most caudal) of the spinal cord with intact strength and sensation. Muscle groups at this level must receive a grade of fair.

Nonreflexive bladder: The bladder is flaccid as a result of a cauda equina or conus medullaris lesion. The sacral reflex arc is damaged.

Paraplegia: A term used to describe injuries that occur at the level of the thoracic, lumbar or sacral spine.

Rhizotomy: A surgical resection of the sensory component of a spinal nerve in order to decrease spasticity and improve function.

Sacral sparing: An incomplete lesion where some of the innermost tracts remain innervated. Characteristics include sensation of the saddle area, movement of the toe flexors, and rectal sphincter contraction.

Spinal shock: A physiologic response that occurs between 30 and 60 minutes after trauma to the spinal cord and can last up to several weeks. Spinal shock presents with total flaccid paralysis and loss of all reflexes below the level of injury.

Tenotomy: A surgical release of a tendon in order to decrease spasticity and improve function.

Tetraplegia (quadriplegia): A term adopted by the American Spinal Cord Injury Association to describe injuries that occur at the level of the cervical spine.

Zone of preservation: A term used to describe poor or trace motor or sensory function for up to three levels below the neurologic level of injury.

Spinal Cord Injury Medications

Acute Medical Management
- **GM-1:** A complex acidic glycolipid that is usually administered in combination with methylprednisolone immediately after spinal cord injury. The medication acts to enhance recovery of white matter and improve motor output.
- **Methylprednisolone:** A corticosteroid that is administered within the first eight hours after injury. The medication can enhance blood flow to the spinal cord, reduce post-traumatic ischemia, and prevent overall decline in white matter.

Antispasticity
- **Baclofen (Lioresal):** Baclofen is usually able to reduce tone in patients with spinal cord injuries with minimal sedative effects. The medication is administered orally or through a pump directly into the lumbar subarachnoid space.
- **Diazepam (Valium):** Diazepam is effective in reducing tone, however it also produces sedative effects.
- **Dantrium (Dantrolene sodium):** Dantrium acts to directly effect the skeletal muscle. It is effective in reducing tone, however can cause a significant increase in generalized weakness of the muscles.

Anticoagulants
- **Coumadin:** Coumadin is administered orally and is used for the treatment of deep vein thrombosis by impairing the synthesis of multiple clotting factors. The medication takes several days to achieve the desired effect of anticoagulation.
- **Heparin:** Heparin is administered parenterally by intravenous injection or through subcutaneous injection. The medication achieves the desired anticoagulant effect almost immediately by enhancing antithrombin II activity, which results in the inactivation of clotting factors.

Ectopic Bone
- **Etidronate (Didronel):** Etidronate is a diphosphonate that is used in the treatment of heterotopic ossification. It inhibits bone resorption and formation, and prevents ossification.

Traumatic Brain Injury

Examination

Types of Injury

Open Injury
An injury of direct penetration through the skull to the brain. Location, depth of penetration, and pathway determine the extent of brain damage. Examples include gunshot wound, knife or sharp object penetration, skull fragments, and direct trauma.

Closed Injury
An injury to the brain without penetration through the skull. Examples include concussion, contusion, hematoma, injury to extracranial blood vessels, hypoxia, drug overdose, near drowning, and acceleration/deceleration injuries.

Primary Injury
Initial injury to the brain sustained by impact. Examples include skull penetration, skull fractures, and contusions to grey and white matter.

Coup lesion – A direct lesion of the brain under the point of impact. Local brain damage is sustained.

Contrecoup lesion – An injury that results on the opposite side of the brain. The lesion is due to the rebound effect of the brain after impact.

Secondary Injury
Brain damage that occurs as a response to the initial injury. Examples include hematoma, hypoxia, ischemia, increased intracranial pressure, and posttraumatic epilepsy.

Epidural hematoma – A hemorrhage that forms between the skull and dura mater.

Subdural hematoma – A hemorrhage that forms due to venous rupture between the dura and arachnoid.

Acute Diagnostic Management

- Glasgow Coma Scale – level of arousal and cerebral cortex function
- CAT Scan – observe intracranial structures
- X-Ray – fractures
- MRI – observe intracranial structures
- Cerebral angiography – observe blood vessels and internal anatomy of the brain
- Evoked potential/electroencephalogram – localizing structural damage
- Positron emission tomography – cerebral metabolism abnormalities
- Ventriculography – radiography used to observe cerebral ventricles following cerebrospinal fluid removal
- Radioisotope imaging – allows for a two dimensional concentrated view of the brain

Levels of Consciousness

Coma: A state of unconsciousness and a level of unresponsiveness to all internal and external stimuli.

Stupor: A state of general unresponsiveness with arousal occurring from repeated stimuli.

Obtundity: A state of consciousness that is characterized by a state of sleep, reduced alertness to arousal, and delayed responses to stimuli.

Delirium: A state of consciousness that is characterized by disorientation, confusion, agitation, and loudness.

Clouding of consciousness: A state of consciousness that is characterized by quiet behavior, confusion, poor attention, and delayed responses.

Consciousness: A state of alertness, awareness, orientation, and memory.

Glasgow Coma Scale

A neurological assessment tool used initially after injury to determine arousal and cerebral cortex function. A total score of 8 or less correlates to coma in 90% of patients. Scores of 9 to 12 indicate moderate brain injuries and scores from 13 to 15 indicate mild brain injuries.

Glasgow Coma Scale:

Eye Opening	E
Spontaneous	4
To speech	3
To pain	2
Nil	1

Best Motor Response	M
Obeys commands	6
Localizes pain	5
Withdraws	4
Abnormal flexion	3
Extensor response	2
Nil	1

Verbal Response	V
Oriented	5
Confused conversation	4
Inappropriate words	3
Incomprehensible sounds	2
Nil	1

Coma Score (E+M+V) = 3 to 15

From Management of Head Injuries by Bryan Jennett and Graham Teasdale, Copyright-1981 by Oxford University Press, Inc. Used by permission of Oxford University Press, Inc.

Memory Impairments

Anterograde memory: The inability to create new memory. Anterograde memory is usually the last to recover after a comatose state. Contributing factors include poor attention, distractibility, and impaired perception of stimuli.

Posttraumatic amnesia: The time between the injury and when the patient is able to recall recent events. The patient does not recall the injury or events up until this point of recovery. Posttraumatic amnesia is used as an indicator of the extent of damage.

Retrograde amnesia: An inability to remember events prior to the injury. Retrograde amnesia may progressively decrease with recovery.

Rancho Los Amigos Levels of Cognitive Functioning

I. **NO RESPONSE**
Patient appears to be in a deep sleep and is completely unresponsive to any stimuli.

II. **GENERALIZED RESPONSE**
Patient reacts inconsistently and nonpurposefully to stimuli in a nonspecific manner. Responses are limited and often the same regardless of stimulus presented. Responses may be physiological changes, gross body movements, and/or vocalization.

III. **LOCALIZED RESPONSE**
Patient reacts specifically but inconsistently to stimuli. Responses are directly related to the type of stimulus presented. May follow simple commands such as closing the eyes or squeezing the hand in an inconsistent, delayed manner.

IV. **CONFUSED-AGITATED**
Patient is in a heightened state of activity. Behavior is bizarre and nonpurposeful relative to the immediate environment. Does not discriminate among persons or objects; is unable to cooperate directly with treatment efforts. Verbalizations frequently are incoherent and/or inappropriate to the environment; confabulation may be present. Gross attention to environment is very brief; selective attention is often nonexistent. Patient lacks short and long-term recall.

V. **CONFUSED-INAPPROPRIATE**
Patient is able to respond to simple commands fairly consistently. However, with increased complexity of commands or lack of any external structure, responses are nonpurposeful, random, or fragmented. Demonstrates gross attention to the environment but is highly distractible and lacks the ability to focus attention on a specific task. With structure, may be able to converse on a social automatic level for short periods of time. Verbalization is often inappropriate and confabulatory. Memory is severely impaired; often shows inappropriate use of objects; may perform previously learned tasks with structure, but is unable to learn new information.

VI. **CONFUSED-APPROPRIATE**
Patient shows goal-directed behavior, but is dependent on external input or direction. Follows simple directions consistently and shows carryover for relearned tasks such as self-care. Responses may be incorrect due to memory problems, but they are appropriate to the situation. Past memories show more depth and detail than recent memory.

VII. **AUTOMATIC-APPROPRIATE**
Patient appears appropriate and oriented within the hospital and home settings; goes through daily routine automatically, but frequently robotlike. Patient shows minimal to no confusion and has shallow recall of activities. Shows carryover for new learning, but at a decreased rate. With structure is able to initiate social or recreational activities; judgment remains impaired.

VIII. **PURPOSEFUL-APPROPRIATE**
Patient is able to recall and integrate past and recent events and is aware of and responsive to environment. Shows carryover for new learning and needs no supervision once activities are learned. May continue to show a decreased ability relative to premorbid abilities, abstract reasoning, tolerance for stress, and judgment in emergencies or unusual circumstances.

From Professional Staff Association, Rancho Los Amigos Hospital, p.87-88, with permission.

Intervention

Guidelines for Treatment of Brain Injury

- Emphasis on motivation
- Promote independence
- Therapy should be goal directed, functional, and recreational
- Focus on orientation
- Focus on behavior modification activities
- The use of repetition may be helpful
- Educate patient in compensatory strategies for success
- Structure is essential depending on the level of the patient
- Avoid overstimulation during therapy
- Use of calm voice and simple commands
- Perform activities that are both familiar and enjoyable for the patient
- Family education and support can enhance and assist in the rehabilitation process
- Allow patient to choose activities on occasion
- Flexibility in treatment is needed based on patient's immediate needs and state of mind

Traumatic Brain Injury Profile

Examination

- Past medical history
- History of current condition
- Social history (caregiver support)
- Medications
- Living environment
- Systems review
- Cognitive and language assessment
- Behavioral assessment
- Safety assessment
- Skin assessment
- Postural tone assessment
- Sensation, proprioception, and kinesthesia
- Range of motion
- Motor assessment
- Endurance assessment
- Mobility skills

Intervention

- Cognitive and orientation training
- Therapeutic exercise
- Positioning
- Sensory integration
- Balance and vestibular training
- Range of motion
- Motor function training
- Wheelchair and adaptive equipment prescription
- Splinting and serial casting
- Mobility training

Goals

- Maximize functional mobility
- Maximize community independence
- Maximize strength
- Maximize range of motion and prevent heterotopic ossification
- Maximize static and dynamic balance
- Maximize endurance
- Maximize patient/caregiver competence with:
  --Positioning
  --Use of adaptive equipment and orthotic/splinting devices
  --Home exercise program

A GUIDE TO SUCCESS

Traumatic Brain Injury Medications

Classification:	Examples:
• **Antibiotics** - Respiratory infections, compound fractures, wounds	Penicillin, Amoxicillin, Ampicillin, Keflex, Duricef, Ceclor, Zithromax
• **Antidepressants** - Reduce disruptive or aggressive behavior	Tricyclics- (Elavil, Marplan, Nardil, Pamelor) Ritalin, Paxil, Prozac, Zoloft
• **Antiepileptics** - Prevent or treat seizures	Tegretol, Clonopin, Phenobarbital
• **Antipsychotics (sedatives)** - Control delirium	Thorazine, Mellaril, Vesprin, Navane, Haldol
• **Antispasticity** - Reduce hypertonicity	Baclofen, Dantrium, Diazepam (Valium), Flexeril, Phenol

4 Cardiopulmonary

Cardiac

Examination

Anatomy of the Heart

Right atrium: Receives venous blood from the superior and inferior vena cava.

Right ventricle: Receives venous blood from the right atrium through the tricuspid valve. Pushes blood into the pulmonary artery and pulmonary circulation.

Tricuspid valve: Prevents right ventricular blood from going back into the right atrium.

Pulmonic valve: Prevents blood from returning to the right ventricle.

Left atrium: Receives arterial blood from the pulmonary veins.

Left ventricle: Receives blood from the left atrium. Pushes blood into the aorta and the systemic circulation.

Mitral valve: Prevents left ventricular blood from returning to the left atrium.

Aortic valve: Prevents the systemic blood from returning to the left ventricle.

Aorta: Largest artery which carries the total cardiac output. Divisions include the carotids, subclavians, and descending aorta.

Cardiac Conduction System

Sinoatrial node (SA): The sinoatrial node is located in the right atrium near the superior vena cava and is the primary pacemaker of the heart.

Atrioventricular node (AV): The atrioventricular node or junctional node is located in the inferior wall of the right atrium close to the tricuspid valve.

Bundle of His: The Bundle of His is a group of fibers that initiates at the atrioventricular node, enters the interventricular system, and splits into both the left and right ventricles. These fibers branch into smaller Purkinje fibers.

Purkinje Fibers: Purkinje fibers compose the last part of the electrical conduction system of the heart. The fibers relay the electrical impulses to the muscle cells of the heart.

Korotkoff's Sounds

S1   "lub" mitral and tricuspid valves closing at the onset of systole

S2   "dub" aortic and pulmonic valves closing at the onset of diastole

S3   (ventricular gallop) abnormal in older adults; noncompliant left ventricle; may be associated with congestive heart failure

S4   Pathological sound of vibration of the ventricular wall with ventricular filling and atrial contraction; may be associated with hypertension or stenosis

Cardiac Facts

Cardiac Output = amount of blood pumped out of the heart per minute
= stroke volume x heart rate
= 5 to 6 liters/minute at rest
= up to 25 liters/minute during intense exercise

Stroke Volume = amount of blood ejected by the ventricle during contraction

Blood Volume = total blood volume in an adult is usually 7 – 8% of body weight; blood is pumped through the body at 30 cm/sec with a total circulation time of 20 seconds

Common Circulatory Pulse Locations

Artery	Location
Carotid	Anterior to sternocleidomastoid muscle
Brachial	Medial aspect of arm midway between shoulder and elbow
Radial	At wrist, lateral to flexor carpi radialis tendon
Ulnar	At wrist, between flexor digitorum superficialis and flexor carpi ulnaris tendons

UNIT FOUR: CARDIOPULMONARY

Artery	Location
Femoral	In femoral triangle (sartorius, adductor longus, and inguinal ligament)
Popliteal	Posterior aspect of knee (deep and hard to palpate)
Posterior tibial	Posterior aspect of medial malleolus
Dorsalis pedis	Between first and second metatarsal bones on superior aspect

From Magee, DJ: Orthopedic Physical Assessment. W.B. Saunders Company, Philadelphia 1997, p.40, with permission.

Diagnostic Tests for Cardiac Dysfunction

Procedure	Description
Cardiac catheterization (for angiography)	The coronary arteries are injected with a contrast material, and the arterial system can be visualized with cinefluoroscopy: narrowing or occlusion of arteries can be evaluated.
Cardiac catheterization	Catheterization is used to measure intracardiac, transvalve, and pulmonary artery pressures and measure blood gas pressures to determine cardiac output and evaluate shunting.
Continuous hemodynamic monitoring	Pulmonary artery catheterization (Swan-Ganz) provides immediate cardiopulmonary pressure measurements. An invasive bedside (intensive care unit) procedure that evaluates left ventricular function. A balloon-tipped, flow-directed catheter, connected to a transducer and a monitor, is used to allow measurements of pulmonary artery pressure; pulmonary capillary wedge pressure; cardiac output; and mixed venous saturation, which evaluates pulmonary vascular resistance and tissue oxygenation.
Echocardiography	
a. Transthoracic (TTE)	The reflections of ultrasound waves from cardiac surfaces are analyzed. It is used to evaluate left ventricular systolic function and the structure and function of cardiac walls, valves, and chambers; it can identify abnormal conditions such as tumors or pericardial effusion.
b. Transesophageal (TEE)	Transesophageal echocardiography is performed through the esophagus and stomach by a modified gastroscopy probe with one or two ultrasound transducers at its tip. TEE provides better image resolution and superior images of posterior cardiac structures. Continuous imaging is possible during operations or invasive procedures.
Electrocardiogram (ECG)	Surface electrodes record the electrical activity of the heart. A 12-lead ECG provides 12 views of the heart; it is used to assess cardiac rhythm, to diagnose the location, extent, and acuteness of myocardial ischemia and infarction; and to evaluate changes with activity.
Exercise stress tests	Numerous protocols for exercise tests have been used to assess responses to increased workloads with steps, treadmills, or bicycle ergometers. In conjunction with ECG and blood pressure recordings, patients are evaluated for exercise capacity, cardiac dysrhythmias, and diagnosis, prognosis, and management of coronary artery disease.
Hemodynamic monitoring	See *Continuous hemodynamic monitoring*
Holter monitoring	Continuous ambulatory ECG monitoring done by tape recording the cardiac rhythm for up to 24 hours. It is used to evaluate cardiac rhythm, efficacy of medications, transient symptoms that may indicate cardiac disease, and pacemaker function; and to correlate symptoms with activity.
Pharmacologic stress tests	A noninvasive assessment for patients with coronary disease who are unable to achieve adequate cardiac stress with exercise.
a. Dipyridamole thallium	This potent vasodilator markedly enhances blood flow to normally perfused myocardium, whereas myocardium fed by stenotic coronary arteries demonstrates relative hypoperfusion and diminished thallium activity.

Procedure	Description
b. Dobutamine echocardiography	An incremental infusion is given causing an increase in the myocardial oxygen demand. Simultaneous evaluation of wall motion abnormalities, ECG, and BP are performed.
Phonocardiography	This test records cardiac sounds. It is used to time the events of the cardiac cycle and to confirm auscultatory findings.
Radionuclide angiography	Red blood cells tagged (marked) with a radionuclide are injected into blood. Ventricular wall motion can be evaluated and the ejection fraction determined; abnormal blood flow with valve and congenital defects can be detected. Techniques include gated-pool equilibrium studies and first-pass techniques.
Technetium-99m scanning (hot spot imaging)	Technetium-99m injected into blood is taken up by damaged myocardial tissue; this identifies and localizes acute myocardial infarctions.
Thallium-201 myocardial perfusion imaging (cold spot imaging)	Thallium-201 injected into blood at peak exercise; scanning identifies ischemic and infarcted myocardium, which does not take up thallium-201. It is used to diagnose coronary artery disease and perfusion, particularly when ECG is equivocal.

From Rothstein J, Roy S, Wolf S: The Rehabilitation Specialist's Handbook. F. A. Davis Company Inc, Philadelphia 1998, p.624-626, with permission.

Electrocardiogram

ECG: Measures the electrical activity of the heart

P wave: Atrial depolarization

PR interval: Time required for conduction from the SA node to the AV node. This is normally .12 to .2 seconds.

QRS complex: Ventricular depolarization.

QT interval: Electrical systole that is measured by the time elapsed from the start of the Q wave to the end of the T wave. This is normally .32 to .40 seconds.

ST segment: Delay before repolarization of the ventricles; useful in assessing myocardial ischemia

T wave: Ventricular repolarization

Pathological Changes in an ECG Denoting Disease

Q Wave: Previous myocardial infarction

ST Segment Elevation: Acute myocardial infarction

Elevated QRS: Hypertrophy of the myocardium

Depressed QRS: Heart failure, ischemia, pericardial effusion, obesity, chronic obstructive pulmonary disease

PAC: Premature atrial contractions occur when an ectopic focus in the atrium fires and supersedes the SA node. The P wave is premature with abnormal configuration. This can be indicative of ischemia or valve pathology.

PVC: Premature ventricular contractions occur when an ectopic focus in the ventricles or Purkinje fibers fires and supersedes normal conduction. The P wave is absent, the ST segment is distorted, and the QRS complex occurs early. PVCs are the most common cardiac arrhythmia. PVCs may be benign, but can also be indicative of cardiac pathology.

Comparisons of Right and Left-Sided Heart Failure

Right	Left

Elevated end-diastolic right ventricular pressure
Systemic congestion:
  -Enlarged liver
  -Ascites
  -Jugular venous distention
  -Dependent (pitting) edema
 	
Fatigue
Oliguria, nocturia
Cyanosis (capillary stasis)
Pleural effusion (R>L)
Anorexia and bleeding
Unexplained weight gain
Etiology:
  -Mitral stenosis
  -Pulmonary parenchymal or vascular disease
  -Pulmonic or tricuspid valvular disease
  -Infective endocarditis
	Elevated end-diastolic left ventricular pressure
	Pulmonary congestion:
	  -Pulmonary edema
	  -Dyspnea, orthopnea
	  -Paroxysmal nocturnal dyspnea
	  -Cough
	  -Bronchospasm
	  -(Cardiac asthma)
	Fatigue
	Oliguria
	Cyanosis (central)
	Tachycardia
	
	Etiology:
	  -Hypertension
	  -Coronary artery disease
	  -Aortic valve disease
	  -Cardiomyopathies
	  -Congenital heart defects
	  -Infective endocarditis
	  -High-output conditions
	  -Various connective tissue disorders

From Rothstein J, Roy S, Wolf S: The Rehabilitation Specialist's Handbook. F. A. Davis Company, Philadelphia 1998, p.654-655, with permission.

Vital Signs

Blood Pressure
- Wrap the cuff above the antecubital area
- Wrap the cuff snugly, false reading if loose
- Ensure proper size cuff for obese patients and children
- Place arrow on cuff over brachial artery
- Palpate the brachial pulse and position the stethoscope
- Inflate the cuff to 20 mm Hg above the point where the pulse disappears
- Slowly deflate the cuff observing the needle gauge
- The first Korotkoff's sound indicates the patient's systolic pressure
- The diastolic pressure reading is noted when the sound disappears

Blood Pressure Standard Values:
Systolic = 120 mm Hg
Diastolic = 80 mm Hg
Hypertension is considered to be 140/90 mm Hg or greater

Heart Rate
- Find the patient's radial pulse
- Use your index and middle fingers to measure heart rate
- Assess and document the rhythm of the heart beat as regular or irregular
- Count the heart rate for 60 seconds
- Assess and document the strength or amplitude of the pulse as strong, medium or weak

Normal heart rate = 60 – 100 beats per minute
Maximal heart rate = 220 – age

Bradycardia: refers to a heart rate below 60 beats per minute.

Tachycardia: refers to a heart rate above 100 beats per minute.

Respiratory Rate
- Observe the patient breathing at rest for 60 seconds
- Determine the number of breaths per minute by observing the patient's chest rise and fall
- Assess and document depth of respiration, even or uneven rhythm, and symmetry of the chest
- Assess and document any accessory muscle use

Normal respirations = 14 – 20 breaths per minute

Borg's Rate of Perceived Exertion Scale and the Revised 10-Grade Scale

RPE:		10-Grade Rating Scale:	
6		0	Nothing at all
7	Very, very light	0.5	Very, very weak (just noticeable)
8		1.0	Very weak
9	Very light	2.0	Weak (light)
10		3.0	Moderate
11	Fairly light	4.0	Somewhat strong
12		5.0	Strong (heavy)
13	Somewhat hard	6.0	
14		7.0	Very strong
15	Hard	8.0	
16		9.0	
17	Very hard	10.0	Very, very strong (almost maximum)
18			Maximal
19	Very, very hard		

From Borg GAV: Psychophysical Bases of Perceived Exertion. Med Sci Sports Exerc 14:377, 1982, American College of Sports Medicine, with permission.

Metabolic Equivalents (METS)

A MET is the amount of oxygen consumed per kilogram of body weight per minute to perform a given activity. At rest a person consumes 3.5 ml/kg/minute. The following list identifies METS associated with common activities of daily living.

Activity	METS
Eating	1
Toileting	1 – 2
Driving a car	1 – 2
Dressing	2
Walking (2 mph)	2 – 2.5
Bathing	2 – 3
Cooking	2 – 3
Light housework	2 – 4
Light gardening	3 – 4
Showering	3.5 – 4
Sexual intercourse	4 – 5
Dancing	4 – 5
Walking (4 mph)	4.5 – 5.5
Swimming	4 – 8
Shoveling snow	6 – 7
Mowing the lawn	6 – 7

Risk Factors for Cardiac Pathology

Modifiable Factors
- Cholesterol – more than 200 mg/dl
- Hypertension
- Smoking
- Atherogenic diet
- Culture
- Physical inactivity

Non-Modifiable Factors:
- Age – risk increases with age
- Sex – male > female (after menopause female equal to male)
- Family history
- Culture

Secondary Factors:
- Alcohol consumption
- Obesity
- Coping with stress
- Diabetes mellitus
- Peripheral vascular disease

Symptoms of Cardiac Pathology

- Chest pain
- Shortness of breath
- Cardiac arrhythmia (palpitation)
- Fainting
- Claudication
- Cyanosis of lips and nailbeds
- Fatigue
- Edema

Symptoms of Myocardial Infarction

- Severe chest pain
- Chest heaviness
- Radiating pain down one or both arms
- Weakness
- Nausea
- Vomiting
- Diaphoresis
- Shortness of breath

Diagnosis of Myocardial Infarction

- Abnormal ECG
- Elevation in enzyme level
  -- Creatine phosphokinase (CPK)
  -- Aspartate aminotransferase (AST)
  -- Lactate dehydrogenase

Intervention

Methods to Determine Exercise Intensity

Target Heart Rate Formula
Target heart rate formula is a method for obtaining an appropriate demand on the heart during exercise. The age adjusted maximum heart rate is determined by subtracting the patient's age from 220. The training heart rate is determined by multiplying the age adjusted maximum heart rate by the appropriate percentage of intensity that the patient should maintain during exercise. Normal training intensity ranges from 60% - 90% of the age adjusted maximum heart rate. A patient with cardiac pathology must have exercise intensity determined from the results of a stress test.

Karvonen's Formula – Heart Rate Reserve Method
The Karvonen formula is a method to obtain an appropriate range for training heart rate. The maximum heart rate is obtained by an exercise stress test (or the age adjusted maximum heart rate) and the resting heart rate is subtracted from it. This number is termed the heart rate reserve. The heart rate reserve is multiplied by both ends of the prescribed range (e.g. HR reserve x 60% and HR reserve x 80%). The resting heart rate is then added to each of the two numbers to identify the upper and lower limits of the prescribed target heart rate.

Cardiac Rehabilitation

Indications for Cardiac Rehabilitation

Patients that are medically stable after:
- Myocardial infarction
- Angina
- Coronary artery bypass graft surgery
- Compensated heart failure
- Cardiac surgery
- Heart transplant
- Peripheral vascular disease

Description of a Cardiac Rehabilitation Program

Phase I
A Phase I program begins with the physician referral to the cardiac rehabilitation program. Patients are referred to the inpatient program when they are medically stable. Phase I consists of patient and family education, self-care evaluation, continuous monitoring of vital signs, group discussions, and low level of exercise. Exercise activities include active range of motion, ambulation, and self-care. Exercise intensity is often prescribed according to heart rate and by rating on a perceived exertion scale. A Phase I program typically

concludes with a low-level exercise test, although this activity may not be appropriate for high-risk clients. The trend toward early hospital discharge following a cardiac event has resulted in Phase I programs averaging 3-5 days.

Phase II
A Phase II program begins immediately after hospitalization and lasts from 2-12 weeks depending on the patient's ability to tolerate the exercise training. Patients are monitored closely during the Phase II program and are supervised during all activities. Goals for a Phase II program include increasing functional capacity through exercise, educating the patient on risk factor modification, and developing independence in self-monitoring. Frequency of visits in a Phase II program average 2-3 times a week. Patients typically progress to a Phase III program when they are clinically stable, independent with self-monitoring techniques, and do not require ECG monitoring.

Phase III
A Phase III program is often viewed as a continuation of a Phase II program and lasts approximately 6-8 weeks. Exercise training, physical fitness, level of endurance, and risk factor modification are the primary emphasis of the program. Phase III programs often include exercise, education, and counseling. A maximal symptom limited exercise test is required to assess fitness level and appropriately plan for exercise intensity. The average frequency of the program is once per week.

Phase IV
A Phase IV program lasts throughout the patient's lifetime and is designed to promote optimal health. Requirements for participation in a Phase IV program include independence with self-monitoring of exercise, stable cardiac status, no contraindications to exercise, and at least a 5 MET capacity for activities.

Therapist Role During Inpatient Cardiac Rehabilitation

- Provide constant monitoring of heart rate, blood pressure, and ECG interpretation before, during, and after each session
- Develop program within the guidelines of the patient's prescribed training heart rate
- Use of exertion scales to identify subjective intensity of exercise
- Promote proper technique and breathing patterns during exercise
- Progress activities based on METs tolerated

Therapist Role During Outpatient Cardiac Rehabilitation

- Initially close monitoring of ECG, heart rate, and blood pressure throughout session
- Constant measurement of vital signs should decrease and self-monitoring of heart rate and perceived exertion by the patient should guide exercise sessions
- Development of an exercise program should be based on a symptom limited treadmill test and determined target heart rate
- Exercise should be gradual in progression; the session should generally include warm-up for 5-10 minutes, aerobic activity for 20-60 minutes, and a cool down for 5-10 minutes
- Warm-up should include stretching as well as low intensity activity which will slowly increase heart rate
- Exercise may include walking, stationary bicycling, as well as isotonic strengthening (low resistance)
- Isometrics are contraindicated

Cardiopulmonary Resuscitation Standards

CPR – Adult (eight years +)

Breathing:	Two initial breaths followed by 12/minute
Compressions:	100/minute
Depth of compressions:	1 ½ to 2 inches
Placement for chest compressions:	Lower half of sternum
One-rescuer ratio of compressions to ventilations:	15:2
Two-rescuer ratio of compressions to ventilations:	15:2

CPR – Child (one to eight years old)

Breathing:	Two initial breaths followed by 20/minute
Compressions:	100/minute
Depth of compressions:	1/3-1/2 the depth of the chest
Placement for chest compressions:	Lower half of sternum
One-rescuer ratio of compressions to ventilations:	5:1
Two-rescuer ratio of compressions to ventilations:	5:1

CPR – Infant (less than one year old)

Breathing:	Two initial breaths mouth to mouth/nose followed by 20/minute
Compressions:	Minimum of 100/minute
Depth of compressions:	1/3-1/2 the depth of the chest
Placement for chest compressions:	Lower half of sternum
One-rescuer ratio of compressions to ventilations:	5:1
Two-rescuer ratio of compressions to ventilations:	5:1

From American Red Cross: BLS Health Care Providers. American Red Cross, 2001

Cardiac Profile

Examination

- Past medical history
- History of current condition
  --Cardiac testing
- Social history (caregiver support)
- Medications
- Living environment
- Risk factors profile
- Systems review
  --Vital signs
  --Auscultation of heart and lung sounds
- Skin assessment
  --Cyanosis
  --Edema
  --Pallor
  --Diaphoresis
- Cognitive assessment
- Pain
- Strength as tolerated
- Endurance
- Mobility skills as tolerated

Intervention

- Patient/caregiver teaching:
  --Risk factor modification
  --Signs and symptoms of pathology
  --Measurement of vital signs
  --Nutrition
- Breathing exercises
- Endurance/exercise training
- Mobility training
- Relaxation techniques

Inpatient Goals

- Maximize self-care skills
- Maximize functional mobility skills
- Maximize endurance
- Maximize patient/caregiver competence with:
  --Safe activity guidelines
  --Modification of risk factors
  --Monitoring of vital signs
  --Breathing exercises
  --Stress management
- Perform low-level exercise test (4-6 METS)
- Maximize energy conservation techniques

Outpatient Goals

- Maximize functional mobility skills
- Maximize endurance
- Maximize aerobic capacity
- Maximize patient/caregiver competence with:
  --Nutritional education
  --Monitoring of vital signs
  --Energy conservation techniques
  --Warning signs of cardiac pathology
  --Home exercise program

Cardiac Pathology

Aneurysm
An aneurysm is a weakening in the wall of a vessel that produces a sac-like area. This can occur from trauma, congenital pathology, atherosclerosis or infection. If an aneurysm ruptures it is a medical emergency.

Angina Pectoris
A transient process that occurs when the coronary arteries are unable to supply the heart with adequate oxygen. Sudden onset is common and primary symptoms include chest pain, chest tightness, and shortness of breath. The four types of angina pectoris are as follows:
- **Nocturnal:** Angina that will wake someone up from his or her sleep with the same characteristics as angina from exertion. This may be related to congestive heart failure.
- **Prinzmetal's:** Angina that occurs while at rest secondary to coronary artery disease or spasm.
- **Stable:** Angina that usually occurs at a predictable level of exertion, exercise or stress and responds to rest or Nitroglycerin.
- **Unstable:** Angina that can occur at rest or with exertion and has changed intensity, frequency, and/or duration.

Atherosclerosis
Progressive accumulation of fatty plaques on the inner walls of vessels that ultimately produces stenosis. This process begins in childhood and usually effects medium sized arteries. Over time the plaque that produces stenosis inside the vessel can also block blood flow. Heart attack or stroke can result from atherosclerosis.

Congestive Heart Failure (CHF)
Congestive heart failure is a condition that usually results from coronary artery disease when the heart is unable to maintain an adequate cardiac output. CHF is characterized by abnormal retention of fluid and results in diminished blood flow to the tissue and congestion of the pulmonary and/or systemic circulation. This is not a disease, but rather a symptom of pathology within the heart muscle itself or the cardiac valves.

Coronary Artery Disease (CAD)
Coronary artery disease is the narrowing or blockage of the coronary arteries that may produce ischemia and necrosis of the myocardium. There is an inability for vasodilation and as a result the arteries cannot meet the metabolic demands. This will produce ischemia and ultimately necrosis. CAD includes thrombus, vasospasms, and atherosclerosis. CAD results from inheritance, environment, culture, nutrition, and smoking.

Endocarditis
Bacterial endocarditis causes inflammation of the endothelium that lines the inner cavity of the heart and can damage the cardiac valves. This can often occur after a person has an invasive medical or dental procedure.

Myocardial Infarction (MI)
A myocardial infarction causes irreversible damage to a segment of heart muscle due to prolonged ischemia. The causative factors include narrowing of coronary arteries due to atherosclerotic occlusion, poor coronary perfusion secondary to hemorrhage or occlusion of one of the major coronary arteries.

Pericarditis
Pericarditis refers to an inflammation of the pericardium. The pericardium is the outer layer of the heart. This condition may be acute or chronic and can be painful or asymptomatic.

Cardiac Medications

There are multiple medications that are administered for various cardiac conditions. General classifications of drugs with example medications are listed. The list is designed to serve as a general overview of major cardiac medications.

Antiarrhythmics
A group of drugs that assist in altering conductivity in order to correct any ectopic stimuli or other electrical abnormalities.
- Quinidine sulfate
- Procainamide
- Lidocaine
- Inderal (beta blocker)
- Verapamil (calcium channel blocker)

Beta Blockers
A group of drugs used in the treatment of angina, hypertension, and arrhythmias. These drugs decrease the heart's oxygen demand by decreasing the heart rate and contractility. Beta blockers attempt to maintain a balance of oxygen supply and demand.
- Tenormin
- Lopressor
- Visken
- Sectral

Calcium Channel Blockers
A group of drugs used in the treatment of hypertension, angina, and arrhythmias. These drugs decrease the heart's oxygen demand by reducing the flow of calcium which is necessary for myocardial contractility. The medication allows for peripheral vasodilation that further reduces demand on the heart. There is decreased contractility, vasomotor tone, and heart rate which allow for a balance in oxygen demand and supply.
- Verapamil - arrhythmias
- Procardia - angina, hypertension
- Cardizem - angina, hypertension

Cardiac Glycosides
A group of drugs used in the treatment of congestive heart failure. Cardiac glycosides increase the amount of calcium in the myocardium which allows for increased contractility and improved cardiac output. They also have a direct effect on improving the efficiency of the electrical activity of the heart. This results in an increase in oxygen throughout the body and a decrease in overall blood volume.
- Digoxin/Lanoxin

Diuretics
A group of drugs used in the treatment of hypertension and congestive heart failure. These drugs directly affect the kidneys and produce an increase in water and sodium excretion. Diuretics are often used in combination with other cardiac medications.
- Diuril, Metahydrin - thiazide diuretic
- Bumex, Lasix - loop diuretic
- Midamor, Aldactone - potassium sparing diuretic

Pulmonary Examination

Pulmonary Function Testing

Expiratory reserve volume (ERV): Maximal volume expired after normal expiration.

Forced expiratory volume (FEV): The amount of air exhaled in the 1st, 2nd, and 3rd second of a forced vital capacity test.

Forced vital capacity (FVC): The amount of air forcefully expired after a maximal inspiration.

Functional residual capacity (FRC): Volume in lungs after normal exhalation.

Inspiratory capacity (IC): The amount of air that can be inspired after a normal exhalation.

Inspiratory reserve volume (IRV): Maximal volume inspired after normal inspiration.

Minute volume (MV): The amount of air expired in one minute.

Residual volume (RV): Lung volume remaining in the lungs at the end of a maximal expiration.

Tidal volume (TV): Total volume inspired and expired per breath.

Total lung capacity (TLC): Lung volume measured at the end of a maximal inspiration.

Vital capacity (VC): Maximal volume forcefully expired after a maximal inspiration.

Pulmonary Function Reference Values

Values are calculated for an individual patient based on variables such as height, weight, sex, and age. A value is usually considered abnormal if it is less than 80% of the reference value.

TV:	5-7 mg/kg of body weight
ERV:	25% of VC
IC:	75% of VC
FEV1:	83% of VC (after one second)
FEV2:	94% of VC (after two seconds)
FEV3:	97% of VC (after three seconds)

Gas Pressure (mm Hg)

Gas	Dry Air	Moist Tracheal Air	Alveolar Gas	Arterial Blood	Mixed Venous Blood
PO_2	159.1	149.2	104.0	100.0	40.0
PCO_2	0.3	0.3	40.0	40.0	46.0
PH_2O	0.0	47.0	47.0	47.0	47.0
PN_2	600.6	563.5	569.0	573.0	573.0
P_{TOTAL}	760.0	760.0	760.0	760.0	760.0

From Rothstein, JM: Rehabilitation Specialist's Handbook. F.A. Davis Company, Philadelphia 1998, p.528, with permission.

Arterial Blood Gases

The study of blood gases is used as a tool to determine the effectiveness of alveolar ventilation. Values are expressed as the partial pressure of the gas. PaO_2, the partial pressure of oxygen within the arterial system, is normally 95 – 100 mm Hg. Supplemental oxygen is usually required for oxygen saturation rates less than 90%. The body cannot carry out vital functions with oxygen saturation less than 70%. $PaCO_2$, the partial pressure of carbon dioxide within the arterial system, is normally 35 – 45 mm Hg. The range for the acid base balance or pH is 7.35 – 7.45. Changes in the $PaCO_2$ directly affect the balance of pH in the body. Prolonged imbalance of the pH in either direction can affect the nervous system and in some cases cause convulsions or coma.

Hypercapnia: an increased amount of CO_2 in the blood.

Hyperkalemia: an increased amount of potassium in the blood.

Hypocapnia: a decreased amount of CO_2 in the blood.

Hypoxemia: when the PaO_2 is less than 80 mm Hg.

Physical Signs Observed in Various Disorders

Condition	Breath Sounds	Adventitious Sounds	Voice Sounds	Inspection	Tactile Fremitus	Percussion
Normal	Nl	None	Muffled, distant, indistinct	Trachea midline, symmetric chest expansion	Nl	Nl
Asthma, acute moderately severe attack	↓, Bronchial, prolonged expiration	Inspiratory plus expiratory wheezes	→	↑ Use of accessory muscles, tachypnea	→	Nl-↑
Atelectasis	↓ Or 0	Crackles	↓ Or 0	Trachea deviated to affected side	→	↓-↓↓
Bronchiectasis	Nl	Crackles	Nl	↓ Expansion AS, tachypnea, clubbing	↑ Rhonchal fremitus	Nl
Bronchitis	Nl, possible prolonged expiration	Crackles, wheezes	Nl	Possible ↓ motion, occasional use of accessory muscles	↓ Bilaterally	↑ Bilaterally
COPD	↓-↓↓, prolonged expiration	None versus crackles and wheezes	↓ Or 0 bilaterally	Barrel-shaped chest, moves as a unit, ↑ use of accessory muscles	↓ Bilaterally	↑ Bilaterally
Consolidation	Bronchial	Crackles	Whispered pectoriloquy	↓ Motion AS	↑	→
Fibrosis • Localized	→	Crackles	→	↓ Motion over area	↓ Or 0	→
• Generalized	→	Crackles	→	↓ Motion bilaterally	↓ Or 0	→
Heart failure	Nl	Dependent crackles	Nl	Nl chest expansion, tachypnea	Nl	Nl
Pleural effusion (moderate to large)	↓ Or 0,* bronchial**	Possible pleural rub	↓*↑**	↓ Motion AS, ↑ RR, trachea deviated to OS	↓ Or 0	↓-↓↓
Pneumothorax (>15%)	↓ Or 0	None	↓ Or 0	↓ Motion AS	↓ Or 0	↑

Nl = normal, ↓ = decreased, ↓↓ = very decreased, ↑ = increased, 0 = absent, AS = on affected side, COPD = chronic obstructive pulmonary disease, RR = respiratory rate, OS = opposite side; *Over the effusion; **Above the fluid.

From Watchie, J: Cardiopulmonary Physical Therapy: A Clinical Manual. W.B. Saunders Company, Philadelphia 1995, p.193, with permission.

Interpretation of Abnormal Acid-Base Balance

Type	pH	PaCO$_2$	HCO$_3$	Causes	Signs and Symptoms
Respiratory alkalosis	↑	↓	WNL	Alveolar hyperventilation	Dizziness, syncope, tingling, numbness, early tetany
Respiratory acidosis	↓	↑	WNL	Alveolar hypoventilation	Early: anxiety, restlessness, dyspnea, headache; late: confusion, somnolence, coma
Metabolic alkalosis	↑	WNL	↑	Bicarbonate ingestion, vomiting, diuretics, steroids, adrenal disease	Vague symptoms: weakness, mental dullness, possibly early tetany
Metabolic acidosis	↓	WNL	↓	Diabetic, lactic, or uremic acidosis, prolonged diarrhea	Secondary hyperventilation (Kussmaul's breathing), nausea and vomiting, cardiac dysrhythmias, lethargy, and coma

From Rothstein, JM: Rehabilitation Specialist's Handbook. F.A. Davis Company, Philadelphia 1998, p.529, with permission.

Intervention

Indications for Chest Physical Therapy

- Patients who have acute or chronic respiratory problems
- The inability to expel pulmonary secretions
- An ineffective cough
- Patients with increased secretions
- Patients with pneumonia
- Patients with atelectasis
- Patients with neurological impairments that cause swallowing difficulties

Contraindications for Chest Physical Therapy

- Recent acute myocardial infarction
- Untreated pneumothorax
- Unstable cardiovascular condition
- Unstable neurological condition
- Rib fracture
- Severe osteoporosis
- Pulmonary embolus
- Bone cancer
- Skin grafts

Guidelines for Chest Physical Therapy

- Treatment should be administered prior to eating or at least one hour after meals.
- Percuss and vibrate over each segment to be treated for at least 3-5 minutes.
- Cough after each segment is treated.
- Allow for a rest period after each segment is treated.
- Review breathing exercises in each drainage position.

Goals for Chest Physical Therapy

- Mobilize secretions
- Expel secretions
- Improve breathing patterns
- Improve ventilation throughout all lobes
- Improve overall function

Bronchial Drainage

Upper Lobes
- **Apical Segment: Left and Right Anterior**
  Sitting: Lean back against a pillow; clap above the clavicles between the neck and shoulder.

- **Apical Segment: Left and Right Posterior**
  Sitting: Lean forward onto a pillow; clap on both sides of the back above the scapula. Fingers should be positioned slightly over the shoulder.

- **Anterior Segment: Left and Right**
  Supine: Lie flat on back with pillow under knees for comfort; clap on both sides just below the clavicles and above the nipple line.

- **Left Posterior Segment**
  Side: Lie on right side with head and shoulders elevated on pillows. Make 1/4 turn forward; clap over the left scapula.

- **Right Posterior Segment**
  Side: Lie on left side. Place a pillow in front from the shoulders to the hips and roll slightly forward onto it; clap over the right scapula.

- **Left Lingula**
  Side: Elevate bottom of bed 14-16 inches. Lie on right side. Place pillow behind from the shoulders to the hips and roll slightly back onto it; clap over left nipple.

Middle Lobe
- **Right Middle Lobe**
  Side: Elevate bottom of bed 14-16 inches. Lie on left side. Place pillow behind from the shoulders to the hips and roll slightly back onto it; clap over selected lobe.

Lower Lobes
- **Superior Segments: Left and Right**
  Prone: Lie flat on stomach; place pillow under the stomach area for added comfort and clap over the middle back at the tip of the scapula.

- **Lateral Basal Segment: Left and Right**
  Side: Elevate bottom of bed 20 inches. Lie on opposing side; clap at lower ribs. A pillow under the waist may help to keep the spine straight.

- **Anterior Basal Segment: Left and Right**
  Supine: Elevate bottom of bed 18-20 inches. Lie on back and place a pillow under the knees; clap at the lower ribs on both sides.

- **Posterior Basal Segment: Left and Right**
  Prone: Elevate bottom of bed 18-20 inches. Lie on stomach and place pillow under the hips; clap at the lower ribs on both sides.

Breathing Exercises

Diaphragmatic breathing:
Diaphragmatic breathing attempts to enhance movement of the diaphragm upon inspiration and expiration and diminish accessory muscle use.
- Position the patient in bed with head and trunk elevated 45 degrees.
- Place dominant hand over the rectus abdominus muscles.
- Place nondominant hand over the sternum.
- Direct the patient to inspire slowly and feel the dominant hand rise.
- Instruct the patient to control both inspiration and expiration.
- The nondominant hand should have only minimal movement.

Incentive spirometry:
Incentive spirometry is used to increase inspiration using a device that provides immediate feedback to the patient regarding performance. This type of intervention is commonly utilized to treat patients status post surgery in order to strengthen weak inspiratory muscles and to prevent alveolar collapse.
- Position the patient in a comfortable setting.
- Instruct the patient to breathe into the spirometer.
- Instruct the patient to perform a maximal exhalation into the spirometer.
- Repeat 7 to 10 times per session and repeat the session 3 – 4 times per day.
- Increase volume expectations on regular intervals until the patient is within normal range.

Low frequency breathing:
Low frequency breathing is slow deep breathing designed to improve alveolar ventilation and oxygenation.
- Instruct the patient to breathe slowly, taking long and deep breaths.
- Ensure that the patient is not at risk for hyperventilation.

Pursed lip breathing:
Pursed lip breathing attempts to improve ventilation by decreasing the respiratory rate and increasing the tidal volume. This technique assists with shortness of breath that is commonly encountered in patients with COPD.
- Position the patient in a comfortable setting.
- Instruct the patient to avoid using the abdominal muscles.
- Instruct the patient to place a hand over the abdominal muscles while breathing.
- Slowly inhale.
- Relax and loosely purse lips during exhalation.
- Expiration should be twice as long as inspiration.

Segmental breathing:
Segmental breathing is used to prevent accumulation of fluid and to increase chest mobility by directing inspired air to predetermined areas.
- Position the patient in a comfortable setting based on the targeted lung segment.
- Place hands on target area and apply pressure downward and inward during exhalation.
- Apply a quick stretch immediately before inspiration.
- Instruct the patient to slowly inspire air into the target lung area under your hands. Give mild resistance during inspiration.
- Observe accessory muscles during exercise in order to limit their use.

Pulmonary Profile

Examination

- Past medical history
- History of current condition
  - --Pulmonary function testing
  - --Arterial blood gases
- Social history (caregiver support)
- Medications
- Living environment
- Systems review
  - --Pulse oximetry
  - --Auscultation of the lungs
  - --Vital signs
  - --Cough
- Observation of breathing/use of accessory muscles
- Postural assessment
- Cognitive assessment
- Pain
- Strength
- Endurance
- Mobility skills

Intervention

- Breathing exercises
- Coughing techniques
- Postural drainage, chest physical therapy
- Endurance/exercise training
- Relaxation techniques
- Patient/caregiver teaching:
  - --Energy conservation
  - --Breathing techniques
  - --Coughing techniques
  - --Stress management
  - --Measurement of vital signs
- Mobility training

Goals

- Maximize independence in secretion clearance
- Maximize self-care skills
- Maximize functional mobility skills
- Maximize aerobic capacity
- Maximize independence with performing and monitoring home exercise program
- Maximize patient/caregiver competence with:
  - --Energy conservation techniques
  - --Breathing techniques
  - --Stress management techniques

Pulmonary Pathology

Asthma
Asthma is an irreversible, obstructive lung condition characterized by increased responsiveness of the trachea and bronchi to stimuli, inflammation, and overproduction of mucous glands with widespread narrowing of the airways. Asthma attacks may be mild or life threatening. Clinical symptoms include increased respiration rate, prolonged expiration time with wheezing, increased use of accessory muscles, episodes of dyspnea, and a nonproductive cough. Immediate medical intervention and the use of bronchodilators may be warranted.

Chronic Bronchitis
Chronic bronchitis is characterized by increased mucus secretions from the bronchioles and structural changes to the bronchi. A productive cough is usually present for three months during two consecutive years. The major impairments include hypertrophy of the mucus secreting gland and insufficient oxygenation of the alveoli due to mucus blockage. Clinical symptoms include increased pulmonary artery pressure, thick sputum, increased use of accessory muscles, persistent cough, wheezing, dyspnea, and cyanosis. Patients with chronic bronchitis are often called "blue bloaters".

Chronic Obstructive Pulmonary Disease (COPD)
Chronic obstructive pulmonary disease is characterized by increased resistance to the passage of air in and out of the lungs due to narrowing of the bronchial tree. COPD symptoms include dyspnea, chronic productive cough, and excessive mucus production. Progression of the disease includes alveolar destruction and subsequent increases in the amount of air that remains in the lungs. Patients with COPD have an overall increased total lung capacity with a significant increase in residual volume. The disease is diagnosed by determining the amount of air forcibly expired from the lungs in one second. Chronic obstructive pulmonary disease includes bronchitis, emphysema, asthma, and bronchiectasis.

Cor Pulmonale
Cor pulmonale is considered to be a medical emergency. There is a sudden dilatation of the right ventricle of the heart secondary to a pulmonary embolus. Right-sided heart failure will occur if the condition is not treated. As the condition progresses symptoms resemble congestive heart failure. Clinical symptoms include chronic cough, chest pain, distal swelling (bilateral), dyspnea, fatigue, and weakness.

Emphysema
Emphysema is a condition that develops from a long history of chronic bronchitis. The alveolar walls present with significant pathology and the air spaces are permanently overinflated. Expiration is difficult and dead space increases within the lungs. Emphysema is categorized as centrilobular, panlobular or paraseptal. Clinical symptoms include dyspnea, chronic cough, orthopnea, barrel chest, increased use of accessory muscles, and increased respiration rate.

Restrictive Pulmonary Disease
Restrictive pulmonary disease is characterized by the lungs' failure to fully expand due to a weakened diaphragm, structural inability of the chest wall to expand, and a decrease in the elasticity of lung tissue. Clinical symptoms include shortness of breath, a persistent nonproductive cough, and increased respiratory rate. There may be chronic inflammation of the alveoli or plaques that develop and result in progressive fibrosis and a decreased lung capacity. Restrictive pulmonary disease results in a decrease in all lung volumes. Restrictive pulmonary diseases include scoliosis, atelectasis, pneumonia, and adult respiratory distress syndrome.

Tuberculosis (TB)
Tuberculosis is a bacterial infection that is transmitted in an airborne fashion (coughing, sneezing, and speaking). The lungs are primarily involved, however TB can occur in kidneys, lymph nodes, and meninges. Lesions in the lungs can be seen with x-ray. Clinical symptoms include fatigue, weight loss, loss of appetite, low-grade fever, productive cough, chest discomfort, and dyspnea. Treatment includes anti-tuberculosis drug therapy. Prevention of TB through immunization is recommended for children.

Pulmonary Medications

Bronchodilators
Medication used to increase the size of the airway and reduce resistance and subsequent obstruction. Bronchodilators promote relaxation of smooth muscle and in some cases increase respiratory strength, increase mucus transport, and decrease overall pressure.

There are three primary families of bronchodilators:
- **Anticholinergic:** Atropine, Atrovent
- **Beta-adrenergic:** Albuterol, Ephedrine, Serevent
- **Xanthine:** Theophylline, Caffeine

Corticosteroids
Medication used to control inflammation in the airway passages and subsequently decrease bronchospasm. Corticosteroids are best delivered in inhaled or nebulized forms.
- Vanceril
- Decadron
- Prednisolone

Cromolyn Sodium
Medication used to prevent bronchospasm. Cromolyn sodium stabilizes the bronchial mast cells so there is no release of histamine. Prophylactic use attempts to prevent inflammatory symptoms, however it is ineffective if used during a bronchospasm attack.

Mucolytics and Expectorants
Mucolytics are medications used to thin mucus secretions by altering the composition of the mucus and its consistency.
- N-acetylcysteine/Mucomyst
- RhDNase

Expectorants increase removal of mucus by increasing mucin (which assists the movement of mucus by the cilia) for transport out of the lungs.
- Guaifenesin/Robitussin
- Iodinated glycerol/organidin
- Terpin hydrate

5 Integumentary

Integumentary System

The integumentary system consists of the dermal and epidermal layers of skin, hair follicles, nails, sebaceous glands, and sweat glands.

Key Functions of the Integumentary System

- Excretion of sweat
- Protection
- Sensation
- Thermoregulation
- Vitamin D synthesis

Burns

Examination

Types of Burns

Thermal burn: Caused by conduction or convection. Examples include hot liquid, fire or steam.

Electrical burn: Caused by the passage of electrical current through the body. Typically there is an entrance and an exit wound. Complications can include cardiac arrhythmias, respiratory arrest, renal failure, neurological damage, and fractures. Lightning is an example of an electrical burn.

Chemical burn: Occurs when certain chemical compounds come in contact with the body. The reaction will continue until the chemical compound is diluted from the site. Compounds that cause chemical burns include sulfuric acid, lye, hydroflouric acid, and gasoline.

Burn Classification

The extent and severity of a burn is dependent on gender, age, duration of burn, type of burn, and affected area. Burns are most appropriately classified according to the depth of tissue destruction.

Superficial Burn: A superficial burn involves only the outer epidermis. The involved area may be red with slight edema. Healing occurs without evidence of scarring.

Superficial Partial-Thickness Burn: A superficial partial-thickness burn involves the epidermis and the upper portion of the dermis. The involved area may be extremely painful and exhibit blisters. Healing occurs with minimal to no scarring.

Deep Partial-Thickness Burn: A deep partial-thickness burn involves complete destruction of the epidermis and the majority of the dermis. The involved area may appear to be discolored with broken blisters and edema. Damage to nerve endings may result in only moderate levels of pain. Healing occurs with hypertrophic scars and keloids.

Full-Thickness Burn: A full-thickness burn involves complete destruction of the epidermis and dermis along with partial damage of the subcutaneous fat layer. The involved area often presents with eschar formation and minimal pain. Patients with full-thickness burns require grafts and may be susceptible to infection.

Subdermal Burn: A subdermal burn involves the complete destruction of the epidermis, dermis, and subcutaneous tissue. Subdermal burns may involve muscle and bone and as a result often require surgical intervention.

Rule of Nines

Allows for a gross approximation of the percentage of the body affected by a burn.

Adult Values

Head and neck	9%
Anterior trunk	18%
Posterior trunk	18%
Bilateral anterior arm, forearm, and hand	9%
Bilateral posterior arm, forearm, and hand	9%
Genital region	1%
Bilateral anterior leg and foot	18%
Bilateral posterior leg and foot	18%
Total	**100%**

Children Values
A child under one year has 9% taken from the lower extremities and added to the head region. Each year of life, 1% is distributed back to the lower extremities until age nine when the head region is considered to be the same as an adult.

Intervention

Positioning and Splinting

Effective management of burns includes proper positioning and splinting. A patient that sustains a burn is prone to develop contractures due to hypertrophic scarring and overall lack of motion. A general rule is to position the affected joint in the opposite direction from which it will contract. The identified position should, if at all possible, be a position of function. Splints are usually left on overnight, worn intermittently during the day, and require frequent observation to ensure proper fit.

Ideal positioning includes placing the neck in extension, upper extremities abducted to 90 degrees, shoulder lateral rotation, and supination of the forearm. The lower extremities should align in neutral hip extension, 20 degrees abduction, full extension of the knee, and ankle dorsiflexion.

Topical Agents Used in Burn Care

Topical Agent	Advantages	Disadvantages
Silver sulfadiazine	Can be used with or without dressings Is painless Can be applied to wound directly Broad-spectrum Effective against yeast	Does not penetrate into eschar
Silver nitrate	Broad-spectrum Nonallergenic Dressing application is painless	Poor penetration Discolors, making assessment difficult Can cause severe electrolyte imbalances Removal of dressings is painful
Povidone-iodine	Broad-spectrum Antifungal Easily removed with water	Not effective against Pseudomonas May impair thyroid function Painful application
Mafenide acetate	Broad-spectrum Penetrates burn eschar May be used with or without occlusive dressings	May cause metabolic acidosis May compromise respiratory function May inhibit epithelialization Painful application
Gentamicin	Broad-spectrum May be covered or left open to air	Has caused resistant strains Ototoxic Nephrotoxic
Nitrofurazone	Bactericidal Broad-spectrum	May lead to overgrowth of fungus and Pseudomonas Painful application

From Trofino, RB: Nursing Care of the Burn-Injured Patient. F.A. Davis Company, Philadelphia 1991, p.46, with permission.

Skin Graft Procedures

Allograft (homograft): A temporary skin graft taken from another human, usually a cadaver, in order to cover a large burned area.

Autograft: A permanent skin graft taken from a donor site on the patient's own body.

Heterograft (xenograft): A temporary skin graft taken from another species.

Mesh graft: A skin graft that is altered to create a mesh-like pattern in order to cover a larger surface area.

Sheet graft: A skin graft that is transferred directly from the donor site to the recipient site.

Split-thickness skin graft: A skin graft that contains only a superficial layer of the dermis in addition to the epidermis.

Full-thickness skin graft: A skin graft that contains the dermis and the epidermis.

Burn Profile

Examination

- Past medical history
- History of current condition
- Social history (caregiver support)
- Medications
- Living environment
- Systems review
- Respiratory assessment
- Neurological assessment
- Edema/girth measurements
- Sensation
- Range of motion
- Flexibility
- Strength
- Pain
- Mobility skills

Intervention

- Positioning
- Splinting
- Edema control
- Scar management
- Passive range of motion
- Massage
- Conditioning exercises
- Endurance training
- Joint mobilization
- Electrotherapeutic modalities
- Compression devices
- Hydrotherapy
- Physical agents
- Mobility training

Goals

- Maximize functional mobility
- Maintain range of motion to all affected joints
- Maximize strength and endurance
- Reduce edema to the affected areas
- Maximize proper positioning and reduce scar contracture
- Maximize patient/caregiver competence with:
    - --Positioning of joints
    - --Use of splinting
    - --Pressure garments
    - --Stretching and strengthening programs

Burn Terminology

Dermis: The vascular layer of skin below the epidermis that contains hair follicles, sebaceous glands, and sweat glands.

Donor site: A site where healthy skin is taken and used as a graft.

Epidermis: The superficial avascular layer of skin that allows for hair follicles, subaceous glands, and sweat glands.

Eschar: The necrotic and nonviable tissue resulting from a deep burn. This skin is hard, dry, and does not possess qualities of normal skin.

Escharotomy: A surgical procedure that removes eschar from a burn site and subsequently enhances circulation.

Hypertrophic scarring: An abnormal and disorganized scar formation characterized by a raised, firm scar with collagen fibers that do not follow any pattern.

Normotrophic scarring: A scar with organized formation of collagen fibers that align in a parallel fashion.

Pressure garments: A custom-made garment that applies sustained pressure in order to improve the structure of a scar. Pressure garments are worn 22-23 hours per day and may be required for up to two years.

Recipient site: A site which has been burned and requires a graft.

Z-plasty: A surgical procedure to eliminate a scar contracture. An incision in the shape of a "z" allows the contracture to change configuration and lengthen the scar.

Patient Care Skills

Patient Management

Body Mechanics

A therapist must consistently use proper body mechanics when treating patients and avoid unnecessary stress and strain by maintaining proper alignment within the musculoskeletal system.

Principles of Proper Body Mechanics:
- Use the shortest lever arm possible
- Stay close to the patient when possible
- Use larger muscles to perform heavy work
- Maintain a wide base of support
- Avoid any rotary movement when lifting
- Attempt to maintain the center of gravity of the therapist and patient within the base of support

Patient Communication

- Verbal commands should focus the patient's attention on specifically desired actions.
- Instruction should remain as simplistic as possible and should not incorporate confusing medical terminology.
- The therapist should detail to the patient the general sequence of events that will occur prior to initiating treatment.
- The therapist should ask the patient questions during treatment in order to establish a rapport with the patient and to provide feedback as to the status of the current treatment.
- The therapist should speak clearly and vary his/her tone of voice as required by the situation.

Infection Control

Asepsis: The elimination of the microorganisms that cause infection and the creation of a sterile field.

Contamination: A term used to describe an area, surface, or item coming in contact with something that is not sterile. Contamination assumes an environment that contains microorganisms.

Handwashing: Handwashing is an important technique for asepsis. Guidelines for acceptable handwashing are as follows:
1. Use warm water
2. Remove all jewelry
3. Wash hands with soap for at least 30 seconds
4. Avoid touching any contaminated surface
5. Rinse thoroughly
6. Use a paper towel as a barrier when turning off the water

Medical Asepsis: A technique that attempts to contain pathogens to a specific area, object, or person. A primary goal is to reduce the spread of pathogens. Example: A patient with tuberculosis is hospitalized and kept in isolation.

Personal protective equipment (PPE): Items that are worn and used as barriers to protect someone who is assisting a patient with a potentially infectious disease. Personal protective equipment includes gowns, lab coats, masks, gloves, goggles, spill kits, and mouthpieces.

Sterile field: A sterile field is used to maintain surgical asepsis. A sterile field is a designated area that is considered void of all contaminants and microorganisms. There are standard and required protocols that must be followed in order to develop and maintain a sterile field.

Surgical Asepsis: A state in which an area or object is without any microorganisms. Example: A sterile field.

Universal precautions: Universal precautions are guidelines created in 1987 and recommended by the Center for Disease Control to protect against blood borne pathogens such as HIV and Hepatitis B. A health care provider must treat all patients as if they are infected with a blood borne disease. The protocol requires gloves, mask, and gown when there is contact or potential contact with blood or body fluids.

Universal precautions require:
- Wash hands before and after each patient contact
- Clean treatment area
- Use of personal protective equipment as needed
- Therapist's should cover any open area on themselves
- Use of medical asepsis
- Place biohazard materials in the appropriate receptacle

Category-Specific Isolation Precautions

ISOLATION CATEGORY	PRIVATE ROOM**	MASKS	GOWNS	GLOVES	COMMON DISEASES PLACED INTO ISOLATION CATEGORY
Strict Isolation	Always	Always	Always	Always	Varicella-zoster (chicken pox); pharyngeal diphtheria; shingles (zoster), localized in an immunocompromised client or disseminated
Contact Isolation	Always	For close contact	If soiling with infective material is likely	If contact with infective material is likely	Acute respiratory tract infection in infants and young children; disseminated herpes simplex; methicillin-resistant Staphylococcus aureus; pediculosis; scabies
Respiratory Isolation	Always	For close contact	No	No	Measles; meningococcal meningitis, pneumonia, or meningococcemia; mumps; pertussis
Acid-fast Bacteria Isolation	Always	Yes	Only to prevent gross contamination	No	Tuberculosis (primary pulmonary or pharyngeal)
Enteric Precautions	Only if the client's hygiene is poor	No	If soiling with infective material is likely	If contact with infective material is likely	Enteroviral infection, including meningitis; infectious gastroenteritis (e.g., giardiasis, salmonellosis, shigellosis,); hepatitis A, Clostridium difficile enterocolitis
Drainage and Secretion Precautions	No	No	If soiling with infective material is likely	If contact with infective material is likely	Minor or limited abscess, wound, burn, skin infection, conjunctivitis
Blood and Body Fluid Precautions	Only if the client's hygiene is poor	If contact with blood or body fluids is likely	If contact with splashes of blood or body fluids is likely	If contact with blood or body fluids is likely	AIDS; hepatitis B; non-A, non-B hepatitis; malaria

**In most instances when a private room is required, clients infected with the same organism may share a room.

From Ignatavicius, DD: Medical-Surgical Nursing: A Nursing Process Approach, Volume One. W.B. Saunders Company, Philadelphia 1995, p.595, with permission

Transfers

Communication During Transfers

The patient should be informed about the transfer itself and his/her responsibility during the transfer. The explanation should be understood by the patient and should occur prior to the transfer.

Commands and counts are used to synchronize the actions of the participants involved in the transfer. The therapist at the head of the patient should give the commands during the transfer when more than one person is involved.

Levels of Physical Assistance

Independent: The patient does not require any assistance to complete the task.

Supervision: The patient requires a therapist to observe throughout completion of the task.

Contact Guard: The patient requires the therapist to maintain contact with the patient to complete the task. Contact guard is usually needed to assist if there is a loss of balance.

Minimal Assist: The patient requires 25% assist from the therapist to complete the task.

Moderate Assist: The patient requires 50% assist from the therapist to complete the task.

Maximal Assist: The patient requires 75% assist from the therapist to complete the task.

Dependent: The patient is unable to participate and the therapist must provide all of the effort to perform the task.

Types of Transfers

Dependent transfers:
- *Three person carry/lift*
  The three person carry or lift is used to transfer a patient from a stretcher to a bed or treatment plinth. Three therapists carry the patient in a supine position; one therapist supports the head and upper trunk, the second therapist supports the trunk, and the third supports the lower extremities. The therapist at the head is usually the one to initiate commands. The therapists flex their elbows that are positioned under the patient and roll the patient on his or her side towards them. The therapists then lift on command and move in a line to the destination surface, lower, and position the patient properly.

- *Two person lift*
  The two person lift is used to transfer a patient between two surfaces of different heights or when transferring a patient to the floor. Standing behind the patient, the first therapist should place his or her arms underneath the patient's axilla. The therapist should grasp the patient's left forearm with his or her right hand and grasp the patient's right forearm with his or her left hand. The second therapist places one arm under the mid to distal thighs and the other arm is used to support the lower legs. The therapist at the head usually initiates the command to lift and transfer the patient out of the chair to the destination surface.

- *Dependent stand/squat pivot transfer*
  The dependent stand or squat pivot transfer is used to transfer a patient who cannot stand independently, but can bear some weight through the trunk and lower extremities. The therapist should position the patient at a 45-degree angle to the destination surface. The patient places his or her upper extremities on the therapist's shoulders, but should not be allowed to pull on the therapist's neck. The therapist should position the patient at the edge of the surface, hold the patient around the hips and under the buttocks, and block the patient's knees in order to avoid buckling while standing. The therapist should utilize momentum, straighten his or her legs, and stand the patient or allow the patient to remain in a squatting position. The therapist should then pivot and slowly lower the patient to the destination surface.

- *Hydraulic lift*
  The hydraulic lift is a device required for dependent transfers when a patient is obese, there is only one therapist available to assist with the transfer, or the patient is totally dependent. The hydraulic lift needs to be locked in position before the transfer. The therapist positions a webbed sling under the patient and attaches the S-ring to the bars on the lift. Once all attachments are checked, the therapist should pump the handle on the device in order to elevate the patient. Once the patient is elevated, the therapist can navigate the lift with the patient to the destination surface. Once transferred, the chains should be removed, however the webbed sling should remain in place in preparation for the return transfer.

Assisted transfers:
- *Sliding board transfer*
  The sliding board transfer is used for a patient who has some sitting balance, some upper extremity strength, and can adequately follow directions. The patient should be positioned at the edge of the wheelchair or bed and should lean to one side while placing one end of the sliding board sufficiently under the proximal thigh. The other end of the sliding board should be positioned on the destination surface. The patient should not hold onto the end of the sliding board in order to avoid pinching the fingers. The patient should place the lead hand four to six inches away from the sliding board and use both arms to initiate a push-up and scoot across the board. The therapist should guard in front of the patient and assist as needed as the patient performs a series of push-ups across the board.

- *Stand pivot transfer*
  The stand pivot transfer is used when a patient is able to stand and bear weight through one or both of the lower extremities. The patient must possess functional balance and the ability to pivot. Patients with unilateral weight bearing restrictions or hemiplegia may utilize this transfer and lead with the uninvolved side. The transfer may also be used therapeutically, leading with the involved side. A patient should be positioned at the edge of the wheelchair or bed to initiate the transfer. The therapist can assist the patient to keep his or her feet flat on the floor while bringing the head and trunk forward. The therapist should assist the patient as needed with his or her feet. The therapist must guard or assist the patient through the transfer and instruct the patient to reach back for the surface before he or she begins to sit down. Once the stand pivot is performed, the therapist should assist as needed to ensure control with lowering the patient to the destination surface.

- *Stand step transfer*
  The stand step transfer is used with a patient who has the necessary strength and balance to weight shift and step during the transfer. The patient requires guarding or supervision from the therapist and performs the transfer as a stand pivot transfer except the patient actually takes a step to maneuver and reposition his or her feet instead of a pivot.

UNIT SIX: PATIENT CARE SKILLS

Wheelchairs

Wheelchair Facts

- Adult standard wheelchair specifications include seat width - 18 inches, seat depth - 16 inches and seat height - 20 inches
- Hemi-height wheelchairs have decreased seat height (17.5 inches) to allow for propulsion using the unaffected foot.
- Rear wheel axles can be positioned two inches posteriorly from normal for patients with amputations to increase the base of support and to compensate for diminished weight in front of the wheelchair.
- Reclining wheelchairs allow intermittent or constant reclined positioning.
- Tilt-in-space wheelchairs allow for a reclined position without losing the required 90 degrees of hip flexion and 90 degrees of knee flexion. The entire chair reclines without any anatomical changes in positioning.

Components of a Wheelchair

Foot Plates/Foot Rests: Heel loops

Legrests:
Stationary
Adjustable/removable
Swing away
Elevating

Seat:
Gel cushion
Air cushion
Foam cushion
No cushion

Armrests:
Fixed versus adjustable
Stationary versus removable
Full length
Desk top

Wheelchair Back:
Fixed versus removable
Sling versus contoured:
- Gel
- Foam

Tall versus low back

Restraints:
Velcro lap belts and chest belts
Airplane seat belts
Automobile seat belts

Wheelchair Frame:
Stationary versus folding
Narrow versus standard versus large

Standard Wheelchair Measurements for Proper Fit

Measurement	Instructions	Average Adult Size
Seat height/leg length	Measure from the user's heel to the popliteal fold and add 2 inches to allow clearance of the footrest.	19.5 to 20.5 inches
Seat depth	Measure from the user's posterior buttock, along the lateral thigh to the popliteal fold; then subtract approximately 2 inches to avoid pressure from the front edge of the seat against the popliteal space.	16 inches
Seat width	Measure the widest aspect of the user's buttocks, hips or thighs and add approximately 2 inches. This will provide space for bulky clothing, orthoses, or clearance of the trochanters from the armrest side panel.	18 inches
Back height	Measure from the seat of the chair to the floor of the axilla with the user's shoulder flexed to 90 degrees and then subtract approximately 4 inches. This will allow the final back height to be below the inferior angles of the scapulae. (Note: This measurement will be affected if a seat cushion is to be used. The person should be measured while seated on the cushion or the thickness of the cushion must be considered by adding that value to the actual measurement.)	16 to 16.5 inches

Measurement	Instructions	Average Adult Size
Armrest height	Measure from the seat of the chair to the olecranon process with the user's elbow flexed to 90 degrees and then add approximately 1 inch. (Note: This measurement will be affected if a seat cushion is to be used. The person should be measured while seated on the cushion or the thickness of the cushion must be considered by adding that value to the actual measurement.)	9 inches above the chair seat

From Pierson, FM: Principles and Techniques of Patient Care. W.B. Saunders Company, Philadelphia 1999, p.149, with permission.

Ambulation

Assistive Devices

Three main indications for using an assistive device during ambulation include:
- Decreased weight bearing on the lower extremities
- Muscle weakness of the trunk or lower extremities
- Decreased balance or impaired kinesthetic awareness

Assistive Device Selection

Parallel bars
Parallel bars provide maximum stability and security for a patient during the beginning stages of ambulation or standing. Proper fit includes bar height that allows for 20–25 degrees of elbow flexion while grasping on the bars approximately four to six inches in front of the body. A patient must progress out of the parallel bars as quickly as possible to increase overall mobility and decrease dependence using the parallel bars.

Walker
A walker can be used with all levels of weight bearing. The walker has a significant base of support and overall good stability. The walker should allow for 20–25 degrees of elbow flexion to ensure proper fit. The standard walker has many variations including the rolling, folding, or adjustable walker with brakes, upper extremity attachments and/or a seat platform.

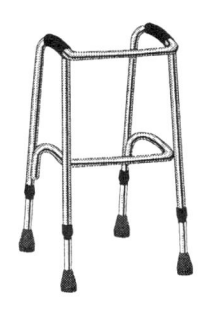

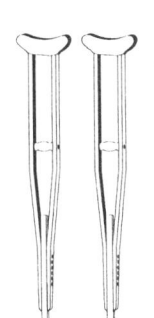

Axillary crutches
Axillary crutches can be used with all levels of weight bearing, however require higher coordination for proper use. Proper fit includes positioning with the crutches six inches in front and two inches lateral to the patient. The crutch height should be adjusted no greater than three finger widths from the axilla. The handgrip height should be adjusted to the ulnar styloid process and allow for 20–25 degrees of elbow flexion while grasping the handgrip. A platform attachment can be utilized with this device.

Lofstrand (forearm) crutches
Lofstrand crutches can be used with all levels of weight bearing, however require the highest level of coordination for proper use. Proper fit includes 20–25 degrees of elbow flexion while holding the hand grip with the crutches positioned six inches in front and two inches lateral to the patient. The arm cuff should be positioned one to one and one half inches below the olecranon process so it does not interfere with elbow flexion. A platform attachment can be utilized with this device if necessary.

Cane
A cane provides minimal stability and support for patients during ambulation activities. The straight cane provides the least support and is used primarily for assisting with balance. A straight cane should not be utilized for patients that are partial weight bearing. The small base and large base quad canes provide a larger base of support and can better assist with limiting weight bearing on an involved lower extremity and improving balance on unlevel surfaces, curbs, and stairs. Proper fit includes standing the cane at the patient's side and adjusting the handle to the level of the wrist crease at the ulnar styloid. The patient should have 20–25 degrees of elbow flexion while grasping the handgrip.

Levels of Weight Bearing

Non-weight bearing (NWB): A patient is unable to place any weight through the involved extremity and is not permitted to touch the ground or any surface. An assistive device is required.

Toe touch weight bearing (TTWB): A patient is unable to place any weight through the involved extremity, however may place the toes on the ground to assist with balance. An assistive device is required.

Partial weight bearing (PWB): A patient is allowed to put a particular amount of weight through the involved extremity. The amount of weight bearing is expressed as allowable pounds of pressure or as a percentage of total weight. A therapist must monitor the amount of actual weight transferred through the involved foot during partial weight bearing. An assistive device is required.

UNIT SIX: PATIENT CARE SKILLS

Weight bearing as tolerated (WBAT): A patient determines the proper amount of weight bearing based on comfort. The amount of weight bearing can range from minimal to full. An assistive device may or may not be required.

Full weight bearing (FWB): A patient is able to place full weight on the involved extremity. An assistive device is not required at this level, but may be used to assist with balance.

Gait Patterns

An appropriate gait pattern is determined by the amount of weight bearing permitted and the severity of the patient's condition.

Commonly used gait patterns include two-point, three-point, four-point, swing-to, and swing-through.

Two-Point Gait
Used to describe a pattern in which a patient uses two crutches or canes. The patient ambulates moving the left crutch forward while simultaneously advancing the right lower extremity and vice-versa. Each step is "one-point" and a complete cycle is two-points.

Three-Point Gait
This pattern can be seen with a walker or crutches. It involves one injured lower extremity that may have decreased weight bearing. The assistive device is advanced followed by the injured lower extremity and then the uninjured lower extremity. The assistive device and each lower extremity are considered separate points.

Four-Point Gait
This pattern is very similar to the two-point pattern. The primary difference is that the patient does not move the lower extremities simultaneously, but rather waits and advances the opposite leg once the crutch/cane has been advanced. This gait pattern may be prescribed when a patient exhibits impaired coordination, balance, or significant strength deficits. Each advancement of the crutch or cane as well as the bilateral lower extremities indicates a single point, thus allowing for a four-point gait pattern.

Swing-to Gait
A style of gait where a patient uses crutches or a walker and advances the lower extremities simultaneously only to the point of the assistive device.

Swing-through Gait
The patient performs the same sequence as a swing-to gait pattern, however advances the lower extremities beyond the point of the assistive device.

Accessibility

Americans with Disabilities Act

The Americans with Disabilities Act is designed to provide a clear and comprehensive national mandate for the elimination of discrimination. The Americans with Disabilities Act (PL101-336) is federal legislation which was signed into law on July 26, 1990.

The Americans with Disabilities Act is divided into five titles:
Title I:	Employment
Title II:	Public Services
Title III:	Public Accommodations
Title IV:	Telecommunications
Title V:	Miscellaneous

The Americans with Disabilities Act applies primarily, but not exclusively, to "disabled" individuals. An individual is "disabled" if he or she meets at least one of the following criteria:
- He or she has a physical or mental impairment that substantially limits one or more of his/her major life activities.
- He or she has a record of such an impairment.
- He or she is regarded as having such an impairment.

The Employment provisions (Title I) apply to employers of fifteen employees or more. The Public Accommodation provisions (Title III) apply to all businesses, regardless of the number of employees.

Employers are required to make reasonable accommodation for qualified individuals with a disability, who are defined by the Americans with Disabilities Act as individuals who satisfy the job-related requirements of a position held or desired, and who can perform the "essential functions" of such position with or without reasonable accommodation. The Americans with Disabilities Act does not require employers to make accommodations that pose an "undue hardship." "Undue hardship" is defined as significantly difficult or expensive accommodations.

Sources of additional information on the Americans with Disabilities Act:

Employment:
Equal Opportunity Commission
1801 L Street, NW
Washington, DC 20507
(800)669-4000
http://www.eeoc.gov

Public Accommodations:
Department of Justice
Office on the Americans with Disabilities Act
Civil Rights Division
P.O. Box 66118
Washington, DC 20035-6118
(202)514-0301
http://www.usdoj.gov

Accessible Design in New Construction and Alterations:
Architectural and Transportation Barriers and Compliance Board
1331 F Street, NW
Suite 1000
Washington, DC 20004-1111
(800)872-2253
http://www.access-board.gov

Transportation:
Department of Transportation
400 Seventh Street, SW
Room 10424
Washington, DC 20590
(202)366-9305
http://www.ffa.dot.gov

Telecommunications:
Federal Communications Commission
1919 M Street, NW
Room 254
Washington, DC 20554
(800)632-7260
http://www.fcc.gov

Accessibility Requirements

Ramps	Grade ≤ 8.3% At least 36 inches width Must have handrails on both sides Twelve inches of length for each inch of vertical rise Handrails required for a rise of six inches or more or for a horizontal run of 72 inches or more.
Doorways	Minimum 32 inch width Maximum 24 inch depth
Thresholds	Less than ¾ inch for sliding doors Less than ½ inch for other doors
Carpet	Requires ½ inch pile or less
Hallway clearance	36 inch width
Wheelchair turning radius (U-turn)	60 inch width 78 inch length
Forward reach in wheelchair	Low reach 15 inches High reach 48 inches
Side reach in wheelchair	Reach over obstruction to 24 inches
Bathroom sink	Not less than 29 inch height Not greater than 40 inches from floor to bottom of mirror or paper dispenser 17 inches minimum depth under sink to back wall
Bathroom toilet	17 - 19 inches from floor to top of toilet Not less than 36 inch grab bars Grab bars should be 1 ¼ - 1 ½ inches in diameter 1 ½ inch spacing between grab bars and wall Grab bar placement 33–36 inches up from floor level
Hotels	Approximately 2% total rooms must be accessible
Parking spaces	96 inches wide 240 inches in length Adjacent aisle must be 60 inches by 240 inches Approximately 2% of the total spaces must be accessible

Laboratory/Diagnostic Testing

Laboratory Testing

Hematocrit
Hematocrit is the percentage of packed red blood cells in total blood volume. Hematocrit is commonly used in the identification of abnormal states of hydration, polycythemia, and anemia. A low hematocrit may result in a feeling of weakness, chills or dyspnea. A high hematocrit may result in an increased risk of thrombus formation.

Hemoglobin
Hemoglobin is the iron containing pigment of the red blood cells. Hemoglobin's function is to carry oxygen from the lungs to the tissues. The laboratory test is commonly used to assess blood loss, anemia, and bone marrow suppression. Low hemoglobin may indicate anemia or recent hemorrhage, while elevated hemoglobin suggests hemoconcentration caused by polycythemia or dehydration.

Partial thromboplastin time
Partial thromboplastin time is most commonly used to monitor oral anticoagulant therapy or to screen for selected bleeding disorders. The test examines all of the clotting factors of the intrinsic pathway with the exception of platelets. Partial thromboplastin time is more sensitive than prothrombin time in detecting minor deficiencies.

Platelet count
Platelet count refers to the number of platelets per milliliter of blood. Platelets play an important role in blood coagulation, homostasis, and blood thrombus formation. Low platelet counts increase the risk of bruising and bleeding. High platelet counts increase the risk of thrombosis.

Prothrombin time
Prothrombin time is most commonly used to monitor oral anticoagulant therapy or to screen for selected bleeding disorders. The test examines extrinsic coagulation factors V, VII, X, prothrombin, and fibrinogen.

White Blood Cell count
White blood cell count refers to the number of white blood cells per milliliter of blood. White blood cell count is commonly used to identify the presence of infection, allergens, bone marrow integrity, or the degree of immunosuppression. An increase in white blood cell count can occur after hemorrhage, surgery, coronary occlusion or malignant growth.

Reference Values in Hematology

		Conventional Units	SI Units
Cell Counts			
Erythrocytes			
Males		4.6-6.2 million/mm^3	4.6-6.2 X 10^{12}/L
Females		4.2-5.4 million/mm^3	4.2-5.4 X 10^{12}/L
Children (varies with age)		4.5-5.1 million/mm^3	4.5-5.1 X 10^{12}/L
Leukocytes			
Total		4500-11,000 mm^3	4.5-11.0 X 10^9/L
Differential	**Percentage**	**Absolute**	**Absolute**
Myelocytes	0	0/mm^3	0/L
Band neutrophils	3-5	150-400/mm^3	150-400 X 10^6/L
Segmented neutrophils	54-62	3000-5800/mm^3	3000-5800 X 10^6/L
Lymphocytes	25-33	1500-3000/mm^3	1500-3000 X 10^6/L
Monocytes	3-7	300-500/mm^3	300-500 X 10^6/L
Eosinophils	1-3	50-250/mm^3	50-250 X 10^6/L
Basophils	0-1	15-50/mm^3	15-50 X 10^6/L
Platelets		150,000-400,000/mm^3	150-400 X 10^9/L
Reticulocytes		25,000-75,000/mm^3 (0.5-1.5% of erythrocytes) 20-165 mg/dL	25-75 X10^9/L 0.20-1.65 g/L
Hematocrit			
Males		40-54 mL/dL	0.40-0.54 volume fraction
Females		37-47 mL/dL	0.37-0.47 volume fraction
Newborns		49-54 mL/dL	0.49-0.54 volume fraction
Children (varies with age)		35-49 mL/dL	0.35-0.49 volume fraction
Hemoglobin			
Males		14.0-18.0 gm/dL	2.17-2.79 mmol/L
Females		12.0-16.0 gm/dL	1.86-2.48 mmol/L
Newborns		16.5-19.5 gm/dL	2.56-3.02 mmol/L
Children (varies with age)		11.2-16.5 gm/dL	1.74-2.56 mmol/L

From Miller-Keane: Encyclopedia and Dictionary of Medicine, Nursing, and Allied Health. W.B. Saunders Company, Philadelphia 1997, p.1843, with permission.

Reference Values for Clinical Chemistry (Blood, Serum, Plasma)

		Conventional Units	SI Units
Cholesterol, serum or EDTA plasma	Desirable range LDL cholesterol HDL cholesterol	<200 mg/dL 60-180 mg/dL 30-80 mg/dL	<5.18 mmol/L 600-1800 mg/L 300-800 mg/L
Oxygen, blood, arterial, room air	Partial pressure (PaO$_2$) Saturation (SaO$_2$)	80-100 mm Hg 95-98%	80-100 mm Hg 95-98%
pH, arterial blood		7.35-7.45	7.35-7.45

From Miller-Keane: Encyclopedia and Dictionary of Medicine, Nursing, and Allied Health. W.B. Saunders Company, Philadelphia 1997, p.1844, with permission.

Diagnostic Tests

Arteriography
Arteriography refers to a radiograph that visualizes injected radiopaque dye in an artery. The test can be used to identify arteriosclerosis, tumors or blockages.

Arthrography
Arthrography is an invasive test utilizing a contrast medium to provide visualization of joint structures through radiographs. Soft tissue disruption can be identified by leakage from the joint cavity and capsule. The test is commonly used at peripheral joints such as the hip, knee, ankle, elbow, and wrist.

Bone Scan
A bone scan is an invasive test that utilizes isotopes to identify stress fractures, infection, and tumors. Bone scans can identify bone disease or stress fractures with as little as 4-7% bone loss.

Computed Tomography
Computed tomography produces cross-sectional images based on x-ray attenuation. A computerized analysis of the changes in absorption produces a detailed reconstructed image. The test is commonly used to diagnose spinal lesions and in diagnostic studies of the brain.

Doppler Ultrasonography
Doppler ultrasonography is a noninvasive test that evaluates blood flow in the major veins, arteries, and cerebrovascular system. The test relies on the transmission and reflection of high frequency sound waves to produce cross-sectional images in a variety of planes. Doppler ultrasonography is safer, less expensive, and requires a shorter time period than more invasive tests such as arteriography and venography.

Electrocardiography
Electrocardiography is the recording of the electrical activity of the heart. The test identifies three distinct waveforms: P wave (atrial depolarization), QRS complex (ventricular depolarization), and the T wave (ventricular repolarization). Electrocardiography is used to help identify conduction abnormalities, cardiac arrhythmias, and myocardial ischemia.

Electroencephalography
Electroencephalography is the recording of the electrical activity of the brain. The electrical activity is collected by examining the difference between the electrical potential of two electrodes placed at different locations on the scalp. Electroencephalography is used to assess seizure activity, metabolic disorders, and cerebellar lesions.

Electromyography
Electromyography is the recording of the electrical activity of a selected muscle or muscle groups at rest and during voluntary contraction. Electromyography is performed by inserting a needle electrode percutaneously into a muscle or through the use of surface electrodes. The test is commonly used to assess peripheral nerve injuries and to differentiate between various neuromuscular disorders.

Fluoroscopy
Fluoroscopy is designed to show motion in joints through x-ray imaging. The technique permits objects placed between a fluorescent screen and a roentgen tube to become visible. Fluoroscopy is not used commonly due to excessive radiation exposure.

Magnetic Resonance Imaging
Magnetic resonance imaging is a noninvasive technique that utilizes magnetic fields to produce an image of bone and soft tissue. The test is valuable in providing images of soft tissue structures such as muscles, menisci, ligaments, tumors, and internal organs. Magnetic resonance imaging requires the patient to remain still for prolonged periods of time and is extremely expensive.

Myelography
Myelography is an invasive test that combines fluoroscopy and radiography to evaluate the spinal subarachnoid space. The test utilizes a contrast medium which is injected into the epidural space by spinal puncture. Myelography is used to

identify bone displacement, disc herniation, spinal cord compression, or tumors.

Venography
Venography refers to a radiograph that visualizes injected radiopaque dye in a vein. The test can be used to identify tumors or blockages in the venous network.

X-ray
X-ray is a radiographic photograph commonly used to assist with the diagnosis of musculoskeletal problems such as fractures, dislocations, and bone loss. X-ray produces planar images and as a result often require images to be taken in multiple planes in order to visualize a lesion's location and size.

Medical Equipment

Tubes, Lines, and Equipment

Arterial Line
An arterial line is a monitoring device consisting of a catheter that is inserted into an artery and attached to an electronic monitoring system. An arterial line is used to measure blood pressure or to obtain blood samples. The device is considered to be more accurate than traditional measures of blood pressure and does not require repeated needle punctures.

External Catheter
An external catheter is applied over the shaft of the penis and is held in place by a padded strap or adhesive tape.

Foley Catheter
A Foley catheter is an indwelling urinary tract catheter that has a balloon attachment at one end. The balloon which is filled with air or sterile water must be must be deflated before the catheter can be removed.

Intravenous System
An intravenous system consists of a sterile fluid source, a pump , a clamp, and a catheter to insert into a vein. An intravenous system can be used to infuse fluids, electrolytes, nutrients, and medication. Intravenous lines are most commonly inserted into superficial veins such as the basilic, cephalic or antecubital.

Nasal Cannula
A nasal cannula consists of tubing extending approximately one centimeter into each of the patient's nostrils. The tubing is connected to a common tube that is attached to an oxygen source. This method of oxygen therapy is capable of delivering up to 6 liters of oxygen per minute.

Nasogastric Tube
A nasogastric tube is a plastic tube inserted through a nostril and extending into the stomach. The device is commonly used for liquid feeding, medication administration or to remove gas from the stomach.

Oximeter
An oximeter is a photoelectric device used to determine the oxygen saturation of blood. The device is most commonly applied to the finger or the ear. Oximetry is often used by therapists to assess activity tolerance.

Suprapubic Catheter
A suprapubic catheter is an indwelling urinary catheter that is surgically inserted directly into the patient's bladder. Insertion of a suprapubic catheter is performed under general anesthesia.

Swan-Ganz Catheter
A Swan-Ganz catheter is a soft, flexible catheter that is inserted through a vein into the pulmonary artery. The device is used to provide continuous measurements of pulmonary artery pressure. Patients utilizing a Swan-Ganz catheter can exercise with the device in place, however the patient should avoid activities that increase pressure on the catheter's insertion site.

Physical Agents

Therapeutic Modalities

Indications for Therapeutic Modalities

Inflammation and repair: Modalities can alter circulation, chemical reactions, flow of body fluids, and cell function throughout all phases of healing. Modalities enhance and accelerate the healing process and reduce the risk of adverse effects associated with inflammation.

Pain: Modalities can control pain by altering the cause of the pain or altering the process of pain perception.

Restriction in motion: Thermal agents are used to enhance extensibility of collagen to allow for greater range of motion and tolerance to stretch.

Abnormal tone: Modalities can influence tonal abnormalities from pain, musculoskeletal or neurological pathology. Alteration in nerve conduction, reduction of pain, and change in muscle biomechanical properties can normalize tone and enhance functional outcome.

Principles of Heat Transfer

Conduction: The gain or loss of heat as a result of direct contact between two materials at different temperatures. Examples include hot pack, paraffin, ice massage, and ice pack.

Convection: The gain or loss of heat as a result of air or water moving in a constant motion across the body. Examples include fluidotherapy and whirlpool.

Conversion: The transfer of heat when nonthermal energy (mechanical, electrical) is absorbed into tissue and transformed into heat. Examples include diathermy and ultrasound.

Evaporation: The transfer of heat as a liquid absorbs energy and changes form to a vapor. An example is a vapocoolant spray.

Radiation: The direct transfer of heat from a radiation energy source of higher temperature to one of cooler temperature. Heat energy is directly absorbed without the need for a medium. An example is an infrared lamp.

Cryotherapy

Therapeutic Effects:
- Decrease temperature
- Initial decrease in blood flow to the treated area
- Decrease metabolism
- Decrease edema
- Increase pain threshold
- Initial vasoconstriction
- Decrease nerve conduction velocity
- Reduce spasticity of muscle
- Produce analgesic effects

Indications:
- Acute or chronic pain
- Muscle spasm
- Myofascial pain syndrome
- Bursitis
- Edema
- Acute or subacute inflammation
- Musculoskeletal trauma
- Reduction of spasticity
- Tendonitis

Contraindications:
- Cold hypersensitivity
- Cryoglobinemia
- Ischemic tissue
- Area of compromised circulation
- Infection
- Cold intolerance
- Raynaud's phenomenon
- Hypertension
- Peripheral vascular disease

Ice Massage

Ice massage is typically performed by freezing water in paper cups and applying the ice directly to the treatment area. Ice massage is ideal for small or contoured areas, allows for observation, and is inexpensive to use.

Treatment Parameters: Ice massage can be administered using a frozen water Popsicle or frozen water in a paper cup. Directly apply ice massage to the area for five to ten minutes.

Cold Pack

A cold pack typically contains silica gel and is available in a variety of shapes and sizes. The cold pack is stored in a refrigeration unit and is usually applied with a moist towel. Cold packs are easy to use, require minimal clinician time, and can cover a large area. Cold packs may not maintain uniform contact with the body and require frequent observation of the skin.

Treatment Parameters: A cold pack requires a temperature of 23 degrees Fahrenheit (–5 degrees Celsius). Apply the cold pack wrapped in a moistened towel to the area for 15 minutes. Application may extend to 30 minutes for reduction in spasticity, however the skin requires observation every ten minutes. Cold packs can be applied every one to two hours for reduction of inflammation and pain control.

Cold Bath

A cold bath is commonly used for immersion of the distal extremities. A basin or whirlpool is most often used to hold the cold water.

Treatment Parameters: A cold bath requires water temperature ranging from 55 to 64 degrees Fahrenheit (13 to 18 degrees Celsius). A whirlpool or container of water with crushed ice can be used. The body part should be immersed for 5 to 15 minutes to attain the desired therapeutic effects.

Vapocoolant Spray

Vapocoolant sprays are often used in conjunction with passive stretching. Fluori-Methane is a commonly used vapocoolant spray that is typically applied from the proximal to distal muscle attachments. Vapocoolant sprays allow for a short duration of cooling to a very localized area of application, however may be harmful to the environment and dangerous if inhaled.

Treatment Parameters: Identify the trigger point and make two to five sweeps with the spray in the direction of the muscle fibers. Keep the spray 12 to 18 inches from the skin and apply at a 30-degree angle. Stretching should begin while applying the spray and continue with steady tension and stretch. Repeated applications during the same treatment are safe if the skin is rewarmed between applications. Chlorofluorocarbons are exempt from the Clean Air Act when used for medical purposes, however may cause environmental and ozone damage.

Superficial Heating Agents

Therapeutic Effects:
- Increase temperature
- Increase blood flow to the treated area
- Decrease nerve conduction latency
- Temporarily decrease muscle strength
- Increase edema
- Increase pain threshold
- Vasodilation
- Increase nerve conduction velocity
- Increase metabolic rate
- Increase muscle elasticity and collagen extensibility
- Decrease muscle tone

Indications:
- Pain control
- Trigger point
- Tissue healing
- Chronic inflammatory conditions
- Muscle spasm
- Decreased range of motion
- Desensitization

Contraindications:
- Circulatory impairment
- Area of malignancy
- Arterial disease
- Thrombophlebitis
- Bleeding or hemorrhage
- Sensory impairment
- Acute musculoskeletal trauma

Fluidotherapy

Fluidotherapy consists of a container that circulates warm air and small cellulose particles. The extremity is placed into the container and dry heat is generated through the energy transferred by forced convection. Fluidotherapy allows for active movement during treatment and constant treatment temperature, however it is expensive and may require the extremity to be placed in a dependent position.

Treatment Parameters: The body part to be treated should be placed into the fluidotherapy unit prior to turning the machine on. The temperature should be set between 100 to 118 degrees Fahrenheit (38 to 48 degrees Celsius) and the degree of agitation should be adjusted to patient comfort. Treatment time is usually 20 minutes. A protective covering is required for any open area.

Hot Pack

A hot pack consists of a canvas or nylon covered pack filled with a hydrophilic silicate gel that provides a moist heat. The size and shape of the hot pack varies depending on the size and contour of the treatment area. A hot pack is easy to use, inexpensive, and can cover large areas. Disadvantages of a hot pack include the need for close monitoring of the skin, the inability to maintain total contact, and the inability to move during treatment.

Treatment Parameters: A hot pack must be stored in hot water between 158 to 167 degrees Fahrenheit (70 to 75 degrees Celsius). Application requires six to eight layers of towels around the hot pack. The hot pack should be applied on top of the patient. If the patient lies on top of the hot pack additional towels are required. Skin checks are required after five minutes for excess redness or signs of a burn. A patient must have a call device to notify the therapist of discomfort. Hot packs require 20 minutes to achieve desired effects.

Infrared Lamp (IR)

An infrared lamp produces superficial heating of tissue through radiant heat. This form of heating is usually limited to penetration of less than one to three millimeters. Infrared does not require contact with the area to be treated and allows for constant observation, however it requires skill to localize a treatment site.

***Treatment Parameters*:** The patient should be positioned approximately 20 inches from the source. A moist towel should be placed over the treatment area and the skin should be monitored intermittently throughout treatment. The standard formula indicates 20 inches in distance should equal 20 minutes of treatment. As the distance decreases, the intensity will increase, and the time of total treatment should decrease.

Paraffin

Paraffin wax is the most commonly used superficial heating agent of the distal extremities. It has the ability to maintain contact over all contoured areas and due to the low specific heat and slower conduction it does not feel as hot as water at the same temperature. Paraffin is easy to use, inexpensive, and can be used at home, however it cannot be used over open areas.

***Treatment Parameters*:** Temperature of the paraffin mixture should be maintained between 113 and 122 degrees Fahrenheit (45 to 50 degrees Celsius). There are three methods of paraffin application: dip-wrap, dip-reimmersion or paint application. The distal extremities rely on the dip-wrap or dip-reimmersion methods. The patient's skin should be dry and clean prior to treatment. The patient is required to maintain a static position as the distal extremity dips into the paraffin bath and is removed. Wait a few seconds for the paraffin to harden and redip five to ten times using the dip-wrap method. Next, place a plastic bag over the extremity with a towel around it to insulate and maintain heating for approximately 15 to 20 minutes. Using the dip-reimmersion method place the distal extremity back into the paraffin bath after the initial 5-10 dips and allow it to remain for the duration of treatment, up to 20 minutes. The paint method is used for body parts that cannot be immersed into the paraffin bath. A layer of paraffin is painted on the body with a brush. After a few seconds, six to ten additional layers are applied and a plastic wrap is placed over the paraffin with a towel on top to insulate the treatment area. Removal of the paraffin is the same for all forms of application. Paraffin should be peeled off after treatment and placed back into the container to melt or to be discarded.

Deep Heating Agents

Diathermy

Diathermy is a deep heating agent that converts high frequency electromagnetic energy into therapeutic heat. Electrical energy produces vibration of molecules within a specific tissue, generates heat, and elevates tissue temperature. Shortwave diathermy can be delivered in a continuous or pulsed mode. A pulsed mode is typically utilized to attain nonthermal effects while a continuous mode is used for thermal effects. The most common frequency used for shortwave diathermy is 27.12 MHz. Shortwave diathermy can utilize a capacitance technique or inductance technique. Capacitive plate applicators produce a high frequency electrical current that alternates between the plates. The patient becomes part of the electrical circuit and the oscillation of ions increases tissue temperature. Inductive coil applicators utilize a coil that generates alternating electric current, creates a magnetic field perpendicular to the coil, and produces eddy currents within the tissues. Eddy currents cause oscillation of ions which increases tissue temperature. Inductive coil applicators are bundled as cables that wrap around an extremity or as a drum applicator.

Indications:
- Decreased collagen extensibility
- Pain
- Tissue healing
- Chronic inflammatory pelvic disease
- Chronic inflammation
- Muscle guarding
- Joint stiffness
- Bursitis
- Peripheral nerve regeneration
- Degenerative joint disease

Contraindications:
- Internal and external metal objects
- Eyes
- Malignant area
- Moist wound dressing
- Low back, abdomen, pelvis of a pregnant woman
- Intrauterine device
- Cardiac pacemaker
- Testes
- Acute inflammation
- Ischemic tissue
- Pain and temperature sensory deficits

***Treatment Parameters*:** A therapist should first select the most appropriate diathermy technique and device based on patient examination. The patient must remove all metal and jewelry in the area surrounding the treatment site. Position the patient and check for clean and dry skin. When using an inductive applicator the therapist must wrap the coils around the extremity that has been covered by a towel. When using a drum the therapist should place the drum directly over the treatment area. When using a capacitive applicator place the two plates over both sides of the treatment area ensuring equal distance from the plates to the skin (two to ten centimeters). The patient must remain in the same position throughout treatment for complete and consistent heating. The patient should have a call bell and should be checked within the first few minutes of treatment. Treatment time varies from 15 to 30 minutes based on diagnosis and desired effects.

Ultrasound

Ultrasound is the most common deep heating agent that transfers heat through conversion, elevates tissue temperature to depths up to five centimeters, and uses inaudible acoustic mechanical vibrations of high frequency to produce thermal and nonthermal effects. The piezoelectric crystal transducer converts electrical energy into sound. Therapeutic ultrasound has a frequency between .75 and 3 MHz. Ultrasound requires the use of a coupling agent and can be applied using the stationary or moving technique. Ultrasound can be administered using a pulsed or continuous mode. Continuous mode ultrasound is more effective in elevating tissue temperature where pulsed mode ultrasound conversely minimizes the thermal effects. Duty cycle indicates the portion of treatment time that ultrasound is generated during the entire treatment. For example, continuous ultrasound generates constant ultrasound waves which correlates to a 100% duty cycle and produces thermal effects at a higher intensity and nonthermal effects at a lower intensity. Pulsed ultrasound that generates ultrasound 20% of the treatment time correlates to a 20% duty cycle and will produce nonthermal effects. A frequency setting of 1 MHz is used for heating of deeper tissues (up to five centimeters) where a setting of 3 MHz produces a higher temperature with a depth of penetration of less than two centimeters.

Phonophoresis describes the use of ultrasound for transdermal delivery of medication. Ultrasound enhances the distribution of the medication through the skin, provides a high concentration of the drug directly to the treatment site, and avoids risks that may be involved with injection of medication. Medications regularly used in phonophoresis include anti-inflammatory agents or analgesics. Phonophoresis is effective with both continuous and pulsed techniques.

Therapeutic Effects:

Thermal

- Increase extensibility of collagen structures
- Decrease joint stiffness
- Decreases muscle spasm
- Pain relief
- Increase blood flow

Nonthermal (through cavitation, microstreaming, or acoustic streaming)

- Stimulation of tissue regeneration
- Increase skin and cell membrane permeability
- Increase macrophage responsiveness
- Soft tissue repair
- Increase blood flow
- Pain relief

Indications:
- Soft tissue repair
- Contracture
- Bone fracture
- Trigger point
- Dermal ulcer
- Scar tissue
- Pain
- Plantar wart
- Muscle spasm

Contraindications:
- Eyes
- Pregnant uterus
- Impaired pain or temperature sensory deficit
- Impaired circulation
- Thrombophlebitis
- Cemented prosthetic joint
- Heart
- Testes
- Epiphyseal areas in children
- Infection
- Over malignancy

Treatment Parameters: Ultrasound can be administered using a stationary or moving technique. For all techniques the therapist should decide the duration, frequency, duty cycle, and intensity of treatment based on diagnosis and desired effects. Apply the coupling medium to the treatment area or place the area to be treated under water if using the immersion technique. Place the transducer on the treatment area or one half-inch parallel to the treatment area under water and then turn on the machine. During the moving technique the transducer should continuously move in a small circular pattern over the treatment area. Maintain contact with the skin and stay within the treatment area. An area two times the size of the transducer typically requires a duration of five to ten minutes of treatment. Intensity for continuous ultrasound is normally set between .5 to 2 W/cm^2 for thermal effects. Pulsed ultrasound is normally set between .5 to .75 W/cm^2 with a 20% duty cycle for nonthermal effects.

Hydrotherapy

Hydrotherapy transfers heat through conduction or convection and is administered in tanks of varying size ranging from extremity whirlpool to Olympic size pools. The specific instrument to be used depends on the treatment objectives and site of the pathology.

Properties of Water:

Buoyancy: Archimedes' principle of buoyancy states that there is an upward force on the body when immersed in water equal to the amount of water that has been displaced by the body. The ability to float in water results from the body possessing a specific gravity less than that of water.

Hydrostatic pressure: Water exerts pressure that is perpendicular to the body and increases in proportion with the depth of immersion.

Viscosity and resistance: Water molecules tend to attract to each other and provide resistance to movement of the body in the water. Resistance by water increases in proportion to speed of motion.

Indications:
- Burn care
- Superficial heating or cooling
- Pain management
- Muscle spasm/spasticity
- Muscle strain
- Arthritis
- Desensitization of residual limb with contrast bath
- Wound care
- Joint stiffness
- Decreased range of motion
- Pool therapy/exercise
- Sprain
- Edema control

Contraindications:
- Peripheral vascular disease
- Advanced cardiovascular or pulmonary disease
- Severe infection
- Gangrene
- Impaired circulation
- Buerger's disease with contrast bath
- Renal infection
- Diminished sensation

Types of Hydrotherapy

Extremity tank: An extremity tank is used for the distal upper or lower extremity. Approximate dimensions for the extremity tank are a depth of 18 to 24 inches, a length of 28 to 32 inches, and a width of 15 inches.

Lowboy tank: A lowboy tank is used for larger parts of the extremities or immersion to waist level. Approximate dimensions for the lowboy tank are a depth of 18 inches, a length of 52 to 65 inches, and a width of 24 inches.

High boy tank: A highboy tank is used for larger parts of the extremities or immersion to waist level. Approximate dimensions for the highboy tank are a depth of 28 inches, a length of 36 to 48 inches, and a width of 20 to 24 inches.

Hubbard tank: The Hubbard tank is used for full body immersion. Approximate dimensions for the Hubbard tank are a depth of four feet, a length of eight feet, and a width of six feet. Contraindications specific to full body immersion include unstable blood pressure and incontinence. Treatment time ranges between 10 to 20 minutes. Temperature should not exceed 100 degrees Fahrenheit (39 degrees Celsius).

Therapeutic pool: A therapeutic pool is used for exercising in a water medium. Temperature should range between 79 to 98 degrees Fahrenheit (26 to 37 degrees Celsius) depending on patient age, health status, and goals.

Treatment Parameters for whirlpool: Prior to treatment the therapist should explain the sensations the patient will experience during treatment. Select the water temperature based on diagnosis and goals and assist the patient into a comfortable position.

Treatment temperature guidelines are as follows:

Temperature	Use
32 - 79 °F (0 - 26 °C)	Acute inflammation of distal extremities
79 - 92 °F (26 - 33 °C)	Exercise
92 - 96 °F (33 - 36 °C)	Wound care, spasticity
96 - 98 °F (36 - 37 °C)	Cardiopulmonary compromise, treatment of burns
99 - 104 °F (37 - 40 °C)	Pain management
104 - 110 °F (40 - 44 °C)	Chronic rheumatoid or osteoarthritis, increased range of motion

Adjust and turn on the turbine. Monitor the patient's vital signs and level of comfort. Treatment time ranges between 10 and 30 minutes. Exercise can be performed during whirlpool as indicated. After treatment dry and inspect the treated area.

Treatment Parameters for pool therapy: In addition to general contraindications for superficial or deep heating, specific contraindications include incontinence, open areas, fear of water, confusion, and significant respiratory pathology. The therapist should assist the patient as needed into the pool and throughout treatment. The therapist must stay with the patient and monitor vital signs and tolerance to activity. Advantages of pool therapy include decreased weight bearing with the assistance of buoyancy, easier handling by the therapist, control over the amount of resistance during exercise, and diminished risk of falling with activity. Recommended populations for pool therapy include patients with arthritis, musculoskeletal injuries, neurological deficits, spinal cord injury, CVA, multiple sclerosis, and selected cardiopulmonary diagnoses. The tank must be thoroughly cleaned after each use with a disinfectant and antibacterial agent.

Contrast Bath

A contrast bath utilizes alternating heat and cold in order to decrease edema in a distal extremity. The alternating vasodilation and vasoconstriction is theorized to stimulate local circulation and systemic circulation to a lesser degree. The technique provides good contact over irregularly shaped areas, allows for movement during treatment, and assists with pain management. Disadvantages include potential intolerance to cold, dependent positioning, and lack of credible research to support the theory of contrast baths and its effect on edema.

Treatment Parameters: The therapist should position the patient so that both baths are accessible to the patient. The treatment should begin with the patient's distal extremity immersed in the hot whirlpool with a temperature between 80

UNIT SEVEN: PHYSICAL AGENTS

to 104 degrees Fahrenheit (27 to 40 degrees Celsius) for three to four minutes. The patient should then place the distal extremity into the cold bath with a temperature between 55 to 67 degrees Fahrenheit (13 to 20 degrees Celsius) for one minute. The patient should repeat this hot/cold sequence for 30 minutes. The patient should end the treatment in the hot whirlpool and then dry off immediately. Contrast baths are utilized primarily with arthritis of the smaller joints, musculoskeletal sprains and strains, RSD, and to desensitize the residual limb of a patient status post amputation.

Mechanical Agents

Traction

Traction is a modality that applies mechanical forces to the body to separate joint surfaces and decrease pressure. The force can be applied manually by the therapist or mechanically by a machine. Traction is indicated for many diagnoses and allows for variation and adjustment of the established protocol based on individual patient need. Traction affects many of the body's systems and requires ongoing monitoring and reassessment of treatment parameters. Mechanical traction, self traction, manual traction, and positional traction are commonly utilized techniques.

Therapeutic Effects:
- Joint distraction
- Soft tissue stretching
- Joint mobility
- Reduction of disc protrusion
- Muscle relaxation

Indications:
- Nerve impingement
- Herniated or protruding disc
- Subacute joint inflammation
- Spondylolisthesis
- Joint hypomobility
- Paraspinal muscle spasm
- Degenerative joint disease
- Osteophyte formation

Contraindications:
- When motion is contraindicated
- Joint instability
- Tumor
- Pregnancy
- Acute inflammatory response
- Acute sprain
- Osteoporosis
- Fracture

Treatment Parameters: Mechanical traction can be performed to the cervical or lumbar spine. All halters and belts should be secured and the patient instructed in what to expect from treatment. The therapist should then set the time of treatment, force of pull, and determine static or intermittent control with hold and relax ratio settings. During treatment the patient should have the ability to stop the machine and call for help. Treatment time varies based on diagnosis and therapeutic goals and falls between five and 20 minutes. To initiate cervical traction the therapist should position the patient in supine with approximately 25-35 degrees of neck flexion or in a sitting position. Cervical traction should start with a force between 10-15 pounds and progress to 7% of the patient's body weight as tolerated for separation of the vertebrae. Application of lumbar traction should be performed in supine or prone. The force of lumbar traction is dependent on the goals of treatment and should be set with a force of less than half of the body weight for the initial treatment. Force of up to 50% of the body weight is required for separation of the vertebrae.

Compression

Compression is a physical agent which applies a mechanical force that increases pressure on the treated body part. Compression works to keep venous and lymphatic flow from pooling into the interstitial space. Static compression utilizes bandaging and compression garments to shape residual limbs, control edema, prevent abnormal scar formation, and reduce the risk of deep vein thrombosis. Intermittent compression with a pneumatic device is primarily used to reduce chronic or posttraumatic edema and requires adjusting the parameters of inflation pressure, on/off ratio, and total treatment time. Compression appliances have coupled compression with therapeutic cold and electrical stimulation.

Therapeutic Effects:
- Control of peripheral edema
- Shaping of residual limb
- Management of scar formation
- Improve lymphatic and venous return
- Prevention of deep vein thrombosis

Indications:
- Lymphedema
- Risk for deep vein thrombosis
- New residual limb
- Edema
- Stasis ulcers
- Hypertrophic scarring

Contraindications:
- Malignancy of treated area
- Deep vein thrombosis
- Unstable or acute fracture
- Heart failure
- Infection of treated area
- Pulmonary edema
- Circulatory obstruction

Treatment Parameters: The therapist must ask the patient to remove all jewelry and ensure appropriate fit of the compression sleeve prior to treatment. The patient should be placed in a comfortable position with the extremity elevated. Blood pressure and girth measurements should be recorded. The therapist should apply the stockinette over the extremity and adjust the compression sleeve. The therapist should set parameters based on desired effect. A 3:1 ratio is generally used for on/off time with inflation between 40 to 100 seconds and deflation between 10 to 35 seconds. Inflation pressure generally ranges from 30 to 80 mm Hg and should not exceed the patient's diastolic blood pressure. Treatment of the upper extremities generally requires between 30 and 60 mm Hg of inflation pressure while treatment of the lower extremities generally requires between 40 and 80 mm Hg of inflation pressure. Treatment time varies based on diagnosis from 2 to 4 hours and is utilized from three times per week to three times per day. The patient should have a call bell and should be monitored for comfort and blood pressure readings throughout treatment. When treatment time is complete the therapist should reassess the extremity, girth measurements, and blood pressure readings.

Additional Physical Agents

Ultraviolet (UV)

Ultraviolet light is a form of energy that is used therapeutically and absorbed one to two millimeters into the skin. Ultraviolet is divided into UV-A, UV-B, and UV-C according to wavelength and place on the electromagnetic spectrum. Treatment parameters and application are based on diagnosis, desired effects, and minimal erythemal dose. Since The most effective use of UV is to treat skin disorders.

Therapeutic Effects:
- Facilitate healing
- Increase pigmentation
- Vitamin D production
- Exfoliation
- Thickening of epidermis
- Bacteriocidal effects
- Tanning

Indications:
- Acne
- Psoriasis
- Tetany
- Vitamin D deficiency
- Chronic ulcer/wound
- Osteomalacia/rickets
- Sinusitis

Contraindications:
- Photosensitive medication
- Lupus erythematosus
- Renal or hepatic pathology
- Herpes simplex
- Tuberculosis
- Diabetes mellitus
- Pellagra

Treatment Parameters: Prior to treatment with UV a therapist must obtain a minimal erythemal dose (MED). This is the time of exposure needed to produce an area of mild redness between eight and 24 hours after treatment. The MED is tested by placing a piece of paper with five one-inch cut outs over a patient's anterior forearm. The patient should have all other nontreatment areas covered as well as wear protective goggles. Once the lamp is warmed up it should be positioned at a 90-degree angle to the area of treatment (for maximum absorption) and at a distance between 24 to 40 inches from the forearm. The squares should be exposed sequentially in 15 second increments for 15, 30, 45, 60, and 75 seconds. Visual inspection after an 8-hour period will determine the MED. Parameters including distance from the lamp, position of the lamp at a 90-degree angle to the treatment site, and MED must remain consistent over the course of treatment. The treatment time should increase each consecutive treatment day since the skin adapts to UV exposure. The therapist should utilize a stopwatch and continue with ongoing visual inspection during all treatment sessions.

Biofeedback

Biofeedback is a modality that uses an electromechanical device to provide visual and/or auditory feedback. Biofeedback can be utilized to receive information related to motor performance, kinesthetic performance, or physiological response. Biofeedback can measure peripheral skin temperature, changes in blood volume through vasodilation and vasoconstriction using finger phototransmission, sweat gland activity, and electrical activity during muscle contraction. Electromyographic biofeedback is the most commonly used biofeedback modality in the clinical setting.

Therapeutic Effects:
- Muscle relaxation
- Improve muscle strength
- Decrease muscle spasm
- Neuromuscular control
- Decrease accessory muscle use
- Decrease pain

Indications:
- Muscle spasm
- Pain
- Spinal cord injury
- Urinary incontinence
- Muscle weakness
- Hemiplegia
- Cerebral palsy
- Bowel incontinence

Contraindications:
- Any condition where muscle contraction is detrimental
- Skin irritation at electrode site

Treatment Parameters: Prior to treatment the therapist should ensure that the patient's skin is clean and dry. The two active electrodes should be placed parallel to the muscle fibers and close to each other. The reference or ground electrode can be placed anywhere on the body, but is often secured between the two active electrodes. The signals are transmitted to a differential amplifier and information is conveyed through visual and audio feedback.

The treatment for muscle reeducation should begin with the patient performing a maximal muscle contraction. The sensitivity of the biofeedback unit should be set at a low sensitivity setting and adjusted so that the patient can perform the repetitions at a ratio of two-thirds of the maximal muscle contraction. Isometric contractions should continue for six to ten seconds with relaxation in between each contraction. Treatment duration for a single muscle group is five to ten minutes. The treatment for muscle relaxation requires a high sensitivity setting and a similar electrode placement with active electrodes initially positioned close to each other. As the patient improves with relaxation, the electrodes should be placed further apart and the sensitivity setting increased. During this treatment, the patient may also benefit from adjunct relaxation techniques such as imagery. Treatment duration of 10 to 15 minutes is usually adequate to attain relaxation.

Massage

Massage is a manual therapeutic modality that produces physiologic effects through different types of stroking, rubbing, and pressure. Massage is capable of producing mechanical and reflexive effects.

Massage Techniques

Effleurage: Effleurage is a massage technique that is usually light in stroke and produces a reflexive response. The technique is performed at the beginning and end of a massage to allow the patient to relax and should be directed towards the heart. Effleurage can be applied as a deep stroke to produce both a mechanical and a reflexive response.

Friction: Friction is a massage technique that incorporates small circular motions over a trigger point or muscle spasm. This is a deep massage technique that penetrates into the depth of a muscle and attempts to reduce edema, loosen adhesions, and relieve muscle spasm. Friction massage is used quite frequently with chronic inflammation or with overuse injuries.

Petrissage: Petrissage is a massage technique described as kneading where the muscle is squeezed and rolled under the therapist's hands. The goal of petrissage is to loosen adhesions, improve lymphatic return, and facilitate removal of metabolic waste from the treatment area. Petrissage must provide a distal to proximal sequence of kneading over the muscle. Petrissage can be performed with two hands over larger muscle groups or with as few as two fingers over smaller muscles.

Tapotement: Tapotement is a massage technique that provides stimulation through rapid and alternating movements such as tapping, hacking, cupping, and slapping. The primary purpose of tapotement is to enhance circulation and stimulate peripheral nerve endings.

Vibration: Vibration is a massage technique that places the therapist's hands or fingers firmly over an area and utilizes a rapid shaking motion that causes vibration to the treatment area. The therapist initiates this motion from the forearm while maintaining firm contact on the treatment area. Vibration is used primarily for relaxation.

Therapeutic Effects:
- Improve circulation
- Increase lymphatic circulation
- Removal of metabolic waste
- Decrease muscle atrophy
- Loosen adhesions
- Facilitate healing
- Stimulate reflexive effects
- Reduction of edema
- Alters the transmission of pain
- Decrease muscle spasm
- Decrease anxiety and tension
- Relaxation

Indications:
- Pain
- Decreased range of motion
- Edema
- Adhesions
- Myositis
- Raynaud's syndrome
- Migrane or general headache
- Trigger point
- Muscle spasm and cramping
- Scar tissue
- Bursitis
- Tendonitis
- Intermittent claudication
- Lactic acid accumulation

Contraindications:
- Infection
- Arteriosclerosis
- Thrombus
- Cellulitis
- Acute injury
- Embolus
- Cancer

Treatment Parameters: The patient should be comfortable and properly draped prior to the initiation of treatment. The therapist's hands must be clean, dry, and warm. The therapist must be positioned in an efficient posture during treatment and maintain the required pressure and rhythm based on the goals of treatment. The massage should start using the effleurage technique. The amount of time required for each treatment is dependent on the body part and therapeutic goal. Generally, the back requires 15 minutes as opposed to a smaller area or joint that requires eight to ten minutes. The intensity should progressively increase and then decrease, using effleurage again to end the treatment session. Lubricant is indicated with all strokes except friction massage.

Electrotherapy

Electrotherapy is utilized in physical therapy for various reasons including facilitation of skeletal muscle contraction, stimulation of denervated muscle, pain management, and wound management.

Therapeutic Effects:
- Relaxation of muscle spasm
- Muscle strengthening
- Improve range of motion
- Decrease pain
- Decrease edema
- Eliminate disuse atrophy
- Muscle reeducation
- Increase local circulation
- Facilitate wound healing
- Facilitate bone repair of a fracture

Indications:
- Muscle spasms
- Muscle weakness
- Pain
- Open wound/ulcer
- Idiopathic scoliosis
- Fracture
- Shoulder subluxation
- Muscle atrophy
- Decreased range of motion
- Bell's palsy
- CVA shoulder subluxation
- Stress incontinence
- Use with labor and delivery
- Facial neuropathy

Contraindications:
- Cardiac pacemaker
- Patient with a bladder stimulator
- Use over carotid sinus
- Phlebitis
- Malignancy
- Cardiac arrhythmia
- Use over a pregnant uterus
- Osteomyelitis

Treatment Parameters

Types of Current

Direct Current (Galvanic)
Direct current is characterized by a constant flow of electrons from the anode to the cathode without interruption. Polarity remains constant and is determined by the therapist based on treatment goals. Iontophoresis requires the use of direct current.

Alternating Current
Alternating current is characterized by polarity that continuously changes from positive to negative with the change in direction of current flow. Alternating current is biphasic, symmetrical or asymmetrical, and is characterized by a waveform that is sinusoidal in shape. Alternating current is used in muscle retraining, spasticity, and stimulation of denervated muscle.

Interferential Current
Interferential current combines two high frequency alternating waveforms that are biphasic. This type of current is used for deep muscle stimulation. Interferential current attempts to reach deeper tissue using the higher frequencies of each waveform and the overall shorter pulse widths. Interferential uses a frequency of 50 – 120 pulses per second and a pulse width of 50 – 150 microseconds for pain management; and a frequency of 20 – 50 pulses per second and a pulse width of 100 – 200 microseconds for muscle contraction.

Russian Current
Russian current is a medium frequency polyphasic waveform. The intensity of this form of alternating current is produced in a 50 burst per second interval with a pulse width range of 50 – 200 microseconds, and an interburst interval of 10 milliseconds. Russian current was originally used to augment muscle strengthening.

Electrode Configuration

Monopolar Technique: The stimulating or active electrode is placed over the target area. A second dispersive electrode is placed at another site away from the target area. Typically the active electrode is smaller than the dispersive electrode. This technique is used with wounds, ionotophoresis, and in the treatment of edema.

Bipolar Technique: Two active electrodes are placed over the target area. Typically the electrodes are equal in size. This technique is used for muscle weakness, neuromuscular facilitation, spasms, and range of motion.

Quadripolar Technique: Two electrodes from two separate stimulating circuits are positioned so that the individual currents intersect with each other. This technique is utilized with interferential current.

Electrode Size

When using a smaller electrode it is particularly important to understand that since the current density is quite high compared to a larger electrode, the patient will be more susceptible to pain and potential tissue damage.

Small Electrodes:
- Increased current density
- Increased impedance
- Decreased current flow

Large Electrodes:
- Decreased current density
- Decreased impedance
- Increased current flow

Neuromuscular Electrical Stimulation

Neuromuscular electrical stimulation or functional electrical stimulation is a technique used to facilitate skeletal muscle activity. Stimulation of an innervated muscle occurs when an electrical stimulus of appropriate intensity and duration is administered to the corresponding peripheral nerve. Electrical stimulation of a denervated muscle can be used in an attempt to maintain the muscle, however there is little documented evidence that supports this treatment option. Functional neuromuscular electrical stimulation is a commonly used therapeutic technique to facilitate the return of controlled functional muscular activity or to maintain postural alignment until recovery occurs.

Treatment Parameters: The patient should be positioned comfortably. The therapist uses a bipolar electrode placement over the target muscle. An interrupted or surged current is utilized with a range of 20 – 40 pulses per second and an on time of one to two seconds followed by an off time of four to ten seconds to avoid immediate motor fatigue. Treatment time ranges from 15 to 20 minutes and can be repeated several times each day.

Transcutaneous Electrical Nerve Stimulation (TENS)

Transcutaneous electrical nerve stimulation is widely used for acute and chronic pain management. Areas of use include obstetrics, temporomandibular joint pain, and postoperative pain. TENS produces pain relief through the gate control theory of Wall and Melzak or the endogenous opiate pain control theory. TENS units are portable and indicated for home use.

Treatment Parameters: The waveforms used are monophasic pulsatile current or biphasic pulsatile current with a spiked square, rectangular or sinewave form. Electrode placement may be based on sites of nerve roots, trigger points, acupuncture sites or key points of pain and sensitivity. Net polarity normally is equal to zero. Sensory level stimulation utilizes a phase duration of 2-50 microseconds, frequency of 50-100 pulses per second, and requires the patient to experience perceptible tingling. Motor level stimulation utilizes a phase duration of more than 150 microseconds, frequency of less than 20 pulses per second, and requires the therapist to identify a visible muscle contraction.

Iontophoresis

Iontophoresis is the process by which medications are induced through the skin into the body by means of continuous direct current electrical stimulation. The medication is separated into ions based on the polarity of the current.

Treatment Parameters: The patient should be positioned comfortably, but should never lie on top of the electrodes. The unit should be set to continuous direct current. Polarity must be set to the same polarity as the ion solution. The ion solution should be massaged into the treatment site or placed into the designated space within the electrode. The therapist must ensure that the negative electrode is twice the size of the positive electrode regardless of which one is the active electrode. The therapist should secure the electrodes and slowly increase the intensity towards a maximum of five milliamperes. Treatment should last 15 to 20. Additional time is required for treatment at an intensity less than five milliamperes. The therapist must monitor the patient during treatment to ensure that the skin is not being burned under the electrode. Upon completion of treatment the therapist must slowly decrease the intensity, remove the electrodes, and provide the area of skin under the negative electrode with a thorough cleaning including the application of lotion to minimize irritation.

Electrical Equipment Care and Maintenance

The use of electrical equipment can be a potential hazard to both therapist and patient. The following is a very abbreviated list of techniques that can minimize the risks of electrical equipment danger.

- Utilize experts to conduct routine inspections to make sure you meet or exceed all local, state, and federal operation standards.
- Never use a piece of electrical equipment until you have a complete understanding of all aspects of its operation.
- Have routine and scheduled service on all electrical equipment at or before the manufacturer's suggested service dates.
- Have repairs performed immediately after the identification of a potential problem.
- Conduct routine inspections of all electrical equipment to identify potential problems.
- Display electrical equipment operation manuals in an accessible location for staff members to use as a resource.

Electrotherapy Terminology

Alternating current (biphasic): Alternating current allows for the constant change in flow of ions.

Ampere: An ampere is a unit of measure used to describe the rate of current.

Amplitude: Amplitude refers to the magnitude of current. Amplitude controls are often labeled intensity or voltage.

Anode: The anode used during direct current electrotherapy is the positively charged electrode that attracts negative ions.

Cathode: The cathode used during direct current electrotherapy is the negatively charged electrode that attracts positive ions.

Chronaxie: Chronaxie is a testing procedure used to measure the amount of time required to produce a small muscle contraction at a particular intensity.

Current: Current describes the flow of electrons from one place to another.

Direct current (monophasic or Galvanic): Direct current refers to the constant unidirectional flow of ions. The direction of the current is dependent on polarity.

Duration of stimulus/Duration of rest: Duration of stimulus/duration of rest refers to the time period of stimulation and the time period of rest between periods of stimulation. The controls that correspond to the periods of stimulation and rest are labeled on-time and off-time.

Duty cycle: Duty cycle refers to the percentage of time that electrical current is on in relation to the entire treatment time.

Electrical impedance: Electrical impedance is the resistance of a tissue to electrical current.

Frequency: Frequency determines the number of pulses delivered through each channel per second. Frequency controls are often labeled rate.

High volt current: High volt current is characterized by a waveform greater than 150 volts with a short pulse duration. High volt is intermittent and is used for deeper tissue penetration.

Interpulse interval: The interpulse interval is the period of time of electrical inactivity between each pulse.

Ion: An ion is a positively or negatively charged atom.

Low volt current: Low volt current is characterized by a waveform of less than 150 volts and is used for neuromuscular stimulation.

Negative ion: A negative ion has gained one or more electrons and possesses a negative charge.

Ohm's law: Ohm's law describes the current of an electrical circuit. There is a direct proportional relationship between current and voltage and an indirect proportional relationship between current and resistance.

Positive ion: A positive ion has lost one or more electrons and possesses a positive charge.

Pulse: A pulse is one individual waveform.

Pulse duration: Pulse duration refers to the duration of pulsatile current. Pulse duration controls are often labeled pulse width.

Pulsed current (interrupted): Pulsed current allows for a noncontinuous flow of either alternating or direct current with periods of no electrical activity.

Ramp: Ramp refers to the number of seconds it takes for the amplitude to gradually increase or decrease to the maximum value set by the amplitude control.

Resistance: Resistance describes the ability of a material to oppose the flow of ions through it.

Rheobase: Rheobase is the minimal intensity used with a long current duration that produces a small muscle contraction.

Volt: A volt is a unit of measure of electrical power or electromotive force.

Waveform: A waveform is the consistent pattern of a current measured on an oscilloscope.

Research

Research Basics

Types of Research

Historical research
Investigating, recording, analyzing, and interpreting the events of the past for the purpose of discovering generalizations that are helpful in understanding the past, the present, and to a limited extent, anticipating the future.

Descriptive research
Recording, analyzing, and interpreting conditions that exist. Descriptive research involves some type of comparison or contrast and attempts to discover relationships between existing and nonmanipulated variables.

Experimental research
A description of what will result when certain variables are carefully controlled or manipulated. The focus is on variable relationships.

Ethical Considerations

Informed consent
Recruitment of volunteers for experimentation must involve the subject's complete understanding of the procedures, risks, and demands that may be made.

Confidentiality
The researcher must hold all information gathered in an experiment in strict confidence, maintaining the subject's anonymity at all times.

Protection from harm or danger
When using treatments that may have a temporary or permanent effect on a subject, the researcher must take all precautions to preserve the subject's well-being.

Knowledge of outcome
Subjects have a right to receive an explanation for the experimental procedures and the results of the investigation.

Reliability

The degree of consistency that a measuring method or device produces.

Intrarater reliability: The consistency of repeated measurements of the same observation by the same rater.

Interrater reliability: The consistency of repeated measurements of the same observation by different raters.

Validity

The degree to which data or results of a study are correct or true.

Concurrent validity: The degree to which the measurement being validated agrees with an established measurement standard administered at approximately the same time. Concurrent validity is a form of criterion validity.

Construct validity: The relationship between an instrument and an established theoretical framework. Construct validity is based on theory and not statistical analysis.

Content validity: The degree to which the indicator provides a complete representation of the domain of interest.

Criterion validity: The degree to which a relationship exists between a measurement being validated and other measures.

External validity: The degree to which results of the research study are generalizable.

Internal validity: The degree to which the reported outcomes of the research study are a consequence of the relationship between the independent and dependent variables and not the result of extraneous factors.

Predictive validity: The ability of an instrument to predict the occurrence of a future behavior or event. Predictive validity is a form of criterion validity.

Variables

Independent variable: The factors in a research study that are manipulated by the researcher.

Dependent variable: The factors in a research study used to measure the effect of the independent variable.

Discrete variable: A variable whose measurements are expressed as integers.

Continuous variable: A variable whose measurements can assume any value along a continuum. Values are not limited to integers and instead are only limited by the degree of accuracy of the measuring instrument.

Levels of Measurement

Nominal
This is the weakest level of measurement. Categories are very broad and each participant of the study will fit into only one of the categories. Each category is independent of the other.
  Example: male vs. female, yes vs. no

Ordinal
This level of measurement is also known as a ranking scale. Data that is collected will be placed into independent categories, however the categories have a qualitative relationship regarding the order of ranking. There is not equality between each category.
  Example: Manual muscle testing, levels of assistance

Interval
A metric measurement scale where the distance between any two numbers is of equal amounts. In this scale the unit of measure and zero are both arbitrary.
  Example: Celsius temperature scale, calendar time

Ratio
A metric measurement scale where the unit of measurement is arbitrary, however there is an absolute zero.
  Example: weight and length scales

Research Design

Controlled trials: Controlled trials require the experimental procedure to be compared with a placebo or another previously accepted procedure. Controlled studies are more likely than uncontrolled studies to determine whether differences are due to the experimental treatment or to some other extraneous factor.

Uncontrolled trials: Uncontrolled trials involve the investigators describing their experience with an experimental procedure, however the experimental procedure is not formally compared with a placebo or another previously accepted procedure.

Quantitative observations: Characteristics measured on a numerical scale.

Qualitative observations: Characteristics measured on a nominal scale.

Single blind study: A study in which the investigator does not know if the subject is in the treatment or the control group.

Double blind study: A study in which neither the investigator nor the subject knows if the subject is in the treatment or the control group.

Sampling

Probability Sampling
Probability sampling requires an investigator to identify the parameters of a population. Every member of the population must have the same probability of being selected for the sample. Probability sampling generates smaller sampling error and therefore is often more desirable when an investigator would like to generalize from a specific population to a larger population.

Probability Sampling Methods:

- *Simple random sampling*
  Subjects have an equal chance of being selected for the sample. The sampling method often relies on a table of random numbers to determine the sample. Sampling can be performed with or without replacement.

- *Systematic sampling*
  Subjects are selected by taking every n^{th} subject from the population. The size of the interval is based on the desired sample size. Systematic sampling is more efficient than simple random sampling and is most commonly employed when a researcher is drawing from a very large sample.

- *Stratified random sampling*
  Subjects are randomly selected from predetermined characteristics related to a particular study. Stratified random sampling enhances the sample representation and lowers sampling error by allowing subgroups to remain homogenous.

- *Cluster sampling*
  Subjects are selected based on a random sample of naturally occurring groups. Cluster sampling allows a random sample without a complete listing of each unit. The sampling technique is less costly and more efficient than simple random sampling.

Nonprobability Sampling
Nonprobability sampling does not require the parameters of a population to be identified and there is an absence of randomization. This type of sampling is often utilized in physical therapy due to the increased difficulty of meeting the more rigid requirements of probability sampling.

Nonprobability Sampling Methods:

- *Convenience sampling*
  Subjects are selected as they become available until the desired sample is reached.

- *Purposive sampling*
  Subjects are deliberately selected based on predefined criteria chosen by the investigators.

- *Snowball sampling*
  Subjects are identified by asking existing subjects to identify the names of other potential participants. Snowball sampling is often used when members of a given sample are difficult to identify.

Research Terminology

Hawthorne effect (placebo effect): An untreated subject experiences a change simply from participating in a research study.

Hypothesis: A statement of belief about population parameters.

Level of significance (alpha): Expresses the probability of rejecting the null hypothesis when it is true. Since it is desirable to limit this probability, traditional values for alpha are .05 and .01. Alpha is synonymous with the probability of a type I error.

Null hypothesis: A statement indicating there is no difference between the population mean and the hypothesized value.

One-tailed test: Used when investigators have a prior expectation about the size of a sample mean and want to test whether it is larger or smaller than the population mean.

Parameter: Numerical measurement describing some characteristic of a population.

Population: Group of all elements to be studied.

Sample: Subgroup of elements drawn from a population.

Sensitivity: The percentage of individuals with a particular diagnosis that are correctly identified as positive.

Specificity: The percentage of individuals without a particular diagnosis that are correctly identified as negative.

Statistic: Numerical measurement describing some characteristic of a sample.

Two-tailed test: Used when investigators do not have a prior expectation about the size of a sample mean and want to test whether it is different from the population mean in either direction.

Type I error (alpha error): Rejecting the null hypothesis when it is in fact true. If the level of significance was set at .01, there would be a 1% chance of a type I error occurring.

Type II error (beta error): Accepting the null hypothesis when it is in fact false. An example of a type II error occurs when a researcher concludes that a given intervention did not have a positive outcome on a dependent variable when it actually did. Type I and Type II errors vary inversely.

Statistics

Types of Statistics

Descriptive statistics: Descriptive statistics summarize or describe important characteristics of a known set of population data. Conditions cannot be extended beyond the known set of population data and any similarity to data outside the known set cannot be assumed.

Inferential statistics: Inferential statistics use sample data to make inferences about a population. This form of statistics is often utilized to determine whether there are significant differences between groups.

Measures of Central Tendency

Mean: The results obtained by adding all of the values and dividing by the total number of values that were added.

Median: The point on a distribution at which 50% of the values fell above and below. The median is identified by first rank ordering the values. If the number of values is odd, the median is the middle value. If the number of values is even, the median is found by determining the mean of the two middle values.

Mode: The value that occurs most frequently. A distribution with two modes is termed bimodal. A distribution with more than two modes is termed multimodal.

Measures of Variation

Range: The difference between the highest and lowest value.

Variance: The sum of the squared deviation from the mean divided by the total number of values.

Standard deviation: The average deviation of values around the mean. Standard deviation is based on the distance of sample values from the mean and equals the square root of the mean of the squared deviation. Expressed differently, the standard deviation is the square root of the variance.

Normal Distribution

A bell shaped curve that is symmetrical around its vertical axis with the values tending to cluster around the mean. The mean, median, and mode have the same value. The curve has no boundaries and only a small fraction of the values fall outside of three standard deviations above or below the mean.

- Approximately 68% of all values fall within one standard deviation above or below the mean.

- Approximately 95% of all values fall within two standard deviations above or below the mean.

- Approximately 99% of all values fall within three standard deviations above or below the mean.

Skewness: Refers to the symmetry or lack of symmetry in the shape of a frequency distribution. Negativity skewed or left skewed data is characterized by the mean and median being to the left of the mode. Positively skewed or right skewed data is characterized by the mean and median being to the right of the mode.

Steps in Testing a Statistical Hypothesis

1. State the research question in terms of statistical hypothesis
   a. null hypothesis
   b. alternative hypothesis
2. Decide on the appropriate test statistic
3. Select the level of significance for the statistical test
4. Determine the value the test statistic must attain to be declared significant
5. Perform the calculations
6. State the conclusion

Parametric Statistics

Parametric statistics assume that samples come from populations that are normally distributed and there is homogeneity of variance. Parametric statistical tests are applied to both interval and ratio level data.

Parametric Statistical Tests:
- *t-test*
  A statistical procedure for comparing a mean with a norm or comparing two means with sample sizes less than or equal to 30.

- *z-test*
  A statistical procedure for comparing a mean with a norm or comparing two means for larger sample sizes greater than 30.

- *Independent t-test*
  A statistical procedure used to compare two independent samples. A sample is independent if the sample selected from one population is not related to the sample selected from the other population.

- *Dependent t-test*
  A statistical procedure used to compare the difference in a numerical variable observed for two paired groups. The test is also used when the same group is subjected to pretest and posttest measurements.

- *Analysis of variance*
  A statistical procedure used to compare differences between two or more population means by analyzing sample variances.

- *One-way analysis of variance*
  A statistical procedure similar to the independent t-test, however the test is designed to accommodate two or more population means. One-way refers to the fact that only one independent variable is examined.

- *Two-way analysis of variance*
  A statistical procedure used to compare two or more population means with two or more independent variables.

Nonparametric Statistics

Nonparametric statistics do not assume that samples come from populations that are normally distributed and do not assume homogeneity of variance. Nonparametric statistical tests are most commonly applied to nominal or ordinal level data.

Nonparametric Statistical Tests:
- *Chi Square*
  A statistical procedure used to determine the probability that group differences result from chance. The nonparametric test uses nominal level data.

- *Kruskal-Wallis test*
  A statistical procedure used to determine if two or more samples come from the same population. The test is the nonparametric version of the one-way analysis of variance.

- *Mann-Whitney test*
  A statistical procedure used to compare two independent samples with ordinal level data. The test is the nonparametric alternative of the independent t-test.

- *Wilcoxon Signed Rank test*
  A statistical procedure used to compare two dependent samples with ordinal level data. The test is the nonparametric alternative of the dependent t-test.

Correlation

The relationship between two variables when one is related to the other.

Correlation coefficient: The measure of the linear relationship between paired variables in a sample.
- A perfect positive correlation indicates that for every unit increase in one variable there is a proportionate unit increase in the other variable. A perfect positive correlation is indicated by +1.0.
- A perfect negative correlation indicates that for every unit increase in one variable there is a proportionate unit decrease in the other variable. A perfect negative correlation is indicated by –1.0.

Pearson Product Moment Correlation (r): A type of correlation statistic that requires interval level data. The test yields a value between –1.0 and +1.0.

Spearman rho: A type of correlation statistic that requires ordinal level data. The test yields a value between –1.0 and +1.0. When interpreting a correlation coefficient it is important to remember that the coefficient does not imply a cause and effect relationship between variables. Attempt to avoid using rates or averages since this type of data reduces variation and may result in an inflated correlation coefficient.

Graphs

Histogram: A graphical display of a frequency distribution. A histogram typically includes the measurement of interest along the x-axis and the number or percentage of observations along the y-axis.

Dotplots: A graphical display in which each piece of data is plotted as a dot along a horizontal scale. When values occur more than once at a given point on the horizontal scale the dots are stacked vertically.

Stem and leaf plots: A graphical display which enables the reader to observe the entire distribution of data without losing any information. Most commonly this is done by organizing data into categories (e.g. 20-29, 30-39), and then dividing a number into two digits. The first digit is placed to the left side of a vertical line (stem) and the second digit is placed on the right side of the vertical line (leaves). The first digit within a category (stem) does not need to be repeated, however the second digit (leaves) should be repeated.

Scatterplot: A graphical display that illustrates the relationship between two measures or variables measured on a numeric scale. Each value is represented by a point or dot on the scatterplot. A scatterplot should not be used to determine if a relationship is significant or occurs due to chance.

Box and whisker plot: A graphical display constructed based on the information in a stem and leaf plot. The graph illustrates both the frequencies and the distribution of the data and is commonly used to illustrate certain locations in the distribution.

9 Administration

Documentation

Purpose of Documentation

- Communicate with other treating professionals
- Assistance with discharge planning
- Reimbursement
- Assistance with utilization review
- A legal document regarding the course of therapy

Records

- An increase in specialization of care and multidisciplinary treatment increases the need for medical records to serve as a means of communication among clinicians.
- Progress notes and referrals related directly to patient care are examples of clinical records.
- Departmental statistics and records are examples of administrative records.

Referrals

Acceptable forms of referral range from a signed prescription form to a highly structured checklist. The referral must include the name of the patient and be signed and dated by the referring physician. Referrals also commonly include some indication as to the number and frequency of treatments desired and any special precautions or instructions.

Progress Notes

- Improvement of patient care is the most important function of progress notes.
- Progress notes allow members of all health services to know what the patient is accomplishing in each given area.
- Progress notes should contain patient identification, the date, and the signature of the therapist.
- Progress notes should be written when the patient is initially treated and at the time of discharge. Additional progress notes should be written when the patient's condition changes during the course of treatment. Specific frequency of progress notes is usually dictated by department policy.
- Appropriate forms of documentation include diagrams, videotapes, and flow sheets as well as many other less frequently used media.

Discharge Summary

A discharge summary should provide a capsule view of the patient's progress during therapy. The discharge summary is usually conducted on the day of the patient's last therapy session.

S.O.A.P. Notes

A commonly used record to write daily notes is the S.O.A.P. note. S.O.A.P. stands for:
- **S:** Subjective
- **O:** Objective
- **A:** Assessment
- **P:** Plan

Subjective
Refers to information the patient communicates to the therapist. This could include social or medical history not previously recorded. It could also include the patient's statements or complaints.

Objective
Refers to information the therapist observes. Common examples include range of motion measurements, muscle strength, and functional abilities. It also includes manual techniques and equipment used during treatment.

Assessment
Allows the therapist to express his/her professional opinion. Short and long-term goals are often expressed in this section as well as changes in the treatment program.

Plan
Includes ideas for future physical therapy sessions. Frequency and expected duration of physical therapy services can also be incorporated into this section.

Guidelines for Physical Therapy Documentation

Preamble

The American Physical Therapy Association (APTA) is committed to meeting the physical therapy needs of society, to meeting the needs and interests of its members and to developing and improving the art and science of physical therapy, including practice, education, and research. To help meet these responsibilities, the APTA Board of Directors has approved the following guidelines for physical therapy documentation. It is recognized that these guidelines do not reflect all of the unique documentation requirements associated with the many specialty areas within the physical therapy profession. Applicable for both handwritten and electronic documentation systems, these guidelines are intended to be used as a foundation for the development of more specific documentation guidelines in specialty areas, while at the same time providing guidance for the physical therapy profession across all practice settings.

It is the position of APTA that physical therapy examination evaluation, diagnosis, and prognosis shall be documented, dated, and authenticated by the physical therapist who performs the service. Intervention provided by the physical therapist or physical therapist assistant is documented, dated, and authenticated by the physical therapist or, when permissible by law, the physical therapist assistant, or both.

Other notations or flow charts are considered a component of the documented record but do not meet the requirements of documentation in, or of, themselves (Position on Authority for Physical Therapy Documentation, HOD 06-98-11-11).

Operational Definitions

Guidelines: APTA defines "guidelines" as approved non-binding statements of advice.

Documentation: Any entry into the client record, such as consultation report, initial examination report, progress note, flow sheet/checklist that identifies the care/service provided, reexamination or summation of care.

Authentication: The process used to verify that an entry is complete, accurate, and final. Indications of authentication can include original written signatures and computer "signatures" on secured electronic record systems only.

I. General Guidelines
   A. All documentation must comply with the applicable jurisdictional/regulatory requirements.
      1. All handwritten entries shall be made in ink and will include original signatures. Electronic entries are made with appropriate security and confidentiality provisions.
      2. Informed consent: The patient/client should be asked to acknowledge understanding and consent before intervention is initiated.

Examples of ways in which to accomplish this documentation:
   Ex 2.1 Signature of patient/client or parent/legal guardian on long or short consent form.
   Ex 2.2 Notation/entry of what was explained by the physical therapist in the official record.
   Ex 2.3 Filing of a completed consent checklist signed by the patient/client or parent/legal guardian.
   3. Charting errors should be corrected by drawing a single line through the error and initializing and dating the chart or through the appropriate mechanism for electronic documentation that clearly indicates that a change was made without deletion of the original record.
   4. Identification
      4.1 Include patient's/client's full name and identification number, if applicable, on all official documents.
      4.2 All entries must be dated and authenticated with the provider's full name and appropriate designation (i.e. PT or PTA).
      4.3 Documentation by graduates or others pending receipt of an unrestricted license shall be authenticated by a licensed physical therapist.
      4.4 Documentation by students (SPT/SPTA) in physical therapist or physic therapist assistant programs must be additionally authenticated by the physical therapist or, when permissible by law, documentation by physical therapist assistant students may be authenticated by a physical therapist assistant.
   5. Documentation should include the referral mechanism by which physical therapy services are initiated.
      Examples include:
         Ex 5.1 Self-referral/direct access.
         Ex 5.2 Request for consultation from a practitioner.

II. Initial Examination and Evaluation/Consultation
   A. Documentation is required at the onset of each episode of physical therapy care.
   B. Documentation of the initial episode of physical therapy care shall include the following elements:
      1. Documentation of appropriate history.
         1.1 History of the presenting problem, current complaints, and precautions (including onset date).
         1.2 Pertinent diagnoses and medical history.
         1.3 Demographic characteristics, including pertinent psychological, social, and environmental factors.
         1.4 Prior or concurrent services related to the current episode of physical therapy care.
         1.5 Comorbidities that may affect the prognosis.
         1.6 Statement of patient's/client's knowledge of the problem.

1.7 Anticipated goals of and expected outcomes for the patient/client (and family members and significant others, if appropriate).
2. Documentation of a systems review:
   2.1 Documentation of physiologic and anatomical status to include the following systems:
      2.1.1 Cardiovascular/pulmonary
      2.1.2 Integumentary
      2.1.3 Musculoskeletal
      2.1.4 Neuromuscular
   2.2 A review of communication, affect, cognition, language, and learning style.
3. Documentation of selection and administration of appropriate tests and measures to determine patient/client status in a number of areas and documentation of findings. The following is a partial list of these areas to be addressed in the documented examination and evaluation, including illustrative tests and measures:
   3.1 Arousal, attention, and cognition
      Examples include examination findings related, but not limited, to the following areas:
         Ex 3.1.1 Level of consciousness
         Ex 3.1.2 Ability to process commands
         Ex 3.1.3 Gross expressive deficits
   3.2 Neuromotor development and sensory integration
      Examples include examination findings related, but not limited, to the following areas:
         Ex 3.2.1 Gross and fine motor skills
         Ex 3.2.2 Reflex movement patterns
         Ex 3.2.3 Dexterity, agility, and coordination
   3.3 Range of motion
      Examples include examination findings related, but not limited, to the following areas:
         Ex 3.3.1 Extent of joint motion
         Ex 3.3.2 Pain and soreness of surrounding soft tissue
         Ex 3.3.3 Muscle length and flexibility
   3.4 Muscle performance (including strength, power, and endurance)
      Examples include examination findings related, but not limited, to the following areas:
         Ex 3.4.1 Force, velocity, torque, work power
         Ex 3.4.2 Manual muscle test grades
         Ex 3.4.3 Amplitude, duration, waveform, and frequency of electromyographic (EMG) signals
   3.5 Ventilation, respiration (gas exchange), and circulation
      Examples include examination findings related, but not limited, to the following areas:
         Ex 3.5.1 Heart rate (HR), respiratory rate (RR), blood pressure (BP)
         Ex 3.5.2 Arterial blood gases
         Ex 3.5.3 Palpation of peripheral pulses
   3.6 Posture
      Examples include examination findings related, but not limited, to the following areas:
         Ex 3.6.1 Static posture
         Ex 3.6.2 Dynamic posture
   3.7 Gait, locomotion, and balance
      Examples include examination findings related, but not limited, to the following areas:
         Ex. 3.7.1 Characteristics of gait
         Ex. 3.7.2 Functional locomotion
         Ex. 3.7.3 Characteristics of balance
   3.8 Self-care and home management
      Examples include examination findings related, but not limited, to the following areas:
         Ex 3.8.1 Activities of daily living
         Ex 3.8.2 Functional capacity
         Ex 3.8.3 Transfers
   3.9 Community and work (job/school/play) integration or reintegration:
      Examples include examination findings related, but not limited, to the following areas:
         Ex 3.9.1 Instrumental activities of daily living
         Ex 3.9.2 Functional capacity
         Ex 3.9.3 Adaptive skills
4. Documentation of evaluation (a dynamic process in which the physical therapist makes clinical judgments based on data gathered during the examination).
5. Documentation of diagnosis (a label encompassing a cluster of signs and symptoms, syndromes or categories that reflects the information obtained from the examination).
6. Documentation of prognosis (determination of the level of optimal improvement that might be attained through intervention and the amount of time required to reach that level. Documentation shall include anticipated goals, expected outcomes, and plan of care).
   6.1 Patient/client (and family members and significant others, if appropriate) is involved in establishing anticipated goals and expected outcomes.
   6.2 All anticipated goals and expected outcomes are stated in measurable terms.
   6.3 Anticipated goals and expected outcomes are related to impairments, functional limitations, and disabilities identified in the examination.
   6.4 All expected outcomes are stated in functional terms.
   6.5 The plan of care:
      6.5.1 Is related to anticipated goals and expected outcomes.
      6.5.2 Includes frequency and duration to achieve the anticipated goals and expected outcomes.
      6.5.3 Includes patient/client and family/caregiver educational goals.
      6.5.4 Involves appropriate collaboration and coordination of care with other professionals/services.
7. Authentication by and appropriate designation of the physical therapist.

III. Documentation of the Continuation of Care
   A. Documentation of intervention or services provided and current patient/client status.
      1. Documentation is required for every visit/encounter.
         1.1 Authentication and appropriate designation of the physical therapist or the physical therapist assistant providing the service under the direction and supervision of a physical therapist.
      2. Documentation of each visit/encounter shall include the following elements:
         2.1 Patient/client self-report (as appropriate)
         2.2 Identification of specific interventions provided, including frequency, intensity and duration as appropriate.
            Examples include:
               Ex 2.2.1 Knee extension, 3 sets, 10 repetitions, 10 lb. weight.
               Ex 2.2.2 Transfer training bed to chair with sliding board.
         2.3 Equipment provided.
         2.4 Changes in patient/client status as they relate to the plan of care.
         2.5 Adverse reaction to interventions, if any.
         2.6 Factors that modify frequency or intensity of intervention and progression toward anticipated goals, including patient/client adherence to patient/client related instructions.
         2.7 Communication/consultation with providers/patient/client/family/significant other.
   B. Documentation of Reexamination
      1. Documentation of reexamination is provided as appropriate to evaluate progress and to modify or redirect intervention.
      2. Documentation of reexamination shall include the following elements:
         2.1 Documentation of elements as identified in III A.2 to update patient's/client's status.
         2.2 Interpretation of findings and, when indicated, revision of anticipated goals, and expected outcomes.
         2.3 When indicated, revision of plan of care as directly correlated with anticipated goals and expected outcomes as documented.
         2.4 Authentication by and appropriate designation of the physical therapist.

IV. Documentation of Summation of Episode of Care
   A. Documentation is required following conclusion of the current episode of the physical therapy intervention sequence.
   B. Documentation of the summation of the episode of care shall include the following elements:
      1. Criteria for discharge.
         Examples include:
            Ex 1.1 Anticipated goals and expected outcomes have been achieved.
            Ex 1.2 Patient/client, caregiver or legal guardian declines to continue intervention.
            Ex 1.3 Patient/client is unable to continue to work toward anticipated goals due to medical or psychosocial complications.
            Ex 1.4 Physical therapist determines that the patient/client will no longer benefit from physical therapy.
      2. Current physical/functional status.
      3. Degree of anticipated goals and expected outcomes achieved and reasons for goals and outcomes not being achieved.
      4. Discharge plan that includes written and verbal communication related to the patient's/client's continuing care.
         Examples include:
            Ex 4.1 Home program.
            Ex 4.2 Referrals for additional services.
            Ex 4.3 Recommendations for follow-up physical therapy care.
            Ex 4.4 Family and caregiver training.
            Ex 4.5 Equipment provided.
      5. Authentication by and appropriate designation of the physical therapist.

Additional references:
1. *Direction and supervision of the Physical Therapist Assistant* (HOD 06-99-30-42).
2. *Comprehensive Accreditation Manual for Hospitals.* Oakbrook Terrace, Ill: Joint Commission on the Accreditation of Healthcare Organizations; 1996.
3. *Glossary of Terms Related to Information Security.* Schaumburg, Ill: Computer-based Patient Record Institute; 1996.
4. *Guidelines for Establishing Information Security Policies at Organizations Using Computer-based Patient Records.* Schaumburg, Ill: Computer-based Patient Record Institute; 1995.
5. *Current Procedural Terminology.* Chicago: American Medical Association (AMA); 2000.
6. *Coding and Payment Guide for the Physical Therapist.* Washington, D.C.: St. Anthony's Publishing; 2000.
7. *Minimal Data Set (MDS) Regulations;* Healthcare Financing Administration (HCFA). Available at: www.hcfa.gov.
8. *HCFA/AMA Documentation Guidelines.* Healthcare Financing Administration (HCFA). Available at: www.hcfa.gov.
9. *Home Health Regulations.* Healthcare Financing Administration (HCFA). Available at: www.hcfa.gov.
10. *State Practice Acts.* Available at: www.fsbpt.org.

Adopted by the Board of Directors, APTA, March 1993.

Amended March 2000, November 1998, March 1997, March 1995, November 1994, June 1993, March 1993.

From American Physical Therapy Association, (Phys. Ther. 2001, Vol. 81, Number 1, 703-705), with permission.

Symbols Commonly Used in Clinical Practice

ā	Before
=	Equal
≠	Unequal
>	Greater than
<	Less than
↑	Increase
↗	Increasing
↓	Decrease
↘	Decreasing
−	Negative, minus, deficiency, alkaline, reaction
±	Very slight trace or reaction, indefinite
+	Slight trace or reaction, positive, plus excess, acid reaction
++	Trace or notable reaction
+++	Moderate amount of reaction
++++	Large amount or pronounced reaction
#	Number, pound, has been given or done
→	Yields, leads to
←	Resulting from or secondary to
1°, 2°	Primary, secondary

From Miller-Keane: Encyclopedia and Dictionary of Medicine, Nursing, and Allied Health. W.B. Saunders Company, Philadelphia 1997, p.1802, with permission.

Military Time

The 24-hour clock (military time) is used to standardize time in the medical record.

Standard Time:	Military Time:
Noon	1200 hours
1:00 PM	1300 hours
2:00 PM	1400 hours
3:00 PM	1500 hours
4:00 PM	1600 hours
5:00 PM	1700 hours
6:00 PM	1800 hours
7:00 PM	1900 hours
8:00 PM	2000 hours
9:00 PM	2100 hours
10:00 PM	2200 hours
11:00 PM	2300 hours
Midnight	2400 hours

Measurement

Length:
1 cm = 0.3937 inch
1 m = 39.37 inches = 3.28 ft = 1.09 yds
1 km = 0.62 mile
1 inch = 2.54 centimeters (cm) = 25.4 millimeters (mm) = 0.0254 meters (m)
1 foot = 30.48 cm = 304.8 mm = 0.304 m
1 mile = 5280 ft = 1760 yds = 1609.35 m = 1.61 kilometers (km)

Weight:
1 ounce (oz) = 0.0625 pounds (lb) = 28.35 grams (g) = 0.028 kilograms (kg)
1 pound (lb) = 16 oz = 454 g = 0.454 kg
1 g = 0.035 oz = 0.0022 lb = 0.001 kg
1 kg = 35.27 oz = 2.2 lb = 1000 g

Energy and Work:
1 kcal = 3086 foot-pounds (ft-lbs) = 426.4 kilogram-meter (kg-m) = kilojoules (kJ)
1 kJ = 1000 joules (J) = 0.23892 kcal
1 liter O_2 consumed = 5.05 kcal = 15.575 ft-lbs = 2153 kg-m = 21.237 kJ
1 MET = 3.5 mL O_2/kg-min = 0.0175 kcal/kg = 0.0732 kJ/kg
1 ft-lb = 0.1383 kg-m
1 kg-m = 7.23 ft-lbs

Temperature:
0°C = 32°F = 273°K
100°C = 212°F
°C = (°F − 32) x 5/9
°F = (°C x 9/5) + 32

Ethics

Ethical Principles

Autonomy: Requires that the wishes of competent individuals must be honored. Autonomy is often referred to as self-determination.

Beneficence: A moral obligation of health care providers to act for the benefit of others.

Nonmaleficence: The obligation of health care providers to above all else, do no harm.

Veracity: Obligation of health care providers to tell the truth.

UNIT NINE: ADMINISTRATION

Management

Quality Management Process

- Review selected patient medical records
- Prioritize adverse event outcomes
- Conduct a thorough review of care
- Identify problematic areas of care
- Develop a plan to change identified aspects of care
- Implement the plan
- Monitor the plan
- Determine if the implemented change results in a measurable difference

Quality Assurance

A form of objective self-examination designed to improve the quality of services.

Agencies Responsible for Quality Assurance
- Joint Commission on Accreditation of Hospitals (JCAH)
- Professional Standards Review Organization (PSRO)

Measures the structure, process, and outcome of physical therapy care. According to the American Physical Therapy Association structure, process, and outcome are defined as follows:

- **Structure**
  A review of structure is an assessment of organization, staffing and staff qualifications, rules and policies governing physical work, records, equipment, and physical facilities. The assessment may include a judgment of the adequacy as well as the presence of the element of structure being examined.

- **Process**
  Process assessment is based on the degree or extent to which the therapist conforms to accepted professional practices in providing services. The various approaches to care, their application, efficacy, adequacy, and timeliness are considered. A process review requires that considerable attention be given to developing and specifying the standards to be used in the assessment.

- **Outcome**
  Outcome assessment is based on the condition of the patient at the conclusion of care in relation to the goals of treatment. Assessment of outcome provides a means of reviewing the practitioner, the services, and events which led to the results of care. The results of outcome assessment ultimately may lead to the evaluation of the basic treatment procedures and modalities of physical therapy and validation of the approaches to patient care. Outcomes are the ultimate manifestations of effectiveness and quality of care.

Legal

Elements of a Risk Management Program

- Management involvement
- Risk management organization
- Incident reporting and investigation
- Inspections
- Communications

Recommendations to Avoid Litigation

- Conduct a thorough examination
- Seek consultation when in doubt
- Check the condition of your equipment
- Instruct patients thoroughly
- Keep the referring physician informed
- Obtain proper consent for treatment
- Do not delegate to unqualified individuals
- Keep accurate and timely written records

Legal Terminology

Abandonment: Unacceptable one-sided termination of services by a health care professional without patient consent or agreement.

Administrative law: Administrative agencies at the federal and state level develop rules and regulations to supplement statutes and executive orders.

Common law: Refers to court decisions in the absence of statutory law. Common law often creates legal precedent in areas where statutes have not been enacted.

Constitutional law: Involves law that is derived from the federal Constitution. The United States Supreme Court is responsible for ultimately interpreting and enforcing the Constitution.

Informed consent: The patient is required to sign a document and give permission to the health care professional to render treatment. This should be obtained from the patient in accordance with the standards of practice prior to initiation of treatment. The patient has the right to full disclosure of treatment procedures, risks, expected outcomes, and goals.

Malpractice: The failure to exercise the skills that would normally be exercised by other members of the profession with similar skills and training. This can include areas of professional negligence, breach of contract issues, and intentional conduct by a health care professional.

Negligence: The failure to do what a reasonable and prudent person would ordinarily have done under the same or similar circumstances for a given situation. In order to prove negligence, the plaintiff must prove all of the following:
- There was a duty owed to the plaintiff by the defendant.
- There was a breach of that duty under conditions that constituted negligence and the negligence was the proximate cause of the breach.
- There was damage to the plaintiff's person or property.

Risk management: The identification, analysis, and evaluation of risks and the selection of the most advantageous method for treating them.

Statutory law: Congress and state legislatures are responsible for enacting statutes. Examples of federal statutes affecting health care include the Americans with Disabilities Act and the Family and Medical Leave Act.

Tort: A private or civil wrong or injury, involving omission and/or commission.

Delegation and Supervision

American Physical Therapy Association Direction, Delegation, and Supervision in Physical Therapy Services

Delegated responsibilities must be commensurate with the qualifications, including experience, education and training, of the individuals to whom the responsibilities are being assigned. When the physical therapist of record delegates patient care responsibilities to physical therapist assistants or other supportive personnel, that physical therapist holds responsibility for supervision of the physical therapy program. Regardless of the setting in which the service is given, the following responsibilities must be borne solely by the physical therapist:

1. Interpretation of referrals when available.
2. Initial examination, evaluation, diagnosis, and prognosis.
3. Development or modification of a plan of care that is based on the initial examination or the reexamination and that includes physical therapy anticipated goals and expected outcomes.
4. Determination of (1) when the expertise and decision-making capability of the physical therapist requires the physical therapist to personally render physical therapy interventions and (2) when it may be appropriate to utilize the physical therapist assistant. A physical therapist determines the most appropriate utilization of the physical therapist assistant that will ensure the delivery of service that is safe, effective, and efficient.
5. Reexamination of the patient/client in light of the anticipated goals, and revision of the plan of care when indicated.
6. Establishment of the discharge plan and documentation of discharge summary/status.
7. Oversight of all documentation for services rendered to each patient.

From Guide to Physical Therapist Practice. American Physical Therapy Association, Alexandria 1999, p.1-11, with permission.

Support Personnel Supervised by Physical Therapists

Physical Therapist Assistants

The physical therapist assistant is a technically educated health care provider who assists the physical therapist in the provision of physical therapy. The physical therapist assistant, under the direction and supervision of the physical therapist, is the only paraprofessional who provides physical therapy interventions. The physical therapist assistant is a graduate of a physical therapist assistant associate degree program accredited by the Commission on Accreditation in Physical Therapy Education (CAPTE).

The physical therapist of record is directly responsible for the actions of the physical therapist assistant. The physical therapist assistant may perform specific components of physical therapy interventions, where allowable by law or regulations, that have been selected by the supervising physical therapist. The ability of the physical therapist assistant to perform the selected interventions should be assessed on an ongoing basis by the supervising physical therapist. The physical therapist assistant may modify an intervention only in accordance with changes in patient/client status and within the scope of the plan of care that has been established by the physical therapist.

Physical Therapy Aides

Aides are any support personnel who may be involved in the provision of physical therapist directed support services. The physical therapy aide is a nonlicensed worker who is specifically trained under the direction and supervision of a physical therapist.

Physical therapist directed support services are limited to those tasks which may include methods and techniques that do not require clinical decision making by the physical therapist or clinical problem solving by the physical therapist assistant. The determination of what tasks are appropriately directed to the aide must be made by the physical therapist or, where allowable by law or regulations, the physical therapist assistant. To make this determination, the physical therapist or physical therapist assistant must have direct contact with the patient/client during each session. The aide may function only with continuous on-site supervision by the physical therapist or, when allowable by law or regulations, the physical therapist assistant.

From Guide to Physical Therapist Practice. American Physical Therapy Association, Alexandria 1999, p.1-10, with permission.

Health Care Professions

Audiologists
Audiologists assess patients with suspected hearing disorders. The audiologist can educate patients on how to make the best use of their available hearing and assist them in selecting and fitting appropriate aids. Audiologists are required to possess a master's degree or equivalent. The vast majority of states require audiologists to obtain a license to practice.

Chiropractors
Chiropractors diagnose and treat patients whose health problems are associated with the body's muscular, nervous, and skeletal systems. Patient care activities include manually adjusting the spine, ordering and interpreting X-rays, performing postural analysis, and administering various physical agents. Chiropractors are required to complete a four-year chiropractic curriculum leading to the Doctor of Chiropractic degree. All states require chiropractors to obtain a license to practice.

Home Health Aides
Home health aides provide health related services to the elderly, disabled, and ill in their homes. Patient care activities include performing housekeeping duties, assisting with ambulation or transfers, and promoting personal hygiene. A registered nurse, physical therapist, or social worker is often the health care professional that assigns specific duties and supervises the home health aide. The federal government has established guidelines for home health aides whose employers receive reimbursement from Medicare. The National Association for Home Care offers voluntary national certification for home health aides.

Licensed Practical Nurses
Licensed practical nurses care for the sick, injured, convalescent, and disabled under the direction of physicians and registered nurses. Patient care activities include taking vital signs, performing transfers, applying dressings, administering injections, and instructing patients and families. In some states licensed practical nurses can administer prescribed medications or start intravenous fluids. Experienced licensed practical nurses may supervise nursing assistants and aides. Educational programs for licensed practical nurses are approximately one year in length and include classroom study and supervised clinical practice. All states require a license to practice.

Medical Assistants
Medical assistants perform routine administrative and clinical tasks in a medical office. Administrative duties include answering telephones, updating patient files, completing insurance forms, and scheduling appointments. Clinical duties include taking medical histories, measuring vital signs, and assisting the physician during treatment. Educational programs for medical assistants are typically 1-2 years in length.

Occupational Therapists
Occupational therapists help people improve their ability to perform activities of daily living, work, and leisure skills. The educational preparation of occupational therapists emphasizes the social, emotional, and physiological effects of illness and injury. Occupational therapists most commonly work with individuals who have conditions that are mentally, physically, developmentally or emotionally disabling. Occupational therapists can enter the field with bachelor's, master's or doctoral degrees. All states require occupational therapists to obtain a license to practice.

Occupational Therapy Aides
Occupational therapy aides work under the direction of occupational therapists to provide rehabilitation services to persons with mental, physical, developmental or emotional impairments. Occupational therapy aides often prepare materials and assemble equipment used during treatment and may be responsible for a variety of clerical tasks. The majority of training for occupational therapy aides occurs on the job.

Occupational Therapy Assistants
Occupational therapy assistants work under the direction of occupational therapists to provide rehabilitation services to persons with mental, physical, developmental or emotional impairments. Occupational therapy assistants perform a variety of rehabilitative activities and exercises as outlined in an established treatment plan. To practice as an occupational therapy assistant individuals must complete an associate's degree or certificate program from an accredited academic institution. Occupational therapy assistants are regulated in the majority of states.

Physical Therapists
Physical therapists provide services to help restore function, improve mobility, relieve pain, and prevent or limit permanent physical disabilities of patients suffering from injuries or disease. Physical therapists engage in examination, evaluation, diagnosis, prognosis, and intervention in an effort to maximize patient outcomes. Physical therapists can enter the field with bachelor's, master's or doctoral degrees. In 2002, all physical therapy programs seeking accreditation will be required to offer a minimum of a master's degree. All states require physical therapists to obtain a license to practice.

Physical Therapist Aides
Physical therapy aides are considered support personnel who may be involved in support services directed by physical therapists. Physical therapy aides receive on the job training under the direction and supervision of a physical therapist and are permitted to function only with continuous on-site supervision by a physical therapist or in some cases a physical therapist assistant. Support services are limited to methods and techniques that do not require clinical decision making by the physical therapist or clinical problem solving by the physical therapist assistant.

Physical Therapist Assistants
Physical therapist assistants perform components of physical therapy procedures and related tasks selected and delegated by a supervising physical therapist. Physical therapist assistants may modify an intervention only in accordance with changes in patient status and within the established plan of care developed by the physical therapist. Physical therapist assistants are the only paraprofessionals that perform physical therapy interventions. Typically physical therapist assistants have an associate's degree from an accredited physical therapist assistant program. The majority of states require physical therapist assistants to obtain a license to practice.

Physicians
Physicians diagnose illnesses and prescribe and administer treatment for people suffering from injury or disease. The term physician encompasses both the Doctor of Medicine (M.D.) and the Doctor of Osteopathic Medicine (D.O.). The role of the M.D. and D.O. are very similar, however the D.O. tends to place special emphasis on the body's musculoskeletal system, preventive medicine, and holistic patient care. All states require physicians to obtain a license to practice.

Physician Assistants
Physician assistants provide health care services with supervision by physicians. The supervising physician and established state law determine the specific duties of the physician assistant. In the vast majority of states physician assistants may prescribe medication. Physician assistants work with the supervision of a physician. All states with the exception of Mississippi require physician assistants to obtain a license to practice.

Psychologists
Psychologists use various techniques including interviewing and testing to advise people how to deal with problems of every day life. In the health care setting psychologists may be involved in counseling programs designed to help people achieve goals such as weight loss or smoking cessation. A doctoral degree is usually required for employment as a licensed clinical or counseling psychologist. All states require psychologists to obtain a license to practice.

Recreational Therapists
Recreational therapists provide treatment services and recreation activities to individuals with disabilities or illness. In acute care hospitals and rehabilitation hospitals recreational therapists work closely with other health care professionals to treat and rehabilitate individuals with specific medical conditions. In long-term care settings recreational therapists function primarily by offering structured group sessions emphasizing leisure activities. Recreational therapists are required to have a bachelor's degree in order to be eligible for certification as certified therapeutic recreation specialists.

Registered Nurses
Registered nurses work to promote health, prevent disease, and help patients cope with illness. Patient care activities are extremely diverse including tasks such as assisting physicians during treatments and examinations, administering medications, recording symptoms and reactions, and instructing patients and families. Registered nurse programs include associate's, bachelor's, and diploma programs. All states require registered nurses to obtain a license to practice.

Respiratory Therapists
Respiratory therapists evaluate, treat, and care for patients with breathing disorders. The vast majority of respiratory therapists are employed in hospitals. Patient care activities include performing bronchial drainage techniques, measuring lung capacities, administering oxygen and aerosols, and analyzing oxygen and carbon dioxide concentrations. Educational programs for respiratory therapists are offered by hospitals, colleges, and universities, vocational-technical institutes, and the military. The vast majority of states require respiratory therapists to obtain a license to practice.

Social Worker
Social workers help patients and their families to cope with chronic, acute or terminal illnesses and attempt to resolve problems that stand in the way of recovery or rehabilitation. A bachelor's degree is often the minimum requirement to qualify for employment as a social worker, however in the health field the master's degree is often required. All states have licensing, certification or registration requirements for social workers.

Speech-Language Pathologists
Speech-language pathologists evaluate speech, language, cognitive-communication, and swallowing skills of children and adults. The majority of practitioners provide direct clinical services to individuals with communication disorders. Speech-language pathologists are required to possess a master's degree or equivalent. The vast majority of states require speech-language pathologists to obtain a license to practice.

Physical Therapy Practice

The Elements of Patient/Client Management Leading to Optimal Outcomes

Examination: The process of obtaining a history, performing a systems review, and selecting and administering tests and measures to gather data about the patient/client. The initial examination is a comprehensive screening and specific testing process that leads to a diagnostic classification. The examination process also may identify possible problems that require consultation with, or referral to, another provider.

Evaluation: A dynamic process in which the physical therapist makes clinical judgments based on data gathered during the examination. This process also may identify possible problems that require consultation with, or referral to, another provider.

Diagnosis: Both the process and the end result of evaluating examination data, which the physical therapist organizes into defined clusters, syndromes or categories to help determine the prognosis (including the plan of care) and the most appropriate intervention strategies.

Prognosis (Including Plan of Care): Determination of the level of optimal improvement that may be attained through intervention and the amount of time required to reach that level. The plan of care specifies the interventions to be used and their timing and frequency.

Intervention: Purposeful and skilled interaction of the physical therapist with the patient/client and, if appropriate, with other individuals involved in the care of the patient/client, using various physical therapy methods and techniques to produce changes in the condition that are consistent with the diagnosis and prognosis. The physical therapist conducts a reexamination to determine changes in patient/client status and to modify or redirect intervention. The decision to reexamine may be based on new clinical findings or on lack of patient/client progress. The process of reexamination also may identify the need for consultation with, or referral to, another provider.

Outcomes: Results of patient/client management, which include the impact of physical therapy interventions in the following domains: pathology/pathophysiology (disease, disorder, or condition); impairments, functional limitations, and disabilities, risk reduction/prevention, health, wellness, and fitness; societal resources; and patient/client satisfaction.

From Guide to Physical Therapist Practice. American Physical Therapy Association, (Phys. Ther. 2001, Vol. 81, Number 1, 43), with permission.

Standards of Practice for Physical Therapy and the Criteria

Preamble
The physical therapy profession is committed to providing an optimum level of service delivery and to striving for excellence in practice. The House of Delegates of the American Physical Therapy Association, as the formal body that represents the profession, attests to this commitment by adopting and promoting the following *Standards of Practice for Physical Therapy*. These *Standards* are the profession's statement of conditions and performances that are essential for provision of high quality physical therapy. The *Standards* provide a foundation for assessment of physical therapy practice.

I. Legal/Ethical Considerations
A. Legal Considerations
The physical therapist complies with all the legal requirements of jurisdictions regulating the practice of physical therapy.

The physical therapist assistant complies with all the legal requirements of jurisdictions regulating the work of the assistant.

B. Ethical Considerations
The physical therapist practices according to the *Code of Ethics* of the American Physical Therapy Association.

The physical therapist assistant complies with the *Standards of Ethical Conduct for the Physical Therapist Assistant* of the American Physical Therapy Association.

II. Administration of the Physical Therapy Service
A. Statement of Mission, Purposes, and Goals
The physical therapy service has a statement of mission, purposes, and goals that reflects the needs and interests of the patients and clients served, the physical therapy personnel affiliated with the service, and the community.

The statement of mission, purposes, and goals:
- Defines the scope and limitations of the physical therapy service.
- Identifies the goals and objectives of the service.
- Is reviewed annually.

B. Organizational Plan
The physical therapy service has a written organizational plan.

The organizational plan:
- Describes relationships among components within the physical therapy service and, where the service

is part of a larger organization, between the service and other components of that organization.
- Ensures that the service is directed by a physical therapist.
- Defines supervisory structures within the service.
- Reflects current personnel functions.

C. **Policies and Procedures**
The physical therapy service has written policies and procedures that reflect the operation of the service and that are consistent with the mission, purposes, and goals of the service.

The written policies and procedures:
- Are reviewed regularly and revised as necessary.
- Meet the requirements for federal and state law and external agencies.
- Apply to, but are not limited to:
  --Clinical education
  --Clinical research
  --Multidisciplinary collaboration
  --Criteria for access to care
  --Criteria for initiation and continuation of care
  --Criteria for referral to other appropriate health care providers
  --Criteria for termination of care
  --Equipment maintenance
  --Environmental safety
  --Fiscal management
  --Infection control
  --Job/position descriptions
  --Competency assessment
  --Medical emergencies
  --Care of patients/clients, including guidelines
  --Rights of patients/clients
  --Personnel-related policies
  --Improvement of quality of care and performance of services
  --Documentation
  --Staff orientation

D. **Administration**
A physical therapist is responsible for the direction of the physical therapy service.

The physical therapist is responsible for the direction of the physical therapy service:
- Ensures compliance with local, state, and federal requirements.
- Ensures compliance with current APTA documents, including Standards of Practice for Physical Therapy and the Criteria, Guide to Physical Therapist Practice, Code of Ethics, Guide for Professional Conduct, Standards of Ethical Conduct for the Physical Therapist Assistant, and Guide for Conduct of the Affiliate Member.
- Ensures that services are consistent with the mission, purposes, and goals of the physical therapy service.
- Ensures that services are provided in accordance with established policies and procedures.
- Reviews and updates policies and procedures.
- Provides training of physical therapy support personnel that ensures continued competence for their job description.
- Provides for continuous inservice training on safety issues and for periodic safety inspection of equipment by qualified individuals.

E. **Fiscal Management**
The director of the physical therapy service, in consultation with physical therapy staff and appropriate administrative personnel, participates in planning for, and allocation of, resources. Fiscal planning and management of the service are based on sound accounting principles.

The fiscal management plan:
- Includes a budget that provides for optimal use of resources.
- Ensures accurate recording and reporting of financial information.
- Ensures compliance with legal requirements.
- Allows for cost-effective utilization of resources.
- Uses a fee schedule that is consistent with the cost of physical therapy services and that is within customary norms of fairness and reasonableness.

F. **Improvement of Quality of Care and Performance**
The physical therapy service has a written plan for continuous improvement of quality of care and performance of services.

The improvement plan:
- Provides evidence of ongoing review and evaluation of the physical therapy service.
- Provides a mechanism for documenting improvement in quality of care and performance.
- Is consistent with requirements of external agencies, as applicable.

G. **Staffing**
The physical therapy personnel affiliated with the physical therapy service demonstrate competence and are sufficient to achieve the mission, purposes, and goals of the service.

The physical therapy service:
- Meets all legal requirements regarding licensure and certification of appropriate personnel.
- Ensures that the level of expertise within the service is appropriate to the needs of the patients/clients served.
- Provides appropriate professional and support personnel to meet the needs of the patient/client population.

H. Staff Development
The physical therapy service has a written plan that provides for appropriate and ongoing staff development.

The staff development plan:
- Includes self-assessment, individual goal setting, and organizational needs in directing continuing education and learning activities.
- Includes strategies for lifelong learning and professional career development.
- Includes mechanisms to foster mentorship activities.

I. Physical Setting
The physical setting is designed to provide a safe and accessible environment that facilitates fulfillment of the mission, purposes, and goals of the physical therapy service. The equipment is safe and sufficient to achieve the purposes and goals of the service.

The physical setting:
- Meets all applicable legal requirements for health and safety.
- Meets space needs appropriate for the number and type of patients and clients served.

The equipment:
- Meets all applicable legal requirements for health and safety.
- Is inspected routinely.

J. Multidisciplinary Collaboration
The physical therapy service collaborates with all appropriate disciplines.

The collaboration when appropriate:
- Uses a multidisciplinary team approach to the care of patients and clients.
- Provides multidisciplinary instruction of patients and clients, and families.
- Ensures multidisciplinary professional development and continuing education.

III. Provision of Services
A. Informed Consent
The physical therapist has sole responsibility for providing information to the patient or client and for obtaining informed consent in accordance with jurisdictional law before initiating intervention.

In obtaining the informed consent of the patient or client, the physical therapist:
- Clearly describes the proposed intervention and delineates the expected benefits and material (decisional) risks as known with the proposed intervention.
- Compares known benefits and risks with and without the proposed intervention, and explains reasonable alternatives to the intervention.

Patient or client informed consent obtained by the physical therapist:
- Requires consent of a competent adult.
- Requires consent of a parent or legal guardian as the surrogate decision maker when the adult patient is not competent or when the patient is a minor.
- Requires the patient, client or legal guardian to acknowledge understanding of the intervention and to give consent before intervention is initiated.

B. Initial Examination and Evaluation
The physical therapist performs and documents an initial examination and evaluates the data to identify problems and determine the diagnosis prior to intervention.

The physical therapist examination:
- Is documented, dated, and appropriately authenticated by the physical therapist who performed it.
- Identifies the physical therapy needs of the patient or client.
- Incorporates appropriate tests and measures to facilitate outcome measurement.
- Produces data that are sufficient to allow evaluation, diagnosis, prognosis, and the establishment of a plan of care.
- May result in recommendations for additional services to meet the needs of the patient or client.

C. Plan of Care
The physical therapist establishes and provides a plan of care for the patient or client based on the evaluation of the examination data and patient or client needs.

The physical therapist involves the patient and appropriate others in the planning, implementation, and assessment of the intervention program.

The physical therapist, in consultation with appropriate disciplines, plans for discharge of the patient or client, taking into consideration the level of goal attainment and provides for appropriate follow-up or referral.

The plan of care:
- Is based on the examination, evaluation, diagnosis and prognosis.
- Identifies anticipated goals and expected outcomes.
- Describes the proposed intervention, including frequency and duration.

- Includes documentation that is dated and appropriately authenticated by the physical therapist who established the plan of care.

D. Intervention
The physical therapist provides, or directs and supervises, the physical therapy intervention in a manner that is consistent with the examination data, the evaluation, and the plan of care.

The physical therapist documents, on an ongoing basis, services provided, responses to the services, and changes in the status of the patient or client relative to the plan of care.

The intervention:
- Is based on the examination, evaluation, diagnosis, prognosis, and plan of care.
- Is provided under the ongoing direction and supervision of the physical therapist.
- Is provided in such a way that directed and supervised responsibilities are commensurate with the qualifications and the legal limitations of the physical therapist assistant.
- Is altered in accordance with changes in response or status.
- Is provided at a level that is consistent with current physical therapy practice.
- Is multidisciplinary when necessary to meet the needs of the patient or client.
- Documentation of the intervention is consistent with the Guidelines for Physical Therapy Documentation.
- Is dated and appropriately authenticated by the physical therapist or when permissible by law, by the physical therapist assistant, or both.

E. Reexamination and Reevaluation
The physical therapist continually reexamines the patient, reevaluates the data, and modifies the plan of care or discontinues the plan accordingly.

The physical therapist reexamination:
- Is documented, dated, and appropriately authenticated by the physical therapist who performs it.
- Includes modifications to the plan of care.

F. Discharge/Discontinuation of Intervention
The physical therapist discharges the patient or client from physical therapy intervention when the goals and projected outcomes have been attained.

Intervention is discontinued when the goals and expected functional outcomes are attained, the patient or client declines to continue care, the patient or client is unable to continue receiving care, or the physical therapist determines that intervention is no longer warranted.

Discharge documentation
- Includes the status of the patient or client at discharge and the goals and functional outcomes attained.
- Is dated and appropriately authenticated by the physical therapist who performed the discharge.
- Includes, when a patient or client is discharged prior to attainment of goals and functional outcomes, the status of the patient or client and the rationale for discontinuation.

IV. Education
The physical therapist is responsible for individual professional development. The physical therapist assistant is responsible for individual career development.

The physical therapist participates in the education of physical therapist students, physical therapist assistant students, and students in other health professions.

The physical therapist educates and provides consultation to consumers and the general public regarding the purposes and benefits of physical therapy.

The physical therapist educates and provides consultation to consumers and the general public regarding the roles of the physical therapist and the physical therapist assistant.

The physical therapist:
- Educates and provides consultation to consumers and the general public regarding the roles of the physical therapist, the physical therapist assistant, and other support personnel.

V. Research
The physical therapist applies research findings to practice and encourages, participates in, and promotes activities that establish the outcomes of patient or client management provided by the physical therapist.

The physical therapist supports collaborative and multidisciplinary research.

The physical therapist:
- Ensures that his or her knowledge of research literature related to practice is current.
- Ensures that the rights of study subjects are protected and the integrity of research is maintained.
- Participates in the research process as appropriate to individual education, experience, and expertise.
- Educates physical therapists, physical therapist assistants, students, other health professionals, and the general public about the outcomes of physical therapist practice.

VI. Community Responsibility

The physical therapist demonstrates community responsibility by participating in community and community agency activities, educating the public, formulating public policy, or providing pro bono physical therapy services.

The physical therapist:
- Participates in community and community agency activities.
- Educates the public, including prevention education and health promotion.
- Helps formulate public policy.
- Provides pro bono physical therapy services.

Adopted by the House of Delegates, APTA, June 1980.
Amended June 2000, June 1999, June 1996, June 1991, June 1985.

From Standards of Practice for Physical Therapy and Criteria. American Physical Therapy Association, (Phys. Ther. 2001, Vol. 81, Number 1, 693-696), with permission.

Code of Ethics

Preamble
This *Code of Ethics* of the American Physical Therapy Association sets forth principles for the ethical practice of physical therapy. All physical therapists are responsible for maintaining and promoting ethical practice. To this end, the physical therapist shall act in the best interest of the patient/client. This *Code of Ethics* shall be binding on all physical therapists.

Principle 1
A physical therapist shall respect the rights and dignity of all individuals and shall provide compassionate care.

Principle 2
A physical therapist shall act in a trustworthy manner toward patients/clients and in all other aspects of physical therapy practice.

Principle 3
A physical therapist shall comply with laws and regulations governing physical therapy and shall strive to effect changes that benefit patients/clients.

Principle 4
A physical therapist shall exercise sound professional judgment.

Principle 5
A physical therapist shall achieve and maintain professional competence.

Principle 6
A physical therapist shall maintain and promote high standards for physical therapy practice, education, and research.

Principle 7
A physical therapist shall seek only such remuneration as is deserved and reasonable for physical therapy services.

Principle 8
A physical therapist shall provide and make available accurate and relevant information to patients/clients about their care and to the public about physical therapy services.

Principle 9
A physical therapist shall protect the public and the profession from unethical, incompetent, and illegal acts.

Principle 10
A physical therapist shall endeavor to address the health needs of society.

Principle 11
A physical therapist shall respect the rights, knowledge, and skills of colleagues and other health care professionals.

Adopted by the House of Delegates, APTA, June 1973.
Amended June 2000, June 1991, June 1987, June 1981, June 1978, June 1977.

From Code of Ethics, American Physical Therapy Association, (Phys. Ther. 2001, Vol. 81, Number 1, 697), with permission.

Guide for Professional Conduct

Purpose
This *Guide for Professional Conduct* (Guide) is intended to serve physical therapists in interpreting the *Code of Ethics* (Code) of the American Physical Therapy Association (Association), in matters of professional conduct. The Guide provides guidelines by which physical therapists may determine the propriety of their conduct. It is also intended to guide the professional development of physical therapist students. The Code and the Guide apply to all physical therapists. These guidelines are subject to change as the dynamics of the profession change and as new patterns of health care delivery are developed and accepted by the professional community and the public. This Guide is subject to monitoring and timely revision by the Ethics and Judicial Committee of the Association.

Interpreting Ethical Principles
The interpretations expressed in this Guide reflect the opinions, decisions, and advice of the Ethics and Judicial Committee. These interpretations are intended to assist a physical therapist in applying general ethical principles to specific situations. They should not be considered inclusive of all situations that could evolve.

Principle 1:
A physical therapist shall respect the rights and dignity of all individuals and shall provide compassionate care.

1.1 Attitudes of a Physical Therapist
A. A physical therapist shall recognize individual differences and shall respect and be responsive to those differences.
B. A physical therapist shall be guided by concern for the physical, psychological, and socioeconomic welfare of patients/clients.
C. A physical therapist shall not harass, abuse or discriminate against others.
D. A physical therapist shall be aware of the patient's health-related needs and act in a manner that facilitates meeting those needs.

Principle 2:
A physical therapist shall act in a trustworthy manner towards patients/clients, and in all other aspects of physical therapy practice.

2.1 Patient/Physical Therapist Relationship
A. To act in a trustworthy manner the physical therapist shall act in the patient/client's best interest. Working in the patient/client's best interest requires knowledge of the patient/client's needs from the patient/client's perspective. Patients/clients often come to the physical therapist in a vulnerable state and normally will rely on the physical therapist's advice, which they perceive to be based on superior knowledge, skill, and experience. The trustworthy physical therapist acts to ameliorate the patient's/client's vulnerability, not to exploit it.
B. A physical therapist shall not exploit any aspect of the physical therapist/patient relationship.
C. A physical therapist shall not engage in any sexual relationship or activity, whether consensual or nonconsensual, with any patient while a physical therapist/patient relationship exists.
D. The physical therapist shall create an environment that encourages an open dialogue with the patient/client.
E. In the event the physical therapist or patient terminates the physical therapist/patient relationship while the patient continues to need physical therapy services, the physical therapist should take steps to transfer the care of the patient to another provider.

2.2 Truthfulness
A physical therapist shall not make statements that he/she knows or should know are false, deceptive, fraudulent or unfair. See Section 8.2.D.

2.3 Confidential Information
A. Information relating to the physical therapist/patient relationship is confidential and may not be communicated to a third party not involved in that patient's care without the prior consent of the patient, subject to applicable law.
B. Information derived from peer review shall be held confidential by the reviewer unless the physical therapist who was reviewed consents to the release of the information.
C. A physical therapist may disclose information to appropriate authorities when it is necessary to protect the welfare of an individual or the community or when required by law. Such disclosure shall be in accordance with applicable law.

2.4 Patient Autonomy and Consent
A. A physical therapist shall not restrict patients' freedom to select their provider of physical therapy.
B. A physical therapist shall communicate to the patient/client the findings of his/her examination, evaluation, diagnosis, and prognosis.
C. A physical therapist shall collaborate with the patient/client to establish the goals of treatment and the plan of care.
D. A physical therapist shall inform the patient/client of the benefits, costs, and substantial risks (if any) of the recommended intervention and treatment alternatives.
E. A physical therapist shall respect the patient's/client's right to make decisions regarding the recommended plan of care, including consent, modification, or refusal.

Principle 3:
A physical therapist shall comply with laws and regulations governing physical therapy and shall strive to effect changes that benefit patients/clients.

3.1 **Professional Practice**
A physical therapist shall provide examination, evaluation, diagnosis, prognosis, and intervention. A physical therapist shall not engage in any unlawful activity that substantially relates to the qualifications, functions or duties of a physical therapist.

3.2 **Just Laws and Regulations**
A physical therapist shall advocate the adoption of laws, regulations, and policies by providers, employers, third party payers, legislatures, and regulatory agencies to provide and improve access to necessary health care services for all individuals.

3.3 **Unjust Laws and Regulations**
A physical therapist shall endeavor to change unjust laws, regulations, and policies that govern the practice of physical therapy. See Section 10.2.

Principle 4:
A physical therapist shall exercise sound professional judgment.

4.1 **Professional Responsibility**
 A. A physical therapist shall make professional judgments that are in the patient/client's best interests.
 B. Regardless of practice setting, a physical therapist has primary responsibility for the physical therapy care of a patient and shall make independent judgments regarding that care consistent with accepted professional standards. See Section 2.4.
 C. A physical therapist shall not provide physical therapy services to a patient/client while his/her ability to do so safely is impaired.
 D. A physical therapist shall exercise sound professional judgment based upon his/her knowledge, skill, education, training, and experience.
 E. Upon accepting a patient/client for physical therapy services, a physical therapist shall be responsible for: the examination, evaluation, and diagnosis of that individual; the prognosis and intervention; re-examination and modification of the plan of care; and the maintenance of adequate records, including progress reports. A physical therapist shall establish the plan of care and shall provide and/or supervise and direct the appropriate interventions. See Section 2.4.
 F. If the diagnostic process reveals findings that are outside the scope of the physical therapist's knowledge, experience, or expertise, the physical therapist shall so inform the patient/client and refer to an appropriate practitioner.
 G. When the patient has been referred from another practitioner, the physical therapist shall communicate the findings of the examination and evaluation, the diagnosis, the proposed intervention, and reexamination findings (as indicated) to the referring practitioner.
 H. A physical therapist shall determine when a patient/client will no longer benefit from physical therapy services.

4.2 **Direction and Supervision**
 A. The supervising physical therapist has primary responsibility for the physical therapy care rendered to a patient/client.
 B. A physical therapist shall not delegate to a less qualified person any activity that requires the unique skill, knowledge, and judgment of the physical therapist.

4.3 **Practice Arrangements**
 A. Participation in a business, partnership, corporation, or other entity does not exempt physical therapists, whether employers, partners, or stockholders, either individually or collectively, from the obligation to promote, maintain and comply with the ethical principles of the Association.
 B. A physical therapist shall advise his/her employer(s) of any employer practice that causes a physical therapist to be in conflict with the ethical principles of the Association. A physical therapist shall seek to eliminate aspects of his/her employment that are in conflict with the ethical principles of the Association.

4.4 **Gifts and Other Considerations**
A physical therapist shall not accept or offer gifts or other considerations that affect or give an appearance of affecting his/her professional judgment.

Principle 5:
A physical therapist shall achieve and maintain professional competence.

5.1 **Scope of Competence**
A physical therapist shall practice within the scope of his/her competence and commensurate with his/her level of education, training, and experience.

5.2 **Self-assessment**
A physical therapist shall engage in self-assessment, which is a lifelong professional responsibility for maintaining competence.

5.3 **Professional Development**
A physical therapist shall participate in educational activities that enhance his/her basic knowledge and skills.

Principle 6:
A physical therapist shall maintain and promote high standards for physical therapy practice, education and research.

6.1 Professional Standards
A physical therapist shall know the accepted professional standards when engaging in physical therapy practice, education and/or research. A physical therapist shall continuously engage in assessment activities to determine compliance with these standards. If a physical therapist is not in compliance with these standards, he/she shall engage in activities designed to reach compliance with the standards. When a physical therapist is in compliance with these standards, he/she shall engage in activities designed to maintain such compliance.

6.2 Practice
A. A physical therapist shall achieve and maintain professional competence. See Section 5.
B. A physical therapist shall demonstrate his/her commitment to quality improvement by engaging in peer and utilization review and other self-assessment activities.

6.3 Professional Education
A. A physical therapist shall support high quality education in academic and clinical settings.
B. A physical therapist participating in the educational process is responsible to the students, the academic institutions, and the clinical settings for promoting ethical conduct. A physical therapist shall model ethical behavior and provide the student with information about the Code of Ethics, opportunities to discuss ethical conflicts, and procedures for reporting unresolved ethical conflicts. See Section 9.

6.4 Continuing Education
A. A physical therapist providing continuing education must be competent in the content area.
B. When a physical therapist provides continuing education, he/she shall ensure that course content, objectives, faculty credentials, and responsibilities of the instructional staff are accurately stated in the promotional and instructional course materials.
C. A physical therapist shall evaluate the efficacy and effectiveness of information and techniques presented in continuing education programs before integrating them into his or her practice.

6.5 Research
A. A physical therapist shall support research activities that contribute knowledge for improved patient care.
B. A physical therapist shall report to appropriate authorities any acts in the conduct or presentation of research that appear unethical or illegal. See Section 9.

Principle 7:
A physical therapist shall seek only such remuneration as is deserved and reasonable for physical therapy services.

7.1 Business and Employment Practices
A. A physical therapist's business/employment practices shall be consistent with the ethical principles of the Association.
B. A physical therapist shall never place his/her own financial interest above the welfare of individuals under his/her care.
C. A physical therapist shall recognize that third-party payer contracts may limit, in one form or another, the provision of physical therapy services. Third-party limitations do not absolve the physical therapist from making sound professional judgments that are in the patient's best interest. A physical therapist shall avoid under utilization of physical therapy services.
D. When a physical therapist's judgment is that a patient will receive negligible benefit from physical therapy services, the physical therapist shall not provide or continue to provide such services if the primary reason for doing so is to further the financial self-interest of the physical therapist or his/her employer. A physical therapist shall avoid over utilization of physical therapy services.
E. Fees for physical therapy services should be reasonable for the service performed, considering the setting in which it is provided, practice costs in the geographic area, judgment of other organizations, and other relevant factors.
F. A physical therapist shall not directly or indirectly request, receive, or participate in the dividing, transferring, assigning or rebating of an unearned fee.
G. A physical therapist shall not profit by means of credit or other valuable consideration, such as an unearned commission, discount, or gratuity, in connection with the furnishing of physical therapy services.
H. Unless laws impose restrictions to the contrary, physical therapists who provide physical therapy services within a business entity may pool fees and monies received. Physical therapists may divide or apportion these fees and monies in accordance with the business agreement.
I. A physical therapist may enter into agreements with organizations to provide physical therapy services if such agreements do not violate the ethical principles of the Association or applicable laws.

7.2 Endorsement of Products or Services
A. A physical therapist shall not exert influence on individuals under his/her care or their families to

use products or services based on the direct or indirect financial interest of the physical therapist in such products or services. Realizing that these individuals will normally rely on the physical therapist's advice, their best interest must always be maintained, as must their right of free choice relating to the use of any product or service. Although it cannot be considered unethical for physical therapists to own or have a financial interest in the production, sale or distribution of products/services, they must act in accordance with law and make full disclosure of their interest whenever individuals under their care use such products/services.

- B. A physical therapist may receive remuneration for endorsement or advertisement of products or services to the public, physical therapists, or other health professionals provided he/she discloses any financial interest in the production, sale, or distribution of said products or services.
- C. When endorsing or advertising products or services, a physical therapist shall use sound professional judgment and shall not give the appearance of Association endorsement unless the Association has formally endorsed the products or services.

7.3 **Disclosure**
A physical therapist shall disclose to the patient if the referring practitioner derives compensation from the provision of physical therapy.

Principle 8:
A physical therapist shall provide and make available accurate and relevant information to patients/clients about their care and to the public about physical therapy services.

8.1 **Accurate and Relevant Information to the Patient**
- A. A physical therapist shall provide the patient/client information about his/her condition and plan of care. See Section 2.4
- B. Upon the request of the patient, the physical therapist shall provide, or make available, the medical record to the patient or a patient-designated third party.
- C. A physical therapist shall inform patients of any known financial limitations that may affect their care.
- D. A physical therapist shall inform the patient when, in his/her judgment, the patient will receive negligible benefit from further care. See Section 7.1.C.

8.2 **Accurate and Relevant Information to the Public**
- A. A physical therapist shall inform the public about the societal benefits of the profession and who is qualified to provide physical therapy services.
- B. Information given to the public shall emphasize that individual problems cannot be treated without individualized examination and plans/programs of care.
- C. A physical therapist may advertise his/her services to the public.
- D. A physical therapist shall not use, or participate in the use of, any form of communication containing a false, plagiarized, fraudulent, deceptive, unfair, or sensational statement or claim.
- E. A physical therapist who places a paid advertisement shall identify it as such unless it is apparent from the context that it is a paid advertisement.

Principle 9:
A physical therapist shall protect the public and the profession from unethical, incompetent and illegal acts.

9.1 **Consumer Protection**
- A. A physical therapist shall provide care that is within the scope of practice as defined by the state practice act.
- B. A physical therapist shall not engage in any conduct that is unethical, incompetent or illegal.
- C. A physical therapist shall report any conduct that appears to be unethical, incompetent, or illegal.
- D. A physical therapist may not participate in any arrangements in which patients are exploited due to the referring sources' enhancing their personal incomes as a result of referring for, prescribing, or recommending physical therapy. See Section 5.

Principle 10:
A physical therapist shall endeavor to address the health needs of society.

10.1 **Pro Bono Services**
A physical therapist shall render pro bono publico (reduced or no fee) services to patients lacking the ability to pay for services, as each physical therapist's practice permits.

10.2 **Community Health**
A physical therapist shall endeavor to support activities that benefit the health status of the community. See Section 3.

Principle 11:
A physical therapist shall respect the rights, knowledge, and skills of colleagues and other healthcare professionals.

11.1 **Consultation**
A physical therapist shall seek consultation whenever the welfare of the patient will be safeguarded or advanced by consulting those who have special skills, knowledge or experience.

11.2 **Patient/Provider Relationships**
A physical therapist shall not undermine the relationship(s) between his/her patient and other healthcare professionals.

11.3 **Disparagement**
Physical therapists shall not disparage colleagues and other healthcare professionals. See Section 9 and Section 2.4.A.

Issued by Ethics and Judicial Committee
American Physical Therapy Association
October 1981
Last Amended January 2001

From Guide to Professional Conduct, American Physical Therapy Association, updated March 2001, with permission.

Health Insurance

There are three major classifications of health insurance companies. They include private health insurance companies, independent health plans, and government health insurance.

Private Health Insurance Companies

Private health insurance companies include stock companies, mutual companies, and nonprofit insurance plans. Reimbursement for physical therapy services is usually on a fee for service basis.

Stock Companies: Operated nationally and are owned by independent stockholders.

Mutual Companies: Operated nationally and are owned by the individual policyholders.

Nonprofit Insurance Plans: Operate in a specific geographic region and are subject to specific state regulations. They are classified as tax exempt due to their nonprofit status.

Independent Health Plans

Independent health plans are organized by various groups. Health maintenance organizations and self insurance plans are examples of independent health plans. Reimbursement is typically based on fee for service or a predetermined fixed fee.

Managed care: A concept of health care delivery where subscribers utilize health care providers that are contracted by the insurance company at a lower cost. Health maintenance organizations (HMO) and preferred provider organizations (PPO) are two examples of a managed care system. This concept attempts to attain the highest quality of care at the lowest cost.

Health maintenance organization: Subscribers to these insurance plans agree to receive all of their health care services through the predetermined providers of the HMO. The primary physician of the subscriber controls health care access through a referral system. Cost containment is a high priority and subscribers cannot receive care from providers outside of the plan except in an emergency.

Preferred provider organization: Subscribers can choose their health care services from a list of providers that contract with the insurance plan. These contracts provide extreme discounts for health care. Subscribers can use a health care provider that is not associated with the PPO, however they will absorb a greater portion of the cost.

Government Health Insurance

Government health insurance such as Medicare and Medicaid is administered by the federal government. The government uses private contractors to manage the payment process of each health plan.

Medicare

Medicare provides health insurance for individuals over 65 years of age and the disabled. Medicare is a nationwide program operated by the Health Care Financing Administration.

Established in 1966, Medicare was the second mandated health insurance program in the United State (Workers' Compensation was the first). In 1972 Medicare coverage was expanded to include certain categories of the disabled, renal dialysis, and transplant patients.

- **Medicare Part A:**
  Provides benefits for care provided in hospitals, outpatient diagnostic services, extended care facilities, and short-term care at home required by an illness for which the patient is hospitalized.

  Enrollment in Medicare Part A is automatic and funding is through payroll taxes.

- **Medicare Part B:**
  Provides benefits for outpatient care, physician services and services ordered by physicians such as diagnostic tests, medical equipment, and supplies.

  Enrollment in Medicare Part B is voluntary and funding is through premiums paid by beneficiaries and general federal tax revenues.

Cost Sharing

The Medicare program requires beneficiaries to share in the costs of health care through deductibles and coinsurance.

- **Deductibles** require beneficiaries to reach a predetermined amount of personal expenditure each 12-month period before Medicare payment is activated.

- **Coinsurance** requires that 20% of the costs for hospitalization is covered by the patient.

Medicare sets limits on the total days of hospital care that will be paid based on a lifetime pool of days limit. Medicare payments for post hospital stays in extended care facilities are limited to 100 days.

Providers are reimbursed for Medicare services through intermediaries such as Blue Cross.

Medicaid

Medicaid provides basic medical services to the economically indigent population who qualify by reason of low income or who qualify for welfare or public assistance benefits in the state of their residence. Medicaid is a jointly funded program through the federal and state governments.

Established in 1965, Medicaid is funded through personal income, corporate and excise taxes. Federal and state support is shared based on the state's per capita income.

Rate setting formulas, procedures, and policies vary widely among states. All state Medicaid operations must be approved by the Health Care Financing Administration. The Medicaid program reimburses providers directly.

The Medicaid program covers inpatient and outpatient hospital services, physician services, diagnostic services, nursing care for older adults, home health care, preventative health screening services, and family planning services.

Workers' compensation

First designed in 1911 to provide protection for employees that were injured on the job. This legislation provides continued income as well as paid medical expenses for employees injured while working. Recently case managers have assisted this process by monitoring the rehabilitation process and controlling potential abuse.

Employers with 10 or more employees or high risk employers must pay a percentage of each employee salary to the worker's compensation board of the state. The exact payment is based on the risk rating of the job or institution.

Fee for Service versus Managed Care

Fee for Service:	Managed Care:
Payers assume primary financial risk	Providers share in financial risk
Provides enrollees with freedom of choice	Services provided by a specific pool of providers
Unlimited access to specialty providers	Primary care provider serves as a gatekeeper
Co-payments often in the form of 80%/20%	Provides services for a fixed, prepaid monthly fee
Limited internal/external cost controls	Formal quality assurance and utilization review
Minimal emphasis on health promotion and education	Health education and preventive medicine emphasized

Special Topics

Obstetrics

Exercise and Pregnancy

Recommended exercise activities
- Swimming
- Walking
- Stretching
- Low impact aerobics
- Golfing
- Stationary cycling

Exercise activities to avoid
- High level balance activities
- Skiing
- Water skiing
- Scuba diving
- Horseback riding
- Contact sports
- Skating
- Strenuous lifting

Pregnant women are encouraged to continue with exercise activity at a moderate rate during a low risk pregnancy. Guidelines permit women to remain at 50% to 60% of their maximal heart rate for approximately thirty minutes per session. Women must monitor their heart rate intermittently to ensure that they are maintaining their target heart rate. Nonweight bearing activities are preferred due to the continuous change in the center of gravity and balance. Loose clothing is advised to allow for adequate heat loss, and adequate fluids are required during exercise. Women should avoid becoming overtired and should not exercise in the supine position after the first trimester.

Physiological changes during pregnancy
- Weight gain between 25 and 35 pounds
- Increased depth of respiration
- Increased tidal volume
- Increased minute ventilation
- Increased oxygen consumption per minute (15-20%)
- Abdominals become overstretched
- Ligaments become lax secondary to hormonal changes
- Joints may become hypermobile
- Increased blood volume (40-50%)
- Anemia may occur
- Hypotension in supine position during late pregnancy from pressure on the inferior vena cava
- Increased cardiac output (30-60%)

Postural changes
- Change in the center of gravity
- Forward head posture
- Increased cervical lordosis
- Increased base of support in standing

Diastasis recti
Diastasis recti is a separation of the rectus abdominis muscle along the linea alba that can occur during pregnancy. The exact cause is unknown, however theories indicate biomechanical and hormonal changes in women may cause the separation. Testing should be performed on all pregnant women for diastasis recti prior to prescribing exercises that require the use of the abdominals. A therapist should place a hand horizontally over the umbilicus as the pregnant woman lies in a hooklying position. A patient is considered to have diastasis recti if the therapist detects a separation greater than the width of two fingers when the woman lifts her head and shoulders off the plinth. The therapist must note how many fingers fit into the separation and modify treatment accordingly. Diastasis recti requires stabilization and support with abdominal strengthening exercises. A newborn can also have diastasis recti secondary to incomplete development, however in infants this condition usually resolves itself without intervention.

Pelvic floor weakness
The pelvic floor is comprised of a group of muscles that stretch between the pubis and coccyx and create the inferior stability of the pelvic cavity. The pubococcygeal muscles can become lax and over stretch during delivery or can become disrupted by an episiotomy. Weakness of the vaginal canal and stress incontinence are two problems that can result from childbirth and may require physical therapy intervention. Pubococcygeal or Kegel exercises should begin during pregnancy for prevention of pubococcygeal muscle weakness. The exercises require a patient to contract or squeeze as if she was stopping the flow of urine. The isometric contraction should be held five to ten seconds with complete relaxation after each contraction. Five to ten contractions should be performed in a series and three to four series should be performed each day.

American College of Obstetricians and Gynecologists (ACOG) Recommendations for Exercise in Pregnancy and Postpartum

1. During pregnancy, women can continue to exercise and derive health benefits even from mild to moderate exercise routines. Regular exercise (at least 3 times per week) is preferable to intermittent activity.
2. Women should avoid exercise in the supine position after the first trimester. Such a position is associated with decreased cardiac output in most pregnant women. Because the remaining cardiac output will be preferentially distributed away from splanchnic beds (including the uterus) during vigorous exercise, such regimens are best avoided during pregnancy. Prolonged periods of motionless standing should also be avoided.
3. Women should be aware of the decreased oxygen available for aerobic exercise during pregnancy. They should be encouraged to modify the intensity of their exercise according to maternal symptoms. Pregnant women should stop exercising when fatigued and not exercise to exhaustion. Weight bearing exercises may under some circumstances be continued at intensities similar to those prior to pregnancy throughout pregnancy. Non-weight bearing exercises, such as cycling or swimming, will minimize the risk of injury and facilitate the continuation of exercise during pregnancy.
4. Morphologic changes in pregnancy should serve as a relative contraindication to types of exercise in which loss of balance could be detrimental to maternal or fetal well-being, especially in the third trimester. Further, any type of exercise involving the potential for even mild abdominal trauma should be avoided.
5. Pregnancy requires an additional 300 kcal/day in order to maintain metabolic homeostasis. Thus, women who exercise during pregnancy should be particularly careful to ensure an adequate diet.
6. Pregnant women who exercise in the first trimester should augment heat dissipation by ensuring adequate hydration, appropriate clothing, and optimal environmental surroundings during exercise.
7. Many of the physiological and morphological changes of pregnancy persist four to six weeks postpartum. Thus, pre-pregnancy exercise routines should be resumed gradually based upon a woman's physical capability.

From American College of Obstetricians and Gynecologists. Exercise During Pregnancy and the Postpartum Period. (Technical Bulletin No. 189). Washington, DC, copyright ACOG, February 1994, with permission.

Contraindications for Exercising During Pregnancy

1. Pregnancy induced hypertension
2. Preterm rupture of membrane
3. Preterm labor during the prior or current pregnancy
4. Incompetent cervix
5. Persistent second to third trimester bleeding
6. Intrauterine growth retardation

From American College of Obstetricians and Gynecologists. Exercise During Pregnancy and the Postpartum Period. (Technical Bulletin No. 189). Washington, DC, copyright ACOG, February 1994, with permission.

Pediatrics

Developmental Gross and Fine Motor Skills

Gross Motor Skills	Fine Motor Skills
Newborn to 1 Month:	
Prone	Regards objects in direct line
Physiological flexion	of sight
Lifts head briefly	Follows moving object to
Head to side	midline
Supine	Hands fisted
Physiological flexion	Arm movements jerky
Rolls partly to side	Movements may be
Sitting	purposeful or random
Head lag in pull to sit	
Standing	
Reflex standing and walking	
2 to 3 Months:	
Prone	Can see further distances
Lifts head 90 degrees briefly	Hands open more
Chest up in prone position with some weight through forearms	Visually follows through 180 degrees
Rolls prone to supine	Grasp is reflexive
Supine	Uses palmar grasp
Asymmetrical tonic neck reflex (ATNR) influence strong	
Legs kick reciprocally	
Prefers head to side	
Sitting	
Variable head lag in pull to sitting position	
Needs full support to sit	
Head upright but bobbing	

Gross Motor Skills	Fine Motor Skills

Standing
  Poor weight bearing
  Hips in flexion, behind shoulders	

4 to 5 Months:	

Prone
  Bears weight on extended arms
  Pivots in prone to reach toys
Supine
  Rolls from supine to side position
  Plays with feet to mouth
Sitting
  Head steady in supported sitting position
  Turns head in sitting position
  Sits alone for brief periods
Standing
  Bears all weight through legs in supported stand
	Grasps and releases toys
	Uses ulnar-palmar group

6 to 7 Months:	

Prone
  Rolls from supine to prone position
  Holds weight on one hand to reach for toy
Supine
  Lifts head
Sitting
  Lifts head and helps when pulled to sitting position
  Gets to sitting position without assistance
  Sits independently
Mobility
  May crawl backward
	Approaches objects with one hand
	Arm in neutral when approaching toy
	Radial-palmar grasp
	"Rakes" with fingers to pick up small objects
	Voluntary release to transfer objects between hands

8 to 9 Months:	

Prone
  Gets into hands-knees position
Supine
  Does not tolerate supine position
Sitting
  Moves from sitting to prone position
  Sits without hand support for longer periods
  Pivots in sitting position
	Develops active supination
	Radial-digital grasp develops
	Uses inferior pincer grasp
	Extends wrist actively
	Points with index finger
	Pokes with index finger
	Release of objects is more refined
	Takes objects out of container

Gross Motor Skills	Fine Motor Skills

Standing
  Stands at furniture
  Pulls to stand at furniture
  Lowers to sitting position from supported stand
Mobility
  Crawls forward
  Walks along furniture (cruising)	

10 to 11 Months:	

Standing
  Stands without support briefly
  Pulls to stand using half-kneel intermediate position
  Picks up object from floor from standing with support
Mobility
  Walks with both hands held
  Walks with one hand held
  Creeps on hands and feet (bear walk)
	Fine pincer grasp developed
	Puts objects into container
	Grasps crayon adaptively

12 to 15 Months:	

Mobility
  Walks without support
  Fast walking
  Walks backward
  Walks sideways
  Bends over to look between legs
  Creeps or hitches upstairs
  Throws ball in sitting position
	Marks paper with crayon
	Builds tower using two cubes
	Turns over small container to obtain contents

16 to 24 Months:	
Squats in play Walks upstairs and downstairs with one hand held—both feet on step Propels ride-on toys Kicks ball Throws ball Throws ball forward Picks up toy from floor without falling	Folds paper Strings beads Stacks six cubes Imitates vertical and horizontal strokes with crayon on paper Holds crayon with thumb and fingers

Gross Motor Skills	Fine Motor Skills
2 Years: Rides tricycle Walks backward Walks on tiptoe Runs on toes Walks downstairs alternating feet Catches large ball Hops on one foot	Turns knob Opens and closes jar Buttons large buttons Uses child-size scissors with help Does 12 to 15 piece puzzles Folds paper or clothes
Preschool Age (3-4 Years): Throws ball 10 feet Walks on a line 10 feet Hops 2-10 times on one foot Jumps distances of up to 2 feet Jumps over obstacles up to 12 inches Throws and catches small ball Runs fast and avoids obstacles	Controls crayons more effectively Copies a circle or cross Matches colors Cuts with scissors Draws recognizable human figure with head and two extremities Draws squares May demonstrate hand preference
Early School Age (5-8 Years): Skips on alternate feet Gallops Can play hopscotch, balance on one foot, controlled hopping, and squatting on one leg Jumps with rhythm, control (jump rope) Bounces large ball Kicks ball with greater control Limbs growing faster than trunk allowing greater speed, leverage	Hand preference is evident Prints well, starting to learn cursive writing Able to button small buttons
Later School Age (9-12 Years): Mature patterns of movement in throwing, jumping, running Competition increases, enjoys competitive games Improved balance, coordination, endurance, attention span Boys may develop preadolescent fat spurt Girls may develop prepubescent and pubescent changes in body shape (hips, breasts)	Develops greater control in hand usage Learns to draw Handwriting is developed
Adolescence (13 Years+): Rapid growth in size and strength, boys more than girls Puberty leads to changes in body proportions: center of gravity rises toward shoulders for boys, lower to hips for girls Balance skills, coordination, eye-hand coordination, endurance may plateau during growth spurt	Develops greater dexterity in fingers for fine tasks (knitting, sewing, art, crafts)

From Ratliffe KT: Clinical Pediatric Physical Therapy: A Guide for the Physical therapy Team. Mosby Company Inc., Philadelphia 1998, p.45-47, with permission.

Concepts of Development

Cephalic to Caudal: A person develops head and upper extremity control prior to trunk and lower extremity control. There is a general skill acquisition from the direction of head to toe.

Gross to Fine: A general trend for large muscle movement acquisition with progression to small muscle skill acquisition.

Mass to Specific: A general trend for a person to acquire simple movements and progress towards complex movements.

Proximal to Distal: A concept that uses the midline of the body as the reference point. Trunk control (midline stability) is acquired first with subsequent gain in distal control (extremities).

Pediatric Therapeutic Positioning

Proper positioning is essential to obtain maximum function for the pediatric population. Positioning is used for many purposes including facilitation of desired patterns of movement, inhibition of abnormal reflexes, normalization of tone, midline orientation, enhancement of respiratory capacity, pulmonary hygiene, maintaining skin integrity, and prevention of contractures.

Ideal Positioning

	Supine	**Prone**	**Sidelying**	**Sitting**
Pelvis and hips	Pelvis in line with trunk. Hips in 30 to 90 degrees of flexion. Neutral rotation of pelvis. Hips symmetrically abducted 10 to 20 degrees.	Pelvis in line with trunk. Hips in extension. Neutral rotation of pelvis. Hips symmetrically abducted 10-20 degrees.	Pelvis in line with trunk. Hips in flexion. Neutral rotation. Hips in 10 to 20 degrees abduction.	Pelvis in line with trunk. Hips at 90 degrees flexion. Neutral rotation of pelvis. Hips symmetrically abducted 10 to 20 degrees.
Trunk	Straight. Shoulders in line with hips. Neutral rotation of trunk.	Straight. Shoulders in line with hips. Neutral rotation.	Straight. Shoulders in line with hips. Slight sidebending okay.	Straight. Shoulders over hips. Not rotated.
Head and neck	Head in neutral position. Facing forward. Slight cervical flexion.	Head in neutral position. Facing to one side. Slight cervical flexion.	Head in neutral position. Facing forward. Slight cervical flexion.	Head in neutral position. Facing forward. Head evenly on shoulders.
Shoulders and arms	Arms fully supported. Arms forward of trunk. Forearms rest on trunk or pillow.	Arms fully supported. Arms forward of trunk. Flexion at shoulders. Flexion at elbows.	Both arms supported. Lower arm forward. Not lying on point of shoulders. Lower arm neutral rotation. Upper arm may have 0 to 40 degrees medial rotation.	Arms fully supported. Elbows in flexion. 0 to 45 degrees internally rotated shoulders.
Legs and feet	Knees supported in flexion. Feet held at 90 degrees.	Knees extended. Feet supported at 90 degrees.	Knees in flexion. Feet positioned at 90 degrees. Pillow between knees.	Knees at 90 degrees. Ankles at 90 degrees. Feet fully supported. Thighs fully supported.

From Ratliffe KT: Clinical Pediatric Physical Therapy: A Guide for the Physical Therapy Team. Mosby Inc., Philadelphia 1998, p.266, with permission.

Infant Reflexes and Possible Effects if Reflex Persists Abnormally

Primitive Reflex	Possible Negative Effect on Movement with Abnormal Persistence of Reflex
Asymmetrical Tonic Neck Reflex (ATNR) **Stimulus:** Head position, turned to one side **Response:** Arm and leg on face side are extended, arm and leg on scalp side are flexed, spine curved with convexity toward face side **Normal age of response:** Birth to 6 months	**Interferes with:** • Feeding • Visual Tracking • Midline use of hands • Bilateral hand use • Rolling • Development of crawling Can lead to skeletal deformities (e.g. scoliosis, hip subluxation, hip dislocation)
Symmetrical Tonic Neck Reflex (STNR) **Stimulus:** Head position, flexion or extension **Response:** When head is in flexion, arms are flexed, legs extended. When head is in extension, arms are extended, legs are flexed **Normal age of response:** 6 to 8 months	**Interferes with:** • Ability to prop on arms in prone position • Attaining and maintaining hands-and-knees position • Crawling reciprocally • Sitting balance when looking around • Use of hands when looking at object in hands in sitting position
Tonic Labyrinthine Reflex (TLR) **Stimulus:** Position of labyrinth in inner ear—reflected in head position **Response:** In the supine position, body and extremities are held in extension; in the prone position, body and extremities are held in flexion **Normal age of response:** Birth to 6 months	**Interferes with:** • Ability to initiate rolling • Ability to prop on elbows with extended hips when prone • Ability to flex trunk and hips to come to sitting position from supine position Often causes full body extension, which interferes with balance in sitting or standing
Galant Reflex **Stimulus:** Touch to skin along spine from shoulder to hip **Response:** Lateral flexion of trunk to side of stimulus **Normal age of response:** 30 weeks of gestation to 2 months	**Interferes with:** • Development of sitting balance Can lead to scoliosis
Palmar Grasp Reflex **Stimulus:** Pressure in palm on ulnar side of hand **Response:** Flexion of fingers causing strong grip **Normal age of response:** Birth to 4 months	**Interferes with:** • Ability to grasp and release objects voluntarily • Weight bearing on open hand for propping, crawling, protective responses
Plantar Grasp Reflex **Stimulus:** Pressure to base of toes **Response:** Toe flexion **Normal age of response:** 28 weeks of gestation to 9 months	**Interferes with:** • Ability to stand with feet flat on surface • Balance reactions and weight shifting in standing
Rooting Reflex **Stimulus:** Touch on cheek **Response:** Turning head to same side with mouth open **Normal age of response:** 28 weeks of gestation to 3 months	**Interferes with:** • Oral-motor development • Development of midline control of head • Optical righting, visual tracking, and social interaction

Moro Reflex
Stimulus: Head dropping into extension suddenly for a few inches
Response: Arms abduct with fingers open, then cross trunk into adduction; cry
Normal age of response: 28 weeks of gestation to 5 months

Interferes with:
- Balance reactions in sitting
- Protective responses in sitting
- Eye-hand coordination, visual tracking

Startle Reflex
Stimulus: Loud, sudden noise
Response: Similar to Moro response but elbows remain flexed and hands closed
Normal age of response: 28 weeks of gestation to 5 months

Interferes with:
- Sitting balance
- Protective responses in sitting
- Eye-hand coordination, visual tracking
- Social interaction, attention

Positive Support Reflex
Stimulus: Weight placed on balls of feet when upright
Response: Stiffening of legs and trunk into extension
Normal age of response: 35 weeks of gestation to 2 months

Interferes with:
- Standing and walking
- Balance reactions and weight shift in standing
- Can lead to contractures of ankles into plantar flexion

Walking (Stepping) Reflex
Stimulus: Supported upright position with soles of feet on firm surface
Response: Reciprocal flexion/extension of legs
Normal age of response: 38 weeks of gestation to 2 months

Interferes with:
- Standing and walking
- Balance reactions and weight shifting in standing
- Development of smooth, coordinated reciprocal movements of lower extremities

From Ratliffe KT: Clinical Pediatric Physical Therapy: A Guide for the Physical Therapy Team. Mosby Inc., Philadelphia 1998, p.266, with permission.

Federal Legislation Affecting Health and Education for Children with Disabilities

Perkins Vocational and Applied Technology Act (enacted 1990)
Reauthorization and modification of the Education for all Handicapped Children (EHA). Provides free appropriate education in the least restrictive environment for individuals with disabilities from age 3 – 21.

IDEA Amendments (enacted 1991)
Reauthorized early intervention; established Federal Interagency Coordination Council.

Rehabilitation Act Amendments (enacted 1992)
Transition planning at high school graduation includes coordination of assistive technology services and rehabilitation system.

IDEA Amendments (enacted 1997)
Restructuring of IDEA into four distinct and individual parts.

Pediatric Assessment Tools

Instrument	Purpose	Other
Alberta Infant Motor Scale	--identify components of motor development --measure gross motor acquisition and skill maturation over time	--use from birth to walking --Piper
Bayley Scale of Infant Development II	--assessment of current developmental status using a mental scale, motor scale, and behavioral scale --includes special populations	--use from 1 month to 42 months --Bayley
Denver II	--screen of four domains: personal-social, fine motor adaptive, language and gross motor --screens for developmental delay and need for further evaluation	--use from 2 weeks to 6 years --Frankenburg
Functional Independence Measure for Children (WeeFim)	--assesses and notes progression of functional independence --a measure of disability --requires consistent performance of a skill	--use from 6 months to 7 years --utilized by Uniform Data System (UDS)
Milani-Comparetti Motor Development Screening Test	--measures functional motor skills and related reflexes --demonstrates age appropriate responses through profile --neuromotor delays	--use from birth to 2 years --Milani-Comparetti, Gidoni
Movement Assessment of Infants	--focus on infants that were treated in neonatal intensive care --categories include muscle tone, reflexes, automatic reactions, and volitional movements --identifies motor dysfunction and establishes baseline	--use from birth to 12 months --Chandler, Swanson
Neonatal Behavioral Assessment	--focus on interactive behavior, competence, and neurological status --predictor of further neurological problems	--use from 3 days to 4 weeks --Brazelton
Peabody Developmental Motor Scales	--provides detailed assessment with instruction programming --gross and fine motor scales --identifies emergency skills --does not require verbal language	--use from birth to 83 months --Folio, Fewell
Pediatric Evaluation of Disability Inventory (PEDI)	--assessment of functional skills --designed for rehabilitation use --includes areas of self care, mobility, social skills, level of assistance, and use of adaptive equipment	--use from 6 months to 7.5 years --Haley

Pediatric Profile

Examination

- Past medical history
- History of current condition
- Social history (caregiver support)
- Medications
- Living environment
- Systems review
- Pediatric assessment tools
- Gross and fine motor skill acquisition
- Pathological reflexes
- Neurological assessment
- Strength
- Range of motion
- Respiratory assessment
- Postural tone assessment
- Reassessment of existing adaptive equipment, orthotics and splinting

Intervention

- Progression through pediatric milestones
- Therapeutic exercise
- Sensory integration
- Postural control
- Therapeutic positioning
- Therapeutic play
- Wheelchair and orthotic prescription
- Chest physical therapy
- Family/caregiver teaching
- Mobility training

Goals

- Maximize functional mobility
- Maximize range of motion
- Maximize strength and postural control
- Maximize patient/caregiver competence with:
    - --Home program
    - --Disease process and its progression
    - --Therapeutic positioning and handling
- Maximize independence with use of equipment

Pediatric Pathology

Cardiopulmonary

Asthma
Asthma is a reversible condition of airway hypersensitivity and bronchoconstriction within the lungs.
- **Causative factors** are extrinsic or intrinsic by nature. Extrinsic factors include allergens such as foods, animals, dust, smoke, and pollen. Intrinsic factors include exercise, stress, viral infections, and overall fatigue.
- **Characteristics** can range from mild to severe depending on the level of airway restriction. A mild asthma attack presents with wheezing, chest tightness, and slight shortness of breath. A severe asthma attack presents with dyspnea, flaring nostrils, diminished wheezing, anxiety, cyanosis, and the inability to speak. A severe attack left untreated will result in respiratory failure.
- **Treatment** includes pharmacological intervention using bronchodilators. Physical therapy management includes caregiver education, bronchial drainage and hygiene, breathing exercises, relaxation, endurance, and strength training.

Cystic Fibrosis
Cystic fibrosis is a disease of the exocrine glands that primarily affects the respiratory and gastrointestinal systems.
- The **causative factor** is a mutation of chromosome seven to include the cystic fibrosistransmembrane conductance regulator (CFTR). Cystic fibrosis is an autosomal recessive genetic disorder and a terminal disease.
- **Characteristics** change with the progression of the disease and include increased secretion of thick mucus, gastrointestinal distress, abnormal bowels, recurrent pulmonary infection, salty tasting skin, wheezing, productive cough, barrel chest, dyspnea, and progressive use of accessory muscles with respiration.
- **Treatment** has improved survival rates from seven years in the late 1960's to a mean age of 30 years today. Pharmacological interventions include antibiotics used to control pulmonary infections, nutritional supplements, pancreatic enzyme replacements, mucus thinning medications, and bronchodilators. Physical therapy treatment is essential and includes bronchial drainage, percussion, vibration, suctioning, breathing techniques, assisted cough, and ventilatory muscle training for optimal pulmonary function. General exercise is indicated to improve overall strength and endurance except with severe lung disease. Family involvement with a home program is vital for the child's ongoing pulmonary needs.

Patent Ductus Arteriosus
Patent ductus arteriosus is a disorder where the ductus arteriosus, which normally shunts blood in utero from the pulmonary artery directly to the descending aorta, fails to close shortly after birth.
- **Causative factors** for this condition include premature birth, respiratory distress syndrome, fetal alcohol syndrome,

Trisomy 13 (Patau's syndrome), and Trisomy 18 (Edwards' syndrome).

- **Characteristics** of this condition depend on the size of the ductus. A small ductus may be asymptomatic where as a large ductus may present with tachycardia, respiratory distress, poor nutrition, weight loss, and congestive heart failure.
- Initial **treatment** attempts to nonsurgically reduce the size of the ductus with use of diuretics and indomethacin when indicated. Surgical repair may be necessary for a large ductus or when initial management fails.

Respiratory Distress Syndrome (RDS)
Respiratory distress syndrome is a pulmonary condition seen in neonates born before 37 weeks of gestation. RDS is also known as hyaline membrane disease and is the leading cause of death in the neonate.

- **Causative factors** are due to the immaturity of the lungs and the inability to produce necessary levels of surfactant. This deficit results in increased alveolar tension, alveolar collapse, atelectasis, and difficulty breathing. Associated factors with RDS include being the second born twin, cesarean delivery, hypoxia, and acidosis.
- **Characteristics** are observed immediately as the infant works hard to breathe and reinflate the collapsed lung. Tachypnea, flaring of the nostrils, use of accessory muscles, and respiratory distress are observed within one to two hours. Untreated, the infant lacks oxygen and presents with metabolic acidosis and acute respiratory failure.
- **Treatment** will vary and can include mechanical ventilation, supplemental oxygen, administration of artificial surfactant, nutritional support, bronchial drainage, and chest physical therapy. As a child recovers from RDS there is an increase in secretions from oxygen therapy and mechanical ventilation that requires short-term chest physical therapy.

Tetralogy of Fallot
Tetralogy of Fallot is the most common cyanotic heart defect where the following four abnormalities exist:
> Ventricular septal defect
> Right ventricular hypertrophy
> Aortic override of the interventricular septum
> Pulmonary stenosis

- The **causative factors** are congenital defect, association with Down syndrome and fetal alcohol syndrome.
- **Characteristics** vary depending on the extent of the defects and include dyspnea, hypoxia, failure to gain weight, cyanosis, and poor development.
- **Treatment** usually includes pharmacological intervention, reopening of the ductus arteriosus, or surgical reconstruction of the defects.

Musculoskeletal

Congenital Hip Dysplasia
Congenital hip dysplasia is a condition also known as developmental dysplasia of the hip. Presentation includes a malalignment of the femoral head with the acetabulum. The condition usually develops during the last trimester in utero.

- **Causative factors** may include cultural predisposition, malposition, and environmental and genetic influences.
- **Characteristics** include asymmetrical hip abduction with tightness and apparent femoral shortening of the involved side. Testing for this condition includes the Ortolani test, Barlow maneuver, and ultrasound.
- **Treatment** is dependent on age, severity, and initial attempts to reposition the femoral head within the acetabulum through the constant use of a harness, bracing, splinting, or traction. Open reduction with subsequent application of a hip spica cast may be required if conservative treatment fails. Physical therapy may be indicated after cast removal for stretching, strengthening, and caregiver education.

Congenital Limb Deficiencies
A congenital limb deficiency is a malformation that occurs in utero secondary to an impaired developmental course. Congenital limb deficiencies are classified as longitudinal or transverse.

- The **causative factor** of a longitudinal limb deficiency is an abnormality present at conception where a bone lacks potential to form. The causative factors of a transverse limb deficiency can include environmental factors, teratogen (thalidomide), trauma or infection.
- The primary **characteristic** of a longitudinal limb deficiency is a missing long bone such as the radius. A transverse limb deficiency is a limb that does not develop beyond a particular point.
- **Treatment** may focus on symmetrical movements, strengthening, range of motion, weight bearing activities, and prosthetic training.

Congenital Torticollis
Congenital torticollis is characterized by a unilateral contracture of the sternocleidomastoid musculature.

- Etiology is unknown, however **causative factors** include malposition in utero, breech position in utero, and birth trauma. An infant is usually diagnosed within the first three weeks after birth.
- **Characteristics** include lateral flexion to the same side as the contracture, rotation toward the opposite side, and facial asymmetries.
- **Treatment** is usually conservative for the first year with emphasis on stretching, active range of motion, positioning, and caregiver education. Surgical management is indicated when conservative options have failed and the child is over one year of age. A surgical release followed by physical therapy may be indicated to attain cervical range of motion and proper alignment.

Legg-Calve-Perthes Disease
Legg-Calve-Perthes disease is characterized by degeneration of the femoral head due to a disturbance in the blood supply (avascular necrosis). The disease is self-limiting and has four distinct stages: condensation, fragmentation, reossification, and remodeling.

- **Causative factors** include trauma, genetic predisposition, synovitis, vascular abnormalities, and infection.
- **Characteristics** include pain, decreased range of motion, antalgic gait, and a positive Trendelenburg sign.
- **Treatment** methods may vary but the primary focus is to relieve pain, maintain the femoral head in the proper position, and improve range of motion. Physical therapy may be required intermittently for stretching, splinting, crutch training, aquatic therapy, traction, and exercise. Orthotic devices and surgical intervention may be indicated depending on classification and severity of the condition.

Osgood-Schlatter Disease
Osgood-Schlatter disease is a condition also known as traction apophysis which results from repetitive traction on the tibial tuberosity apophysis.
- The **causative factor** is the repeated tension to the patella tendon over the tibial tuberosity in young athletes, which results in a small avulsion of the tuberosity and swelling.
- **Characteristics** of this self-limiting condition include point tenderness over the patella tendon at the insertion on the tibial tubercle, antalgic gait, and pain with increasing activity.
- **Treatment** is usually conservative with focus on education, icing, flexibility exercises, and eliminating activities that place strain on the patella tendon such as squatting, running, or jumping.

Osteogenesis Imperfecta
Osteogenesis imperfecta is a connective tissue disorder that affects the formation of collagen during bone development. There are four classifications of osteogenesis imperfecta that vary in levels of severity.
- The **causative factor** is genetic inheritance with type I and IV considered autosomal dominant traits, and types II and III considered autosomal recessive traits.
- **Characteristics** of this condition include pathological fractures, osteoporosis ("brittle bones"), hypermobile joints, bowing of the long bones, weakness, scoliosis, and impaired respiratory function.
- **Treatment** begins at birth with caregiver education on proper handling and facilitation of movement. Use of orthotics, active and symmetrical movements, positioning, functional mobility, and fracture management are essential areas of treatment. In severe cases where ambulation is not realistic, wheelchair prescription and training is indicated.

Scoliosis
Scoliosis is a lateral curvature of the spine. The three types of scoliosis are idiopathic, neuromuscular, and congenital.
- **Causative factors** include altered development of the spine in utero, association with cerebral palsy, muscular dystrophy or other neuromuscular conditions.
- **Characteristics** indicate whether a scoliosis is a structural or nonstructural curve. A structural curve cannot be corrected with active or passive movement and there is rotation of the vertebrae towards the convexity of the curve. This results in a rib hump over the thoracic region on the convex side of the curve. Asymmetries will be visually noted at the shoulders, scapulae, pelvis, and skinfolds. A nonstructural curve will correct with lateral bending towards the apex of the curve. This type of curve is typically nonprogressive with minimal vertebral rotation. The primary causative factor for a nonstructural curve is a leg length discrepancy.
- **Treatment** is based on the type and severity of the curve, age, and previous management. Generally, curves that are less than 25 degrees require monitoring; curves between 25 and 40 degrees are treated with orthotic management and physical therapy intervention for posture, flexibility, respiratory function, and body mechanics. Curves that progress beyond 40 degrees require surgical intervention to improve spinal stability.

Talipes Equinovarus
Talipes equinovarus is a deformity of the ankle and foot also known as "clubfoot."
- **Causative factors** are unclear, however theories postulate familial tendency, positioning in utero, or defect in the ovum. This condition accompanies other neuromuscular abnormalities including spina bifida and arthrogryposis, and may result from the lack of movement that assists with repositioning in utero.
- **Characteristics** of this deformity involve adduction of the forefoot, various positioning of the hindfoot, and equinus at the ankle. Severe cases can include deformity of the lower leg.
- **Treatment** begins soon after birth and includes splinting and serial casting. The goal of intervention is to restore proper positioning of the foot and ankle. Failed management or severe involvement will require surgical intervention and subsequent casting.

Neurological

Arthrogryposis Multiplex Congenita
Arthrogryposis multiplex congenita is a nonprogressive neuromuscular disorder that is estimated to occur during the first trimester in utero. The restriction in utero allows for fibrosis of muscles and structures within the joints.
- An exact etiology is unknown, but **causative factors** include poor movement during early development due to myopathic, neuropathic or joint abnormalities. The causative factor for a small percentage of children with this condition is genetic inheritance as an autosomal dominant trait.
- **Characteristics** include cylinder-like extremities with minimal definition, significant and multiple contractures, dislocation of joints, and muscle atrophy.
- The goal of **treatment** is to attain the maximum level of developmental skills through positioning, stretching, strengthening, splinting, and the use of adaptive equipment. Significant family involvement is required for the home program. Surgical intervention may be indicated.

Cerebral Palsy

Cerebral palsy is an umbrella term used to describe movement disorders due to brain damage that are nonprogressive and are acquired in utero, during birth or infancy. The brain damage decreases the brain's ability to monitor and control nerve and voluntary muscle activity.

- **Causative factors** before or during birth include a lack of oxygen, maternal infections, drug and alcohol abuse, placental abnormalities, toxemia, prolonged labor, prematurity, and Rh incompatibility. Causative factors that are seen in acquired cerebral palsy include meningitis, CVA, seizures, and head injury.
- **Characteristics** vary from mild and undetectable to severe loss of control accompanied by profound mental retardation. All types of cerebral palsy demonstrate abnormal muscle tone, impaired modulation of movement, presence of abnormal reflexes, and impaired mobility.
  - **--Cerebral Palsy Primary Motor Patterns (mixed motor patterns exist):**
    Spastic - indicating a lesion in the motor cortex of the cerebrum
    Athetoid - indicating a lesion involving the basal ganglia
    Ataxic - indicating a lesion involving the cerebellum
  - **--Distribution of Involvement**
    Monoplegia - one extremity
    Diplegia - primarily bilateral lower extremity involvement, however upper extremities may be affected
    Hemiplegia - unilateral involvement of the upper and lower extremities
    Quadriplegia - involvement of the entire body
- **Treatment** of cerebral palsy is a lifelong process. Intervention includes ongoing family and caregiver education, normalization of tone, stretching, strengthening, motor learning and developmental milestones, positioning, weight bearing activities, and mobility skills. Splinting, assistive devices, and specialized seating may be indicated. Surgical intervention may be required for orthopedic management or reduction of spasticity.

Down Syndrome

Down syndrome is a genetic abnormality consisting of an extra twenty first chromosome, usually termed trisomy 21.

- **Causative factors** include incomplete cell division of the 21st pair of chromosomes due to nondisjunction, translocation or mosaic classification. Advanced maternal age increases the risk of genetic imbalance.
- **Characteristics** of this syndrome include mental retardation, hypotonia, joint hypermobility, flattened nasal bridge, narrow eyelids with epicanthal folds, small mouth, feeding impairments, flat feet, scoliosis, congenital heart disease, and visual and hearing loss.
- **Treatment** should emphasize exercise and fitness, stability, maximizing respiratory function, and education for caregivers. Surgical intervention may be indicated for cardiac abnormalities.

Duchenne Muscular Dystrophy

Duchenne muscular dystrophy is a progressive disorder caused by the absence of the gene required to produce the muscle proteins dystrophin and nebulin. Without dystrophin and nebulin, cell membranes weaken, myofibrils are destroyed, and muscle contractility is lost. Fat and connective tissue eventually replace muscle, and death usually occurs from cardiopulmonary failure prior to age 25.

- The **causative factor** for this disorder is inheritance as an X-linked recessive trait. The child's mother is a silent carrier and only male offspring will manifest the disease.
- **Characteristics** usually manifest between two and five years of age. Progressive weakness, disinterest in running, falling, toe walking, excessive lordosis, and pseudohypertrophy of muscle groups are common symptoms. Progressive impairment with ADLs and mobility begins around age five and the inability to ambulate follows.
- **Treatment** focuses on family and caregiver education, respiratory function, submaximal exercise, mobility skills, splinting, orthotics, and adaptive equipment. Medical management includes the use of immunosuppressants, steroids, and surgical intervention for orthopedic impairments.

Prader-Willi Syndrome

Prader-Willi syndrome is a genetic condition that is diagnosed by physical attributes and patterns of behavior rather than genetic testing.

- The **causative factor** is a partial deletion of chromosome 15.
- **Characteristics** include physical and behavioral attributes such as small hands, feet, and sex organs, hypotonia, almond shaped eyes, obesity, and a constant desire for food. This child will present with coordination impairments and mental retardation.
- **Treatment** includes postural control, exercise and fitness, and gross and fine motor skills training.

Spina Bifida

Spina bifida is a developmental abnormality due to insufficient closure of the neural tube by the 28th day of gestation. This defect usually occurs in the low thoracic, lumbar or sacral regions and affects the central nervous, musculoskeletal, and urinary systems.

- A single etiology has not been identified, however **causative factors** include genetic predisposition, environmental influence, low levels of maternal folic acid, maternal hyperthermia, and certain classifications of drugs.
  - **--Types of Spina Bifida**
    Spina Bifida Occulta - An impairment and nonfusion of the spinous processes of a vertebrae, however the spinal cord and meninges remain intact. There is usually no associated disability.
    Spina Bifida Cystica - Presents with a cyst-like protrusion through the nonfused vertebrae, which results in impairment.

--Forms of Spina Bifida Cystica
Meningocele - Herniation of meninges and cerebrospinal fluid into a sac that protrudes through the vertebral defect. The spinal cord remains within the canal.

Myelomeningocele - A severe form characterized by herniation of meninges, cerebrospinal fluid, and the spinal cord extending through the defect in the vertebrae. The cyst may or may not be covered by skin.

- **Characteristics** and associated impairments of myelomeningocele include motor loss below the level of defect in the spinal cord, sensory deficits, hydrocephalus, Arnold-Chiari Type II malformation, osteoporosis, clubfoot, scoliosis, tethered cord syndrome, latex allergy, bowel and bladder dysfunction, and learning disabilities.
- Initial **treatment** for this population prioritizes significant family teaching regarding positioning, handling, range of motion, and therapeutic exercise. Ongoing treatment in physical therapy includes range of motion, facilitation of developmental milestones, skin care, strengthening, balance and mobility training, adaptive equipment, splinting, orthotic prescription, and wheelchair prescription. Physical therapy is ongoing through adolescence and is based on the severity of impairments and needs of the child.

Spinal Muscular Atrophy (SMA)
Spinal muscular atrophy is a condition of progressive degeneration of the anterior horn cell.

--Categories of Spinal Muscular Atrophy
Acute Infantile SMA (Werdnig-Hoffmann disease) - Occurs between birth and two months of age. Motor degeneration progresses quickly and life expectancy is less that one year.

Chronic Childhood SMA (type II muscular atrophy, chronic Werdnig-Hoffmann disease) - Usually presents after six months to one year and is slower in progression than infantile SMA. Progression is steady, however children can survive into adulthood.

Juvenile SMA (Kugelberg-Welander SMA) - Occurs later in childhood from 4-17 years of age. This population can also survive into adulthood.

- The **causative factor** of spinal muscular atrophy is an autosomal recessive genetic inheritance. Certain types of this disease involve a mutation on chromosome 5. Characteristics for all categories of the disease are the same, and vary in onset and speed of progression.
- **Characteristics** include progressive muscle weakness and atrophy, diminished or absent deep tendon reflexes, normal intelligence, intact sensation, and end stage respiratory compromise.
- **Treatment** includes positioning, vestibular and visual stimulation, and access to play. Treatment for the slower progressing categories of SMA is primarily supportive including educating caregivers, mobility training, and use of assistive devices and adaptive equipment.

Oncology

Astrocytoma
An astrocytoma is a classification that accounts for approximately fifty percent of pediatric brain tumors. The etiology of pediatric cancers is usually unknown.
- **Causative factors** include genetic predisposition, environmental influence, radiation and toxin exposure, and association with certain childhood disorders.
- There are two types of astrocytoma with **characteristics** as follows:
    Cerebellar - clumsiness, ataxic gait, headache, change in personality, and vomiting
    Supratentorial - headache, seizures, change in personality, visual impairments, and vomiting
- **Treatment** for *cerebellar* tumors consists of surgical resection with an 80-90% cure rate. Treatment for *supratentorial* tumors requires surgery to resect the tumor with radiation and/or chemotherapy.

Leukemia
Leukemia is a cancer of the blood that occurs when leukocytes change into malignant cells. These immature cells proliferate, accumulate in bone marrow, and ultimately cease the production of normal cells. This process will spread to lymph nodes, liver, spleen, and other areas of the body.
- The exact etiology is unknown, however **causative factors** include environmental, chemical or toxin exposure, genetic predisposition, and viral association. There are many types of leukemia with acute lymphoblastic leukemia (ALL), and acute myelogenous leukemia (AML) occurring most frequently in children.
- **Characteristics** of these types include an abrupt onset with high fever, bleeding, enlarged lymph nodes and spleen, progressive weakness, fatigue, and painful joints. Blood work will indicate anemia, thrombocytopenia, and leukocyte count greater than 500,000 mm^3.
- **Treatment** will vary based on the type and degree of leukemia. Options include immunotherapy, cytotoxic agents, chemotherapy or radiation, and bone marrow transplant if indicated. Over 90% of patients with ALL achieve complete remission with treatment, while patients with AML achieve complete remission at a rate of 70-80%.

Neuroblastoma
A neuroblastoma is a tumor that initiates from primitive ectodermal cells of the neural plate and is found within the sympathetic nervous system, primarily seen in the adrenal glands or paraspinal ganglions. This is the most common malignant tumor seen in children. The etiology remains unknown, but **causative factors** include genetic predisposition, familial incidence, environmental influence, radiation and toxin exposure or viral association. **Characteristics** vary with the site and include an abdominal mass, change in personality, anemia, sweating, pain, and diarrhea. **Treatment** includes surgical resection, chemotherapy, and radiation. Prognosis is best for children diagnosed in the first year of life. In rare instances a neuroblastoma will spontaneously regress.

Non-Hodgkin's Lymphoma
Non-Hodgkin's lymphoma is a cancer of the lymphatic system with peak incidence between seven to ten years of age.
- The etiology is unknown, however a likely **causative factor** is viral infection.
- **Characteristics** can differ from adults and include abdominal pain, swallowing issues, anemia, and swelling. Nodular histologies are rare in children.
- **Treatment** is dependent on the site and extent of the cancer and includes surgical resection, chemotherapy, and radiation.

Osteogenic Sarcoma
An osteogenic sarcoma is a cancer that occurs at the epiphyses of long bones. Osteogenic sarcoma is the most common form of bone cancer in children with a peak incidence between the ages of 10 to 20.
- **Causative factors** are unknown, however there is a correlation between immunoincompetence and rate of tumor progression. Osteogenic sarcoma can metastasize quickly.
- **Characteristics** include presence of a mass, rapid metastases, and associated pain. Diagnosis can be made with a biopsy.
- **Treatment** includes amputation with proximal resection to ensure proper removal of affected tissue or surgical procedures which attempt to resect the tumor and salvage the limb. Chemotherapy is beneficial, however radiation is not effective with this type of tumor.

Wilms' Tumor
Wilms' tumor is an embryonal adenomyosarcoma found in the kidney. Most cases are diagnosed between one and four years of age.
- **Causative factors** include genetic inheritance as an autosomal dominant disease or a noninherited form with an unknown etiology.
- **Characteristics** include an abdominal mass, pain, hematuria, fever, nausea, and vomiting.
- **Treatment** includes resection of the kidney and the associated lymphatic tissue followed by chemotherapy and/or radiation. Dactinomycin is also administered due to the drug's antitumor properties. The five-year cure rate is approximately 75%.

Rheumatory

Juvenile Rheumatoid Arthritis
Juvenile rheumatoid arthritis (JRA) is the most common chronic rheumatic disease in children and presents with inflammation of the joints and connective tissues.
- The exact etiology is unknown, however it is theorized that **causative factors** include an external source such as a virus, infection or trauma that may trigger an autoimmune response producing JRA in a child with a genetic predisposition.
- **Characteristics** depend on the classification of JRA. *Systemic juvenile rheumatoid arthritis* occurs in 10% to 20% of children with JRA and presents with acute onset, high fevers, rash, enlargement of the spleen and liver, and inflammation of the lungs and heart. *Polyarticular juvenile rheumatoid arthritis* accounts for 30-40% of children with JRA and presents with high female incidence, RF+ majority, and arthritis in more than five joints with symmetrical joint involvement. *Oligoarticular (Pauciarticular) juvenile rheumatoid arthritis* accounts for 40-60% of children with JRA and affects less than five joints with asymmetrical joint involvement. General characteristics include inflammation, malaise, pain with palpation and movement, stiffness, iritis, fever, and rash.
- **Treatment** includes pharmacological management to relieve inflammation and pain through NSAIDs, corticosteroids, and antirheumatic and immunosuppressive agents. Physical therapy management includes passive and active range of motion, positioning, splinting and orthotic prescription, strengthening, endurance, weight bearing activities, postural training, and functional mobility. Pain management includes use of modalities such as paraffin, ultrasound, warm water, and cryotherapy. A realistic home program must be a constant priority. Surgical intervention may be indicated secondary to pain, contractures or irreversible joint destruction.

Models of Disability

The Nagi Model

Originally designed in 1965 by a social worker named Saad Nagi as an alternative to the medical model of disease. It describes health status as a product of the relationship between health and function and is defined by four primary concepts:

- **Pathology** - An interruption or interference in the body's normal processes and the simultaneous efforts of the systems to regain homeostasis. Pathology occurs at the cellular level.

- **Impairment** - The loss or abnormality at the tissue, organ or body system level. This can be of an anatomic, physiologic, mental or emotional nature. Each pathology will present with an impairment, however impairments can exist without pathology (e.g. congenital defects). Impairments occur at the organ level.

- **Functional limitation** - The inability to perform an action or skill in a normal manner due to an impairment. Functional limitations are at the level of the whole person.

- **Disability** - Any restriction or inability to perform a socially defined role within a social or physical environment due to an impairment. Environmental barriers impose disability.

Example:
A patient with progressive weakness presents with paralysis of the trunk and lower extremities. The patient is diagnosed with

a T12 spinal cord tumor. The patient utilizes a wheelchair for mobility and requires assistance with self-care. Prior to hospitalization the patient worked as a delivery man.

Pathology - Spinal cord tumor at T12
Impairment - Loss of motor function below T12
Functional limitation - Unable to ambulate
Disability - Cannot continue to work as a delivery man

The International Classification of Impairment, Disabilities, and Handicaps (ICIDH) Model

The World Health Organization (WHO) developed this model in 1980 with the focus on the long-term impact of nonfatal or chronic diseases. The model is defined by four primary concepts:

- **Disease** - A biomechanical, physiological or anatomical abnormality within the body.

- **Impairment** - The loss or abnormality of psychological, physiological or anatomical structure or function. Impairments occur at the organ level.

- **Disability** - The inability to perform an activity in a normal manner due to an impairment. Disability occurs at the level of the whole person.

- **Handicap** - The inability to perform in a social role due to social or environmental restrictions. Handicap occurs in a person-to-person or person-to-environment level. Handicap clearly separates environmental barriers and the person's ability to interact with the environment.

Example:
A 36-year-old female is diagnosed with multiple sclerosis. The patient resides alone and has recently utilized a wheelchair for mobility secondary to weakness and hypertonicity in her upper and lower extremities. She is no longer able to visit her brother who lives in a second floor apartment two blocks away.

Disease - Demyelination secondary to multiple sclerosis
Impairment - Weakness and tonal abnormalities in lower extremities
Disability - Unable to ambulate
Handicap - Unable to visit her brother who resides in the second floor apartment

Disablement Model

This model was designed by physical therapists appointed by the House of Delegates as the framework for the Guide to Physical Therapist Practice. This model rejects the medical model of disease and focuses on disablement using guidelines from the Nagi model. This model defines three primary concepts as they relate to physical therapy intervention.

- **Impairment** - The loss or abnormality of physiological, psychological, or anatomical structure or function.

- **Functional limitation** - A restriction of the ability to perform in a competent manner. This occurs at the level of the whole person.

- **Disability** - The inability to engage in roles in a particular social context and physical environment.

Example:
A 45-year-old right hand dominant female fell down a flight of stairs and sustained a compound fracture of the right humerus. She is currently casted and has difficulty with many self-care skills. She is employed in the data entry department of a local hospital.

Impairment - Fracture of the humerus
Functional limitation - Unable to get dressed
Disability - Cannot use the computer at work

Outcome Measurement Tools

Balance

Berg Functional Balance Scale
A tool designed to assess a patient's risk for falling. There are fourteen tasks, each scored on an ordinal scale from 0-4. These tasks include static, transitional, and dynamic activities in sitting and standing positions. The maximum score is a 56 with a score less than 45 indicating an increased risk for falling. This tool is used as a one-time examination or as an ongoing tool to monitor a patient who may be at risk for falls.

Functional Reach
A single task screening tool used to assess standing balance and risk of falling. A person is required to stand upright with a static base of support. A yardstick is positioned to measure the forward distance that a patient can reach without moving the feet. Three trials are performed and averaged together. The following are age related standard measurements for functional reach:
20 - 40 years – 14.5 - 17 inches
41 - 69 years – 13.5 - 15 inches
70 - 87 years – 10.5 - 13.5 inches
A patient that falls below the age appropriate range for functional reach has an increased risk for falling. The outcome measure demonstrates high test-retest correlation and intrarater reliability.

"Get Up and Go" Test
A functional performance screening tool used to assess a person's level of mobility and balance. The person initially sits in a supported chair with a firm surface, transfers to a

standing position, and walks a few feet. The patient must then turn around without external support, walk back towards the chair, and return to a sitting position. The patient is scored based on amount of postural sway, excessive movements, reaching for support, side stepping, or other signs of loss of balance. The 5-point ordinal rating scale designates a score of one as normal and a score of five as severely abnormal. In an attempt to increase overall reliability the use of time was implemented. Patients who require over 20 seconds to complete the process may be at an increased risk for falling.

Romberg Test
An assessment of balance that positions the patient in unsupported standing, feet together, upper extremities folded, and eyes closed. A patient receives a grade of "normal" if they are able to maintain the position for 30 seconds.

Tinetti Performance Oriented Mobility Assessment
A tool used to screen patients and identify if there is an increased risk for falling. The first section assesses balance through sit to stand and stand to sit from an armless chair, immediate standing balance with eyes open and closed, tolerating a slight push in the standing position, and turning 360 degrees. A patient is scored from 0-2 in most categories with a maximum score of 16. The second section assesses gait at normal speed and at a rapid, but safe speed. Items scored in this section include initiation of gait, step length and height, step asymmetry and continuity, path, stance during gait, and trunk motion. A patient is scored either 0 to 1 or 0 to 2 with a maximum score of 12. The tool has a combined maximum total of 28 with the risk of falling increasing as the total score decreases.

Cognitive Assessment

Mini Mental State Examination
A tool designed to screen patients for cognitive impairment, psychoses or affective disorders. Each of the five sections: orientation, registration, attention and calculation, recall and language, and motor skills have multiple questions that receive one point for the correct answer or zero for the incorrect answer. There is a maximum score of 30 with a progressive level of cognitive impairment noted when a score of 24 or less is obtained.

Short Portable Mental Status Questionnaire
A ten item screening tool used to assess cognitive impairment primarily in the geriatric population. Orientation, short and long-term memory, practical skills, and mathematical tasks are tested. The maximum score is ten with a score below eight indicating cognitive impairment. The lower the score below eight the more significant the cognitive impairment.

Coordination and Manual Dexterity

Frenchay Arm Test
A tool used to assess coordination and dexterity by performing five activities based on functional movement patterns. The activities include stabilizing and drawing lines with a ruler, manipulating a cylinder without dropping it, drinking from a glass, placing and removing a clothespin, and combing hair. A patient receives three attempts to complete each task. A score of one is noted for successful completion; a score of zero is noted for failure to complete the task.

Jebsen Hand Function Test
A tool designed to assess hand function using seven timed activities. These activities include writing a 24-letter sentence, turning cards, placing six small objects into a container, using a teaspoon to pick up five small items, stacking items, moving large lightweight items, and large heavy objects. Each activity is timed and the results are compared to normative data.

Peg Test
There are multiple tools that utilize a peg board to assess dexterity including the Purdue Pegboard test, the nine hole peg test, and the ten hole peg test. These tools use the element of time for completion of the task and compare results to normative data.

Endurance

Borg Rating of Perceived Exertion Scale
A tool designed to measure perceived exertion, dyspnea, and exercise intensity. The original scale measures 6 to 20 points and the revised scale measures 0 to 10 points. The patient is instructed that a 6 (original) or 0 (new) corresponds to walking at a normal pace without fatigue. A score of 20 (original) or 10 (new) indicates high intensity exercise that cannot be completed due to exhaustion. After an activity a patient's score can indicate cardiopulmonary fatigue versus muscle fatigue. The score correlates with exercise intensity, heart rate, oxygen consumption, and blood lactate levels. Cardiopulmonary training effects can be seen with exercise intensity beginning at a 14 (original) or 4 to 5 (new) respectively. The scale is commonly used for patients with cardiovascular impairments.

Dyspnea Levels
A tool designed by Rancho Los Amigos Medical Center that attempts to rate the intensity and level of dyspnea that a patient experiences with activity. This ordinal scale consists of ratings from 0 to 4. A patient at level 0 is able to perform an activity and count to 15 without any additional breaths required. Levels 1, 2, and 3 require progressive extra breaths to count to 15. Level 4 indicates that the patient is unable to count while performing an activity. The test has not been shown to be valid, however can be used to measure progress or decline during a course of rehabilitation.

Six-Minute Walk Test
A tool used to determine a patient's functional exercise capacity. The patient walks as far as he or she can for a timed six minutes with rest periods permitted as necessary. The tool is commonly used upon admission, discharge, and to monitor progress or decline throughout physical therapy. It allows for observation of heart rate and oxygen consumption during activity. This tool is administered to various populations including those with cardiac impairments, pulmonary disease, geriatrics with chronic conditions, and patients recovering from orthopedic surgical procedures.

Motor Recovery

Fugl-Meyer Assessment
An ordinal scale used to measure recovery post CVA. The framework is based on Brunnstrom's sequence of recovery. The five areas of assessment are joint movement and pain, balance, upper extremity motor function, sensation, and lower extremity motor function. Each item tested within an area is assigned a score from 0-3. The maximum combined score for upper extremity and lower extremity motor function is 100 and can be interpreted as a percentage of motor recovery. A score of 63 indicates approximately 63% return of motor function. This tool utilizes cumulative scoring for the entire assessment.

Montreal Evaluation
A tool that determines a patient's level of mobility by examining six specific areas in the following order: mental clarity, muscle tone, reflex activity, voluntary movement, automatic reactions, and pain. The construction of this tool utilized Bobath's NDT approach to neurological recovery. An ordinal scale of 0 to 3 is used for each item in each category. Muscle tone and active movements are examined separately, but scoring is cumulative for all areas. Each scored item includes multiple factors for a single score. This makes comparison of the individual scored items difficult.

Rivermead Motor Assessment
A tool based on the NDT approach to neurological recovery. The Rivermead Motor Assessment is divided into three major sections: gross function, leg and trunk, and arm. Each section is comprised of a subscale of tasks. These tasks increase in difficulty and are graded with a score of one for completion or zero for inability to perform the activity. The assessment possesses a high level of sensitivity when examining higher level patients and is reliable within one point.

Pain

McGill Pain Questionnaire
A pain assessment tool that is divided into four parts with a total of 70 questions.
  Part 1 Patient marks on a drawing of the body to indicate area and type of pain (internal or external)
  Part 2 Patient chooses one word that best describes the pain from each of the twenty categories
  Part 3 Patient describes pattern of pain, factors that increase and relieve pain
  Part 4 Patient rates the intensity of pain on a scale of zero to five

This tool can be used to establish a baseline, evaluate particular treatment regimens, and monitor progress. It is valid, reliable, and the most widely used pain assessment scale.

Numerical Rating Scale
A tool used to assess pain intensity by rating pain on a scale of 0-10 or 0-100. The 0 represents no discernable pain and the 10 or 100 represent the worst pain ever. The information is used as a baseline and should be reassessed at regular intervals in order to monitor progress. This scale is easy to administer, assess, and monitor.

Visual Analogue Scale
A tool used to assess pain intensity using a 10-15 cm line with the left anchor indicating "no pain" and the right anchor indicating "the worst pain you can have." The level of perceived pain is indicated on the line and is reassessed frequently over the course of physical therapy to record changes and progress, and to predict patient outcome. This scale can be highly sensitive if small increments such as millimeters are used to measure the patient's point of pain on the scale. The visual analogue scale is a valid tool if measurements are taken accurately.

Self-Care and ADL

Barthel Index
A tool designed to measure the amount of assistance needed to perform ten different activities with a total maximum score of 100. These activities include bowel management, bladder management, grooming, toilet use, feeding, transfers, mobility, dressing, stairs, and bathing. A score of 75-95 denotes mild impairment, 50-70 moderate impairment, 20-45 severe impairment, and below 20 indicates a very severe impairment. The index does not account for cognitive or safety issues and is not sensitive to higher level patients regarding their level of disability. It remains one of the oldest and most widely used tools that is reliable and possesses predictive validity.

Functional Independence Measure (FIM)
A tool that is primarily used in rehabilitation hospitals in order to determine a patient's level of disability and burden of care. This tool is part of the Uniform Data System for Medical Rehabilitation (UDS). A seven point scale is utilized to examine 18 areas, which include self-care, sphincter control, transfers, locomotion, communication, and social cognitive activities. These items were designed based on the World Health Organization's Model of Disability. Scoring between a 1 and 5 denotes a level of dependence and between 6 and 7 a level of independence for a specific item. This tool is both valid and reliable and is used as a predictor of disability for

the CVA population. The FIM is utilized on a larger scale to assess change within rehabilitation programs over time.

Katz Index of Activities of Daily Living
A nominal scale index used to identify self-care problems and the level of assistance required with the six areas of bathing, dressing, toileting, transfers, continence, and feeding. The score for each area is combined and the total score correlates with a letter grade scale (A through G). Each letter represents a level of ability with A representing independence in all six areas, the following letters representing increasing dependence, and G representing dependence in all six areas. This tool was originally intended only for inpatient and nursing home settings, however it is now utilized with patients that require outpatient and community based services. It is a simple and quick assessment tool used to efficiently gather self-care information and predict outcome and need for ongoing assistance.

Pharmacology

Pharmacological Categories

Nonsteroidal Anti-inflammatory Drugs (salicylates)
Salicylates are commonly used to treat muscle and joint pain in acute and chronic conditions. Aspirin is the most frequently used salicylate.
- **Examples:** Bufferin, Bayer, Doan's pills
- **Side Effects:** gastrointestinal irritation

Nonsteroidal Anti-inflammatory Drugs (nonsalicylates)
Nonsalicylates are primarily utilized for analgesic and anti-inflammatory effects. They possess many similarities to aspirin, however may have diminished side effects.
- **Examples:** Advil, Motrin, Naprosyn
- **Side Effects:** gastrointestinal irritation, dizziness, drowsiness

Acetaminophen
Acetaminophen is commonly used as an analgesic and antipyretic, however does not possess anti-inflammatory properties.
- **Examples:** Tylenol
- **Side Effects:** minimal side effects

Opioids
Opioids are a class of analgesic used to treat moderate-severe pain.
- **Examples:** Codeine, Morphine
- **Side Effects:** addictive, CNS depression

Skeletal Muscle Relaxants
Skeletal muscle relaxants are commonly used to treat spasticity and muscle spasm. The class of medication is divided into two general categories: centrally acting and direct acting agents.
- **Examples:** Flexeril, Baclofen, Diazepam
- **Side Effects:** drowsiness, dry mouth, blurred vision, dizziness

Diuretics
Diuretics promote an increase in the renal excretion of sodium and water therefore diminishing the volume within the vascular system. They are commonly used to treat hypertension and congestive heart failure.
- **Examples:** Diuril, Lasix, Aldactone
- **Side Effects:** fluid depletion, electrolyte imbalance

Digitalis Preparations
Digitalis preparations serve to increase the force of contractions and slow heart rate through actions on the autonomic nervous system. This action allows for increased ventricular filling and a resultant increase in cardiac output.
- **Examples:** Digitoxin, Digoxin
- **Side Effects:** toxicity, nausea, diarrhea, vomiting

Nitrates
Nitrates cause smooth muscle relaxation of both the venous, and to a lesser extent, the arterial systems. As a result they serve to reduce oxygen demand and the symptoms associated with angina.
- **Examples:** Nitroglycerin, Isosorbide dinitrate
- **Side Effects:** headache, dizziness, hypotension

Beta Blockers
Beta adrenergic blockers are commonly utilized to treat hypertension, angina, and arrhythmia.
- **Examples:** Sectral, Lopressor, Toprol
- **Side Effects:** fatigue, depression, excessive decrease in heart rate

Angiotensin-Converting Enzyme (ACE) Inhibitors
ACE inhibitors serve to decrease peripheral vascular resistance. They can be used to treat hypertension and congestive heart failure.
- **Examples:** Captopril, Enalapril, Lisinopril
- **Side Effects:** hypotension, angioedema, hyperkalemia, cough, skin rash

Calcium-Channel Blockers
Calcium-channel blockers inhibit the entry of calcium into smooth muscle cells lining arterial walls so that those muscles cannot contract and produce vasoconstriction. Calcium-channel blockers are useful in treating hypertension and angina.
- **Examples:** Cardizem, Procardia, Calanix, Cardene, Dynacirc
- **Side Effects:** headache, dizziness, flushing, peripheral edema

Benzodiazepines
The Benzodiazepines are among the most frequently prescribed classes of drugs. Central nervous system effects of the benzodiazepines include sedation, decreased anxiety, and muscle relaxation.
- **Examples:** Halcion, Restoril, Dalmane, Ativan, Serax
- **Side Effects:** drowsiness, lethargy, confusion

Antidepressants
Depression is believed to result from increased sensitivity of the postsynaptic receptors for norepinephrine. Antidepressants act to increase norepinephrine transmission and overstimulate the receptor site.
- **Examples:** Prozac, Buspar, Elavil, Ludiomil
- **Side Effects:** tachycardia, arrhythmia, orthostatic hypotension, increased appetite, dry mouth, blurred vision

Review of Systems: Side Effects/Subjective Complaints (In Order of Most Common Occurrence)

Gastrointestinal Distress: dyspepsia, heartburn, nausea, vomiting, abdominal pain, constipation, diarrhea, bleeding
- Salicylates
- Skeletal muscle relaxants
- Antiarrhythmic agents
- Theophylline
- Calcium-channel blockers
- Cholesterol-lowering agents
- Antidepressants (TCAs and MAOIs, lithium)
- Opioids
- ACE inhibitors
- Neuroleptics
- NSAIDs
- Diuretics
- Estrogens and progestins
- β-Blockers
- Nitrates
- OCAs
- Corticosteroids
- Digoxin
- Antiepileptic agents

Pulmonary: bronchospasm, shortness of breath, respiratory depression
- Salicylates
- NSAIDs
- Opioids
- β-Blockers
- ACE inhibitors

Central Nervous System: dizziness, drowsiness, insomnia, headaches, hallucinations, confusion, anxiety, depression, muscle weakness
- NSAIDs
- Nitrates
- Antiepileptic agents
- Corticosteroids
- Antianxiety agents
- Opioids
- Digoxin
- Estrogens and progestins
- Calcium-channel blockers
- Neuroleptics
- β-Blockers
- Antidepressants (TCAs and MAOIs)
- Skeletal muscle relaxants
- ACE inhibitors
- OCAs

Dermatologic: skin rash, itching, flushing of face
- NSAIDs
- Nitrates
- Antiepileptics
- ACE inhibitors
- Estrogens and progestins
- β-Blockers
- Antiarrhythmic agents
- Corticosteroids
- Cholesterol-lowering agents
- Calcium-channel blockers
- OCAs
- Opioids
- MAOIs and lithium

Musculoskeletal: weakness, fatigue, cramps, arthritis, decreased exercise tolerance, osteoporosis
- Corticosteroids
- Antianxiety agents
- ACE inhibitors
- Neuroleptic agents
- Calcium-channel blockers
- Antidepressants
- Digoxin
- Diuretics
- β-Blockers
- Antiepileptic agents

Cardiac: bradycardia, ventricular irritability, AV block, CHF, PVCs, ventricular tachycardia
- Opioids
- TCAs
- Calcium-channel blockers
- β-Blockers
- Oral antiasthmatic agents
- Antiarrhythmic agents
- Digoxin
- Diuretics
- Neuroleptics

Vascular: claudication, hypotension, peripheral edema, cold extremities
- NSAIDs
- Nitrates
- Corticosteroids
- Antidepressants (TCAs and MAOIs)
- Diuretics
- Neuroleptics
- β-Blockers
- OCAs
- Calcium-channel blockers
- Estrogens and progestins
- ACE inhibitors

Genitourinary: sexual dysfunction, urinary retention, urinary incontinence
- Opioids
- OCAs
- Neuroleptics
- β-Blockers
- Diuretics
- Antidepressants (TCAs and MAOIs)
- Estrogens and progestins
- Antiarrhythmic agents

HEENT: tinnitus, loss of taste, headache, light-headedness, dizziness
- Salicylates
- Calcium-channel blockers
- Antiepileptic agents
- Nitrates
- Antidepressants (TCAs and MAOIs)
- Opioids
- Digoxin
- NSAIDs
- ACE inhibitors
- β-Blockers
- Antianxiety agents
- Skeletal muscle relaxants
- Antiarrhythmic agents

**Abbreviations: ACE, angiotensin-converting enzyme; MAOIs, monoamine oxidase inhibitors; NSAIDs, nonsteroidal anti-inflammatory drugs; OCAs, oral contraceptive agents; TCAs, tricyclic antidepressants.

From Boissonnault, WG: Examination in Physical Therapy Practice: Screening for Medical Disease. W.B. Saunders Company, Philadelphia 1995, p.350-351, with permission.

Vitamins

Vitamins are essential non-caloric nutrients that are required in small amounts for certain metabolic functions and cannot be manufactured by the body. Vitamins are most often classified as fat-soluble or water-soluble.

Fat-Soluble Vitamins

Fat-soluble vitamins include vitamins A, D, E, and K. After being absorbed by the intestinal tract, the vitamins are stored in the liver and fatty tissues. Fat-soluble vitamins require protein carriers to move through body fluids and excesses are stored in the body. Since they are not water-soluble, it is possible that the vitamins may reach toxic levels.

Vitamin A
Vitamin A is essential to the eyes, epithelial tissue, normal growth and development, and reproduction.

- **Common food sources** containing Vitamin A include green, orange, and yellow vegetables, liver, butter, egg yolks, and fortified margarine.
- **Symptoms of deficiency** include night blindness, rough and dry skin, and growth failure.
- **Symptoms of toxicity** include appetite loss, hair loss, and enlarged liver and spleen.

Vitamin D
Vitamin D increases the blood flow levels of minerals, notably calcium and phosphorus.

- **Common food sources** containing Vitamin D include fortified milk, fish oils, and fortified margarine.
- **Symptoms of deficiency** include faulty bone growth, rickets, and osteomalacia.
- **Symptoms of toxicity** include calcification of soft tissues and hypercalcemia.

Vitamin E
Vitamin E functions as an antioxidant in cell membranes and is especially important for the integrity of cells that are constantly exposed to high levels of oxygen such as the lungs and red blood cells.

- **Common food sources** containing Vitamin E include vegetable oils, wheat germ, nuts, and fish.
- **Symptoms of deficiency** include the breakdown of red blood cells, however this is relatively rare in adults.
- **Symptoms of toxicity** include decreased thyroid hormone levels and increased triglycerides.

Vitamin K
Vitamin K is necessary for the synthesis of at least two of the proteins involved in blood clotting.

- **Common food sources** containing Vitamin K include dark green leafy vegetables, cheese, egg yolks, and liver.
- **Symptoms of deficiency** include hemorrhage and defective blood clotting.
- **Toxicity** has not been reported.

Water-Soluble Vitamins

Water-soluble vitamins are not stored in the body in any significant amount and therefore need to be included in the diet on a daily basis. Toxicity is less common than with fat-soluble vitamins.

Vitamin B$_2$ (Riboflavin)
Vitamin B$_2$ facilitates selected enzymes involved in carbohydrate, protein, and fat metabolism.

- **Common food sources** containing Vitamin B$_2$ include milk, green leafy vegetables, eggs, and peanuts.
- **Symptoms of deficiency** include inflammation of the tongue, sensitive eyes, and scaling of the skin.
- **Toxicity** has not been reported.

Vitamin B$_3$ (Niacin)
Vitamin B$_3$ facilitates several enzymes that regulate energy metabolism.

- **Common food sources** containing Vitamin B$_3$ include meats, whole grains, and white flour.
- **Symptoms of deficiency** include pellagra and gastrointestinal disturbances.
- **Symptoms of toxicity** include abnormal glucose metabolism, nausea, vomiting, and gastric ulceration.

Vitamin B$_6$ (Pyridoxine)
Vitamin B$_6$ is essential in the metabolism of proteins, amino acids, carbohydrates, and fat.

- **Common food sources** containing Vitamin B$_6$ include liver, red meats, whole grains, and potatoes.
- **Symptoms of deficiency** include peripheral neuropathy, convulsions, and depression.
- **Symptoms of toxicity** include sensory damage, numbness of the extremities, and ataxia.

Vitamin B$_{12}$ (Cobalamin)
Vitamin B$_{12}$ is essential for the functioning of all cells and aids in hemoglobin synthesis.

- **Common food sources** containing Vitamin B$_{12}$ include meats, whole eggs, and egg yolks.
- **Symptoms of deficiency** include pernicious anemia and various psychological disorders.
- **Toxicity** has not been reported.

Vitamin C
Vitamin C assists the body to combat infections and facilitates wound healing. The vitamin is necessary for the development and maintenance of bones, cartilage, connective tissue, and blood vessels.

- **Common food sources** containing Vitamin C include citrus fruits, tomatoes, and cantaloupe.
- **Symptoms of deficiency** include anemia, swollen gums, loose teeth, and scurvy.
- **Symptoms of toxicity** include urinary stones, diarrhea, and hypoglycemia.

Biotin
Biotin is necessary for the action of many enzyme systems.

- **Common food sources** containing biotin include liver, meats, and milk.
- **Symptoms of deficiency** include anemia, depression, and muscle pain.
- **Toxicity** has not been reported.

Choline
Choline is a component of compounds necessary for nerve function and lipid metabolism.

- Choline is synthesized from methionine which is an amino acid.
- **Symptoms of deficiency** only occur when intake of methylamine is low.
- **Toxicity** has not been reported.

Folacin (Folic acid)
Folacin is involved in the formation of red blood cells and in the functioning of the gastrointestinal tract.

- **Common food sources** containing folacin include yeast, dark green leafy vegetables, and whole grains.
- **Symptoms of deficiency** include impaired cell division and alteration of protein synthesis.
- **Toxicity** has not been reported.

Pantothenic acid
Pantothenic acid is an integral component of complex enzymes involved in the metabolism of fatty acids.

- **Common food sources** containing pantothenic acid include liver, eggs, and whole grains.
- **Symptoms of deficiency** include headache, fatigue, and poor muscle coordination.
- **Symptoms of toxicity** include diarrhea.

Minerals

Minerals are organic elements that fulfill essential roles in metabolism.

Major Minerals

Calcium (Ca)
Calcium facilitates muscle contraction and relaxation, builds strong bones and teeth, and aids in coagulation.

- **Common food sources** containing calcium include milk, green leafy vegetables, and soy products.
- **Calcium deficiency** may lead to poor bone growth, rickets, osteomalacia, and osteoporosis.
- **Symptoms of toxicity** include kidney stones.

Chloride (Cl)
Chloride facilitates the maintenance of fluid and acid-base balance.

- **Common food sources** containing chloride include table salt, fish, and vegetables.
- **Chloride deficiency** may lead to a disturbance of acid-base balance.
- **Toxicity** has not been reported.

Magnesium (Mg)
Magnesium builds strong bones and teeth, activates enzymes, and helps regulate heartbeat.

- **Common food sources** containing magnesium include raw dark vegetables, nuts, soybeans, milk, and cheese.
- **Symptoms of deficiency** include confusion, apathy, muscle weakness, and tremors.
- **Symptoms of toxicity** include increased calcium excretion.

Phosphorus (P)
Phosphorus strengthens bones, assists in the oxidation of fats and carbohydrates, and aids in maintaining acid-base balance.

- **Common food sources** containing phosphorus include milk and milk products, meats, whole grains, and soft drinks.
- **Symptoms of deficiency** include weakness, stiff joints, and fragile bones.
- **Symptoms of toxicity** include muscle spasms.

Potassium (K)
Potassium maintains fluid and acid-base balance.

- **Common food sources** containing potassium include apricots, bananas, oranges, grapefruit, and milk.
- **Symptoms of deficiency** include impaired growth, hypertension, and diminished heart rate.
- **Symptoms of toxicity** include hyperkalemia and cardiac disturbances.

Sodium (Na)
Sodium facilitates the maintenance of acid-base balance, transmits nerve impulses, and helps control muscle contractions.

- **Common food sources** containing sodium include salt and milk.
- **Deficiency and toxicity** have not been reported.

Sulfur (S)
Sulfur facilitates enzyme activity and energy metabolism.

- **Common food sources** containing sulfur include meat, eggs, milk, and cheese.
- **Deficiency** is extremely rare.
- **Toxicity** has not been reported.

Trace Minerals

Chromium (Cr)
Chromium controls glucose metabolism.

- **Common food sources** containing chromium include whole grains, meats, and cheese.
- **Symptoms of deficiency** include weight loss and central nervous system abnormalities.
- **Symptoms of toxicity** include liver damage.

Cobalt (Co)
Cobalt is an essential component of vitamin B_{12} and functions to activate enzymes.

- **Common food sources** containing cobalt include figs, cabbage, and spinach.
- **Symptoms of deficiency** include pernicious anemia.
- **Symptoms of toxicity** include polycythemia and increased blood volume.

Copper (Cu)
Copper facilitates hemoglobin synthesis and lipid metabolism.

- **Common food sources** containing copper include shellfish, liver, meat, and whole grains.
- **Symptoms of deficiency** include anemia, central nervous system abnormalities, and abnormal electrocardiograms.
- **Symptoms of toxicity** include Wilson's disease.

Fluorine (F)
Fluorine aids in the formation of bones and teeth and prevents osteoporosis.

- **Common food sources** containing fluorine include fish and water.
- **Symptoms of deficiency** include increased susceptibility of dental cavities.
- **Symptoms of toxicity** include fluorosis.

Iodine (I)
Iodine assists with the regulation of cell metabolism and basal metabolic rate.

- **Common food sources** containing iodine include iodized salt and seafood.
- **Symptoms of deficiency** may include goiters.
- **Toxicity** has not been reported.

Iron (Fe)
Iron assists in the oxygen transport and cell oxidation.

- **Common food sources** containing iron include red meats and liver.
- **Symptoms of deficiency** include anemia.
- **Symptoms of toxicity** include hemochromatosis.

Manganese (Mn)
Manganese facilitates proper bone structure and functions as an enzyme component in general metabolism.

- **Common food sources** containing manganese include cereals and whole grains.
- There are no known **symptoms of deficiency.**
- **Toxicity** has not been reported.

Molybdenum (Mo)
Molybdenum is a component of three enzymes necessary for normal cell functioning.
- **Common food sources** containing molybdenum include meats, whole grains, and dark green vegetables.
- **Symptoms of deficiency** include vomiting and tachypnea.
- **Toxicity** has not been reported

Selenium (Se)
Selenium is a synergistic antioxidant with Vitamin E.
- **Common food sources** containing selenium include meat, eggs, milk, seafood, and garlic.
- **Symptoms of deficiency** include Keshan's disease.
- **Symptoms of toxicity** include physical defects of fingernails and toenails, nausea, and abdominal pain

Zinc (Zn)
Zinc aids in immune function and cell division.
- **Common food sources** containing zinc include seafood, liver, milk, cheese, and whole grains.
- **Symptoms of deficiency** include depressed immune functions and impaired skeletal growth.
- **Symptoms of toxicity** include anemia, nausea, and vomiting.

11 Education

Psychology

Maslow's Hierarchy of Needs

Maslow's hierarchy of needs hypothesizes that there is a hierarchy of biogenic and psychogenic needs which individuals must progress through. In order to move to a higher level of needs an individual must attain the objectives associated with the previous level. In essence an individual must achieve basic or fundamental needs before moving to upper level needs.

Self-Actualization needs: The need to realize one's full potential as a human being.

Esteem needs: The need to feel good about oneself and one's capabilities; to be respected by others, and to receive recognition and appreciation.

Affiliative needs: The need for security, stability, and a safe environment.

Physiological needs: The need for basic things necessary in order to survive such as food, water, and shelter.

Classical Conditioning (Pavlov)

When an unconditioned stimulus (food) is repeatedly preceded by a neutral stimulus (bell), the neutral stimulus serves as a conditioned stimulus and the learned reaction that results is termed the conditioned response. In order to maintain a conditioned response the conditioned and unconditioned stimuli must occasionally be paired.

Operant Conditioning (B.F. Skinner)

Learning that occurs when an individual engages in specific behaviors in order to receive certain consequences.

Positive reinforcement: Administering desirable consequences to individuals who perform a specific behavior.

Negative reinforcement: Removing undesirable consequences from individuals who perform a specific behavior.

Extinction: Removing selected variables that reinforce a specific behavior.

Punishment: Administering negative consequences to individuals who perform undesirable behaviors.

Reinforcement frequency and schedules:
- *Continuous reinforcement*
  A behavior is reinforced every time it occurs.

- *Partial reinforcement*
  A behavior is reinforced intermittently.

- *Fixed-interval schedule*
  The period of time between the occurrences of each instance of reinforcement is fixed or set.

- *Variable-interval schedule*
  The amount of time between reinforcements varies around a constant average.

Social Learning Theory

A theory that takes into account the influence of thoughts and feelings in learning.

Vicarious learning: Learning that occurs when one person learns a behavior by observing another person perform the behavior.

Self-control: Self-discipline that allows a person to learn to perform a behavior even though there is no external pressure to do so.

Self-reinforcers: Consequences or rewards that individuals can supply to themselves.

Patient Education

Adult Learning

- Therapists must strive to make patient education sessions practical and useful for the patient.
- Failure to identify the relevance of the presented information will promote disinterest and decrease compliance.

Guidelines to Promote Adult Learning

- Design learning activities that will incorporate the patient's past experiences.
- Encourage the learner to play an active role in his/her educational program.
- Attempt to demonstrate the relevance of selected learning activities.
- Provide ample opportunities for practice and feedback.
- Recognize skill acquisition or objective improvement in patient performance.

Domains of Learning

Domains of learning are educational terms that describe various aspects of human behavior. The three most commonly recognized domains of learning are the cognitive, psychomotor, and affective domains. Recognizing the various levels of each of the domains can assist therapists to plan appropriate patient learning activities.

Cognitive domain: The cognitive domain is primarily concerned with knowledge and understanding. The domain consists of six specific levels: knowledge, comprehension, application, analysis, synthesis, and evaluation.

Psychomotor domain: The psychomotor domain is primarily concerned with physical action or motor skill. The domain consists of seven specific levels: perception, set, guided response, mechanism, complex overt response, adaptation, and origination.

Affective domain: The affective domain is primarily concerned with attitudes, values, and emotions. The domain consists of five specific levels: receiving, responding, valuing, organization, and characterization.

Learning Style

Therapists can often obtain information related to a patient's preferred learning style by asking a few basic questions.

1. Do you prefer to learn new information by observing, reading, listening or experiencing?
2. Are you more comfortable learning in an active or passive manner?
3. What increases your motivation to learn?

Teaching Methods

Individual:
- Therapists most commonly instruct patients on an individual basis.
- The individual approach allows the therapist to focus on the needs of the learner and is the model of choice when the objectives of the session are unique to an individual patient.
- The individual approach allows the therapist to strengthen the patient/therapist bond and provides additional opportunities for specific feedback.

Group:
- Therapists often instruct patients in a group.
- Group teaching may occur with patients, family members, staff, and support persons.
- Group teaching can be difficult if patients are not supportive of each other or if the learning needs of the group are diverse.
- Some patients may be intimidated by selected group members and tend to withdraw, while others may attempt to take control of the group.
- Since individuals typically receive less individual attention in a group it is critical for the therapist to regularly assess individual patient progress.
- Group teaching allows participants to support each other in the educational process and permits therapists to effectively use scarce resources such as time or money.
- Patients participating in group activities often feel a sense of camaraderie interacting with others who have similar personal experiences.

Guidelines for Effective Patient Education

- Attempt to establish a positive rapport with the patient.
- Assess the patient's readiness and motivation to learn.
- Attempt to identify the patient's preferred learning style and available resources.
- Identify potential barriers to patient progress.
- Design an individualized education program for the patient based on his/her medical condition and personal goals.
- Coordinate education with the other members of the health care team.
- Focus the majority of available time on the most important concepts.
- Provide clear and succinct communication to the patient.
- Use repetition to improve patient learning.
- Provide frequent feedback to the patient.
- Utilize appropriate teaching resources to facilitate patient learning.
- Assess the effectiveness of patient education.
- Modify the patient education program based on the assessment results.

Principles of Motivation

- Readiness to learn significantly influences motivation.
- Individuals respond differently to selected motivational strategies.
- Success is more motivating than failure.
- Internal motivation has a greater potential to contribute to meaningful and lasting change than external motivation.
- Positive patient/therapist relationship enhances motivation.
- Limited anxiety may serve to motivate, while excessive anxiety may debilitate.
- Affiliation and approval can be motivating.

Cultural Influences

- Understanding cultural differences in patients can assist therapists to function as more effective educators.
- Patient culture is influenced and shaped by society, community, family, personal values, and attitudes.
- Language barriers, nonverbal communication, and limited personal experience can serve as obstacles when educating patients with significant cultural differences.
- Therapists should embrace cultural diversity and avoid efforts to make patients conform to any particular norm or standard.
- Therapists must be cautious when interpreting specific language or behavior and avoid labeling patients as unmotivated or disinterested.
- Therapists should use available resources such as experienced staff members, interpreters, or consultants as necessary to achieve desired outcomes.

Designing Effective Patient Education Materials

- Design the materials to convey only the necessary information.
- Emphasize essential information.
- Utilize active instructions such as "you" and avoid passive terms such as "patient."
- Larger print may be more desirable than smaller print.
- Avoid long sentences or complex medical terminology.
- Pictures or graphics should be used where appropriate to complement written information.
- Incorporate answers to frequently asked questions.
- Written materials should flow in a logical sequence.
- Written materials should utilize a reading level appropriate for the target audience.

Teaching Guidelines for Specific Patient Categories

Therapists often vary their approach when educating patients of various ages and ability. It is difficult to develop recommendations that apply to all patients in a given category, however the following represent general guidelines for therapists to consider when treating selected patient categories.

Infants/Children:
- Therapists should try to make therapy sessions with infants/children interactive.
- Sessions should include structured play and should be of relatively short duration.
- Frequent breaks and positive reinforcement will serve to increase the patient's level of participation.

Adolescents:
- Therapists should try to assume the role of an advocate when working with adolescents.
- It is important for therapists to establish patients' trust and incorporate patient goals into the plan of care.
- Adolescents prefer to be treated like adults and may resent the presence of parents during therapy sessions.
- Therapists should provide patients with clear and concise instructions and offer frequent positive reinforcement.

Adults:
- Therapists should involve adults in determining education outcomes.
- The education program should be compatible with the patient's daily routine and goals.
- Emphasizing the relevance of educational activities will serve to increase patient compliance.
- Therapists should be aware of the available patient support system and identify any barriers to progress.

Elderly:
- Therapists may find it necessary to introduce new information gradually when working with the elderly.
- Special attention should be paid to identify signs of hearing loss or visual impairments.
- The elderly population often benefits from the social benefits of group activities.
- Education sessions for the elderly should not be longer in duration, however the achievement of selected outcomes may require additional sessions.

Terminally Ill:
- Therapists should incorporate patient goals as an integral component of any educational session for patients with terminal illness.
- Family members and other support personnel should be encouraged to participate in the educational session, however it is important to provide the patient with the opportunity to make independent decisions whenever possible.

- Goals for the terminally ill patient often include maximizing function, safety, and comfort.
- Therapists may alter their teaching methods based on the current mental and physical well-being of the patient.

Cognitively Impaired:
- The therapist should focus on the education of the caregiver and incorporate the patient whenever possible.
- When incorporating the patient in the session, instructions should be clear and concise and should be summarized though demonstration and pictures.
- Therapists should encourage the patient to compensate for any memory deficit.

Illiteracy:
- Therapists should attempt to determine the literacy level of their patients.
- If a patient is determined to be illiterate the therapist may elect to modify language to use basic wording and short sentences.
- Demonstration, repetition, and pictures should be incorporated into educational sessions.
- Therapists may include more detailed written information in educational sessions if the patient has adequate support at home.

Stages of Dying

Elizabeth Kubler-Ross identified five stages in coming to terms with death after interviewing 500 terminally ill patients. The stages Kubler-Ross identified were denial, anger, bargaining, depression, and acceptance.

Denial: The denial stage is characterized by a failure of the individual to believe that his/her condition is terminal. Therapists should attempt to establish trust with a patient in this stage and avoid trying to make the patient accept his/her condition.

Anger: The anger stage is characterized by frustration and negative emotional feelings often directed at anyone the individual comes in contact with. Individuals often ask "Why me?" Therapists should avoid taking the anger personally and recognize that expressing anger is often a useful step for the individual to move beyond this stage.

Bargaining: The bargaining stage is characterized by the individual trying to negotiate with fate. The individual may try to make a deal with a higher being based on good behavior, compliance with an exercise program, or dedication of his/her life to a specific cause. Therapists should facilitate discussion with the patient and serve as a good listener.

Depression: The depression stage is characterized by the individual expressing the depths of his/her anguish. The individual is often deeply depressed and may show little interest in any form of medical intervention. Therapists should listen to the individual and exhibit a great deal of patience during this stage.

Acceptance: The acceptance stage is characterized by the individual coming to terms with his/her fate. The individual may attempt to resolve any unfinished business and may experience a sense of inner peace. Therapists should encourage the individual and family to ask questions and attempt to spend meaningful time with the individual.

Education Concepts

Practice

Practice refers to repeated performance of an activity in order to learn or perfect a skill. There are several commonly used terms that describe various types of practice.

Massed practice: The practice time in a trial is greater than the amount of rest between trials.

Distributed practice: The amount of rest time between trials is equal to or is greater than the amount of practice time for each trial.

Constant practice: Practice of a given task under a uniform condition.

Variable practice: Practice of a given task under differing conditions.

Random practice: Varying practice amongst different tasks.

Blocked practice: Consistent practice of a single task.

Whole training: Practice of an entire task.

Part training: Practice of an individual component or selected components of a task.

Feedback

Therapists should provide patients with specific and timely feedback in a manner that will promote attainment of the learning objective.

Summary feedback: Provided at the end of a defined number of activities or at the conclusion of the entire session.

Immediate feedback: Provided at the conclusion of a given activity.

Intrinsic feedback: Provided by the individual's internal sensory system as a result of the normal production of movement.

Extrinsic feedback: Provided by an external source such as a therapist, spouse or physician.

Team Models

Unidisciplinary: A single discipline provides patient care services.

Multidisciplinary: Several different disciplines are involved in providing patient care, however the disciplines tend to function independently and communication occurs primarily through the medical record.

Interdisciplinary: Several different disciplines are involved in providing patient care. The disciplines function independently, however routinely report to each other and may coordinate patient care.

Transdisciplinary: Numerous disciplines function as a collective unit to provide patient care services. Team goals are established rather than individual discipline goals and as a result, discipline specific boundaries tend to erode.

Clinical Application Templates

Template 1	Achilles Tendon Rupture	171
Template 2	Alzheimer's Disease	173
Template 3	Amputation due to Arteriosclerosis Obliterans	175
Template 4	Amyotrophic Lateral Sclerosis	177
Template 5	Ankylosing Spondylitis	179
Template 6	Anterior Cruciate Ligament Sprain – Grade III	181
Template 7	Breast Cancer	183
Template 8	Carpal Tunnel Syndrome	185
Template 9	Cerebrovascular Accident	187
Template 10	Cystic Fibrosis	189
Template 11	Duchenne Muscular Dystrophy	191
Template 12	Emphysema	193
Template 13	Huntington's Disease	195
Template 14	Medial Collateral Ligament Sprain – Grade II	197
Template 15	Multiple Sclerosis	199
Template 16	Myocardial Infarction	201
Template 17	Parkinson's Disease	203
Template 18	Patellofemoral Syndrome	205
Template 19	Plantar Fasciitis	207
Template 20	Restrictive Lung Disease	209
Template 21	Rheumatoid Arthritis	211
Template 22	Rotator Cuff Tendonitis	213
Template 23	Scoliosis	215
Template 24	Spina Bifida - Myelomeningocele	217
Template 25	Spinal Cord Injury – C7 Tetraplegia	219
Template 26	Systemic Lupus Erythematosus	221
Template 27	Thoracic Outlet Syndrome	223
Template 28	Total Hip Replacement	225
Template 29	Total Knee Replacement	227
Template 30	Urinary Stress Incontinence	229

Clinical Application Templates

Introduction

Clinical application templates provide candidates with a unique study tool designed to broaden their exposure to a variety of commonly encountered medical conditions. By utilizing the templates candidates can improve their decision-making skills when answering challenging multiple-choice questions and as a result improve their performance on the Physical Therapist Examination. The clinical application template was adapted from a document by the Academy of Specialty Boards entitled "Preparing Items that Measure More than Recall." The document was originally designed to help item writers develop sample questions for the Physical Therapy Specialty Examinations.

The clinical application template allows candidates to explore all of the elements of patient/client management for any medical condition. Although candidates have been exposed to a variety of medical conditions during their clinical education experiences it is unlikely they have been exposed to the vast number of medical conditions commonly encountered on the examination. By utilizing the clinical application templates students can broaden their experience base and as a result be better prepared to answer examination questions involving selected subject matter.

This clinical application template section presents 30 different templates. Candidates are encouraged to review the templates and carefully reflect on each of the elements of patient/client management. The clinical scenarios presented at the conclusion of each template provide candidates with an opportunity to compare and contrast the presented medical condition with other related conditions.

Candidates should not rely solely on the presented clinical application templates and instead should utilize the template format to review a variety of other medical conditions. This type of active learning is best performed by a small group of candidates with a given candidate acting as the facilitator. In this manner students can share their collective clinical experiences with the group and at the same time benefit from the knowledge of their classmates.

Achilles Tendon Rupture

Diagnosis:

What condition produces a patient's symptoms?
A patient will present with symptoms secondary to the rupture and discontinuity of the Achilles tendon. Rupture of the Achilles tendon normally occurs within two to six centimeters above the tendinous insertion on the calcaneus.

An injury was most likely sustained to which structure?
Theories suggest that an Achilles tendon rupture usually occurs in an Achilles tendon that has undergone degenerative changes. The degenerative changes will begin with hypovascularity in the Achilles tendon area. The impaired blood flow in combination with repetitive microtrauma creates degenerative changes within the tendon and as a result makes the tendon more susceptible to injury.

Inference:

What is the most likely contributing factor in the development of this condition?
An Achilles tendon rupture occurs most frequently when pushing off of a weight bearing extremity with an extended knee, unexpected dorsiflexion while weight bearing or a forceful eccentric contraction of the plantar flexors. A person over 30 years of age is at a higher risk for rupture secondary to the decrease in blood flow to the area of the tendon associated with aging.

Confirmation:

What is the most likely clinical presentation?
A patient with an Achilles tendon rupture will present with swelling over the distal tendon, a palpable defect in the tendon above the calcaneal tuberosity, and pain and weakness with plantar flexion. A patient in a prone position will not present with passive plantar flexion with squeezing of the affected calf muscle.

What laboratory or imaging studies would confirm the diagnosis?
Confirmation of an Achilles tendon rupture should utilize x-ray to rule out an avulsion fracture or bony injury. Magnetic resonance imaging can be used to locate the presence and severity of the tear.

What additional information should be obtained to confirm the diagnosis?
Diagnosis of an Achilles tendon rupture relies on patient history of the event and a positive Thompson's test. Patient history usually reveals a popping sound and a release from the back of the ankle. Physical examination and palpation reveal a discontinuity within the tendon.

Examination:

What history should be documented?
Important areas to explore include mechanism of present injury, past medical history, medications, current health status, social history and habits, occupation, living environment, and social support system.

What test/measures are most appropriate?
- **Anthropometric characteristics:** circumferential measurements for edema, palpation to determine ankle effusion
- **Arousal attention, and cognition:** examine mental status, learning ability, memory, and motivation
- **Assistive and adaptive devices:** potential utilization of crutches
- **Gait, locomotion, and balance:** safety with/without an assistive device during gait
- **Integumentary integrity:** assessment of sensation
- **Joint integrity and mobility:** special tests such as Thompson's test
- **Muscle performance:** strength assessment, characteristics of muscle contraction
- **Pain:** pain perception assessment scale
- **Range of motion:** active and passive range of motion
- **Sensory integration:** assessment of proprioception and kinesthesia
- **Self-care and home management:** assessment of functional capacity

What additional findings are likely with this patient?
A typical patient that is diagnosed with an Achilles tendon rupture is usually between 30 and 40 years of age and participates in recreational sports. An Achilles tendon rupture is more common in men and in people that do not consistently exercise. An avulsion fracture is another additional finding that is occasionally observed with an Achilles rupture.

Management:

What is the most effective management of this patient?
Management of a ruptured Achilles tendon incorporates immobilization through casting or a surgical approach for repair or reconstruction. Postsurgically a patient will require a cast or brace for six to eight weeks. Physical therapy intervention includes range of motion, stretching, icing, assistive device training, endurance programming, gait training, strengthening, plyometrics, and skill specific training. Modalities, pool therapy, and other cardiovascular equipment may assist in the recovery of functional motion and endurance.

What home care regimen should be recommended?
A home care regimen is vital to the success of a patient's recovery. A program must be based on a patient's postoperative impairments and follow the physician's postsurgical protocol. A home program generally incorporates icing and elevation early in the rehabilitation process. A patient is required to continue a home program throughout the six to seven months of rehabilitation. Other areas of focus include range of motion, gait, therapeutic exercise, endurance activities, and high level skill and sport specific tasks.

Outcome:

What is the likely outcome of a course in physical therapy?
Physical therapy should begin after surgical intervention. Assuming an unremarkable recovery, a patient should return to his/her previous functional level within six to seven months.

What are the long-term effects of the patient's condition?
A patient that manages the Achilles tendon rupture without surgery and allows the tendon to heal on its own has a higher rate of rerupture than a patient that has surgical repair of the tendon. An advantage to nonsurgical management is a reduced risk of infection from surgery, however it may result in an incomplete return of functional performance. A patient that has surgical intervention has a decreased risk for reinjury and a higher rate of return to full athletic activities.

Comparison:

What are the distinguishing characteristics of a similar condition?
Achilles tendonitis can be an acute or chronic condition due to repetitive microtrauma that builds scar tissue in the area over time. A patient initially feels an aching sensation after activity and progresses to pain with walking. There may be localized tenderness and swelling in the area. In the acute stage a patient should rest for two to three weeks and utilize anti-inflammatory medications and a heel lift. In the chronic stage the symptoms and pain may last beyond six weeks. Examination often reveals a thickened and nodular Achilles tendon. Surgical intervention may be warranted at this stage.

Clinical Scenarios:

Scenario One
A 32-year-old female is playing soccer in a recreational league. A physical therapist that assists the team observes her kick the ball and then fall to the ground. The therapist examines the patient in the training room and finds that the patient has some plantar flexion in a non-weight bearing position, but is unable to plantar flex the foot while weight bearing. The patient states that something popped while running and palpation indicates a separation in the Achilles tendon.

Scenario Two
A 46-year-old male is referred to physical therapy status postsurgical reconstruction of a left Achilles tendon rupture. The patient has been casted for one week and has been using axillary crutches for household mobility. The patient has no significant past medical history. He is employed as a truck driver and resides in a one story home. The patient sustained the injury while playing tennis.

Alzheimer's Disease

Diagnosis:

What condition produces a patient's symptoms?
Alzheimer's disease is a progressive neurological disorder that results in deterioration and irreversible damage within the cerebral cortex and subcortical areas of the brain.

An injury was most likely sustained to which structure?
Neurons that are normally involved with acetylcholine transmission deteriorate within the cerebral cortex. Postmortem biopsy reveals neurofibrillary tangles within cytoplasm, amyloid plaques, and cerebral atrophy.

Inference:

What is the most likely contributing factor in the development of this condition?
The exact etiology of Alzheimer's disease is unknown, however hypothesized causes include lower levels of neurotransmitters, higher levels of aluminum within brain tissue, genetic inheritance, autoimmune disease, and virus. The risk of developing Alzheimer's disease increases with age and there is a higher incidence in women. Approximately 20% of people over 80 years of age demonstrate symptoms of Alzheimer's disease.

Confirmation:

What is the most likely clinical presentation?
Alzheimer's disease is initially characterized by subtle changes in memory, impaired concentration, and difficulty with new learning. These symptoms progress in the early stages and there is a loss of orientation, emotional lability, depression, poor judgment, and impaired ability to perform self-care skills. During the middle stages of Alzheimer's disease the patient will present with neurological symptoms such as aphasia, apraxia, perseveration, agitation, and violent or socially unacceptable behavior. End stage Alzheimer's disease is characterized by severe intellectual and physical destruction. Patients in this stage will present with vegetative symptoms including incontinence, functional dependence, the inability to speak, and seizure activity.

What laboratory or imaging studies would confirm the diagnosis?
Alzheimer's disease presently cannot be confirmed until a postmortem biopsy reveals the neurofibrillary tangles and amyloid plaques. Magnetic resonance imaging can be used to assess any abnormalities or signs of atrophy within the brain or to rule out other medical conditions. Blood work, urine, and spinal fluid may be required to rule out other diseases that may cause signs of dementia.

What additional information should be obtained to confirm the diagnosis?
A physical examination, neurological examination, and neuropsychological testing are required for diagnosis of probable Alzheimer's disease. Family history and symptoms may provide insight into the expected speed of progression of the disease.

Examination:

What history should be documented?
Important areas to explore include past medical history, family history, history of current symptoms, current health status, living environment, social history and habits, occupation, and social support system.

What test/measures are most appropriate?
- **Aerobic capacity and endurance:** assessment of vital signs at rest and with activity
- **Arousal, attention, and cognition:** examine mental status, learning ability, memory, and motivation, Mini Mental State Examination, level of consciousness
- **Assistive and adaptive devices:** analysis of components and safety of a device
- **Environmental, home, and work barriers:** analysis of current and potential barriers or hazards
- **Gait, locomotion, and balance:** static and dynamic balance in sitting and standing, safety during gait with/without an assistive device, Functional Ambulation Profile
- **Motor function:** equilibrium and righting reactions, coordination, physical performance scales
- **Muscle performance:** strength assessment
- **Posture:** analysis of resting and dynamic posture
- **Range of motion:** active and passive range of motion

- **Reflex integrity:** assessment of deep tendon and pathological reflexes (e.g. Babinski, ATNR)
- **Self-care and home management:** assessment of functional capacity, Functional Independence Measure (FIM), Barthel ADL Index

What additional findings are likely with this patient?
A patient with end stage Alzheimer's disease may experience complications from a persistent vegetative state such as contractures, decubiti, fracture, and pulmonary compromise.

Management:
What is the most effective management of this patient?
Management of Alzheimer's disease may include pharmacological intervention during the early stages of the disease process. Medications are administered to inhibit acetylcholinesterase, alleviate cognitive symptoms, and control behavioral changes. Tacrine (Cognex), hydrochloride (Aricept), and rivastigmine (Exelon) are common pharmacological agents used to treat Alzheimer's disease. Physical therapy management should focus on maximizing the patient's remaining function and providing family and caregiver education. The therapist should attempt to create an emotional and physical environment that provides the patient with the opportunity to experience success. Modifying the layout of the patient's living space in order for the patient to easily find items is one example of creating an environment that encourages success. Safety with functional mobility and gait training may be indicated in the early stages of the disease. Later stages may require ongoing caregiver education regarding assistance with mobility, range of motion, and positioning.

What home care regimen should be recommended?
During the early stages of Alzheimer's disease a patient should continue with activity as tolerated and utilize a memory book or other compensatory strategies at home. As the disease progresses, a patient will rely on caregiver and family support to assist with a daily exercise program.

Outcome:
What is the likely outcome of a course in physical therapy?
Physical therapy may be indicated intermittently throughout the course of the disease, however will not alter or cease the progression of the disease process.

What are the long-term effects of the patient's condition?
Alzheimer's disease is a chronic and progressive disorder. It can progress slowly over ten to fifteen years or can steadily progress to end stage within a few years.

Comparison:
What are the distinguishing characteristics of a similar condition?
Multi-infarct dementia produces symptoms in a step-like manner secondary to ongoing cerebral infarcts. This form of dementia is usually found in patients that are over 70 years of age and is more common in males. Hypertension is a primary risk factor. Depression is common and in the later stages a patient will experience neurological deficits such as hemiplegia and emotional lability.

Clinical Scenarios:
Scenario One
A 65-year-old female is referred to physical therapy for gait disturbances. The patient resides alone and drives on a regular basis. During the initial examination the patient reveals that she is sometimes confused when she is driving and forgets how to get to certain places. The patient complains that she has difficulty managing her time around the house and requires an extended amount of time to get ready in the morning.

Scenario Two
A 79-year-old male is seen by a physical therapist in an Alzheimer's residential facility. The physician recommends gait training with a walker. The patient enjoys walking around the unit, however has fallen several times within the last month.

Amputation due to Arteriosclerosis Obliterans

Diagnosis:

What condition produces a patient's symptoms?
Arteriosclerosis obliterans is a form of peripheral vascular disease that produces thickening, hardening, and eventual narrowing and occlusion of the arteries. Arteriosclerosis obliterans results in ischemia and subsequent ulceration of the affected tissues. The affected area may become necrotic, gangrenous, and require amputation.

An injury was most likely sustained to which structure?
Injury will occur to all structures that receive blood supply from vessels that have become occluded. Prolonged ischemia results in tissue death and infection.

Inference:

What is the most likely contributing factor in the development of this condition?
Risk factors associated with arteriosclerosis obliterans include age, diabetes, sex, hypertension, high serum cholesterol and low density lipid levels, smoking, obesity, and sedentary lifestyle. Unsuccessful management of peripheral vascular disease may ultimately lead to uncontrolled infection, gangrene, necrosis, and amputation.

Confirmation:

What is the most likely clinical presentation?
The patient that requires amputation secondary to arteriosclerosis obliterans will present with intermittent claudication that produces cramps and pain in the affected areas. Other characteristics include resting pain, decreased pulses, pallor skin, and decreased skin temperature.

What laboratory or imaging studies would confirm the diagnosis?
Arteriosclerosis obliterans can be diagnosed using a Doppler ultrasonography, MRI or arteriography. These diagnostic tests examine the degree of blood flow throughout the extremities. A patient with arteriosclerosis obliterans would typically demonstrate poor results including blockage, tissue damage, and tissue death.

What additional information should be obtained to confirm the diagnosis?
The physician should examine the limb for temperature, skin condition, presence of hair, sensation, and palpable pulses when determining the need for amputation. The physician may perform a selected noninvasive test such as a claudication test that examines the presence of intermittent claudication that can occur with prolonged ambulation.

Examination:

What history should be documented?
Important areas to explore include past medical history, medications, current health status, social history and habits, occupation, living environment, and social support system.

What test/measures are most appropriate?
- **Aerobic capacity and endurance:** palpation of pulses, pulse oximetry, vital signs at rest and with activity
- **Anthropometric characteristics:** residual limb circumferential measurements, length of limb
- **Arousal, attention, and cognition:** examine mental status, learning ability, memory, and motivation
- **Assistive and adaptive devices:** analysis of components and safety of a device
- **Gait, locomotion, and balance:** analysis of wheelchair mobility, static and dynamic balance in sitting and standing, safety during gait with an assistive device
- **Integumentary integrity:** examine presence of hair growth, color, temperature, assessment of sensation
- **Muscle performance:** strength assessment
- **Orthotic, protective, and supportive devices:** analysis of components and wearing of a device
- **Pain:** phantom pain, pain perception assessment scale
- **Range of motion:** active and passive range of motion
- **Self-care and home management:** assessment of functional capacity, Barthel ADL Index, Functional Independence Measure (FIM)
- **Sensory integrity:** assessment of proprioception and kinesthesia

What additional findings are likely with this patient?
A patient may have a decrease in cardiovascular status depending on the frequency of intermittent claudication the patient experienced prior to the amputation. The patient may initially experience diminished balance secondary to the loss of the limb. Other issues that directly affect the residual limb include phantom pain, decreased range of motion, poor skin integrity, and hypersensitivity. The presence of any of these findings can have a negative influence on a patient's ability to utilize a prosthesis.

Management:
What is the most effective management of this patient?
A patient should be a candidate for inpatient physical therapy services immediately after the amputation. Preprosthetic intervention should focus on strength, range of motion, functional mobility, use of assistive devices, desensitization, and patient education for care of the residual limb. Intervention should focus on proper positioning in order to avoid the risk of contractures. If the patient does not experience complications he/she should be able to return home either independently or with support. The patient may receive continued short-term physical therapy for prosthetic intervention once the residual limb has fully healed.

What home care regimen should be recommended?
A home care regimen for a patient status post amputation should include exercises and stretching. Since ambulation with a prosthesis increases the energy cost, the patient should be encouraged to perform cardiovascular activities on a frequent basis. In order to be successful, the patient will need to consistently monitor the residual limb and wrap the limb to ensure proper shaping until the prosthesis is tolerated.

Outcome:
What is the likely outcome of a course in physical therapy?
Physical therapy for both preprosthetic and prosthetic intervention is typically necessary. A patient should be able to achieve the established goals and function with a prosthesis and an assistive device if warranted. The general health, cognition, motivation, and social support system of the patient will influence the patient's functional outcome.

What are the long-term effects of the patient's condition?
Arteriosclerosis obliterans is a chronic disease that a patient should continue to manage. The current amputation should not permanently alter a patient's level of functional mobility. The patient should be able to manage all aspects of self-care and functional mobility after prosthetic training with the permanent prosthesis unless hindered by other ailments.

Comparison:
What are the distinguishing characteristics of a similar condition?
There will be many similar characteristics regardless of the level of amputation to the lower or upper extremity. Intervention will include desensitization, phantom pain education, proper compression and shaping, strength improvement, proper positioning, and self-care and mobility with all patients. In most cases patients and therapists share the common goal of functional prosthetic utilization.

Clinical Scenarios:
Scenario One
A two-year-old female born with a congenital malformation of the ankle joint and without a foot is referred to physical therapy. The child is in good health, active, and has no other past medical history. The child has become increasingly frustrated with her alternate means of mobility. Her parents are supportive and carry her for community mobility. She prefers to scoot and crawl around the house since she cannot bear weight through the affected lower extremity.

Scenario Two
An 83-year-old male, status post right transfemoral amputation secondary to insulin dependent diabetes mellitus, is admitted to a skilled nursing facility for rehabilitation. The patient is obese and presents with cardiopulmonary insufficiency. The patient previously resided alone with intermittent home health care and requires two liters of oxygen with activity.

Amyotrophic Lateral Sclerosis

Diagnosis:

What condition produces a patient's symptoms?
Amyotrophic lateral sclerosis (ALS) is a chronic degenerative disease that produces both upper and lower motor neuron impairments. This disease is also referred to as Lou Gehrig's disease.

An injury was most likely sustained to which structure?
Rapid degeneration and demyelination occurs in the corticospinal tract, cell bodies of the lower motor neurons in the gray matter, anterior horn cells, and within the precentral gyrus of the cortex. The rapid degeneration causes denervation of muscle fibers, muscle atrophy, and weakness.

Inference:

What is the most likely contributing factor in the development of this condition?
The exact etiology of ALS is unknown, however there are multiple theories of causative factors that include genetic inheritance as an autosomal dominant trait, a slow acting virus, metabolic disturbances, and toxicity of lead and aluminum. Risk for ALS is higher in men and onset usually occurs between 40 and 70 years of age.

Confirmation:

What is the most likely clinical presentation?
Early clinical presentation of ALS includes muscle weakness, cramping, and atrophy of the hands. The weakness spreads throughout the body over the course of the disease. A patient will exhibit fatigue, oral motor impairment, fasciculations, spasticity, and eventual respiratory paralysis. Mental capacity usually remains intact.

What laboratory or imaging studies would confirm the diagnosis?
There are multiple tests used to assist with diagnosing ALS. Electromyography assesses fibrillation and muscle fasciculation. Muscle biopsy verifies lower motor neuron involvement rather than muscle disease. A spinal tap may reveal a higher protein content in some patients with ALS. Computed tomography will appear normal until late in the disease process.

What additional information should be obtained to confirm the diagnosis?
Diagnosis relies heavily on symptoms that determine both upper and lower motor neuron involvement. Motor impairment without sensory impairment is a primary indication of ALS. Definitive diagnosis first requires a physician to rule out other neurological conditions such as multiple sclerosis, spinal cord tumors, progressive muscular dystrophy, and syringomyelia.

Examination:

What history should be documented?
Important areas to explore include past medical history, family history, history of current symptoms, current health status, living environment, social history and habits, occupation, and social support system.

What test/measures are most appropriate?
- **Aerobic capacity and endurance:** assessment of vital signs at rest and with activity, perceived exertion scale
- **Arousal, attention, and cognition:** examine mental status, learning ability, memory, and motivation
- **Assistive and adaptive devices:** analysis of components and safety of a device
- **Environmental, home, and work barriers:** analysis of current and potential barriers or hazards
- **Gait, locomotion, and balance:** static and dynamic balance in sitting and standing, safety during gait with/without an assistive device
- **Motor function:** motor assessment scales, coordination, equilibrium and righting reactions
- **Muscle performance:** strength assessment, muscle endurance, muscle tone assessment, degree of muscle atrophy
- **Neuromotor development and sensory integration:** analysis of reflex movement patterns, assessment of involuntary movements, sensory integration tests, gross and fine motor skills
- **Posture:** analysis of resting and dynamic posture

- **Range of motion:** active and passive range of motion
- **Reflex integrity:** assessment of deep tendon and pathological reflexes (e.g. Babinski, ATNR)
- **Self-care and home management:** assessment of functional capacity, Functional Independence Measure (FIM), Barthel ADL Index
- **Ventilation, respiration, and circulation:** respiratory muscle strength, accessory muscle utilization

What additional findings are likely with this patient?
During the beginning stages of the disease ALS affects various areas of the body. As the disease progresses the brain and the spinal cord become involved resulting in paralysis of vocal cords, swallowing impairment, contractures, decubiti, and breathing difficulty that may require ventilatory support.

Management:
What is the most effective management of this patient?
Effective management of ALS is based on supportive care. Pharmacological intervention may include antispasticity and antidepressant medications. Surgical intervention is rare but tracheostomy and gastrostomy may be indicated. Physical, occupational, and speech therapies may be warranted. Physical therapy intervention should focus on the quality of life. A low level exercise program, range of motion, mobility training with an assistive device, energy conservation techniques, and family teaching and support are important aspects of treatment.

What home care regimen should be recommended?
A home care regimen for a patient with ALS must consider the rate of disease progression and the level of respiratory involvement. Goals should focus on maximizing the patient's functional capacity. Low level exercise may be indicated as long as the patient does not exercise to fatigue. Family involvement is encouraged to support the patient through the course of the disease and assist with mobility, energy conservation techniques, and overall safety.

Outcome:
What is the likely outcome of a course in physical therapy?
Physical therapy intervention may assist with current issues, however does not hinder the progression of ALS.

What are the long-term effects of the patient's condition?
ALS is usually a rapidly progressing neurological disease with an average course of two to five years. Death usually occurs from respiratory failure.

Comparison:
What are the distinguishing characteristics of a similar condition?
Progressive spinal muscle atrophy, also known as Aran-Duchenne muscle atrophy, is a motor neuron disease that primarily affects the anterior horn cell. Characteristics include muscle weakness that begins in the hands and progresses proximally. Life expectancy can be 20 to 25 years after being diagnosed.

Clinical Scenarios:
Scenario One
A 56-year-old male diagnosed with ALS presents with mild atrophy of the hand musculature. The patient owns his own business as a painter and wants to continue working for as long as he can. The patient is referred to physical therapy for instruction in a home exercise program.

Scenario Two
A 60-year-old female is hospitalized and referred to physical therapy secondary to left CVA with right hemiparesis. The patient was diagnosed with ALS five years ago. The patient requires the use of a wheelchair for mobility and occasionally chokes when eating. The patient has assistance at home from her husband who is in good health.

Ankylosing Spondylitis

Diagnosis:

What condition produces a patient's symptoms?
Ankylosing spondylitis (Marie-Strumpell disease) is a systemic condition that is characterized by inflammation in the spine and larger peripheral joints. The chronic inflammation causes destruction and fibrosis of the affected areas.

An injury was most likely sustained to which structure?
Ankylosing spondylitis primarily affects the sacroiliac joint, intervertebral disks, spine, adjacent connective tissue, and larger peripheral joints. Ossification can occur within all affected joints resulting in deformity.

Inference:

What is the most likely contributing factor in the development of this condition?
Ankylosing spondylitis is a progressive systemic disorder with an unclear etiology. Research supports a possible etiology of genetic inheritance combined with environmental influence. A person born with a histocompatibility antigen HLA-B27 has a high risk for the disease. Men are at greater risk than women and onset is typically seen between ten and thirty years of age.

Confirmation:

What is the most likely clinical presentation?
A patient with early ankylosing spondylitis will present with recurrent episodes of low back pain, morning stiffness, impaired spinal extension, and limited range of motion in the affected joints. As the disease progresses pain will extend to the midback and sometimes towards the neck. The natural lumbar curve will flatten due to muscle spasm and late manifestations include fixed flexion at the hips, spinal kyphosis, fatigue, weight loss, and peripheral joint involvement. If the costovertebral joints are affected a patient will present with impaired chest mobility and decreased vital capacity.

What laboratory or imaging studies would confirm the diagnosis?
X-ray of the spine will reveal areas of erosion, demineralization, calcification, and syndesmophyte formation (ossification of the outside of the intervertebral disks). In the later stages of the disease x-ray will reveal fusion of the sacroiliac joint, calcification of apophyseal joints and spinal ligaments, and a bamboo appearance of the spine. The majority of patients with ankylosing spondylitis possess the HLA- B27 antigen and approximately 40% have an elevated erythrocyte sedimentation rate.

What additional information should be obtained to confirm the diagnosis?
Physical examination may reveal joint tenderness, pain, and/or limitation of the sacroiliac joint and the spine. Family inheritance and a thorough history of a patient's symptoms assist with the diagnosis of ankylosing spondylitis.

Examination:

What history should be documented?
Important areas to explore include past medical history, medications, current health status, family inheritance, living environment, leisure activities, social history and habits, and social support system.

What test/measures are most appropriate?
- **Anthropometric characteristics:** baseline height measurement
- **Arousal, attention, and cognition:** examine mental status, learning ability, memory, and motivation
- **Assistive and adaptive devices:** analysis of components and safety of a device
- **Community and work integration:** analysis of community, work, and leisure activities
- **Environmental, home, and work barriers:** analysis of current and potential barriers or hazards
- **Ergonomics and body mechanics:** analysis of dexterity and coordination
- **Gait, locomotion, and balance:** assessment of static and dynamic balance in sitting and standing, safety during gait, Functional Ambulation Profile, analysis of wheelchair management
- **Joint integrity and mobility:** assessment of hypomobility and limitation of a joint, Wright-Schober test
- **Muscle performance:** strength assessment
- **Pain:** pain perception assessment scale
- **Posture:** analysis of resting and dynamic posture

- **Range of motion:** active and passive range of motion
- **Reflex integrity:** assessment of deep tendon and pathological reflexes (e.g. Babinski, ATNR)
- **Self-care and home management:** assessment of functional capacity
- **Sensory integrity:** assessment of sensation
- **Ventilation, respiration, and circulation:** analysis of thoracolumbar movement and chest expansion during breathing, measurement of vital capacity

What additional findings are likely with this patient?
Iritis and cardiac pathology can occur in severe longstanding cases of ankylosing spondylitis. Pericarditis, pulmonary fibrosis, cardiac arrhythmias, and aortic insufficiency have been noted as potential complications.

Management:
What is the most effective management of this patient?
Management of ankylosing spondylitis includes pharmacological intervention using analgesics, NSAIDs, and specifically Indomethacin to relieve pain. Physical therapy intervention should include postural exercises emphasizing extension, general range of motion, pain management, and energy conservation techniques. Swimming is a highly recommended activity. Surgical intervention is rarely indicated to correct or stabilize a musculoskeletal deformity.

What home care regimen should be recommended?
A home care regimen for a patient with ankylosing spondylitis should include a daily therapeutic exercise program. Exercise should focus on spinal movement in all directions. The supine position is a preferred position during sleep to avoid a prolonged flexed posture and is an important component of a home program.

Outcome:
What is the likely outcome of a course in physical therapy?
Physical therapy cannot modify the progression of ankylosing spondylitis, however it may assist to alleviate pain and improve a patient's functional capacity. A patient may require physical therapy on an intermittent basis throughout the disease process.

What are the long-term effects of the patient's condition?
Ankylosing spondylitis progresses slowly over a fifteen to twenty five year period and may remain isolated to the spine and sacroiliac joint or spread to larger peripheral joints. Stiffness and joint limitation are common long-term effects of ankylosing spondylitis that can negatively impact a patient's functional mobility.

Comparison:
What are the distinguishing characteristics of a similar condition?
Cervical spondylosis is a complication of osteoarthritis that is characterized by osteophyte formation within the cervical vertebrae. There is narrowing of the intervertebral foramina and subsequent compression of the corresponding nerves. Symptoms include stiffness, neck pain, and discomfort into the hand. Cervical spondylosis can produce long-term chronic disability.

Clinical Scenarios:
Scenario One
A 28-year-old male is seen in physical therapy shortly after being diagnosed with ankylosing spondylitis. The patient complains of sacroiliac pain and tenderness. The patient has a negative family history and is currently employed as a high school maintenance technician.

Scenario Two
A 60-year-old female is seen in physical therapy with advanced ankylosing spondylitis. The patient has bilateral hip flexion contractures and kyphosis. The patient resides alone, however receives daily assistance from her two sisters who live locally. The patient has previously refused recommendations to utilize an assistive device.

Anterior Cruciate Ligament Sprain – Grade III

Diagnosis:

What condition produces a patient's symptoms?
The anterior cruciate ligament (ACL) extends from the anterior intracondylar region of the tibia to the medial aspect of the lateral femoral condyle in the intracondylar notch. The ligament prevents anterior translation of the tibia on the fixed femur and posterior translation of the femur on the fixed tibia. Injuries to the anterior cruciate ligament most commonly occur during agility activities, rapid deceleration or landing in an off balance position.

An injury was most likely sustained to which structure?
A grade III ACL sprain refers to a complete tear of the ligament with excessive laxity. Tears of the anterior cruciate ligament most often occur in the midsubstance of the ligament and not at the ligament's attachment on the femur or tibia. Laxity rarely occurs solely in a straight plane and instead is often classified as anterolateral or anteromedial.

Inference:

What is the most likely contributing factor in the development of this condition?
Participation in athletic activities requiring high levels of agility increases the incidence of an ACL injury. Recent studies indicate that women involved in selected athletic activities experienced significantly higher ACL injury rates than their male counterparts. There are many hypothesized reasons for this finding, however to date a definitive answer has not been identified.

Confirmation:

What is the most likely clinical presentation?
A grade III ACL sprain is characterized by significant pain, effusion, and edema that significantly limits range of motion. The patient may be unable to bear weight on the involved extremity resulting in dependence on an assistive device. Ligamentous testing reveals visible laxity in the involved knee and may exacerbate the patient's pain level.

What laboratory or imaging studies would confirm the diagnosis?
Magnetic resonance imaging is the preferred imaging tool to identify the presence of an ACL tear and possible disruption of other soft tissue structures such as ligaments and menisci. X-rays may be used to rule out the possibility of a fracture.

What additional information should be obtained to confirm the diagnosis?
Subjective reports such as hearing a loud pop or feeling as though the knee buckled is often associated with a complete tear of the anterior cruciate ligament. Special tests such as the Lachman, anterior drawer, and pivot shift test can be used to confirm the diagnosis. It is important to perform all special tests bilaterally.

Examination:

What history should be documented?
Important areas to explore include mechanism of present injury, current symptoms, past medical history, medications, living environment, social history and habits, and social support system.

What test/measures are most appropriate?
- **Anthropometric characteristics:** determine the amount of knee effusion, lower extremity circumferential measurements
- **Arousal, attention, and cognition:** examine mental status, learning ability, memory, and motivation
- **Assistive and adaptive devices:** analysis of components and safety of a device, potential utilization of crutches
- **Gait, locomotion, and balance:** safety during gait with an assistive device
- **Integumentary integrity:** assessment of sensation (pain, temperature, tactile), skin assessment
- **Joint integrity and mobility:** special tests for ligaments and menisci, Lachman test, reverse Lachman test, anterior drawer test, palpation of structures, joint play, soft tissue restrictions, joint pain
- **Muscle performance:** strength assessment, assessment of active movement, resisted isometrics, muscle contraction characteristics, muscle endurance
- **Orthotic, protective, and supportive devices:** potential utilization of bracing, taping or wrapping
- **Pain:** pain perception assessment scale
- **Range of motion:** active and passive range of motion
- **Self-care and home management:** assessment of functional capacity
- **Sensory integrity:** assessment of proprioception and kinesthesia

What additional findings are likely with this patient?
Approximately two thirds of the time the anterior cruciate ligament is torn there is an accompanying meniscal tear. The collateral ligaments can also be involved although not as commonly as the menisci.

Management:
What is the most effective management of this patient?
Management of a patient following a grade III ACL sprain includes controlling edema, improving range of motion and strength, and improving the fluidity of gait. For patients electing to have surgery the patellar tendon is the most commonly utilized graft for intraarticular reconstruction. Patients often initially present with a knee immobilizer and crutches to protect the reconstructed ligament. Specific management parameters are difficult to identify since many orthopedic surgeons utilize very specific protocols. Management in the immediate postoperative phase includes protecting the integrity of the graft, controlling edema, and improving range of motion. Specific intervention activities include pain modulation, patellar mobility, active range of motion exercises, gait activities, and quadriceps exercises. As patients progress in their rehabilitation program treatment begins to focus on strengthening activities emphasizing closed chain exercises and selected functional activities. Closed chain exercises are considered more desirable than open chain exercises since they minimize anterior translation of the tibia. Patients should be required to complete a functional progression prior to returning to unrestricted athletic activities. For patients opting for a conservative (nonoperative) approach it is necessary to begin an aggressive strengthening program once the acute phase of the injury has subsided.

What home care regimen should be recommended?
The home care regimen should consist of range of motion, strengthening, palliative care, and functional activities as warranted based on the results of the patient examination.

Outcome:
What is the likely outcome of a course in physical therapy?
It is possible that with an aggressive strengthening program and/or activity modification patients may be able to participate in light to moderate athletic activities without formal surgical reconstruction. Patients electing to have surgery can expect to return to their previous functional level in four to six months.

What are the long-term effects of the patient's condition?
Patients that sustain a complete tear of the anterior cruciate ligament and elect not to have reconstructive surgery will likely be at increased risk for instability and subsequent deterioration of joint surfaces.

Comparison:
What are the distinguishing characteristics of a similar condition?
A grade III posterior cruciate ligament (PCL) sprain is less common than an anterior cruciate ligament sprain. The most common mechanism of injury for a posterior cruciate ligament sprain is a "dashboard" injury or with the knee in forced hyperflexion with the foot plantar flexed. A grade III posterior cruciate ligament injury will typically produce effusion, posterior tenderness, and a positive posterior drawer test. Knee extension is often limited due to the effusion and stretching of the posterior capsule and gastrocnemius. The rehabilitation program typically emphasizes strengthening of the quadriceps muscles. Individuals with an isolated posterior cruciate ligament sprain may not exhibit any functional performance limitations and as a result surgical intervention is far less common than with an anterior cruciate ligament sprain. A posterior cruciate ligament sprain alters the arthrokinematics of the knee joint and as a result a patient will be susceptible to future degenerative changes such as arthritis.

Clinical Scenarios:
Scenario One
A 16-year-old gymnast sustains a grade I ACL injury after landing awkwardly on her left leg during a vault. The patient is two days status post injury and has mild effusion in the involved knee. The patient describes diffuse pain in the knee during prolonged periods of immobilization or prolonged weight bearing. The patient is a competitive gymnast and needs to compete in a regional meet in slightly less than four weeks.

Scenario Two
A 35-year-old male is referred to physical therapy after injuring his knee in a softball game. The patient reports tearing the anterior cruciate ligament ten years ago in a skiing accident. The patient describes himself as active, however reports an increasing number of instability episodes in recent years. A note from the patient's physician describes significant arthritic changes in the involved knee including diminished joint space.

Breast Cancer

Diagnosis:

What condition produces a patient's symptoms?
Breast cancer's primary symptom is a painless mass within the breast tissue. This mass is composed of malignant altered cells that proliferate and spread without control. There may or may not be generalized discomfort in the area of the mass.

An injury was most likely sustained to which structure?
Injury occurs initially at the cellular level within the breast tissue. Breast cancer can spread into the lymphatic system and will commonly metastasize to the brain, lungs, bones, and liver.

Inference:

What is the most likely contributing factor in the development of this condition?
Breast cancer has an unknown etiology, however estrogen is believed to have some relationship to the disease process. Risk factors include young menarche, late menopause, family history of breast cancer, high alcohol intake, high fat diet, radiation exposure or past history of cancer.

Confirmation:

What is the most likely clinical presentation?
A patient with breast cancer will present with a lump in the breast that is noticed by a physician or by the patient through self-examination. Breast cancer is initially otherwise asymptomatic. As the disease progresses the breast may become painful, change shape, bleed from the nipple, and dimple over the area of the mass.

What laboratory or imaging studies would confirm the diagnosis?
Mammography is used to detect the location and growth of a mass, however definitive diagnosis of breast cancer is only made after microscopic examination of a suspected mass by needle or excision biopsy.

What additional information should be obtained to confirm the diagnosis?
Additional information such as family history of cancer, past medical history, and history of self-examination is helpful in support of a definitive diagnosis. This information is usually obtained prior to mammography and biopsy.

Examination:

What history should be documented?
Important areas to explore include past medical history, family history of cancer, medications, current health status, social history and habits, hand dominance, occupation, living environment, and social support system.

What test/measures are most appropriate?
- **Aerobic capacity and endurance:** assessment of vital signs at rest and with activity
- **Anthropometric characteristics:** upper extremity circumferential measurements
- **Arousal, attention, and cognition:** examine mental status, learning ability, memory, and motivation
- **Community and work integration:** analysis of community, work, and leisure activities
- **Gait, locomotion, and balance:** assessment of static and dynamic balance in sitting and standing, safety during gait
- **Integumentary integrity:** assessment for potential infection of surgical incision
- **Muscle performance:** strength assessment
- **Pain:** pain perception assessment scale, visual analog scale
- **Range of motion:** active and passive range of motion
- **Self-care and home management:** assessment of self-care and home management skills, assessment of functional capacity, Barthel ADL Index
- **Sensory integrity:** assessment of superficial and combined sensations, proprioception and kinesthesia

What additional findings are likely with this patient?
Additional findings are dependent on the course of treatment. If a patient has undergone surgical resection or mastectomy the patient may experience pain, edema, fatigue, and psychological issues. Patients that are diagnosed with advanced breast cancer may experience pleural effusion, pathological fractures, and spinal compression.

Management:
What is the most effective management of this patient?
Breast cancer is managed based on the size and the stage of the mass and corresponding involvement of the lymph nodes. Surgical management may range from excision of the mass to total mastectomy with axillary dissection. Chemotherapy, radiation therapy, and immunotherapy may be used in isolation or after a surgical procedure. Physical therapy may be indicated to assist with lymphedema management, postsurgical breathing exercises, positioning, range of motion exercises, massage, intermittent compression, and patient education.

What home care regimen should be recommended?
A home care regimen should include education, positioning, and techniques to manage lymphedema. Range of motion exercises, energy conservation techniques, as well as general exercises should continue on a regular basis at home.

Outcome:
What is the likely outcome of a course in physical therapy?
Physical therapy may be indicated for postsurgical management to assist with impairments and promote independence with self-care and functional skills.

What are the long-term effects of the patient's condition?
The long-term effects of breast cancer are varied. The risk of recurrence is always present and should be monitored closely. Post-surgical lymphedema may persist and require ongoing home management. Overall prognosis for women that do not have lymph node involvement is over 80% for a ten year survival rate. The survival rate decreases as the tumor progresses and lymph nodes become involved.

Comparison:
What are the distinguishing characteristics of a similar condition?
Fibrocystic breast disease usually occurs in both breasts and is characterized by nodular lumps within the breast tissue. The cysts are benign and become tender immediately prior to menstruation. Other symptoms include aching and burning within the breast. Symptoms normally disappear after menstruation is over. Although benign, fibrocystic breast disease increases a patient's risk for breast cancer later in life.

Clinical Scenarios:
Scenario One
A 65-year-old female is seen by a physical therapist 24 hours after total mastectomy. The patient was active prior to the surgery walking two miles every day. The patient's past medical history is positive for diabetes mellitus and skin cancer. The patient reports pain with coughing.

Scenario Two
A 45-year-old female is referred to outpatient physical therapy with lymphedema secondary to radical mastectomy. The patient is fatigued and anxious about the increased size of her arm and limitation in range of motion. The patient runs a daycare center out of her home and is active in her church.

Carpal Tunnel Syndrome

Diagnosis:

What condition produces a patient's symptoms?
The carpal tunnel is created by the transverse carpal ligament on the volar side, the scaphoid tuberosity and trapezium on the radial side, the hook of the hamate and pisiform on the ulnar side, and the volar radiocarpal ligament and volar ligamentous extensions between the carpal bones on the dorsal side. The median nerve, four flexor digitorum profundus tendons, four flexor digitorum superficialis tendons, and the flexor pollicis longus tendon pass through the carpal tunnel. Carpal tunnel syndrome occurs as a result of compression of the median nerve where it passes through the carpal tunnel.

An injury was most likely sustained to which structure?
The median nerve is injured with compression and results in sensory and motor disturbances in the median nerve distribution of the hand.

Inference:

What is the most likely contributing factor in the development of this condition?
Any condition such as edema, inflammation, tumor or fibrosis may cause compression of the median nerve within the tunnel and result in nerve ischemia. The exact etiology of carpal tunnel syndrome is unclear, however conditions that produce inflammation to the carpal tunnel such as repetitive use, rheumatoid arthritis, pregnancy, diabetes, trauma, tumor, hypothyroidism, and wrist sprain or fracture can contribute to carpal tunnel syndrome. Other etiologies include a congenital narrow tunnel and vitamin B6 deficiency.

Confirmation:

What is the most likely clinical presentation?
A patient with carpal tunnel syndrome will initially present with sensory changes and paresthesias along the median nerve distribution in the hand. Symptoms include night pain, weakness of the hand, muscle atrophy, and decreased joint mobility in the wrist. Initial muscle atrophy is often noted in the abductor pollicis brevis muscle and later progresses to all of the thenar muscles.

What laboratory or imaging studies would confirm the diagnosis?
Electromyographic and electroneurographic studies can be used to diagnose a motor conduction delay along the median nerve within the carpal tunnel.

What additional information should be obtained to confirm the diagnosis?
Physical examination, history, and review of symptoms are extremely important when diagnosing carpal tunnel syndrome. A positive Tinel's sign (tingling produced by tapping over the median nerve) and a positive Phalen's test (produces symptoms of tingling and numbness after holding a position of wrist flexion for one minute) along with the other symptoms will assist to confirm the diagnosis.

Examination:

What history should be documented?
Important areas to explore include past medical history, medications, history of symptoms, current health status, occupation, living environment, social history and habits, leisure activities, and social support system.

What test/measures are most appropriate?
- **Anthropometric characteristics:** wrist and hand circumferential measurements
- **Arousal, attention, and cognition:** examine mental status, learning ability, memory, and motivation
- **Community and work integration:** analysis of community, work, and leisure activities
- **Environmental, home, and work barriers:** analysis of current and potential barriers or hazards
- **Ergonomics and body mechanics:** analysis of dexterity and coordination
- **Integumentary integrity:** skin and nailbed assessment, assessment of sensation
- **Joint integrity and mobility:** assessment of hypomobility of a joint, soft tissue swelling, inflammation, and sprain
- **Muscle performance:** strength assessment
- **Orthotic, protective, and supportive devices:** potential utilization of bracing or splinting
- **Pain:** pain perception assessment scale
- **Range of motion:** active and passive range of motion
- **Self-care and home management:** assessment of functional capacity

What additional findings are likely with this patient?
Advanced carpal tunnel syndrome can present with muscle atrophy of the hand, radiating pain in the forearm and shoulder, and permanent nerve damage with motor and sensory loss. The patient may present with ape hand deformity caused by atrophy of the thenar muscles and first two lumbricals.

Management:
What is the most effective management of this patient?
A patient with carpal tunnel syndrome will initially receive conservative management including local corticosteroid injections to reduce inflammation, splinting, and physical therapy management. Physical therapy intervention at this stage includes splinting, carpal mobilization, and gentle stretching. Biomechanical analysis and adaptation of a patient's occupation, work place, leisure activities, and living environment may be necessary. If conservative treatment fails the patient may require surgical intervention to release the carpal ligament and decompress the median nerve. Postsurgical physical therapy intervention should include the use of moist heat with electrical stimulation, iontophoresis, cryotherapy, light massage, desensitization of the scar, tendon gliding exercises, and active range of motion. A patient should initially avoid wrist flexion and a forceful grasp. After four weeks a patient can progress with active wrist flexion, gentle stretching, putty exercises, light progressive resistive exercise training, and continued modification of posture and body mechanics. Radial deviation against resistance should be avoided due to the tendency for irritation and inflammation with this movement. Postsurgical rehabilitation usually lasts six to eight weeks.

What home care regimen should be recommended?
A home care regimen for a patient with carpal tunnel syndrome should consist of continued stretching and strengthening exercises. The patient must be competent with donning/doffing a splint and monitoring the splint's use.

Outcome:
What is the likely outcome of a course in physical therapy?
Physical therapy intervention should improve a patient's condition and decrease symptoms of carpal tunnel syndrome within four to six weeks. If conservative treatment fails and the patient requires surgical intervention rehabilitation may last six to eight weeks.

What are the long-term effects of the patient's condition?
Carpal tunnel syndrome can have minor effects on some patients while having debilitating effects on others. The overall long-term effects are dependent on the degree of involvement, the amount of permanent damage, and the level of success with conservative or surgical management. It is possible to have no long-term effects from this condition if the patient responds positively to physical therapy. Other patients may be left with permanent motor and sensory impairments along the median nerve distribution.

Comparison:
What are the distinguishing characteristics of a similar condition?
Compression in the tunnel of Guyon occurs with inflammation to the ulnar nerve between the hook of the hamate and the pisiform. This condition occurs from tasks such as leaning during extended handwriting, leaning on bike handles while riding, repetitive griping activities or trauma. The patient will present with paresthesia along the ulnar distribution, weakness and atrophy of the hypothenar musculature, decreased mobility of the pisiform, and impaired grip strength. This condition can be treated with conservative management or surgical intervention.

Clinical Scenarios:
Scenario One
A 26-year-old female is seen in physical therapy with a diagnosis of carpal tunnel syndrome. The patient has not been treated previously for carpal tunnel syndrome. The patient is employed as a telephone sales specialist and types on the computer throughout the day. The patient complains of pain in her hands, numbness when sleeping and while performing at work, and muscle soreness.

Scenario Two
A 45-year-old male is referred to physical therapy ten days after surgical decompression due to carpal tunnel syndrome. The patient's postoperative routine includes resting the hand, using a splint, icing, and keeping the extremity elevated. Minimal edema is noted at the wrist. The patient has no other significant past medical history and is anxious to return to his previous activities.

Cerebrovascular Accident

Diagnosis:

What condition produces a patient's symptoms?
Cerebrovascular accident (CVA) occurs when there is an interruption of cerebral circulation that results in cerebral insufficiency and subsequent neurological deficit. The ischemia occurs from either a stroke in evolution (the infarct slowly progresses over one to two days) or as a completed stroke (an abrupt infarct with immediate neurological deficits).

An injury was most likely sustained to which structure?
CVA results from prolonged ischemia to an artery in the brain. This condition can cause subsequent neurological damage relative to the size and location of the infarct.

Inference:

What is the most likely contributing factor in the development of this condition?
The primary risk factors for CVA include hypertension, atherosclerosis, heart disease, diabetes, previous transient ischemic attacks, smoking, and coronary artery disease. Secondary risk factors include age, physical inactivity, alcohol abuse, and obesity.

Confirmation:

What is the most likely clinical presentation?
The clinical presentation is determined by the location and extent of the infarct. Typical characteristics include flaccidity or weakness of one side of the body, sensory impairment, balance impairment, dysphagia, cognitive deficit, perceptual impairment, and visual impairment.

What laboratory or imaging studies would confirm the diagnosis?
Computed tomography can confirm an area of infarct in the brain and its vascular origin, however it can present as negative for up to a few days after the event. Diagnosis is usually based upon patient history, symptoms, and laboratory testing. Angiography may be utilized to identify a clot and determine if surgical intervention is necessary.

What additional information should be obtained to confirm the diagnosis?
A chest x-ray may be warranted to rule out lung disease while an electrocardiogram is used to examine potential cardiac abnormalities. Blood and urine tests are routinely administered before confirming the diagnosis.

Examination:

What history should be documented?
Important areas to explore include past medical history, medications, current health status, social history and habits, occupation, living environment, and social support system.

What test/measures are most appropriate?
- **Arousal, attention, and cognition:** examine mental status, learning ability, memory, and motivation, Mini Mental State Exam, Boston Diagnostic Aphasia Examination
- **Assistive and adaptive devices:** analysis of components and safety of a device
- **Gait, locomotion, and balance:** static and dynamic balance in sitting and standing, safety during gait with an assistive device, Berg Functional Balance Scale, Tinetti Performance Oriented Mobility Assessment, Functional Ambulation Profile
- **Integumentary integrity:** skin assessment
- **Motor function:** equilibrium and righting reactions, coordination, motor assessment scales
- **Muscle performance:** muscle tone assessment, assessment of active movement
- **Neuromotor development and sensory integration:** assessment of involuntary movements, sensory integration tests, gross and fine motor skills, reflex movement patterns
- **Orthotic, protective, and supportive devices:** analysis of components of a device, analysis of movement while wearing a device
- **Posture:** analysis of resting and dynamic posture
- **Pain:** pain perception assessment scale

- **Range of motion:** active and passive range of motion
- **Reflexes:** assessment of pathological reflexes (e.g. Babinski, ATNR)
- **Self-care and home management:** assessment of functional capacity, Rankin Scale, NIH Stroke Scale, Functional Independence Measure (FIM)
- **Sensory integrity:** assessment of proprioception and kinesthesia

What additional findings are likely with this patient?
A patient with a left CVA may present with weakness or paralysis to the right side, impaired processing, heightened frustration, aphasia, dysphagia, motor apraxia, and right hemianopsia. A patient with a right CVA may present with weakness or paralysis to the left side, poor attention span, impaired awareness and judgment, memory deficits, left inattention, emotional lability, impulsive behavior, and left hemianopsia.

Management:
What is the most effective management of this patient?
The patient will initially require physical therapy services while in the hospital. The acute phase focuses on positioning, pressure relief, sensory awareness and integration, ROM, weight bearing, facilitation, muscle reeducation, balance, and postural control. There are many approaches to neurological rehabilitation that include but are not limited to motor control, Bobath, Brunnstrom, Rood, and PNF. Many therapists integrate facets from multiple approaches based on the patient's response to selected interventions.

What home care regimen should be recommended?
Approximately 75% of patients that have experienced a CVA return home at various levels of functional mobility. The majority of patients require ongoing therapy services either on an outpatient basis or through a home health agency as part of their home care regimen. A therapeutic program should be designed for a patient to continue at home independently or with the required level of assistance.

Outcome:
What is the likely outcome of a course in physical therapy?
A patient that experiences neurological deficits due to a CVA may require physical therapy to assist with motor reeducation, sensory stimulation, and functional mobility. The outcome is dependent on the patient's overall health, level of cognition, level of motivation, motor recovery, and family support.

What are the long-term effects of the patient's condition?
The effects of a CVA can be quite diverse ranging from spontaneous recovery to permanent disability requiring compensatory strategies and techniques in order to function. The first three months of recovery are usually a good indicator of the long-term outcome, however individuals can continue to make progress over time.

Comparison:
What are the distinguishing characteristics of a similar condition?
A transient ischemic attack (TIA) has a similar characteristic of diminished blood supply to the brain. Although the patient may present with similar symptoms, the symptoms last for only a brief period of time. Unlike a CVA, the TIA does not cause permanent residual neurological deficits.

Clinical Scenarios:
Scenario One
A 43-year-old male diagnosed with left hemorrhagic CVA due to an aneurysm of the middle cerebral artery is referred to physical therapy. Medical history reveals moderate hypertension (uncontrolled) and an appendectomy. The patient is a supervisor at a hardware store and resides with his wife and two teenage sons.

Scenario Two
A 79-year-old female is diagnosed with a right CVA involving the anterior cerebral artery. The patient appears to be functioning at a very low level. Past medical history includes multiple TIAs, history of PVCs, cataract in the left eye, and angina. The patient was residing in an independent living facility where she had her own apartment, but had meals provided for her in the dining area.

Cystic Fibrosis

Diagnosis:

What condition produces a patient's symptoms?
Cystic fibrosis is an inherited disease that affects the exocrine glands. The disease can cause overproduction and obstruction by thick mucus, overproduction of secretions, and/or overproduction of sodium and chloride. Cystic fibrosis is the major cause of severe chronic lung disease in children.

An injury was most likely sustained to which structure?
Cystic fibrosis affects multi-systems within the body, however the respiratory and gastrointestinal systems are the most involved in the disease process.

Inference:

What is the most likely contributing factor in the development of this condition?
Cystic fibrosis is an autosomal recessive genetic disorder and presents as a mutation of chromosome seven.

Confirmation:

What is the most likely clinical presentation?
Cystic fibrosis can be diagnosed shortly after birth, however is sometimes not diagnosed for a few years. Symptoms vary and may include meconium ileus at birth, salty tasting sweat, dehydration, weight loss, failure to thrive, wheezing, digital clubbing, repeated upper respiratory infections, dyspnea, and a persistent cough.

What laboratory or imaging studies would confirm the diagnosis?
Neonates' meconium can be tested as a screening tool for increased albumin. The quantitative pilocarpine iontophoresis sweat test is the sole diagnostic tool in determining the presence of cystic fibrosis. Sodium and chloride amounts greater than 60 mEq/l diagnose the disease.

What additional information should be obtained to confirm the diagnosis?
Additional information in the diagnosis of cystic fibrosis is found through a positive family history, a previous diagnosis of failure to thrive, and in the manifestation of symptoms. (See clinical presentation)

Examination:

What history should be documented?
Important areas to explore include past medical history (if diagnosed after birth), medications, current health status, living environment, and social support system.

What test/measures are most appropriate?
- **Aerobic capacity and endurance:** assessment of vital signs at rest and with activity, perceived exertion scale
- **Arousal, attention, and cognition:** examine mental status, learning ability, memory, and motivation
- **Assistive and adaptive devices:** analysis of components and safety of a device
- **Integumentary integrity:** skin assessment
- **Muscle performance:** strength assessment through active movement
- **Range of motion:** active and passive range of motion
- **Self-care and home management:** assessment of functional capacity
- **Ventilation, respiration, and circulation:** assessment of cough and clearance of secretions, pulmonary function testing, pulse oximetry, auscultation of the lungs, accessory muscle utilization and vital capacity

What additional findings are likely with this patient?
A patient with cystic fibrosis will present with obstructive pulmonary disease. Pulmonary function testing results in a decreased forced expiratory volume (FEV_1) and forced vital capacity (FVC). The functional residual capacity (FRC) and residual volume (RV) become increased. Hypoxemia and hypercapnia develop due to the alteration in perfusion.

Management:

What is the most effective management of this patient?
A patient with cystic fibrosis requires pharmacological intervention to treat infections, thin mucus secretions, replace enzymes, and assist with breathing. Nutritional and psychological counseling are indicated as needed. Physical therapy intervention is essential for management of the disease. Treatment includes bronchial drainage, percussion, vibration, breathing and assistive cough techniques, and ventilatory muscle training. General exercise is indicated to optimize overall function. Family and patient education is vital.

What home care regimen should be recommended?
A home care regimen for a patient with cystic fibrosis requires an ongoing routine emphasizing postural drainage and chest physical therapy. Family members are trained to provide this ongoing support at home.

Outcome:

What is the likely outcome of a course in physical therapy?
A patient with cystic fibrosis will require intermittent physical therapy throughout his or her life. The goals of physical therapy are to maximize secretion clearance from the lungs, optimize pulmonary function, and maximize the patient's quality of life.

What are the long-term effects of the patient's condition?
Cystic fibrosis is a terminal disease, however the median age of death has increased to over 30 years of age due to early detection and comprehensive management. The most common cause of death for patients with cystic fibrosis is respiratory failure.

Comparison:

What are the distinguishing characteristics of a similar condition?
There is no other respiratory disease that is similar to the etiology of cystic fibrosis, however chronic obstructive pulmonary disease (COPD) has similar lung characteristics. COPD is characterized by altered pulmonary function tests, difficulty with expiration, cough, sputum production, and physical damage to specific portions of the lungs.

Clinical Scenarios:

Scenario One
A four-week-old infant is referred to physical therapy after being diagnosed with cystic fibrosis. The infant has a pleasant disposition and does not have any observable findings of distress or discomfort, however the parents are very anxious and concerned. The patient has three siblings that do not present with the disease.

Scenario Two
A 26-year-old female with cystic fibrosis is referred to physical therapy after hospitalization for a severe respiratory infection. The patient recently moved into an apartment with her boyfriend and works 30 hours per week in a hair salon. Prior to the infection the patient was living at home and able to manage the disease with occasional assistance from family members. The physical therapy referral is for chest physical therapy.

Duchenne Muscular Dystrophy

Diagnosis:

What condition produces a patient's symptoms?
Duchenne muscular dystrophy is a progressive degenerative disorder that manifests symptoms once fat and connective tissue begin to replace muscle that has been destroyed by the disease process.

An injury was most likely sustained to which structure?
A patient with Duchenne muscular dystrophy is born without the gene that is required for synthesis of the muscle proteins dystrophin and nebulin. The absence of these two proteins cause cell membranes to weaken, destruction of myofibrils, and loss of muscle contractility. The disease process affects all muscles.

Inference:

What is the most likely contributing factor in the development of this condition?
The etiology of Duchenne muscular dystrophy is inheritance as an X-linked recessive trait. The mother is the silent carrier and only male offspring will manifest the disease.

Confirmation:

What is the most likely clinical presentation?
Diagnosis of Duchenne muscular dystrophy usually occurs between two and five years of age. The first symptoms include a waddling gait, proximal muscle weakness, clumsiness, weakness, toe walking, pseudohypertrophy of the calf and other muscle groups, excessive lordosis, and difficulty climbing stairs.

What laboratory or imaging studies would confirm the diagnosis?
Electromyography is used to examine the electrical activity within the muscles. A muscle biopsy can be performed to determine the absence of dystrophin and evaluate the muscle fiber size. DNA analysis and the serum creatine kinase levels in the blood also assist with confirming the diagnosis.

What additional information should be obtained to confirm the diagnosis?
Clinical examination, current symptoms, and family history are used to diagnose the type and progression of the disease.

Examination:

What history should be documented?
Important areas to explore include past medical history, family history, medications, current symptoms, current health status, living environment, and social support system.

What test/measures are most appropriate?
- **Aerobic capacity and endurance:** assessment of vital signs at rest and with activity
- **Arousal, attention, and cognition:** examine mental status, learning ability, memory, and motivation
- **Assistive and adaptive devices:** analysis of components and safety of a device
- **Environmental, home, and work barriers:** analysis of current and potential barriers or hazards
- **Gait, locomotion, and balance:** static and dynamic balance in sitting and standing, safety during gait with/without an assistive device
- **Joint integrity:** assessment of hypermobility and hypomobility of a joint, assessment of deformity
- **Muscle performance:** assessment of active movement
- **Pain:** pain perception assessment scale
- **Posture:** analysis of resting and dynamic posture
- **Range of motion:** active and passive range of motion, contracture assessment
- **Ventilation, respiration, and circulation:** breathing patterns, respiratory muscle strength, accessory muscle utilization, pulmonary function testing

What additional findings are likely with this patient?
Additional findings occur with progression of the disease. Disuse atrophy, contractures, scoliosis, inability to ambulate, and cardiac impairment are the most common findings.

Management:
What is the most effective management of this patient?
A patient with Duchenne muscular dystrophy may utilize immunosuppressant and steroid medications as part of the medical management. Orthopedic surgical intervention may be warranted secondary to scoliosis or contractures. Physical therapy is initially indicated to assist a young child with progression through the developmental milestones. Once a child presents with impairments, physical therapy should focus on maintaining available strength, encouraging mobility with an assistive device when necessary, adapting to the loss of function, and promoting family involvement in a home program. As Duchenne muscular dystrophy progresses important aspects of care will include range of motion, prevention of contractures through splinting and positioning, breathing exercises, and the use of a wheelchair. Emotional support for the child and the family is necessary.

What home care regimen should be recommended?
Family involvement is required for an ongoing home care regimen. Proper positioning, range of motion, submaximal exercise, and breathing exercises are all important aspects that assist a child to maintain function for as long as possible. As the child continues to lose function the family must assist with all aspects of the home program.

Outcome:
What is the likely outcome of a course in physical therapy?
Physical therapy is an important aspect in the care of a child with Duchenne muscular dystrophy, however it will not alter the degenerative process of the disease. The goal of physical therapy throughout the course of the disease is to maintain present function, adapt to the progressive loss of mobility skills, and educate the patient and family.

What are the long-term effects of the patient's condition?
Duchenne muscular dystrophy is a progressive disorder that affects the cardiac muscle in the later stages of the disease. Death occurs primarily from cardiopulmonary problems or other complications of the disease usually during the teenage years.

Comparison:
What are the distinguishing characteristics of a similar condition?
Landouzy-Dejerine dystrophy (LDMD) is a form of muscular dystrophy that is also inherited, but the exact genetic origin is presently unclear. This disease presents later in a child's life, usually between seven and twenty years of age. Characteristics include facial and shoulder girdle weakness, weakness lifting the arms over the head, and difficulty closing the eyes. Life span remains normal with this form of muscular dystrophy.

Clinical Scenarios:
Scenario One
A three-year-old male was recently diagnosed with Duchenne muscular dystrophy. The mother reports that the child can ambulate, however prefers to be carried. The child crawls up the stairs and has been falling more frequently over the last six months. The patient has two sisters at home and resides in a two story home. At present, both parents work full time and the child is enrolled in a home daycare.

Scenario Two
A 12-year-old male diagnosed with Duchenne muscular dystrophy is referred to physical therapy secondary to increased weakness and frequent falls. The patient is currently ambulating with bilateral Lofstrand crutches. There is evidence of pseudohypertrophy and a mild plantar flexion contracture. The patient's mother is concerned that he is at risk for serious injury while ambulating at school.

Emphysema

Diagnosis:

What condition produces a patient's symptoms?
Emphysema results from a long history of chronic bronchitis or recurrent alveolar inflammation. Emphysema may also result from genetic predisposition of a congenital alpha 1-antitrypsin deficiency.

An injury was most likely sustained to which structure?
Emphysema results from a nonreversible injury to the alveolar walls and enlargement of the air spaces distal to the terminal bronchioles within the lungs. Progression of the disease includes further destruction of the alveolar walls, collapse of the peripheral bronchioles, and impaired gas exchange.

Inference:

What is the most likely contributing factor in the development of this condition?
The primary risk factors for the development of emphysema include chronic bronchitis, lower respiratory infections, cigarette smoking, and genetic predisposition. Environmental influence includes air pollution and other airborne toxins. The risk of acquiring emphysema increases with age.

Confirmation:

What is the most likely clinical presentation?
Emphysema can be asymptomatic until middle age. Symptoms worsen with the progression of the disease and include a persistent cough, wheezing, difficulty breathing especially with expiration, and an increased respiration rate. Advanced disease symptoms include increased use of accessory muscles, severe dyspnea, cor pulmonale, and cyanosis.

What laboratory or imaging studies would confirm the diagnosis?
X-ray is utilized to visually evaluate the shape and spacing of the lungs. Other imaging studies include a planogram to detect bullae and a bronchogram to evaluate mucus ducts and enlargement of the bronchi.

What additional information should be obtained to confirm the diagnosis?
Pulmonary function testing will result in impaired forced expiratory volume (FEV_1), vital capacity (VC), and forced vital capacity (FVC). Total lung capacity (TLC), residual volume (RV), and functional residual capacity (FRC) will be increased. Arterial blood gases may indicate a decreased PaO_2.

Examination:

What history should be documented?
Important areas to explore include past medical history, medications, current health status, social history and habits, occupation, living environment, and social support system.

What test/measures are most appropriate?
- **Aerobic capacity and endurance:** assessment of vital signs at rest and with activity, perceived exertion scale, Six Minute Walk Test, Three Minute Step Test
- **Arousal, attention, and cognition:** examine mental status, learning ability, memory, and motivation
- **Assistive and adaptive devices:** analysis of components and safety of a device
- **Environmental, home, and work:** analysis of current and potential barriers or hazards
- **Gait, locomotion, and balance:** static and dynamic balance in sitting and standing, safety during gait with/without an assistive device
- **Muscle performance:** strength assessment, assessment of active movement and muscle endurance
- **Posture:** analysis of resting and dynamic posture
- **Self-care and home management:** assessment of functional capacity
- **Ventilation, respiration, and circulation:** assessment of thoracoabdominal movement, auscultation of vesicular sounds and potential rhonchi, pulse oximetry, pulmonary function testing, accessory muscle utilization

What additional findings are likely with this patient?
A patient with emphysema may present with a barrel chest appearance and utilize pursed lip breathing to assist with ventilation. Complications from emphysema such as the formation and rupture of bullae and blebs in the lungs can lead to pneumothorax. Cor pulmonale is a serious complication that can occur with advanced emphysema.

Management:

What is the most effective management of this patient?
A patient with emphysema is managed with pharmacological intervention, oxygen therapy, and physical therapy. Physical therapy intervention is based on the severity of the disease process and can include general exercise and endurance training, breathing exercises, ventilatory muscle strengthening, chest wall exercises, and patient education on posture, airway secretion clearance, and energy conservation techniques. Chest physical therapy is required during advanced stages of emphysema.

What home care regimen should be recommended?
The home care regimen should include breathing strategies and exercises, energy conservation, pacing techniques, and general strength and endurance training.

Outcome:

What is the likely outcome of a course in physical therapy?
A patient with emphysema may require physical therapy intermittently as the disease progresses. The goals of physical therapy are to maximize the patient's functional abilities and optimize pulmonary function.

What are the long-term effects of the patient's condition?
Emphysema is a chronic progressive disease process. Life expectancy decreases to less than five years with severe expiratory slowing measured at a rate of <1L of air during forced expiratory volume (FEV_1).

Comparison:

What are the distinguishing characteristics of a similar condition?
Bronchiectasis is inherited or acquired and is characterized by chronic inflammation and dilation of the bronchi and destruction of the bronchial walls. Characteristics include a chronic cough with sputum, hemoptysis, wheezing, dyspnea, and recurrent pneumonia or respiratory infections.

Clinical Scenarios:

Scenario One
A 65-year-old male is referred to physical therapy after recently being diagnosed with emphysema. The patient works in an oil refinery part time and manages a small dairy farm. The patient's past medical history is negative for smoking and consists of recurrent respiratory infections and chronic cough. The patient complains of shortness of breath with exertion, however pulmonary function testing indicates only minimal impairment in lung volumes.

Scenario Two
A 75-year-old female requires physical therapy for management of emphysema. The patient has a history of smoking cigarettes for over 40 years and continues to smoke approximately one pack per day. The patient has an oxygen saturation rate of 94% at rest and requires two liters of oxygen with exertion. The patient has moderate impairment in pulmonary function testing and a persistent cough. The patient presently resides in a two story home and assists with the care of her disabled husband.

Huntington's Disease

Diagnosis:

What condition produces a patient's symptoms?
Huntington's disease (also known as Huntington's chorea) is characterized by degeneration of the basal ganglia and cerebral cortex within the brain.

An injury was most likely sustained to which structure?
Huntington's disease affects the basal ganglia and cerebral cortex of the brain. There appears to be an overall decrease in gamma-aminobutyric acid (GABA) and acetylcholine neurons that are produced in these areas. The identified neurotransmitters become deficient and are unable to modulate movement. The thalamus is also believed to contribute to the movement disorders associated with the disease process.

Inference:

What is the most likely contributing factor in the development of this condition?
Huntington's disease is genetically transmitted as an autosomal dominant trait with the defect linked to chromosome four. The disease is usually perpetuated by a person that has children prior to the normal onset of symptoms and without knowledge that he/she possesses the defective gene. Genetic testing is able to identify the defective gene for Huntington's disease prior to the onset of symptoms.

Confirmation:

What is the most likely clinical presentation?
A patient with Huntington's disease will initially develop symptoms between 35 and 50 years of age. The patient will initially present with involuntary choreic movements and a mild alteration in personality. As the disease progresses gait will become ataxic and a patient will experience choreoathetoid movement of the extremities and the trunk. Speech disturbances and mental deterioration are common. Late stage Hungtington's disease is characterized by a decrease in IQ, dementia, depression, dysphagia, inability to ambulate or transfer, and progression from choreiform movement to rigidity.

What laboratory or imaging studies would confirm the diagnosis?
Magnetic resonance imaging or computed tomography may indicate atrophy or abnormalities within the cerebral cortex as well as the basal ganglia. Positron-emission tomography may be used to augment other testing and obtain information regarding blood flow, oxygen uptake, and metabolism of the brain. A DNA marker study may be administered to determine if the autosomal dominant trait is present for Huntington's disease.

What additional information should be obtained to confirm the diagnosis?
A physical examination, review of symptoms, and family history are important components in the diagnosis of Huntington's disease.

Examination:

What history should be documented?
Important areas to explore include past medical history, medications, family history, current symptoms, current health status, social history and habits, occupation, living environment, and social support system.

What test/measures are most appropriate?
- **Aerobic capacity and endurance:** assessment of vital signs at rest and with activity
- **Arousal, attention, and cognition:** examine mental status, learning ability, memory, and motivation
- **Gait, locomotion, and balance:** static and dynamic balance in sitting and standing, safety during gait with/without an assistive device, Functional Reach, Tinetti Performance Oriented Mobility Assessment, Functional Ambulation Profile
- **Motor function:** equilibrium and righting reactions, coordination, posture and balance in sitting, physical performance scales
- **Muscle performance:** strength assessment, muscle tone assessment, tremor assessment
- **Neuromotor development and sensory integration:** analysis of reflex movement patterns, assessment of involuntary movements

- **Posture:** analysis of resting and dynamic posture
- **Range of motion:** active and passive range of motion
- **Self-care and home management:** assessment of functional capacity, Functional Independence Measure (FIM), Barthel ADL Index

What additional findings are likely with this patient?
Dementia and other psychological changes usually occur after neurological symptoms appear. The emotional disorder worsens with progression of the disease and may require admission to a psychiatric facility for severe depression and/or suicidal attempts.

Management:
What is the most effective management of this patient?
Pharmacological management of a patient with Huntington's disease is usually initiated once choreiform movement impairs a patient's functional capacity. Commonly utilized drugs include Perphenazine, Haloperidol (Haldol), and Reserpine. Physical, occupational, and speech therapy intervention may be warranted intermittently throughout the course of the disease. Physical therapy should maximize endurance, strength, and functional mobility. Intervention should focus on motor control and utilize techniques including coactivation of muscles, trunk stabilization, the use of biofeedback, and relaxation to maintain a patient's status. As the disease progresses, the degree of dementia will influence treatment and goals. The physical therapist must emphasize family involvement and caregiver teaching. As the patient continues to lose function the caregiver will require education regarding assistance with transfers, mobility, and the use of adaptive equipment.

What home care regimen should be recommended?
A home care regimen should include an exercise routine, functional mobility skills, relaxation techniques, range of motion and stretching exercises, and endurance activities. Participation in a home care regimen can assist a patient to maintain an optimal quality of life.

Outcome:
What is the likely outcome of a course in physical therapy?
Physical therapy is recommended on an intermittent basis throughout the course of the disease. Physical therapy will not prevent further degeneration, however it will maximize the patient's functional potential and safety and maintain an optimal quality of life.

What are the long-term effects of the patient's condition?
Huntington's disease is a chronic progressive genetic disorder that is fatal within 15 to 20 years after clinical manifestation. Late stages of the disease result in total physical and mental incapacitation. The patient usually requires an extended care facility due to the significant burden of care.

Comparison:
What are the distinguishing characteristics of a similar condition?
Athetoid (dyskinetic) cerebral palsy is a nonprogressive motor disorder caused by central nervous system damage specifically to the basal ganglia. Clinical manifestations include slow and involuntary movements, choreiform movements, severe dysarthria, and an increased risk of aspiration pneumonia. The involuntary movements will increase with stress and fatigue and subside with sleep. Physical therapy intervention should focus on motor control and mobility deficits in order for the patient to attain the highest level of functioning.

Clinical Scenarios:
Scenario One
A 48-year-old attorney is referred for physical therapy home services. The patient was diagnosed with Huntington's disease two years ago and resides in a two story home. The patient has a significant other and they reside together. The patient's primary complaint is a loss of balance while ambulating. The patient has a walker, but refuses to use it.

Scenario Two
A 45-year-old female is referred to physical therapy. The woman was diagnosed with Huntington's disease seven years ago and has recently fallen multiple times. According to family members the patient is short-tempered, irritable, and occasionally demonstrates poor judgment. The physician requests physical therapy for an evaluation and home program.

Medial Collateral Ligament Sprain – Grade II

Diagnosis:

What condition produces a patient's symptoms?
The medial collateral ligament connects the medial epicondyle of the femur to the medial tibia and as a result resists medially directed force at the knee. A common mechanism of injury is a direct blow against the lateral surface of the knee causing valgus stress.

An injury was most likely sustained to which structure?
A grade II injury of the medial collateral ligament is characterized by partial tearing of the ligament's fibers resulting in joint laxity when the ligament is stretched. Often the medial capsular ligament is involved in a grade II sprain of the medial collateral ligament.

Inference:

What is the most likely contributing factor in the development of this condition?
Individuals participating in contact activities requiring a high level of agility are particularly susceptible to a medial collateral ligament injury. Muscle weakness resulting in poor dynamic stabilization may also increase the incidence of this type of injury.

Confirmation:

What is the most likely clinical presentation?
A patient with a grade II medial collateral ligament injury will likely present with an inability to fully extend and flex the knee, pain along the medial aspect of the knee, diminished strength, and an antalgic gait. There is typically discernable laxity with valgus testing and slight swelling around the knee. More severe swelling may be indicative of meniscus or cruciate ligament involvement.

What laboratory or imaging studies would confirm the diagnosis?
Magnetic resonance imaging is a noninvasive imaging technique that can be utilized to view soft tissue structures such as ligaments. The imaging technique is extremely expensive and therefore may not be commonly employed on an individual with a suspected medial collateral ligament injury without other extenuating circumstances.

What additional information should be obtained to confirm the diagnosis?
A valgus stress test is a technique designed to detect medial instability in a single plane. The examiner applies a valgus stress at the knee while stabilizing the ankle in slight lateral rotation. The test is often performed initially in full extension and then in 30 degrees of flexion. A patient with a grade II medial collateral ligament sprain may exhibit 5-15 degrees of laxity with valgus stress at 30 degrees of flexion.

Examination:

What history should be documented?
Important areas to explore include mechanism of present injury, current symptoms, past medical history, medications, living environment, social history and habits, and social support system.

What test/measures are most appropriate?
- **Anthropometric characteristics:** palpation to determine knee effusion, lower extremity circumferential measurements
- **Arousal, attention, and cognition:** examine mental status, learning ability, memory, and motivation
- **Assistive and adaptive devices:** analysis of components and safety of a device, potential utilization of crutches
- **Gait, locomotion, and balance:** safety during gait with an assistive device
- **Integumentary integrity:** assessment of sensation (pain, temperature, tactile), skin assessment
- **Joint integrity and mobility:** special tests for ligaments and menisci, valgus stress test, palpation of structures, joint play, soft tissue restrictions, joint pain
- **Muscle performance:** strength assessment, assessment of active movement, resisted isometrics, muscle contraction characteristics, muscle endurance
- **Orthotic, protective, and supportive devices:** potential utilization of bracing, taping or wrapping

- **Pain:** pain perception assessment scale
- **Range of motion:** active and passive range of motion
- **Self-care and home management:** assessment of functional capacity
- **Sensory integrity:** assessment of proprioception and kinesthesia

What additional findings are likely with this patient?
Anterior cruciate ligament and/or meniscal damage often accompanies a grade II medial collateral ligament injury. As a result it is often prudent to perform special tests directed at these particular structures.

Management:
What is the most effective management of this patient?
The patient may utilize a full length knee immobilizer and crutches to limit weight bearing through the involved lower extremity for up to one week. Intervention should be directed towards increasing range of motion in the involved extremity and beginning light resistive exercises. Range of motion exercises may include heel slides or stationary cycling without resistance. Resistive exercises should be directed towards the quadriceps and may include isometrics and closed kinetic chain exercises. Functional activities such as gait and stair climbing should be incorporated into the treatment program. Superficial modalities and electrical stimulation may be utilized to combat pain and inflammation. A patient should be required to complete a functional progression prior to returning to unrestricted activity.

What home care regimen should be recommended?
The home care regimen should consist of range of motion, strengthening, palliative care, and functional activities as warranted based on the results of the patient examination.

Outcome:
What is the likely outcome of a course in physical therapy?
A patient should be able to return to his/her previous functional level within four to eight weeks following the injury.

What are the long-term effects of the patient's condition?
If the patient has residual laxity from the injury the patient may be susceptible to reinjury.

Comparison:
What are the distinguishing characteristics of a similar condition?
A grade II lateral collateral ligament injury differs from a medial collateral ligament injury in several ways. The lateral collateral ligament connects the lateral epicondyle of the femur to the head of the fibula and as a result resists laterally directed force. Lateral collateral ligament injuries are far less common than medial collateral ligament injuries. Management should focus on the same general goals (range of motion, strengthening, palliative care, and functional activities) as those outlined for the medial collateral ligament injury.

Clinical Scenarios:
Scenario One
A 17-year-old male is diagnosed with a left grade III medial collateral ligament sprain and a small tear in the medial meniscus. The patient was playing football when he was tackled and hit at the knee. The patient has no significant past medical history and plans to participate in football at the collegiate level.

Scenario Two
A 20-year-old college field hockey player complains of knee pain after being diagnosed with a grade I medial collateral ligament sprain. The patient is mildly tender to palpation over the medial joint line and exhibits trace effusion. The patient has no significant past medical history and would like to return to athletic competition as soon as possible.

Multiple Sclerosis

Diagnosis:

What condition produces a patient's symptoms?
Multiple sclerosis (MS) produces patches of demyelination that decreases the efficiency of nerve impulse transmission. Symptoms vary based on the location of the affected area and the extent of demyelination.

An injury was most likely sustained to which structure?
Multiple sclerosis is characterized by demyelination of the myelin sheaths that surround nerves within the brain and spinal cord. Myelin breakdown results in plaque development, decreased nerve conduction velocity, and eventual failure of impulse transmission.

Inference:

What is the most likely contributing factor in the development of this condition?
The exact etiology of MS is unknown. It is theorized that a slow acting virus initiates the autoimmune response in people that have genetic factors and environmental influence for the disease. There is a higher incidence of MS in geographical areas that are further from the equator, in the caucasian population, and in women. Diagnosis is usually made between the ages of 15 and 40.

Confirmation:

What is the most likely clinical presentation?
The clinical presentation of MS varies based on the extent and location of demyelination and sclerosis. Initial symptoms include visual problems, paresthesias, clumsiness, weakness, ataxia, fatigue, and urinary incontinence. The symptoms can be transient based on the course of the disease process. The clinical course of MS consists of exacerbations and remissions. The frequency and intensity of exacerbations may indicate the speed and course of the disease process.

What laboratory or imaging studies would confirm the diagnosis?
There is not a sole testing procedure to diagnose MS early in the disease process. Magnetic resonance imaging (MRI) may assist with observation and establishing a baseline for lesions, however other disease processes may contribute to an abnormal finding. Evoked potentials may demonstrate slowed nerve conduction. Cerebrospinal fluid can be analyzed for an elevated concentration of gamma globulin and protein levels. The tests should be evaluated in combination with the clinical presentation when determining a diagnosis of MS.

What additional information should be obtained to confirm the diagnosis?
Clinical presentation and reliable patient history of symptoms are vital in the diagnosis of MS. Guidelines indicate that a definitive diagnosis can be made if a person experiences two separate attacks and shows evidence of two separate lesions.

Examination:

What history should be documented?
Important areas to explore include past medical history, history of symptoms, medications, current health status, social history and habits, occupation, living environment, and social support system.

What test/measures are most appropriate?
- **Aerobic capacity and endurance:** assessment of vital signs at rest and with activity
- **Arousal, attention and cognition:** examine mental status, learning ability, memory, and motivation
- **Assistive and adaptive devices:** analysis of components and safety of a device
- **Community and work integration:** analysis of community, work, and leisure activities
- **Gait, locomotion, and balance:** static and dynamic balance in sitting and standing, safety with gait, Tinetti Performance Oriented Mobility Assessment, Berg Functional Balance Scale
- **Motor function:** assessment of dexterity and coordination; assessment of postural, equilibrium, and righting reactions; gross and fine motor skills
- **Muscle performance:** strength assessment, muscle tone and tremor assessment, muscle endurance
- **Neuromotor development and sensory integration:** analysis of reflex movement patterns
- **Pain:** pain perception assessment scale

CLINICAL APPLICATION TEMPLATES

- **Posture:** resting and dynamic posture, examine potential contractures
- **Range of motion:** active and passive range of motion
- **Self-care and home management:** Barthel ADL Index, assessment of functional capacity and safety assessments
- **Sensory integrity:** assessment of proprioception and kinesthesia

What additional findings are likely with this patient?
A low percentage of patients experience benign MS and have little to no long-term disability. The majority of patients with MS experience progressive degeneration through periods of exacerbations and remissions. As the disease advances exacerbations leave greater ongoing disability and the length of remissions decrease. Some patients will experience a clinical course of ongoing progression, no periods of remission, and death within one to two years. Ongoing symptoms can include emotional lability, depression, dementia, spasticity, weakness, paralysis, and loss of bowel and bladder control.

Management:
What is the most effective management of this patient?
Management of MS includes medical, pharmacological, and therapeutic intervention. MS is treated by attempting to lessen the length of exacerbations and maximize the health of the patient. Physical, occupational, and speech therapies are indicated throughout the clinical course of the disease. Nutritional and psychological counseling are also recommended. Physical therapy intervention includes regulation of activity level, relaxation and energy conservation techniques, decreasing tone, balance activities, gait training, proximal stability and control, and adaptive and assistive device training as needed.

What home care regimen should be recommended?
A home care regimen for a patient with MS should include a moderate exercise and endurance program. A patient should exercise in the morning when he or she is rested and avoid exercising to the point of fatigue. Ongoing ambulation and mobility activities are important to maintain endurance and prevent disuse atrophy.

Outcome:
What is the likely outcome of a course in physical therapy?
Physical therapy is indicated intermittently throughout the clinical course of MS with the goal of maximizing functional capacity and the quality of life. Physical therapy will not alter the progression of the disease process.

What are the long-term effects of the patient's condition?
MS is generally a progressive degenerative disease process that creates permanent damage and disability. Factors that influence exacerbations include heat, stress, and trauma. Most patients live with MS for many years and die from secondary complications such as disuse atrophy, pressure sores, contractures, pathological fractures, renal infection, and pneumonia.

Comparison:
What are the distinguishing characteristics of a similar condition?
Guillain-Barre syndrome is a rapidly progressive demyelinating polyneuropathy that results from an autoimmune response to an infection. This disease is reversible with 90% of patients eventually making a full recovery. Characteristics of Guillain-Barre include peripheral weakness and paresthesias that progress proximally, absent deep tendon reflexes, and potential motor and respiratory paralysis. Spontaneous recovery can occur and may take patients up to three years to return to their previous level of function.

Clinical Scenarios:
Scenario One
A 28-year-old female has had visual difficulty, urinary urgency, tingling, and upper extremity weakness on two separate occasions over the past year. The patient has an aunt with multiple sclerosis, however has no other significant medical history. The patient was recently referred to physical therapy by her primary physician.

Scenario Two
A 42-year-old male diagnosed with MS is referred to physical therapy. The patient has experienced several exacerbations and remissions with full recovery over the past two years. The patient presently appears to have an exacerbation of symptoms and complains of excessive fatigue. He lives alone and works in a library.

Myocardial Infarction

Diagnosis:

What condition produces a patient's symptoms?
Myocardial infarction occurs when there is poor coronary artery perfusion due to atherosclerosis, coronary spasm or a clot and as a result a segment of the myocardium becomes ischemic.

An injury was most likely sustained to which structure?
Myocardial infarction produces ischemia and subsequent necrosis to a portion of the myocardium. The extent of the damage to the myocardium is dependent on the duration of ischemia and on the thickness of the tissue involved. A transmural myocardial infarction involves the full thickness of the myocardium while a nontransmural myocardial infarction involves the subendocardial area.

Inference:

What is the most likely contributing factor in the development of this condition?
The primary risk factors for myocardial infarction include patient or family history of heart disease, smoking, inactivity, stress, hypertension, elevated cholesterol, diabetes mellitus, and obesity.

Confirmation:

What is the most likely clinical presentation?
A patient that is experiencing a myocardial infarction will initially present with deep pain or pressure in the substernal area. The pain may radiate to the jaw and down the left arm. The patient cannot alleviate the pain with rest or nitroglycerin. The patient is usually anxious, pale, sweaty, fatigued, and may present with nausea and vomiting.

What laboratory or imaging studies would confirm the diagnosis?
The primarily tool to detect a myocardial infarction is a 12-lead electrocardiogram. A blood serum analysis can be utilized to determine the level of selected cardiac enzymes. The level of selected enzymes such as creatine phosphokinase (CPK), aspartate transferase (AST), and lactic dehydrogenase (LDH) can be dramatically altered by a myocardial infarction. A complete blood count (CBC), chest radiograph, radionuclide imaging, and amylase level may be ordered to assist with the diagnosis.

What additional information should be obtained to confirm the diagnosis?
Additional information in the diagnosis of a myocardial infarction is found through the manifestation of symptoms. (See clinical presentation)

Examination:

What history should be documented?
Important areas to explore include past medical history, family history, medications, current health status, living environment, social history and habits, occupation, and social support system.

What test/measures are most appropriate?
- **Aerobic capacity and endurance:** assessment of vital signs at rest and during activity, palpation of pulses, perceived exertion scale, electrocardiogram analysis, auscultation of the heart and lungs, pulse oximetry
- **Arousal, attention, and cognition:** examine mental status, learning ability, memory, and motivation
- **Assistive and adaptive devices:** analysis of components and safety of a device
- **Environmental, home, and work:** analysis of current and potential barriers or hazards
- **Gait, locomotion, and balance:** assessment of static and dynamic balance in sitting and standing, safety during gait with/without an assistive device
- **Muscle performance:** strength assessment through active movement
- **Pain:** pain perception assessment scale, visual analog scale
- **Posture:** analysis of resting and dynamic posture
- **Self-care and home management:** assessment of functional capacity, Barthel ADL Index

What additional findings are likely with this patient?
A patient status post myocardial infarction is at risk for complications that include dysrhythmias, hypotension, impaired cardiac output, pulmonary edema, congestive heart failure, pericarditis, cardiogenic shock, and sudden death.

Management:

What is the most effective management of this patient?
A patient will initially require pharmacological intervention to hinder the evolution of the myocardial infarction. Anticoagulants, beta blockers, angiotensin-converting enzyme inhibitors, vasodilators, and estrogen (in women) may be used. Once stable, the patient is managed through a cardiac rehabilitation program. Patient education regarding reduction of risk factors, return to activity, and commitment to fitness and health are the focus of physical therapy intervention.

What home care regimen should be recommended?
A home care regimen for a patient status post myocardial infarction should follow the guidelines indicated for each phase of cardiac rehabilitation. A patient must continue a safe exercise program and integrate risk factor reduction, recognition of symptoms, and nutritional strategies into his/her daily routine.

Outcome:

What is the likely outcome of a course in physical therapy?
Cardiac rehabilitation is recommended status post myocardial infarction. The patient should start as an inpatient in the coronary care unit (CCU) and progress through each of the phases of cardiac rehabilitation. The goal of physical therapy is successful completion of all phases of the cardiac rehabilitation program.

What are the long-term effects of the patient's condition?
A patient that has experienced a myocardial infarction may be able to return to all previous activities after successful completion of a cardiac rehabilitation program. A patient must continue to reduce the modifiable risk factors and maintain an appropriate level of exercise in order to limit the possibility of subsequent myocardial infarction. Long-term outcome is dependent on prior functional ability and the initial extent of the damage to the heart.

Comparison:

What are the distinguishing characteristics of a similar condition?
Angina pectoris is a myocardial ischemic disorder that occurs when there is oxygen deficit to the coronary arteries. Angina is classified as stable, nocturnal or variant. Symptoms often occur during exertion and include chest pain or pressure that may radiate. Rest or nitroglycerin normally provides relief of the symptoms.

Clinical Scenarios:

Scenario One
A 51-year-old male is referred to a phase I cardiac rehabilitation program after a transmural myocardial infarction two days ago. The patient has hypertension, high cholesterol, smokes one pack of cigarettes, and is moderately obese. The patient currently supervises the operations of a local automobile dealership and indicates that it is a high stress position.

Scenario Two
A 78-year-old female is status post nontransmural myocardial infarction. The patient is very active and plays golf three times per week. The patient's past medical history includes a cardiac arrhythmia that is treated by medication. The patient's history is negative for smoking, obesity, and diabetes mellitus. The physician referred the patient to physical therapy for outpatient cardiac rehabilitation.

Parkinson's Disease

Diagnosis:

What condition produces a patient's symptoms?
Parkinson's disease is characterized by a decrease in production of dopamine within the corpus striatum portion of the basal ganglia. The degeneration of the dopaminergic pathways creates an imbalance between dopamine and acetylcholine and the resulting imbalance produces the symptoms of Parkinson's disease.

An injury was most likely sustained to which structure?
Injury occurs within the basal ganglia of the brain. The basal ganglia is responsible for modulation and control of voluntary movement. Degeneration of dopamine production within the basal ganglia is progressive and irreversible.

Inference:

What is the most likely contributing factor in the development of this condition?
Primary Parkinson's disease has an unknown etiology and accounts for the majority of patients with Parkinsonism. Contributing factors that can produce symptoms of Parkinson's disease include genetic defect, toxicity from carbon monoxide, manganese, carbon disulfide, structural lesions or tumors of the basal ganglia, vascular impairment of the striatum, encephalitis, and other neurodegenerative diseases such as Huntington's or Alzheimer's disease.

Confirmation:

What is the most likely clinical presentation?
A patient with Parkinson's disease will initially notice a resting tremor in the hands or feet that disappears with movement or sleep. A patient's symptoms slowly progress and often include hypokinesia, sluggish movement, difficulty with initiating and stopping movement, festinating and shuffling gait, poor posture, dysphagia, and rigidity in all skeletal muscles. A patient with Parkinson's disease may have a mask-like appearance with little facial expression.

What laboratory or imaging studies would confirm the diagnosis?
There are no laboratory or imaging studies that initially diagnose Parkinson's disease. Computed tomography or magnetic resonance imaging may be used to rule out other neurodegenerative disease processes and obtain a baseline for potential future comparison.

What additional information should be obtained to confirm the diagnosis?
Definitive diagnosis is difficult in the early stages of the disease. The course of Parkinson's disease is believed to progress slowly over 25 to 30 years prior to the onset of pharmacological intervention. Diagnosis is made from patient history, history of symptoms, and differential diagnosis to rule out other potential disorders. There are standardized evaluation tools that are utilized to classify a patient by stage of the disease process.

Examination:

What history should be documented?
Important areas to explore include past medical history, medications, current symptoms, current health status, social history and habits, occupation, living environment, and social support system.

What test/measures are most appropriate?
- **Aerobic capacity and endurance:** assessment of vital signs at rest and with activity
- **Arousal, attention, and cognition:** examine mental status, learning ability, memory, motivation, and Mini Mental State Examination
- **Gait, locomotion, and balance:** static and dynamic balance in sitting and standing, Functional Reach, Tinetti Performance Oriented Mobility Assessment, Berg Functional Balance Scale, outcome measurement tools, safety with/without an assistive device during gait
- **Joint integrity and mobility:** analysis of quality of movement, examine joint hypermobility and hypomobility
- **Motor function:** assessment of dexterity, coordination and agility, assessment of postural, equilibrium, and righting reactions
- **Muscle performance:** strength assessment, muscle tone assessment, and tremor assessment
- **Posture:** analysis of resting and dynamic posture

- **Range of motion:** active and passive range of motion
- **Self-care and home management:** assessment of functional capacity, Barthel ADL Index, safety assessments
- **Sensory integration:** assessment of combined sensation, assessment of proprioception and kinesthesia
- **Ventilation, respiratory, and circulation:** assessment of chest wall mobility, expansion, and excursion

What additional findings are likely with this patient?
Since Parkinson's disease is a progressive condition there are ongoing physical and cognitive impairments. A patient may develop a stooped posture and an increased risk for falling. Progression of the disease process may result in dysphagia, difficulty with speech, and impairment in pulmonary function. Many patients with Parkinson's disease die from complications of bronchopneumonia.

Management:
What is the most effective management of this patient?
Management of a patient with Parkinson's disease relies heavily on pharmacological intervention. Dopamine replacement therapy, (Levodopa), antihistamines, anticholinergics, and antidepressants are utilized to slow and reduce the effects of the disease process. Physical, occupational, and speech therapies may be warranted intermittently throughout the course of the disease. Physical therapy intervention should include maximizing endurance, strength, and functional mobility. Family teaching, balance activities, gait training, assistive device training, relaxation techniques, and respiratory therapy are all important components in the treatment of this condition. Psychological and nutritional counseling are recommended. Surgical intervention is rare but may be indicated to alleviate tremors or rigidity if pharmacological intervention fails.

What home care regimen should be recommended?
A home care regimen should include an exercise routine, functional mobility skills, relaxation techniques, range of motion, stretching exercises, and endurance activities.

Outcome:
What is the likely outcome of a course in physical therapy?
Physical therapy is recommended on an intermittent basis throughout the course of the disease. Physical therapy will not prevent further degeneration, however it will assist the patient to maximize their quality of life.

What are the long-term effects of the patient's condition?
As the disease progresses there will be an exacerbation of all symptoms and significant loss of mobility. The inactivity and deconditioning allows for complications and eventual death.

Comparison:
What are the distinguishing characteristics of a similar condition?
Wilson's disease is inherited as an autosomal recessive trait and causes a defect in the metabolism of copper. The accumulation of copper within erythrocytes, the liver, the brain, and kidneys produces the associated degenerative changes. The patient presents with hepatic insufficiency, tremor, choreoathetoid movements, dysarthria, and progressive rigidity.

Clinical Scenarios:
Scenario One
A 35-year-old female is sent to physical therapy shortly after being diagnosed with Parkinson's disease. The woman presently is having difficulty maintaining a grasp on items from an assembly line at work and complains of frequently dropping her paperwork and tripping in the office. The patient had not been to a physician in over ten years.

Scenario Two
A 42-year-old male was diagnosed with Parkinson's disease four years ago. The patient requires physical therapy services to reassess gait and prescribe an assistive device. The caregiver states that the patient sits a great deal at home and lacks the necessary motivation to engage in exercise on a regular basis.

Patellofemoral Syndrome

Diagnosis:

What condition produces a patient's symptoms?
Abnormal tracking of the patella between the femoral condyles causes patellofemoral syndrome. The tracking problem most commonly occurs when the patella is pulled too far laterally during knee extension.

An injury was most likely sustained to which structure?
Damage occurs to the articular cartilage of the patella. The damage can range from softening of the cartilage to complete destruction resulting in exposure of subchondral bone.

Inference:

What is the most likely contributing factor in the development of this condition?
Patellofemoral syndrome is extremely common during adolescence and is more prevalent in females than males. In an older population patellofemoral syndrome is often associated with osteoarthritis. Additional factors associated with patellofemoral syndrome include patella alta, insufficient lateral femoral condyle, weak vastus medialis obliquus, excessive pronation, and tightness in selected lower extremity muscles such as the iliotibial tract, hamstrings, gastrocnemius, and vastus lateralis.

Confirmation:

What is the most likely clinical presentation?
A patient with patellofemoral syndrome often describes a gradual onset of anterior knee pain following an increase in physical activity. The pain may be exacerbated with activities that increase patellofemoral compressive forces and with prolonged static positioning. Point tenderness is common over the lateral border of the patella and crepitus may be elicited when the patella is manually compressed into the trochlear groove. Visible quadriceps atrophy may be noted in the involved lower extremity particularly along the vastus medialis obliquus.

What laboratory or imaging studies would confirm the diagnosis?
Laboratory or imaging studies are not commonly used to diagnose patellofemoral syndrome. X-rays are often ordered to rule out a fracture and examine the configuration of the patellofemoral joint. Arthrogram and arthroscopy can be used to examine the articular cartilage.

What additional information should be obtained to confirm the diagnosis?
Special tests such as Clarke's sign can be useful when attempting to confirm the diagnosis. The test is performed by a therapist applying pressure immediately proximal to the upper pole of the patella. The therapist then asks the patient to isometrically contract the quadriceps. A positive test is indicated by a failure to fully contract the quadriceps or by the presence of retropatellar pain. The test should be performed at varying degrees of flexion and extension.

Examination:

What history should be documented?
Important areas to explore include past medical history, history of symptoms, medications, current health status, social history and habits, occupation, living environment, and social support system.

What test/measures are most appropriate?
- **Anthropometric characteristics:** determine the amount of knee effusion, lower extremity circumferential measurements
- **Arousal, attention, and cognition:** examine mental status, learning ability, memory, and motivation
- **Assistive and adaptive devices:** analysis of components and safety of a device, potential utilization of crutches
- **Gait, locomotion, and balance:** safety during gait with an assistive device
- **Integumentary integrity:** assessment of sensation (pain, temperature, tactile), skin assessment
- **Joint integrity and mobility:** Clarke's sign, patella grind test (active and passive), dynamic patella tracking, patella glide test, palpation of structures, joint play, soft tissue restrictions, joint pain
- **Muscle performance:** strength assessment, assessment of active movement, resisted isometrics, muscle contraction characteristics, muscle endurance
- **Orthotic, protective, and supportive devices:** potential utilization of bracing, taping or wrapping
- **Pain:** pain perception assessment scale
- **Range of motion:** active and passive range of motion

- **Self-care and home management:** assessment of functional capacity
- **Sensory integrity:** assessment of proprioception and kinesthesia

What additional findings are likely with this patient?
Patients diagnosed with patellofemoral syndrome often have an increased Q angle. The normal Q angle is 13 degrees in males and 18 degrees in females. The Q angle is measured using the anterior superior iliac spine, the midpoint of the patella, and the tibial tubercle.

Management:
What is the most effective management of this patient?
Management of a patient with patellofemoral syndrome includes controlling edema, stretching, strengthening, improving range of motion, and activity modification. The patient may be instructed to take anti-inflammatory medication by the referring physician. Mobilization activities to increase medial glide can be beneficial to increase the flexibility of the lateral fascia. Strengthening activities emphasizing the vastus medialis obliquus in non-weight bearing and weight bearing positions are recommended. Biofeedback can be a useful tool in order to selectively train the muscle. Stretching activities should emphasize the hamstrings, iliotibial band, tensor fasciae latae, and rectus femoris. Strengthening activities may include quadriceps setting exercises, straight leg raising and mini-squats incorporating the hip adductors. Exercises such as deep squats should be avoided since they will tend to aggravate the patient's condition. Patellar taping to improve the position and tracking of the patella during dynamic activities can be useful to limit irritation. Some patients may benefit from a patellofemoral support device designed to avoid direct pressure on the patella and prevent lateral subluxation.

What home care regimen should be recommended?
The home care regimen should consist of range of motion, strengthening, stretching, palliative care, and functional activities as warranted based on the results of the patient examination.

Outcome:
What is the likely outcome of a course in physical therapy?
A patient with patellofemoral syndrome may be able to return to his/her previous level of functioning within two to four weeks.

What are the long-term effects of the patient's condition?
Failure to adequately address the cause of the patellofemoral syndrome will likely result in a patient's condition further deteriorating. The patient may experience increased irritation of the patellofemoral joint that further impacts his/her ability to participate in activities of daily living. Periodic exacerbations of the condition most commonly due to an increased activity level may require further physical therapy intervention.

Comparison:
What are the distinguishing characteristics of a similar condition?
Patellar tendonitis is an overuse condition characterized by inflammatory changes of the patellar tendon. The condition is most prevalent in athletes who participate in activities requiring repetitive jumping such as basketball or volleyball. The patient's primary complaint is often pain over the anterior portion of the superior tibia with activities such as jumping or ascending and descending stairs. Patients may also experience pain after prolonged sitting or during resisted knee extension and often exhibit point tenderness at the superior pole of the patella tendon. Management of patellar tendonitis incorporates many of the same interventions as patellofemoral syndrome such as range of motion, stretching, and palliative care. Strengthening activities may emphasize eccentric activities of the quadriceps in an attempt to increase the tensile strength of the patellar tendon. Some patients may experience a reduction of pain during activities when using a strap attached perpendicular to the patellar tendon.

Clinical Scenarios:
Scenario One
A 14-year-old female is referred to physical therapy diagnosed with patellofemoral syndrome. The patient has mild edema and is sensitive to light touch over the anterior surface of the knee. The patient reports gaining ten pounds over the last three months and expresses that she is willing to do "anything" to improve her present condition.

Scenario Two
A 45-year-old male is referred to physical therapy after experiencing anterior knee pain for the last week. The patient is 19 weeks status post anterior cruciate ligament reconstruction and has recently returned to playing in a softball league. The patient reports an insidious onset of pain and insists that he has been faithful to his home strengthening program. A note from the referring physician confirms that the integrity of the graft is fine and that he believes the patient's pain is related to patellofemoral syndrome.

Plantar Fasciitis

Diagnosis:

What condition produces a patient's symptoms?
Plantar fasciitis is produced by inflammation of the plantar aponeurosis at its origin on the calcaneus. Plantar fasciitis is a chronic overuse condition that develops when there is excessive foot pronation during the loading phase of gait resulting in stress at the calcaneal origin of the plantar fascia.

An injury was most likely sustained to which structure?
Injury can occur to the plantar fascia itself and cause microtearing, inflammation, and pain. The abductor hallucis, flexor digitorum brevis, and quadratus plantae muscles share the same origin on the medial tubercle of the calcaneus and may also become inflamed and irritated.

Inference:

What is the most likely contributing factor in the development of this condition?
Factors that contribute to the development of plantar fasciitis include excessive pronation during gait, obesity, and possessing a high arch. A person participating in endurance sports such as running and dancing or with an occupation that requires prolonged walking or standing has an increased risk for plantar fasciitis.

Confirmation:

What is the most likely clinical presentation?
A patient with plantar fasciitis presents with severe pain in the heel when first standing up in the morning. Pain typically subsides for a few hours during the day, but increases with prolonged activity or when the patient has been non-weight bearing and resumes a weight bearing posture. A patient will typically experience point tenderness and pain with palpation over the calcaneal insertion of the plantar fascia.

What laboratory or imaging studies would confirm the diagnosis?
Plantar fasciitis is initially treated based on symptoms and physical examination. If pain persists after six to eight weeks of physical therapy intervention, magnetic resonance imaging may be used to confirm the diagnosis. Other diagnostic tools may include x-ray and bone scan to rule out a stress fracture, rheumatology work up to rule out systemic etiology, and EMG testing to rule out nerve entrapment.

What additional information should be obtained to confirm the diagnosis?
A thorough history and biomechanical assessment of the foot, observation of the fat pad, examination for Achilles tendon tightness, errors in athletic training programs, analysis of footwear, and gait disturbances all assist in obtaining the diagnosis.

Examination:

What history should be documented?
Important areas to explore include mechanism of current injury, training routine (if appropriate), past medical history, medications, social history and habits, occupation, living environment, and social support system.

What test/measures are most appropriate?
- **Arousal, attention, and cognition:** examine mental status, learning ability, memory, and motivation
- **Community and work integration:** analysis of community, work, and leisure activities
- **Gait, locomotion, and balance:** biomechanical analysis of gait during walking and running (if appropriate)
- **Integumentary inspection:** assessment of sensation, skin assessment
- **Joint integrity and mobility:** assessment of swelling, inflammation, and joint restriction
- **Muscle performance:** strength assessment, muscle endurance
- **Pain:** pain perception assessment scale, visual analog scale
- **Orthotic, protective, and supportive devices:** potential utilization of taping or use of cushions
- **Range of motion:** active and passive range of motion
- **Self-care and home management:** assessment of functional capacity

What additional findings are likely with this patient?
Bony hypertrophy can occur at the origin of the plantar fascia resulting in a heel spur. Gastrocnemius/soleus complex tightness is common.

Management:
What is the most effective management of this patient?
A patient with plantar fasciitis may require local corticosteroid injections or anti-inflammatory medications to reduce inflammation within the plantar fascia. Physical therapy consists of ice massage, shoe modification, heel insert application, foot orthotics, modification of activities to include non-weight bearing endurance activities, and gentle stretching of the Achilles tendon and plantar fascia. Muscle strengthening exercises for the intrinsic and extrinsic muscles should be implemented once the acute symptoms have subsided.

What home care regimen should be recommended?
A home care regimen for a patient with plantar fasciitis should include ongoing strengthening and stretching exercises, maintenance of a fitness program, and use of foot orthotics and heel inserts. Night tension splints may be indicated if symptoms persist.

Outcome:
What is the likely outcome of a course in physical therapy?
Physical therapy on an outpatient basis should allow the patient to return to his or her previous level of function within eight weeks.

What are the long-term effects of the patient's condition?
A patient previously diagnosed with plantar fasciitis is at an increased risk for recurrence, however with successful conservative management, ongoing compliance with a home program, and proper footwear the patient may not have any negative long-term effects. If conservative management fails the patient may require surgical intervention, however this option is relatively rare.

Comparison:
What are the distinguishing characteristics of a similar condition?
Tarsal tunnel syndrome is characterized by pain that is experienced with weight bearing, but not with direct palpation to the plantar fascia. Characteristics of tarsal tunnel syndrome include complaints of numbness, burning pain, tingling paresthesias at the heel, and a positive Tinel sign. Etiology consists of entrapment and compression of the posterior tibial nerve or plantar nerves within the tarsal tunnel.

Clinical Scenarios:
Scenario One
A 19-year-old male athlete is referred to physical therapy with bilateral heel pain. The physician has ruled out systemic disorders and diagnosed bilateral mechanical plantar fasciitis. The athlete is a swimmer and began running cross-country last fall. The patient is otherwise healthy, but wants to return to athletic activities as soon as possible.

Scenario Two
A 56-year-old female is referred to physical therapy with left plantar fasciitis. The patient is mildly obese and works the night shift at a paper mill. She stands at her station throughout the shift and is required to walk between the two buildings every hour. The patient has a history of mild asthma and a cardiac murmur.

Restrictive Lung Disease

Diagnosis:

What condition produces a patient's symptoms?
Restrictive lung disease is caused by a pulmonary or extrapulmonary restriction that produces an impairment in lung expansion. There are multiple conditions that result in restrictive lung disease.

An injury was most likely sustained to which structure?
Pulmonary restriction of the lungs include tumor, interstitial pulmonary fibrosis, scarring within the lungs, and pneumonia. Extrapulmonary restrictions of the lungs include pleural effusion, chest wall stiffness, structural abnormality, postural deformity, respiratory muscle weakness or central nervous system injury.

Inference:

What is the most likely contributing factor in the development of this condition?
There are varying etiologies for the group of disorders that cause restrictive lung disease. Musculoskeletal etiology includes scoliosis, pectus excavatum, ankylosing spondylitis, and kyphosis. Pulmonary etiology includes idiopathic pulmonary fibrosis, pneumonia, pleural effusion, hyaline membrane disease, and tumor within the lungs. Other etiologies include inhalation of toxic fumes, asbestos, muscular dystrophy, spinal cord injury, and obesity.

Confirmation:

What is the most likely clinical presentation?
Restrictive lung disease is characterized by a reduction of lung volumes due to impaired lung expansion. A patient with restrictive lung disease will present with decreased chest mobility, shortness of breath, respiratory muscle weakness, ineffective cough, and increased use of accessory muscles.

What laboratory or imaging studies would confirm the diagnosis?
X-ray is utilized to evaluate lung structure and evidence of fibrosis, infiltrates, tumor, and deformity. Arterial blood gas analysis may indicate a decrease in PaO_2.

What additional information should be obtained to confirm the diagnosis?
Pulmonary function testing will result in impaired vital capacity (VC), forced vital capacity (FVC), and total lung capacity (TLC). The patient will usually present with normal residual volume (RV) and expiration flow rates. Expiratory reserve volume (ERV) and functional residual capacity (FRC) are often decreased. Arterial blood gas analysis examines the presence of hypoxemia and hypocapnia.

Examination:

What history should be documented?
Important areas to explore include past medical history, medications, current health status, social history and habits, occupation, living environment, and social support system.

What test/measures are most appropriate?
- **Aerobic capacity and endurance:** assessment of vital signs at rest and with activity, perceived exertion scale, pulse oximetry, auscultation of the lungs
- **Arousal, attention, and cognition:** examine mental status, learning ability, memory, and motivation
- **Assistive and adaptive devices:** analysis of components and safety of a device
- **Environmental, home, and work barriers:** analysis of current and potential barriers or hazards
- **Gait, locomotion, and balance:** static and dynamic balance in sitting and standing, safety during gait with/without an assistive device, Berg Functional Balance Scale, Tinetti Performance Oriented Mobility Assessment, Functional Ambulation Profile
- **Muscle performance:** strength assessment, active movement
- **Posture:** analysis of resting and dynamic posture
- **Range of motion:** active and passive range of motion
- **Self-care and home management:** assessment of functional capacity
- **Ventilation, respiration, and circulation:** thoracoabdominal movement, auscultation of breath sounds, pulmonary function testing, perceived exertion scale, assessment of cough and clearance of secretions

What additional findings are likely with this patient?
A patient with restrictive lung disease may become incapable of deep inspiration due to poor lung expansion. Prolonged restrictive disease can lower oxygen saturation with exercise.

Management:
What is the most effective management of this patient?
Management of restrictive lung disease includes treatment of the underlying cause through pharmacological intervention, physical therapy, and surgical intervention. Physical therapy is based on the severity of the condition with a common goal of maximizing gas exchange and functional capacity. Intervention may include body mechanics, posture training, diaphragm and ventilatory muscle strengthening, and energy conservation with functional mobility. Breathing exercises, coughing techniques, and airway secretion clearance are often components of a comprehensive care plan.

What home care regimen should be recommended?
A home care regimen should include breathing strategies and exercises, energy conservation and pacing techniques, and postural awareness with mobility. Low level general strengthening and endurance training are indicated as tolerated.

Outcome:
What is the likely outcome of a course in physical therapy?
Physical therapy intervention is specific to the underlying cause of the restrictive lung disease. Outcome is based on cause and patient response to physical therapy intervention.

What are the long-term effects of the patient's condition?
Long-term effects from restrictive lung disease are also specific to the underlying cause. Some disorders require surgical intervention that alleviate the condition while other conditions are progressive. Idiopathic pulmonary fibrosis has a high mortality rate within four to six years of diagnosis. Many conditions that cause restrictive lung disease are alleviated through appropriate management.

Comparison:
What are the distinguishing characteristics of a similar condition?
Tuberculosis can result in restrictive lung disease. Tuberculosis is a chronic pulmonary and extrapulmonary disease that causes fibrosis within the lungs. The disease is transmitted through airborne droplets that are inhaled. Pulmonary symptoms include fatigue, weakness, an initial nonproductive cough, and dyspnea with exertion. The disease also affects other systems within the body. Pharmacological intervention is the primary means of treating a patient with tuberculosis.

Clinical Scenarios:
Scenario One
A 32-year-old male shows signs of restrictive lung disease. The patient is slightly short of breath with activity, has difficulty with deep inspiration, and complains of a nonproductive cough. The patient had prolonged exposure to asbestos at his last place of employment and is under a physician's care. The physician referred the patient to physical therapy to improve the patient's general pulmonary status.

Scenario Two
A 65-year-old female is seen in physical therapy for restrictive lung disease secondary to the removal of a benign tumor from the left lung. The patient reports having difficulty breathing, limited inhalation capability, and a productive cough.

Rheumatoid Arthritis

Diagnosis:

What condition produces a patient's symptoms?
Rheumatoid arthritis is a systemic autoimmune disorder of the connective tissue that is characterized by chronic inflammation within synovial membranes, tendon sheaths, and articular cartilage. The acute and chronic inflammatory changes produce the symptoms of this condition.

An injury was most likely sustained to which structure?
Smaller peripheral joints are usually the first to be affected by rheumatoid arthritis, however all connective tissue may become involved. Inflammation is present within the synovial membrane and granulation tissue forms as a result of the synovitis. The granulation tissue erodes articular cartilage resulting in adhesions and fibrosis within the joint.

Inference:

What is the most likely contributing factor in the development of this condition?
The etiology of rheumatoid arthritis is unknown, however there appears to be evidence of genetic predisposition with viral or bacterial triggers. The incidence of rheumatoid arthritis in women is three times greater than the incidence in men.

Confirmation:

What is the most likely clinical presentation?
Rheumatoid arthritis will vary in onset and progression. This condition is characterized by periods of exacerbations and occurs most frequently between 30 and 50 years of age. Early characteristics include fatigue, bilateral involvement, tenderness of smaller joints, and low grade fever. Patients often experience pain with motion, stiffness, and progression of symptoms to larger synovial joints. In late stages of the disease the heart can become affected and deformities, subluxations, and contractures can occur.

What laboratory or imaging studies would confirm the diagnosis?
Blood work assists with the diagnosis of rheumatoid arthritis through evaluation of the rheumatoid factor (RF), white blood cell count, erythrocyte sedimentation rate, hemoglobin, and hematocrit values. A synovial fluid analysis evaluates the content of synovial fluid within a joint. X-rays can be used to evaluate the joint space and the extent of decalcification.

What additional information should be obtained to confirm the diagnosis?
Physical examination and patient history of symptoms are required to confirm the diagnosis. The American Rheumatoid Association has designed diagnostic criteria for rheumatoid arthritis that can be used as a guide to determine a definite, possible, probable, or classic diagnosis of the disease.

Examination:

What history should be documented?
Important areas to explore include past medical history, family history, medications, current symptoms, current health status, living environment, social history and habits, occupation, and social support system.

What test/measures are most appropriate?
- **Aerobic capacity and endurance:** assessment of vital signs at rest and with activity
- **Anthropometric characteristics:** affected joint circumferential measurements
- **Arousal, attention, and cognition:** examine mental status, learning ability, memory, and motivation
- **Community and work integration:** analysis of community, work, and leisure activities
- **Ergonomics and body mechanics:** analysis of dexterity and coordination
- **Gait, locomotion, and balance:** safety during gait with/without an assistive device, Functional Ambulation Profile
- **Joint integrity and mobility:** assessment of joint hypomobility, soft tissue inflammation, presence of deformity
- **Muscle performance:** strength assessment
- **Orthotic, protective, and supportive devices:** potential utilization of bracing
- **Pain:** pain perception assessment scale
- **Range of motion:** active and passive range of motion
- **Self-care and home management:** assessment of functional capacity
- **Sensory integrity:** assessment of sensation, proprioception, and kinesthesia

What additional findings are likely with this patient?
A patient with late stage rheumatoid arthritis may present with swan neck and/or boutonniere deformities, tearing of tendons and musculature, muscle atrophy, carpal tunnel syndrome, pericarditis, and valvular lesions.

Management:
What is the most effective management of this patient?
A patient with rheumatoid arthritis requires pharmacological intervention to decrease inflammation and retard the progression of the disease. NSAIDs, corticosteroids, and disease modifying medications such as methotrexate are indicated. Physical therapy management during the acute stage or exacerbation includes patient education regarding regular rest, pain relief, relaxation, positioning, joint protection techniques, splinting, energy conservation, and body mechanics. Treatment may include gentle massage, hydrotherapy, hot pack, paraffin or cold modalities, gentle isometrics, and instruction in the use of assistive devices. Treatment during the acute stage should avoid resistive exercise, deep heating modalities, and any form of active stretching since these activities will further exacerbate the arthritis. Physical therapy management during the chronic stage or remission focuses on improving overall functional capacity, endurance, and strength. Treatment consists of low impact conditioning through swimming or the stationary bicycle. Gentle stretching may be indicated to maintain available range of motion, however aggressive stretching is contraindicated.

What home care regimen should be recommended?
A home care regimen for a patient with rheumatoid arthritis must continue with a balance between activity and rest. The patient should perform low level exercise, utilize relaxation and energy conservation techniques, and use splints as needed. The patient should recognize when total rest is indicated due to an acute exacerbation.

Outcome:
What is the likely outcome of a course in physical therapy?
Physical therapy cannot halt the progression of rheumatoid arthritis, however it can improve a patient's ability to function. Physical therapy may be indicated intermittently throughout the disease process. Goals focus on pain relief, relaxation, improving motion, and preventing deformity.

What are the long-term effects of the patient's condition?
Rheumatoid arthritis is a chronic disease process that progresses at a varied rate, creates deformity, and results in disability. As the disease progresses there is bilateral and symmetrical involvement of joints. Systemic effects include insomnia, fatigue, and organ involvement including the heart and lungs.

Comparison:
What are the distinguishing characteristics of a similar condition?
Osteoarthritis is a chronic degenerative condition that usually develops secondary to repetitive trauma, disease or obesity. The hyaline cartilage in the joint softens and breaks apart allowing bone-to-bone contact which produces joint deformity, crepitus, impaired range of motion, and pain. Pain typically increases with prolonged activity. Joints become swollen and tender and joint deformity develops. Men and women are equally affected by osteoarthritis. Surgical intervention including osteotomy and joint replacement may be indicated if conservative treatment is unsuccessful.

Clinical Scenarios:
Scenario One
A 38-year-old female diagnosed with rheumatoid arthritis is seen in an outpatient clinic. The patient history reveals fatigue and malaise for two to three weeks and pain in the fingers and wrists. The patient has difficulty caring for herself at home and is on medical leave from her job as an office manager. The patient does not have any other significant past medical history and resides alone.

Scenario Two
A 74-year-old male diagnosed with rheumatoid arthritis is treated by a physical therapist. The patient presents with multi-joint involvement, deformities of the hands and feet, poor endurance, stiffness, and pain. The patient is ambulatory, however is currently in a wheelchair secondary to pain from an exacerbation. The patient is oriented and has a history of COPD.

Rotator Cuff Tendonitis

Diagnosis:

What condition produces a patient's symptoms?
Repetitive overhead activities result in impingement of the supraspinatus tendon immediately proximal to the greater tubercle of the humerus. The impingement is caused by an inability of a weak supraspinatus muscle to adequately depress the head of the humerus in the glenoid fossa during elevation of the arm. As a result the humerus translates superiorly due to the disproportionate action of the deltoid muscle.

An injury was most likely sustained to which structure?
The supraspinatus muscle is the most commonly involved tendon in rotator cuff tendonitis. The muscle originates on the supraspinatus fossa of the scapula and inserts on the greater tubercle of the humerus.

Inference:

What is the most likely contributing factor in the development of this condition?
Individuals participating in activities requiring excessive overhead activity such as swimming, tennis, and baseball are at increased risk for rotator cuff tendonitis. Excessive use of the upper extremity following a prolonged period of inactivity often produces this condition. Statistically individuals from 25 to 40 years of age are the most likely to develop this condition.

Confirmation:

What is the most likely clinical presentation?
A patient with rotator cuff tendonitis often reports difficulty with overhead activities and a dull ache following periods of activity. The patient may identify the presence of a painful arc of motion most commonly occurring between 60 and 120 degrees of active abduction. Pain often increases at night resulting in difficulty sleeping on the affected side.

What laboratory or imaging studies would confirm the diagnosis?
Magnetic resonance imaging can be used to identify the presence of rotator cuff tendonitis, however due to the high cost it is not commonly employed prior to the initiation of formal treatment. X-rays with the shoulder laterally rotated can be used to identify the presence of calcific deposits or other bony abnormalities.

What additional information should be obtained to confirm the diagnosis?
A number of specific special tests including the empty can test, Neer impingement test, and Hawkins-Kennedy impingement test can be used to confirm the presence of rotator cuff tendonitis or impingement.

Examination:

What history should be documented?
Important areas to explore include past medical history, family history, medications, history of symptoms, current health status, living environment, social history and habits, occupation, and social support system.

What test/measures are most appropriate?
- **Anthropometric characteristics:** upper extremity circumferential measurements
- **Arousal, attention, and cognition:** examine mental status, learning ability, memory, and motivation
- **Assistive and adaptive devices:** analysis of components and safety of a device
- **Community and work integration:** analysis of community, work, and leisure activities
- **Ergonomics and body mechanics:** analysis of dexterity and coordination
- **Integumentary integrity:** skin assessment, assessment of sensation
- **Joint integrity and mobility:** soft tissue swelling and inflammation, assessment of joint play, palpation of the joint, empty can test, Neer impingement test, Hawkins-Kennedy impingement test
- **Motor function:** posture and balance
- **Muscle performance:** strength assessment
- **Pain:** pain perception assessment scale
- **Posture:** analysis of resting and dynamic posture

- **Range of motion:** active and passive range of motion
- **Reflex integrity:** assessment of deep tendon and pathological reflexes (e.g. Babinski, ATNR)
- **Self-care and home management:** assessment of functional capacity

What additional findings are likely with this patient?
Rotator cuff tendonitis often presents in association with impingement syndrome. Impingement syndrome typically involves the supraspinatus tendon, glenoid labrum, long head of the biceps, and subacromial bursa. It is extremely difficult to determine through examination the level of involvement of each of the identified structures.

Management:
What is the most effective management of this patient?
Intervention should include cryotherapy, activity modification, range of motion, and rest. The patient will likely be instructed to take an anti-inflammatory medication by the physician. As the acute phase subsides the patient is often instructed in strengthening exercises. Since the rotator cuff muscles are dependent on adequate blood supply and oxygen tension it is essential that all range of motion and strengthening exercises are pain free. Range of motion exercises using a pulley system or a cane can serve as an effective intervention. Strengthening exercises are initiated with the arm at the patient's side in order to prevent the possibility of impingement. Elastic tubing or hand held weights are often the preferred equipment of choice. It is important for the entire rotator cuff to be strong prior to initiating overhead activities. Shoulder shrugs and push-ups with the arms abducted to 90 degrees can effectively be used to strengthen the upper trapezius and serratus anterior and therefore promote elevation of the acromion without direct contact with the rotator cuff.

What home care regimen should be recommended?
The home care regimen should consist of range of motion, strengthening, palliative care, and functional activities as warranted based on the results of the patient examination.

Outcome:
What is the likely outcome of a course in physical therapy?
A patient with rotator cuff tendonitis should be able to return to his/her previous level of functioning within four to six weeks.

What are the long-term effects of the patient's condition?
Failure to adequately treat rotator cuff tendonitis may necessitate significant activity modification or more aggressive surgical management such as subacromial decompression. Prolonged inflammation of the rotator cuff tendon may facilitate eventual tearing of the rotator cuff.

Comparison:
What are the distinguishing characteristics of a similar condition?
A rotator cuff tear is usually the result of repetitive microtrauma. Partial tears often occur in a younger population while complete tears more commonly occur in older individuals. The mechanism of injury is often a fall on an outstretched arm or a sudden strain applied to the shoulder during pushing or pulling activities. Surgical repair of the rotator cuff is often required. Heavy lifting may be restricted for up to six to twelve months following surgery.

Clinical Scenarios:
Scenario One
A 23-year-old female diagnosed with rotator cuff tendonitis is referred to physical therapy after experiencing pain while swimming the breaststroke in a competitive swim meet one week ago. The patient participates on a school swim team and a private club and practices four to six times a week. A few days after experiencing the shoulder pain the patient was back in the pool, however was unable to return to her previous training regimen.

Scenario Two
A 45-year-old male employed as a pipe fitter is referred to physical therapy after having subacromial decompression. The patient is one week status post surgery and is anxious to "test" his involved shoulder. Prior to surgery the patient was placed on "light duty." It has been six months since the patient was able to perform his job without restrictions. The patient presently denies any pain in the involved shoulder.

Scoliosis

Diagnosis:

What condition produces a patient's symptoms?
A patient with scoliosis presents with lateral curvature of the spine. The curvature is usually found in the thoracic or lumbar vertebrae.

An injury was most likely sustained to which structure?
The injury or deformity begins when the vertebrae of the spine deviate from the normal vertical position. The curvature disrupts normal alignment of the ribs and muscles and can create compensatory curves that attempt to keep the body in proper alignment.

Inference:

What is the most likely contributing factor in the development of this condition?
Nonstructural scoliosis is a reversible curve that can change with repositioning. This type of curve is nonprogressive and is usually caused by poor posture or by a leg length discrepancy. Structural scoliosis cannot be corrected with movement. This type of curve includes rotation of the vertebrae towards the convexity of the curve. The exact etiology of scoliosis is unknown, however contributing factors of a structural curve include altered development of the spine in utero, association with neuromuscular diseases such as cerebral palsy and muscular dystrophy, congenital defect of the vertebrae, and inheritance as an autosomal dominant trait.

Confirmation:

What is the most likely clinical presentation?
A patient with a structural curve will present with asymmetries of the shoulders, scapulae, pelvis, and skinfolds. The thoracic curve is most commonly convex towards the right and compensatory curves develop above and below. As the curve progresses there will be a rib hump posteriorly over the thoracic region on the convex side of the curve. The patient does not typically experience pain or other subjective symptoms until the curve has progressed.

What laboratory or imaging studies would confirm the diagnosis?
X-rays should be taken in an anterior and lateral view with the patient standing and with the patient bending over. A device called a scoliometer can be used to measure the angle of trunk rotation. The Cobb method can be used to determine the angle of curvature.

What additional information should be obtained to confirm the diagnosis?
Physical examination allows visual inspection of the curvature and physical asymmetries. The examination can determine if the scoliosis is nonstructural or structural.

Examination:

What history should be documented?
Important areas to explore include past medical history, medications, current health status, living environment, school activities, and social support system.

What test/measures are most appropriate?
- **Arousal, attention, and cognition:** examine mental status, learning ability, memory, and motivation
- **Ergonomics and body mechanics:** analysis of dexterity and coordination
- **Integumentary integrity:** skin assessment, assessment of sensation
- **Joint integrity and mobility:** assessment of hypermobility and hypomobility of a joint
- **Muscle performance:** strength assessment
- **Orthotic, protective, and supportive devices:** analysis of components of a device, analysis of movement while wearing a device
- **Pain:** assessment of muscle soreness
- **Posture:** analysis of resting and dynamic posture
- **Range of motion:** active and passive range of motion
- **Self-care and home management**: assessment of functional capacity

What additional findings are likely with this patient?
If a progressive scoliosis is untreated the deformity can cause a decrease in lung capacity, significant pain, and degenerative changes including arthritis and disc pathology.

Management:
What is the most effective management of this patient?
Management of scoliosis is based on the type and severity of the curve, patient age, and previous management. A patient with scoliosis that is less than 25 degrees should be monitored every three months. Breathing exercises and a strengthening program for the trunk and pelvic muscles are indicated. A patient with scoliosis that ranges between 25 and 40 degrees requires a spinal orthosis and physical therapy intervention for posture, flexibility, strengthening, respiratory function, and proper use and wearing of the spinal orthosis. A patient with scoliosis that is greater then 40 degrees usually requires surgical spinal stabilization. One method to surgically correct scoliosis is through posterior spinal fusion and stabilization with a Harrington rod. Physical therapy intervention after surgical fusion is indicated for breathing exercises, posture, flexibility, muscle strengthening, and respiratory muscle strengthening once the patient's spine is stable.

What home care regimen should be recommended?
A home care regimen is based on the type and severity of the curve. Exercise, stretching, posture, and flexibility are important components of an exercise program.

Outcome:
What is the likely outcome of a course in physical therapy?
Physical therapy intervention should improve a patient's condition through patient education and therapeutic exercise. Physical therapy may be indicated for implementation of a home program, to assist with posture and wearing tolerance of a corrective orthosis or following surgical stabilization.

What are the long-term effects of the patient's condition?
Prognosis for structural scoliosis is based on the age of onset and the severity of the curve. Early intervention results in the best possible outcome. Scoliosis does not usually progress significantly once bone growth is complete.

Comparison:
What are the distinguishing characteristics of a similar condition?
Torticollis is a deformity of the neck that is caused by shortened or spastic sternocleidomastoid muscles. The patient presents with a bending of the neck towards the affected side and rotation of the head towards the unaffected side. Causative factors include malpositioning in utero, damage to the sternocleidomastoid muscle with scarring, spasms secondary to central nervous system impairment, or psychogenic origin. Conservative treatment for congenital torticollis includes stretching and positioning. Treatment for acquired torticollis includes heat, traction, massage, stretching, and bracing. Surgical intervention may be indicated if conservative management fails.

Clinical Scenarios:
Scenario One
An 11-year-old female is seen in physical therapy with a diagnosis of a 30-degree right thoracic scoliosis. The physician has prescribed a spinal orthosis and physical therapy intervention. The patient denies any pain, but states that she has soreness in her back. The patient is in the marching band and plays basketball. There is no significant past medical history and her parents are very supportive.

Scenario Two
A seven-year-old boy is referred to physical therapy with a 12-degree right thoracic scoliosis. The physical therapy prescription requests evaluation for a home exercise program. The patient has insulin dependent diabetes and a low I.Q. The mother is present for the evaluation and appears to be supportive.

Spina Bifida - Myelomeningocele

Diagnosis:

What condition produces a patient's symptoms?
Spina bifida with myelomeningocele is a developmental abnormality that occurs in the low thoracic, lumbar or sacral spine due to insufficient closure of the neural tube by the 28th day of gestation.

An injury was most likely sustained to which structure?
There are two forms of spina bifida. Spina bifida with meningocele is characterized by herniation of meninges and cerebrospinal fluid into a sac that protrudes through the vertebral defect. The spinal cord remains within the canal. Spina bifida with myelomeningocele is characterized by herniation of meninges, cerebrospinal fluid, and the spinal cord through the defect in the vertebrae. The cyst may not be covered by skin.

Inference:

What is the most likely contributing factor in the development of this condition?
A single etiology for spina bifida with myelomeningocele has not been identified, however causative factors include genetic predisposition, environmental influence, low levels of maternal folic acid, alcohol, maternal hyperthermia, and certain classifications of drugs.

Confirmation:

What is the most likely clinical presentation?
Myelomeningocele is a severe condition that is characterized by a sac that is seen on an infant's back protruding from a specific area of the spinal cord. Impairments associated with myelomeningocele including motor and sensory loss below the vertebral defect, hydrocephalus, Arnold-Chiari Type II malformation, clubfoot, scoliosis, bowel and bladder dysfunction, and learning disabilities.

What laboratory or imaging studies would confirm the diagnosis?
Prior to birth a fetal ultrasound may identify the myelomeningocele defect in the spine. Alpha-fetoprotein blood testing will show an elevation in levels at approximately week 16 of gestation. At birth a sac will be present over the spinal defect. Other tests such as magnetic resonance imaging, myelography, and bowel and bladder testing can determine the extent of damage.

What additional information should be obtained to confirm the diagnosis?
Diagnosis is confirmed through prenatal testing or upon visual observation at birth. Past medical history of the mother, history of the pregnancy, and family history of neural tube defects may be noted.

Examination:

What history should be documented?
Important areas to explore include past medical history, current symptoms and health status, level of injury, medications, past surgical procedures, living environment, and social support system.

What test/measures are most appropriate?
- **Aerobic capacity and endurance:** assessment of vital signs at rest and with activity
- **Arousal, attention, and cognition:** examine mental status, learning ability, memory, and motivation
- **Assistive and adaptive devices:** education in use of appropriate devices, analysis of components and safety of a device
- **Environmental, home, and work barriers:** analysis of current and potential barriers or hazards
- **Ergonomics and body mechanics:** analysis of dexterity and coordination
- **Gait, locomotion, and balance:** developmental milestones assessment, static and dynamic balance in prone and sitting, analysis of wheelchair management, standing with standing frame or gait with assistive device
- **Integumentary integrity:** skin assessment, assessment of sensation
- **Motor function:** equilibrium and righting reactions, motor assessment scales, balance in sitting
- **Muscle performance:** assessment of active movement, muscle tone assessment
- **Orthotic, protective, and supportive devices:** analysis of components of a device, analysis of movement while wearing a device
- **Range of motion:** active and passive range of motion
- **Reflex integrity:** assessment of deep tendon and pathological reflexes (e.g. Babinski, ATNR)
- **Self-care and home management:** assessment of functional capacity

What additional findings are likely with this patient?
Immediately after birth an infant with myelomeningocele has an increased risk of meningitis, hemorrhage, and hypoxia, however surgical intervention may significantly reduce the risks. Ongoing additional findings with myelomeningocele include neuropathic fracture, osteoporosis, kyphosis, hip dislocations, and latex allergy.

Management:
What is the most effective management of this patient?
A patient with myelomeningocele will require immediate surgical intervention to repair and close the defect and for placement of a shunt to alleviate hydrocephalus. Orthopedic surgical intervention may be warranted throughout a patient's life to correct deformities such as clubfoot, hip dysplasia, and scoliosis. Pharmacological intervention may include medications that assist in the management of bowel and bladder dysfunction. Physical and occupational therapy are important components in the management of myelomeningocele. Physical therapy is initiated immediately and focuses on family education regarding positioning, handling techniques, range of motion, and therapeutic play. Long-term physical therapy attempts to maximize functional capacity and may include range of motion, facilitation of developmental milestones, therapeutic exercise, skin care, strengthening, balance, and mobility training. Physical therapy will also assist with wheelchair prescription, assistive and adaptive device selection, and the use of orthotics and splinting.

What home care regimen should be recommended?
Successful management of myelomeningocele requires a patient to continue a home care regimen that includes an exercise program, range of motion, and mobility training. Family and caregiver involvement are important in assisting a patient through a daily exercise program. The home program will require modification as the child matures.

Outcome:
What is the likely outcome of a course in physical therapy?
Physical therapy is ongoing through adolescence and is based on the severity of impairments and the needs of the child.

What are the long-term effects of the patient's condition?
A patient with myelomeningocele has a near normal life expectancy as long as the patient receives consistent and thorough health care. Functional outcome of the patient depends on the level of injury, the amount of associated impairments, and the caregiver support that is provided.

Comparison:
What are the distinguishing characteristics of a similar condition?
Anencephaly is a condition that presents from failed closure of the cranial end of the neural tube. The cerebral hemispheres do not form and some neural tissue may protrude through the defect. This type of neural tube defect cannot be repaired. Many infants with this condition are stillborn, while others only survive a short time after birth.

Clinical Scenarios:
Scenario One
A six-month-old boy in an acute care hospital is seen in physical therapy after revision of a ventriculoperitoneal shunt. The parents state that the child has been responsive at home and has been doing well. The child can position himself in prone on elbows and sits with support.

Scenario Two
An 11-year-old girl with a T12 spinal cord lesion is seen in outpatient physical therapy. The patient presently uses a wheelchair for mobility, however indicates that her goal is to walk in her home. The patient's upper body strength is good and intellect is normal.

Spinal Cord Injury – C7 Tetraplegia

Diagnosis:

What condition produces a patient's symptoms?
Compression, flexion or extension of the spine with or without rotation causes the majority of traumatic spinal cord injuries. Traumatic injury to the spinal cord produces a physiological and biochemical chain of events that result in vascular impairment and permanent tissue and nerve damage.

An injury was most likely sustained to which structure?
A patient with C7 tetraplegia sustained damage to the spinal cord and surrounding tissues at the C7 level. C7 is therefore the most distal segment of the spinal cord that both the motor and sensory components remain intact.

Inference:

What is the most likely contributing factor in the development of this condition?
Statistics from the National Spinal Cord Injury Database (NSCID) indicate that motor vehicle accidents, violence, and falls are the top causes of spinal cord injury. Statistics indicate a higher ratio of injury in men and Caucasians. The highest incidence of age of injury (over 50%) occurs between 15 to 30 years of age.

Confirmation:

What is the most likely clinical presentation?
Spinal shock presents immediately following injury to the spinal cord. Presentation includes total flaccid paralysis and loss of all reflexes and sensation below the level of the lesion. Spinal shock may last hours or days.

What laboratory or imaging studies would confirm the diagnosis?
X-rays are commonly taken of the cervical spine to observe the positioning and damage to the involved vertebrae. The results of imaging determine subsequent medical intervention including stabilization of the spine. A myelogram or tomogram may be useful to confirm the extent of surrounding damage at the level of the injury.

What additional information should be obtained to confirm the diagnosis?
Other information commonly obtained in order to confirm the diagnosis includes interviews regarding the mechanism of injury and a full neurological examination by a physician.

Examination:

What history should be documented?
Important areas to explore include past medical history, medications, mechanism of injury, precautions, current health status, social history and habits, occupation or school responsibilities, living environment, and social support system.

What test/measures are most appropriate?
- **Aerobic capacity and endurance:** autonomic responses to positional changes, assessment of vital signs at rest and with activity
- **Arousal, attention, and cognition:** examine mental status, learning ability, memory, and motivation
- **Assistive and adaptive devices:** analysis of components and safety of a device, wheelchair prescription, adaptive devices, environmental controls
- **Integumentary integrity:** skin assessment, American Spinal Injury Association (ASIA) - Standard Neurological Classification of Spinal Cord Injury Sensory Examination
- **Motor function:** posture and balance in sitting
- **Muscle performance:** ASIA - Standard Neurological Classification of Spinal Cord Injury Motor Examination, muscle tone assessment
- **Neuromotor development and sensory integration:** analysis of reflex movement patterns
- **Pain:** dysesthetic pain (deafferentation pain), nerve root pain, or musculoskeletal pain
- **Posture:** assessment of positioning, analysis of resting and dynamic posture
- **Range of motion:** active and passive range of motion
- **Reflex integrity:** assessment of deep tendon reflexes and pathological reflexes

- **Self-care and home management:** assessment of functional capacity, Functional Independence Measure (FIM)
- **Sensory integrity:** assessment of proprioception and kinesthesia
- **Ventilation, respiration, and circulation:** assessment of cough and clearance of secretions, breathing patterns, respiratory muscle strength, accessory muscle utilization, and vital capacity

What additional findings are likely with this patient?
There are many additional findings that can exist with a patient with a C7 spinal cord injury. The most common complications that can occur indirectly from the injury include orthostatic hypotension when assuming a vertical position, pressure sores, spasticity, heterotopic ossification, and autonomic dysreflexia.

Management:
What is the most effective management of this patient?
Once a patient is medically stable, physical therapy intervention is initiated. Inpatient rehabilitation should initially focus on range of motion, upright positioning, and respiratory issues such as cough, clearance of secretions, and incentive spirometry. Ongoing intervention should include mat activities, strengthening, self-range of motion, pressure relief, transfer skills, wheelchair skills, and patient education.

What home care regimen should be recommended?
A home care regimen should include breathing exercises, incentive spirometry, stretching, and mobility skills. Outpatient physical therapy intervention may be indicated for continuation of community skills.

Outcome:
What is the likely outcome of a course in physical therapy?
A patient diagnosed with C7 tetraplegia will require extensive physical therapy with projected outcomes based upon the C7 level of motor and sensory innervation. Typical outcomes at this level include independence with feeding, grooming, and dressing, self-range of motion, manual wheelchair propulsion for mobility, transfers, and driving with an adapted automobile. A patient may be able to live independently with adaptive equipment.

What are the long-term effects of the patient's condition?
At this time there is no cure for a complete spinal cord injury. A patient with a complete C7 injury will not regain innervation below this level. The triceps, latissimus dorsi, and pronator teres will remain the lowest innervated muscles. There will be ongoing musculoskeletal and cardiopulmonary deficits that can increase the risk for other health issues. The latest research suggests, however that approximately 40% of the spinal cord injured population have a life expectancy over 45 years of age.

Comparison:
What are the distinguishing characteristics of a similar condition?
Brown-Sequard syndrome is a condition that results from injury to one side of the spinal cord. Characteristics include motor and sensory loss. Motor function, proprioception, and vibration are lost ipsilateral to the lesion and vibration, pain, and temperature sensations are absent contralateral to the lesion.

Clinical Scenarios:
Scenario One
A patient is diagnosed with a T12 spinal cord injury after a motor vehicle accident. X-rays reveal a burst fracture of the vertebrae with fragmentation. Neurological examination in the emergency room reveals no active movement or sensation below the T12 level. The patient is a chemistry teacher at a local high school and coaches basketball. He is in good health with no significant past medical history.

Scenario Two
A 25-year-old male was injured when he was tackled from behind during a rugby game. The blow produced cervical hyperextension and bleeding within the central gray matter of the spinal cord. The patient was ultimately diagnosed with central cord syndrome and referred to physical therapy. The patient has a history of insulin dependent diabetes mellitus and mild hypertension. The patient resides alone in a second floor apartment and is a full time graduate student.

Systemic Lupus Erythematosus

Diagnosis:

What condition produces a patient's symptoms?
Systemic lupus erythematosus (SLE) is a connective tissue disorder caused by an autoimmune reaction in the body. The chronic inflammatory disorder produces varied symptoms depending on the severity and extent of involvement.

An injury was most likely sustained to which structure?
The autoimmune disorder creates high levels of autoantibodies (antinuclear antibodies) that attack various cells and tissues within the body. The autoantibodies form immune complexes that produce an inflammatory response and cause further tissue destruction.

Inference:

What is the most likely contributing factor in the development of this condition?
The exact etiology of SLE is unknown, however it is described as an immunoregulatory disturbance from genetic, environmental, viral, and hormonal contributing factors. Environmental factors associated with SLE include ultraviolet light exposure, infection, the use of antibiotics (specifically penicillin and sulfa drugs), extreme stress, and pregnancy. SLE can occur at any age, but the most common age group is 20 to 40. The disorder is eight to ten times more common in women.

Confirmation:

What is the most likely clinical presentation?
A patient with SLE will have diverse symptoms based on the involvement of the connective tissue throughout the body. Symptoms will come and go through exacerbations and remissions throughout the course of the disease. A patient may initially see a physician for symptoms that include fever, malaise, rash, arthralgias, headache, and weight loss. Common clinical presentation throughout the course of SLE includes a red butterfly rash across the cheeks and nose, a red rash over light exposed areas, arthralgias, alopecia, pleurisy, kidney involvement, seizures, depression, fibromyalgia, and cardiac involvement.

What laboratory or imaging studies would confirm the diagnosis?
Microscopic fluorescent techniques are indicated to detect the presence of the antinuclear antibody (ANA) within the blood. A positive ANA test warrants an additional test for antideoxyribonucleic acid antibodies. These two tests in combination with physical presentation support the presence of SLE. Other testing including erythrocyte sedimentation rate, CBC, and urinalysis should be performed on a regular basis when monitoring a patient during a period of remission.

What additional information should be obtained to confirm the diagnosis?
The American Rheumatism Association has designated criteria to confirm the diagnosis of SLE. A patient requires at least four of fourteen characteristics that occur during the same period of time. A patient evaluation including a thorough history and current symptoms assists with confirming a diagnosis of SLE.

Examination:

What history should be documented?
Important areas to explore include past medical history, family history, medications, current symptoms, current health status, living environment, social history and habits, occupation, and social support system.

What test/measures are most appropriate?
- **Aerobic capacity and endurance:** assessment of vital signs at rest and with activity, auscultation of the lungs and heart
- **Arousal, attention, and cognition:** examine mental status, learning ability, memory, and motivation
- **Assistive and adaptive devices:** analysis of components and safety of a device
- **Community and work integration:** analysis of community, work, and leisure activities
- **Environmental, home, and work barriers:** analysis of current and potential barriers or hazards
- **Ergonomics and body mechanics:** analysis of dexterity and coordination
- **Gait, locomotion, and balance:** static and dynamic balance in sitting and standing, safety during gait with/without an assistive device, Berg Functional Balance Scale, Tinetti Performance Oriented Mobility Assessment, Functional Ambulation Profile, analysis of wheelchair management
- **Integumentary integrity:** skin assessment, assessment of sensation, presence and assessment of rash
- **Joint integrity and mobility:** soft tissue swelling and inflammation, presence of deformity
- **Muscle performance:** strength assessment

- **Neuromotor development and sensory integration:** analysis of reflex movement patterns, assessment of involuntary movements, sensory integration tests, gross and fine motor skills
- **Orthotic, protective, and supportive devices:** potential utilization of bracing
- **Pain:** pain perception assessment scale
- **Range of motion:** active and passive range of motion
- **Reflex integrity:** assessment of deep tendon and pathological reflexes (e.g. Babinski, ATNR)
- **Self-care and home management:** assessment of functional capacity

What additional findings are likely with this patient?
Depending on its clinical course SLE can produce skeletal deformities such as ulnar deviation and subluxed interphalangeal joints. Kidney involvement and cardiovascular impairments such as endocarditis, myocarditis, and pericarditis can occur during an exacerbation. Patients that experience nephritis or myocarditis have an overall poorer prognosis.

Management:
What is the most effective management of this patient?
A patient with mild SLE will utilize pharmacological intervention including salicylates, indomethacin, or NSAIDs. Antimalarial medications may be used for a rash or to assist the other medications in controlling the disease. Corticosteroids may be added to control myalgia and polyarthritis. A patient with severe SLE requires immediate corticosteroid intervention and immunosuppressive drug therapy. General management of SLE includes good nutrition, ongoing medical supervision, and avoidance of ultraviolet exposure and certain antibiotics that may aggravate the disease process.

What home care regimen should be recommended?
A home program may be indicated during an acute exacerbation of SLE. The program should include relaxation and energy conservation techniques, therapeutic exercise as tolerated, and pain management.

Outcome:
What is the likely outcome of a course in physical therapy?
Physical therapy cannot cease or alter the clinical course of SLE, however it may assist in controlling the debilitating effects during an acute phase or exacerbation of the disease. Physical therapy goals focus on pain relief, relaxation, strengthening, and preventing deformity.

What are the long-term effects of the patient's condition?
The clinical course of SLE is highly unpredictable. A patient may only exhibit symptoms for skin and joint involvement or may exhibit multi-system involvement. Periods of remission may last years and the prognosis depends on the severity and the extent of the disease process. The overall prognosis for SLE is good, although in rare cases the disease process can remain acute and become fatal within a short period of time. There is a high ten year survival rate with SLE. Death is usually attributed to kidney failure or secondary infections.

Comparison:
What are the distinguishing characteristics of a similar condition?
Scleroderma, also termed progressive systemic sclerosis, is a chronic disease that primarily affects the skin, but can involve articular structures and internal organs. There is long-term hardening and shrinking of the affected connective tissues. Etiology is unknown and the disease varies in course and progression.

Clinical Scenarios:
Scenario One
A 25-year-old female is referred to physical therapy for a therapeutic exercise program. The patient was diagnosed last year with SLE and has not exercised since that time. The patient is currently taking corticosteroids and antimalarial medications to manage a recent exacerbation.

Scenario Two
A 43-year-old female was seen in outpatient physical therapy to assist with pain management. The patient was diagnosed five years ago with SLE and has recently experienced increased difficulty using her hands secondary to deformity and pain. The patient's goal is to reduce the pain in her hands.

Thoracic Outlet Syndrome

Diagnosis:

What condition produces a patient's symptoms?
Thoracic outlet syndrome is a term used to describe a group of disorders that present with symptoms secondary to neurovascular compression. Compression occurs to the nerves and blood supply as they pass over the first rib.

An injury was most likely sustained to which structure?
Thoracic outlet syndrome results from compression and damage to the brachial plexus nerve trunks, subclavian vascular supply and/or the axillary artery.

Inference:

What is the most likely contributing factor in the development of this condition?
Contributing factors in the development of thoracic outlet syndrome include the presence of a cervical rib, an abnormal first rib, postural deviations, chronic hyperabduction of the arm, hypertrophy or spasms of the scalene muscles, degenerative disorders, and an elongated cervical transverse process.

Confirmation:

What is the most likely clinical presentation?
A patient with thoracic outlet syndrome will present with symptoms based on nerve and/or vascular compression. Typical symptoms include diffuse pain in the arm, paresthesias in the fingers and through the upper extremities, weakness and muscle wasting, poor posture, edema, and discoloration.

What laboratory or imaging studies would confirm the diagnosis?
X-ray will confirm the presence of a cervical rib or other bony abnormality. Otherwise, diagnosis relies solely on a thorough history of patient symptoms and a physical examination.

What additional information should be obtained to confirm the diagnosis?
A patient can be diagnosed with thoracic outlet syndrome following a thorough history of symptoms, physical examination, and orthopedic special tests that include Adson's maneuver, Wright's maneuver, Roo's test, Halsted's test, and the hyperabduction test.

Examination:

What history should be documented?
Important areas to explore include past medical history, family history, medications, history of symptoms, current health status, living environment, social history and habits, occupation, and social support system.

What test/measures are most appropriate?
- **Anthropometric characteristics:** upper extremity circumferential measurements
- **Arousal, attention, and cognition:** examine mental status, learning ability, memory, and motivation
- **Community and work integration:** analysis of community, work, and leisure activities
- **Cranial nerve integrity:** assessment of muscles innervation by the cranial nerves, dermatome assessment
- **Ergonomics and body mechanics:** analysis of dexterity and coordination
- **Integumentary integrity:** skin assessment, assessment of sensation
- **Joint integrity and mobility:** soft tissue swelling and inflammation, assessment of joint play, palpation of the joint
- **Motor function:** posture and balance
- **Muscle performance:** strength assessment
- **Pain:** pain perception assessment scale
- **Posture:** analysis of resting and dynamic posture
- **Range of motion:** active and passive range of motion
- **Reflex integrity:** assessment of deep tendon and pathological reflexes (e.g. Babinski, ATNR)
- **Self-care and home management:** assessment of functional capacity

What additional findings are likely with this patient?
A patient with thoracic outlet syndrome may have difficulty sleeping due to excessive pillows or malpositioning of the arm. The patient may have difficulty at work with carrying items on the affected side or with driving a car. Thoracic outlet most commonly affects the population between 30 and 40 years of age with women being affected two to three times more than men.

Management:
What is the most effective management of this patient?
A patient with thoracic outlet syndrome requires physical therapy intervention to assist with modification of posture, breathing patterns, positioning in bed, and the work site. Physical therapy should focus on strengthening, joint mobilization, body mechanics, flexibility, and postural awareness. A therapist may utilize modalities such as transcutaneous nerve stimulation, ultrasound, and biofeedback to attain goals. Work site analysis and subsequent activity modification may be necessary to relieve the pain and other symptoms. A patient may benefit from anti-inflammatory agents in combination with physical therapy. If physical therapy management fails, the patient may require surgical decompression of bony or fibrotic abnormalities.

What home care regimen should be recommended?
A home care regimen for a patient with thoracic outlet syndrome must include stretching, strengthening, and postural awareness. The patient should utilize these strategies on an ongoing basis at work and with recreational activities in order to promote pain free movement and limit undesirable symptoms associated with the condition.

Outcome:
What is the likely outcome of a course in physical therapy?
Most patients with thoracic outlet syndrome have positive results from physical therapy intervention and are able to return to their previous level of function within four to eight weeks.

What are the long-term effects of the patient's condition?
If a patient has positive results from physical therapy intervention there will not be any long-term impairments, however if the patient's symptoms persist for three to four months surgical intervention may be warranted.

Comparison:
What are the distinguishing characteristics of a similar condition?
A radial nerve lesion may be caused by direct trauma, excessive traction, entrapment or compression. A patient presents with an inability to extend the wrist, thumb, and fingers. The patient will also present with impaired grip strength and coordination. Splinting is recommended to maintain proper positioning. Passive range of motion is necessary to prevent secondary impairments such as contractures within the hand.

Clinical Scenarios:
Scenario One
A 35-year-old female is seen in physical therapy secondary to pain and paresthesias throughout the left upper extremity. The patient's work history reveals that she works as a telemarketer and is required to hold the phone between her ear and shoulder throughout her shift. The patient carries a five-pound brief case with a shoulder strap as she walks one-half mile to work. The patient has a one-year-old child.

Scenario Two
A 45-year-old female is referred to physical therapy by her physician secondary to pain when reaching overhead and carrying objects. The patient recently complains of waking up during the night with pain and paresthesias in the involved arm. The patient is very anxious and concerned because she is required to carry items and place them above her head as part of her job at a local production mill.

Total Hip Replacement

Diagnosis:

What condition produces a patient's symptoms?
Progressive and severe arthritis in the hip joint produces the pain and disability that warrants a total hip replacement. Total hip replacement may also be required with trauma to the hip, avascular necrosis or a nonunion fracture.

An injury was most likely sustained to which structure?
Arthritis causes the hip joint to undergo a degenerative process including destruction of articular cartilage resulting in bone-to-bone contact.

Inference:

What is the most likely contributing factor in the development of this condition?
The destruction of articular cartilage found in arthritis may come from repetitive microtrauma, obesity, nutritional imbalances, or abnormal joint mechanics. Indications for total hip replacement include osteoarthritis, rheumatoid arthritis, avascular necrosis, developmental dysplasia, osteomyelitis, and failed fixation of a fracture.

Confirmation:

What is the most likely clinical presentation?
A patient that requires total hip replacement will present with decreased range of motion, impaired mobility skills, and persistent pain that worsens with motion and weight bearing.

What laboratory or imaging studies would confirm the diagnosis?
X-ray, computed tomography, and magnetic resonance imaging procedures may be used to view the integrity of the joint. These procedures are also used to rule out a fracture or a tumor.

What additional information should be obtained to confirm the diagnosis?
Patient history, current functional status, and level of pain and disability are important factors in determining the need for surgical intervention. A standardized pain assessment scale and the Arthritis Impact Measurement tool may be used to establish an objective baseline.

Examination:

What history should be documented?
Important areas to explore include past medical history, family history, medications, current symptoms, current health status, living environment, social history and habits, occupation, and social support system.

What test/measures are most appropriate?
- **Aerobic capacity and endurance:** assessment of vital signs at rest and with activity, perceived exertion scale
- **Anthropometric characteristics:** hip circumferential measurements, leg length measurements
- **Arousal, attention, and cognition:** examine mental status, learning ability, memory, and motivation
- **Assistive and adaptive devices:** analysis of components and safety of a device
- **Environmental, home, and work barriers:** analysis of current and potential barriers or hazards
- **Gait, locomotion, and balance:** safety during gait with/without an assistive device, Functional Ambulation Profile
- **Joint integrity and mobility:** soft tissue swelling and inflammation
- **Muscle performance:** strength assessment, assessment of active movement
- **Pain:** pain perception assessment scale
- **Range of motion:** active and passive range of motion
- **Self-care and home assessment:** assessment of functional capacity, Barthel ADL Index
- **Sensory integrity:** assessment of sensation

What additional findings are likely with this patient?
A patient that requires a total hip replacement may also have arthritis in other areas of the body. The patient may present with low endurance and may be deconditioned secondary to inactivity from the effects of arthritis.

Management:
What is the most effective management of this patient?
A total hip replacement that utilizes a posterolateral approach allows the abductor muscles to remain intact, however there may be a higher incidence of postoperative joint instability due to the interruption of the posterior capsule. This type of surgical approach requires a patient to avoid excessive hip flexion greater than 90 degrees, hip adduction, and hip medial rotation. A patient with a hip replacement that utilizes an anterolateral approach should avoid hip flexion and lateral rotation.

A patient status post total hip replacement may require anticoagulant therapy and pain medication. The patient's postoperative care includes hip precautions, use of an abduction pillow (with posterolateral approach), initiation of hip protocol exercises, and physical therapy intervention. The hip protocol exercises usually include ankle pumps, quadriceps sets, gluteal sets, heel slides, and isometric abduction. Physical therapy should emphasize patient education regarding hip precautions and weight bearing status. A cemented hip replacement usually allows for partial weight bearing initially and a noncemented hip replacement requires toe touch weight bearing for up to six weeks. Physical therapy encourages early ambulation training in order to avoid deconditioning and the risk of deep vein thrombosis. A patient must practice all mobility skills using the proper hip precautions. Outpatient physical therapy may be indicated to assist with progression to a cane.

What home care regimen should be recommended?
The patient should be instructed in a home care regimen that includes range of motion, strengthening, and progressive ambulation. The patient must adhere to the hip precaution guidelines until a physician determines that the hip is adequately stable.

Outcome:
What is the likely outcome of a course in physical therapy?
A patient status post total hip replacement will benefit from physical therapy and should attain an improved functional capacity. The patient should have diminished to no pain, increased strength and endurance, and improved mobility within six to eight weeks after surgery.

What are the long-term effects of the patient's condition?
A total hip replacement is a highly successful surgical procedure. The current life span of the prosthesis is less than 20 years and as a result some patients may require a subsequent replacement. The patient must follow established hip precautions to decrease the risk of subluxation or dislocation.

Comparison:
What are the distinguishing characteristics of a similar condition?
A hemiarthroplasty or hemireplacement of the hip is a replacement of the femoral head due to a subcapital fracture of the femur or degeneration of the femoral head. This type of surgical intervention is sometimes used as an alternative to a total hip replacement if a patient has a shortened expected life span.

Clinical Scenarios:
Scenario One
A patient is seen in physical therapy after total hip replacement surgery. The surgeon performed an anterolateral approach and used a noncemented prosthesis. The patient is mildly obese and has a lengthy cardiac history. The patient has osteoarthritis and had progressive pain and difficulty with mobility prior to surgery. The patient complains of soreness in the hip and is anxious to get home.

Scenario Two
A 75-year-old male is seen in physical therapy status post reduction of a dislocated right hip prosthesis. The patient had a total hip replacement three weeks ago and dislocated the hip two days ago while bending over to tie his shoes. The patient is currently using a walker for mobility and is toe touch weight bearing.

Total Knee Replacement

Diagnosis:

What condition produces a patient's symptoms?
The most common primary symptom that warrants a total knee replacement is progressive and disabling pain within the knee joint. The pain is most often due to severe degenerative arthritic changes that occur within the knee.

An injury was most likely sustained to which structure?
Arthritis causes the knee joint to undergo a degenerative process including destruction of articular cartilage resulting in bone-to-bone contact. The knee presents with decreased joint space and osteophyte formation.

Inference:

What is the most likely contributing factor in the development of this condition?
Osteoarthritis is the most common indication for a total knee replacement. A patient that has a history of participation in high impact sports or has experienced trauma to the knee is at a higher risk for arthritis and subsequent total knee replacement. Obesity and a varus/valgus deformity at the knee are also contributing factors.

Confirmation:

What is the most likely clinical presentation?
A patient that requires a total knee replacement will present with severe knee pain that worsens with motion and weight bearing, impaired range of motion, possible deformity of the knee, and impaired mobility skills. The patient has often attempted more conservative treatment measures to address the condition without success.

What laboratory or imaging studies would confirm the diagnosis?
X-ray and magnetic resonance imaging are used to determine the extent of deterioration and bony abnormalities within the knee. Radiographic images can be utilized postoperatively to ensure proper fit and obtain baseline information.

What additional information should be obtained to confirm the diagnosis?
Patient history, current functional status, and level of pain and disability are important factors in determining the need for surgical intervention. A standard pain assessment scale and the Arthritis Impact Measurement tool may be used to establish an objective baseline.

Examination:

What history should be documented?
Important areas to explore include past medical history, family history, medications, current symptoms, social history and habits, occupation, and social support system.

What test/measures are most appropriate?
- **Aerobic capacity and endurance:** assessment of vital signs at rest and with activity, perceived exertion scale
- **Anthropometric characteristics:** knee circumferential measurements
- **Arousal, attention, and cognition:** examine mental status, learning ability, memory, and motivation
- **Assistive and adaptive devices:** analysis of components and safety of a device
- **Environmental, home, and work barriers:** analysis of current and potential barriers or hazards
- **Gait, locomotion, and balance:** safety during gait with an assistive device, Functional Ambulation Profile
- **Joint integrity and mobility:** soft tissue swelling and inflammation
- **Muscle performance:** strength assessment, assessment of active movement
- **Pain:** pain perception assessment scale
- **Range of motion:** active and passive range of motion
- **Self-care and home assessment:** assessment of functional capacity, Barthel ADL Index
- **Sensory integrity:** assessment of sensation

What additional findings are likely with this patient?
A patient that requires total knee replacement may have arthritis in other joints, previous replacement surgeries, or previous trauma to the knee joint.

Management:

What is the most effective management of this patient?
A patient status post total knee replacement will require anticoagulant and pain medications. The patient's postoperative care includes a knee immobilizer, elevation of the limb, intermittent range of motion using a continuous passive motion (CPM) machine and initiation of knee protocol exercises. Physical therapy should emphasize ankle pumps, quad sets, and hamstrings sets as well as range of motion and stretching. A goal of 90 degrees of knee flexion and 0 degrees knee extension is often established prior to discharge from the hospital or rehabilitation facility. A cemented knee prosthesis allows for partial weight bearing to weight bearing as tolerated after surgery based on the individual physician's discretion. A noncemented knee prosthesis requires toe touch weight bearing for up to six weeks. Physical therapy should focus on mobility training with the proper weight bearing status and an appropriate assistive device. Outpatient therapy may be recommended to progress the patient from an assistive device. Intervention including strengthening with closed chain exercises, stationary bicycling, and stair training is indicated once the physician progresses the patient to weight bearing as tolerated.

What home care regimen should be recommended?
A home care regimen would typically include range of motion, strengthening, and progressive ambulation exercises.

Outcome:

What is the likely outcome of a course in physical therapy?
A patient status post total knee replacement will benefit from physical therapy and should attain an improved functional capacity. The patient should experience relief of pain that will allow for a full return to previous functional activities within three months.

What are the long-term effects of the patient's condition?
A total knee replacement is a highly successful surgical procedure that should significantly reduce pain and increase function. After successful completion of a rehabilitation protocol a patient may have only minor limitations in knee range of motion. A knee replacement may loosen over time and require revision, however the life expectancy of the prosthesis is between 15 and 20 years.

Comparison:

What are the distinguishing characteristics of a similar condition?
A patellectomy (surgical removal of the patella) is a surgical procedure that is indicated for a comminuted facture of the patella that cannot be repaired with internal fixation. A patellectomy can include the entire patella or just the inferior or superior pole of the patella. The retinaculum and extensor mechanism are repaired with the surgical procedure and the patient is immobilized for six to eight weeks. Once rehabilitation is initiated the patient starts with range of motion and closed chain exercises. Full rehabilitation may take six to eight months.

Clinical Scenarios:

Scenario One
An 80-year-old female in an acute care hospital is two days status post left total knee replacement. The patient presents with partial hearing loss and moderate dementia. The patient's past medical history includes a right CVA with no residual impairment and hypertension that is controlled by medication. The patient resides with her sister in a ranch style home with three steps to enter.

Scenario Two
A 49-year-old male is referred to outpatient physical therapy seven weeks after surgery. The patient received a noncemented knee prosthesis and has recently advanced to weight bearing as tolerated. The patient has 85 degrees of passive knee flexion, –10 degrees of passive knee extension, and moderate edema around the knee. The patient is otherwise independent with axillary crutches. No significant past medical history is noted.

Urinary Stress Incontinence

Diagnosis:

What condition produces a patient's symptoms?
Urinary stress incontinence may occur when there is an increase in abdominal pressure through straining, sneezing, coughing, or lifting. Urine will leak when the pressure within the bladder becomes greater than the urethral closure pressure.

An injury was most likely sustained to which structure?
Urinary stress incontinence usually occurs from loss of strength and/or integrity of the contractile and noncontractile tissues that maintain bladder control. Urinary stress incontinence is caused by weakness of the pelvic floor musculature (pubococcygeus muscle), weakness of the urogenital diaphragm muscles, shortening with malposition of the urethra or sphincter incompetence.

Inference:

What is the most likely contributing factor in the development of this condition?
Risk factors for the development of urinary stress incontinence include pregnancy, vaginal delivery, episiotomy, prostate surgery, aging, diabetes mellitus, central nervous system and peripheral system dysfunction, and recurrent urinary infection.

Confirmation:

What is the most likely clinical presentation?
Urinary stress incontinence is manifested solely by the involuntary loss of urine with any form of exertion or increased abdominal pressure. The amount of urine that leaks is typically less than 50 milliliters with coughing, sneezing or straining.

What laboratory or imaging studies would confirm the diagnosis?
A voiding cystourethrography can be utilized to observe leakage of contrast material with increased abdominal pressure. Urodynamic testing observes the stability of the bladder and electromyography observes formal bladder contractions.

What additional information should be obtained to confirm the diagnosis?
Diagnosis is usually determined without extensive imaging studies. Urinary stress incontinence can be determined through history, pelvic examination, and noted loss of urine with straining activities. The Marshall-Marchetti test utilizes finger elevation of the paraurethral vaginal tissues at the neck of the bladder in order to stop the leakage of urine during coughing, sneezing or straining. Baseline examination should include the amount of time that a patient can hold urine, repetitions performed of a holding contraction, and the amount of pelvic floor contractions that a patient is able to perform.

Examination:

What history should be documented?
Important areas to explore include past medical history, medications, current health status, fluid intake, social history and habits, occupation, living environment, and social support system.

What test/measures are most appropriate?
- **Aerobic capacity and endurance:** assessment of vital signs at rest and with activity, perceived exertion scale
- **Arousal, attention, and cognition:** examine mental status, learning ability, memory, and motivation
- **Environmental, home, and work barriers:** analysis of current and potential barriers or hazards
- **Integumentary integrity:** skin assessment, examination of the pelvic floor
- **Muscle performance:** strength assessment of the pelvic floor muscles, muscle tone assessment
- **Pain:** pain perception assessment scale
- **Self-care and home management:** assessment of functional capacity

What additional findings are likely with this patient?
A patient with urinary stress incontinence may be at increased risk for a urinary tract infection with subsequent skin breakdown. Pelvic floor weakness, uterine prolapse, and kidney infection may all relate to urinary stress incontinence. A patient may demonstrate noncompliance with a physical therapy exercise program related to another diagnosis if urinary stress incontinence is uncontrolled.

Management:
What is the most effective management of this patient?
Urinary stress incontinence is initially managed with pharmacological agents and physical therapy. Physical therapy intervention for pelvic floor muscle weakness that is tested as 0/5 – 2/5 includes biofeedback, electrical stimulation, bladder retraining, and therapeutic exercise. Pelvic floor muscle strengthening at this level includes facilitation and tapping of the pelvic floor muscles, overflow exercises using the buttocks, adductors, and lower abdominals, and implementation of Kegel exercises. Physical therapy intervention for pelvic floor muscle weakness that is tested as 3/5 – 5/5 includes continued biofeedback and bladder retraining, weighted vaginal cones for resistance training, and implementation of pelvic floor muscle exercise during functional activities. If the patient does not respond to conservative treatment surgical intervention may be warranted.

What home care regimen should be recommended?
A home care regimen for a patient with urinary stress incontinence should emphasize an active exercise program that includes pelvic floor strengthening in order to regain control of the flow of urine. Patients are encouraged to perform the recommended exercises throughout the day and integrate the activity into their daily routine.

Outcome:
What is the likely outcome of a course in physical therapy?
Outpatient physical therapy for urinary stress incontinence should alleviate pelvic floor weakness and involuntary leakage of urine within eight to twelve weeks. If a patient requires surgical intervention or presents with multiple impairments then physical therapy may be warranted for a longer period of time.

What are the long-term effects of the patient's condition?
The long-term effects of urinary stress incontinence depend on the exact cause for the incontinence and the responsiveness to therapeutic intervention. Some patients do not have any long-term effects upon successful completion of physical therapy while other patients do not benefit from physical therapy intervention.

Comparison:
What are the distinguishing characteristics of a similar condition?
Bowel incontinence can occur from birth defects, trauma to the rectum, spinal cord injuries, fecal impaction, and tumor. Conservative treatment is preferred and includes diet, pharmacological agents, and strengthening of the sphincter muscles through exercise, electrical stimulation, and biofeedback. Surgical intervention may be warranted.

Clinical Scenarios:
Scenario One
A 32-year-old female is referred to physical therapy with a diagnosis of incontinence. The patient gave birth to her fourth child six weeks ago. The patient reports involuntary leakage of urine with exertion. The patient has no significant past medical history, however reports that she is very anxious about participating in physical therapy.

Scenario Two
A 68-year-old female complains to her doctor during her annual examination that she has difficulty controlling her bladder since a kidney infection six months ago. The patient states that she is unable to hold her urine if she sneezes or coughs and cannot perform any activity of exertion without wearing feminine pads due to leakage. The physician referred the patient to physical therapy for Kegel exercises.

Sample Examinations

Exam One	Licensing Exam One	233
	Answer Sheets	257
	Exam One Explanations and Resources	259
Exam Two	Licensing Exam Two	271
	Answer Sheets	295
	Exam Two Explanations and Resources	297
Exam Three	Licensing Exam Three	309
	Answer Sheets	333
	Exam Three Explanations and Resources	335
Exam Four	Licensing Exam Four	347
	Answer Sheets	371
	Exam Four Explanations and Resources	373

Sample Examinations

Introduction

The sample examination section of *A Guide to Success* is divided into four, 200 question sample examinations. The actual Physical Therapist Examination is 225 questions, however 25 of the questions serve as pretest items and therefore have no impact on a candidate's score. The pretest items are arranged in a manner that makes it impossible to differentiate between scored and pretest items. Since candidate performance is based solely on the number of scored items answered correctly, each examination in *A Guide to Success* consists of 200 questions. Candidates will have a maximum of four hours to complete each examination. All examination questions have four possible answers: one best answer and three plausible options.

A detailed answer key follows each of the sample examinations. The answer key includes the correct answer, an explanation supporting the correct answer, and a cited resource with page number. The resources utilized were selected since they are often required textbooks in physical therapy academic programs. When consulting specific page numbers candidates should make sure that the edition of a given textbook they are using is consistent with the edition referenced in the bibliography of *A Guide to Success*.

Scoring

Scoring can be calculated using the formula:

$$\% \text{ Correct} = \frac{\text{Number of Questions Correct}}{200} * 100$$

Candidates should strive to achieve a score of greater than or equal to 80% correct on each of the sample examinations. The examinations provide candidates with an ideal self-assessment activity. Candidates should carefully review the results of the examination and attempt to identify any areas of weakness. The academic review section of *A Guide to Success*, textbooks, and lecture notes can serve as valuable resources when designing a plan for remediation. Special emphasis should be placed on distinguishing between academic and test taking mistakes.

An exact passing score for the Physical Therapist Examination is impossible to predict since the minimum scoring requirement fluctuates based on the difficulty of each examination. Criterion-referenced passing scores typically range from 138-152. Candidates should avoid using their score on a given sample examination as a predictor of success or failure on the actual examination.

Directions

- Each of the sample examinations consists of 200 multiple-choice questions.

- Choose the **best** answer to each question. Each question has only one correct answer.

- Candidates will have a maximum of four hours to complete each sample examination.

- Utilize the sample examination explanation section that immediately follows each of the examinations.

Sample Examination: One

1. A patient prepares for discharge from a rehabilitation hospital after completing three months of therapy. The patient has made significant progress in his rehabilitation, however expresses concern that his previous employer may not want him to return to work due to his injury. The most appropriate action is to:

   1. explain to the patient that to return to work after a serious injury is very difficult
   2. inform the patient of his rights according to the Americans with Disabilities Act
   3. request that the patient consider vocational retraining
   4. refer the patient to a psychologist to assist with the transition back to work

2. A physical therapist employed in an acute care hospital attempts to identify a standardized instrument that measures level of consciousness. The most appropriate standardized instrument is the:

   1. Glasgow Coma Scale
   2. Rankin Scale
   3. Barthel Index
   4. Sickness Impact Profile

3. A patient status post medial meniscus repair is referred to physical therapy. Which of the following would be the responsibility of the physician postoperatively?

   1. specify the parameters for superficial modality application
   2. specify the frequency and duration of range of motion exercises
   3. determine weight bearing status
   4. select an appropriate resistive exercise program

4. A physical therapist completes a family training session with a patient rehabilitating from a spinal cord injury. During the training the family asks a question regarding the functional ability of the patient following rehabilitation. The most appropriate therapist response is to:

   1. explain to the family that it is difficult to predict since all patients progress differently
   2. provide information on the expected prognosis based on the nature and severity of the injury
   3. refer the family to the director of rehabilitation
   4. refer the family to the patient's referring physician

5. A physical therapist completes an examination on a patient diagnosed with complete C7 tetraplegia. The patient problem list includes the following: inability to complete an independent bed to wheelchair transfer, decreased passive lower extremity range of motion, tissue breakdown over the ischial tuberosities, and decreased upper extremity strength. Which of the following treatment activities should be given the highest priority?

   1. pressure relief activities
   2. transfer training using a sliding board
   3. self range of motion activities
   4. upper extremity strengthening exercises

6. A physical therapist reviews the medical record of a patient admitted to the hospital. A recent entry in the medical record indicates the patient has a lesion affecting the facial motor nucleus. Based on the patient's diagnosis, the most probable clinical presentation is:

   1. facial muscle weakness ipsilateral to the lesion
   2. facial muscle weakness contralateral to the lesion
   3. impaired facial sensation ipsilateral to the lesion
   4. impaired facial sensation contralateral to the lesion

7. A 32-year-old male of Portuguese descent is referred to physical therapy for instruction in a home exercise program. The physician referral indicates that the patient is approved for one visit. What is the likelihood the patient will comprehend the home exercise program in the allotted time?

   1. the patient will require external assistance such as the use of an interpreter to comprehend the home exercise program
   2. the patient will comprehend the home exercise program
   3. the patient will not be able to comprehend the home exercise program
   4. the physical therapist cannot make a prediction based on the supplied information

8. A physical therapist and a physical therapist assistant are employed in a skilled nursing facility. Which of the following activities would be the most appropriate for the physical therapist assistant?

1. fitting of an assistive device
2. development of a plan of care
3. reexamination of a patient
4. establishment of a discharge plan

9. A physical therapist treats a patient with emphysema. As part of the treatment session the therapist teaches the patient to perform diaphragmatic breathing exercises. The primary goal for diaphragmatic breathing is to:

1. decrease tidal ventilation
2. increase respiration rate
3. decrease accessory muscle use
4. decrease oxygenation

10. A physical therapist attempts to reduce a child's genu recurvatum using an ankle-foot orthosis. Which ankle setting would be the most effective to achieve the therapist's objective?

1. 5-10 degrees of dorsiflexion
2. neutral
3. 5-10 degrees of plantar flexion
4. 15-20 degrees of plantar flexion

11. A physical therapist compares the significance of the mean vertical leap difference between samples of 12 athletes and 10 non-athletes. How many degrees of freedom are there in the study?

1. 20
2. 21
3. 22
4. 23

12. Physical therapists utilize a variety of sampling designs when conducting research. Which design is most likely to result in the greatest degree of sampling error?

1. simple random sample
2. systematic sample
3. cluster sample
4. stratified random sample

13. A physical therapy program designs a study that uses performance on the scholastic aptitude test as a predictor of grade point average in a physical therapy academic program. The results of the study identify that the overall correlation between the variables is r =.87. Which statement is most accurate based on the results of the study?

1. grade point average in a physical therapy program is a function of performance on the scholastic aptitude test
2. a student that performs well on the scholastic aptitude test is likely to have a high grade point average in a physical therapy academic program
3. there is no relationship between grade point average in a physical therapy program and performance on the scholastic aptitude test
4. there is an inverse relationship between grade point average in a physical therapy program and performance on the scholastic aptitude test

14. A physical therapist places a patient's hip in the resting position prior to assessing joint play. Which of the following would be considered the resting position of the hip?

1. 10 degrees flexion, 15 degrees abduction, slight medial rotation
2. 30 degrees flexion, 30 degrees abduction, slight lateral rotation
3. 30 degrees flexion, 30 degrees adduction, 20 degrees lateral rotation
4. 10 degrees extension, 20 degrees adduction, 20 degrees medial rotation

15. A patient is referred to physical therapy with a C6 nerve root injury. Which of the following clinical findings would not be expected with this type of injury?

1. diminished sensation on the anterior arm and the index finger
2. weakness in the biceps and supinator
3. diminished brachioradialis reflex
4. paresthesias of the long and ring fingers

16. A physical therapist completes a vertebral artery test on a patient diagnosed with a cervical strain. Which component of the vertebral artery test is most likely to assess the patency of the intervertebral foramen?

1. rotation
2. lateral flexion
3. flexion
4. extension

234 A GUIDE TO SUCCESS

17. A 22-year-old male status post traumatic brain injury receives physical therapy services in a rehabilitation hospital. The patient is presently functioning at Rancho Los Amigos level VI. The patient has progressed well in therapy, however has been bothered by diplopia. Which treatment strategy would be the most appropriate to address diplopia?

   1. provide verbal and nonverbal instructions within the patient's direct line of sight
   2. place a patch over one of the patient's eyes
   3. ask the patient to turn his head to one side when he experiences diplopia
   4. instruct the patient to carefully focus on a single object

18. A patient diagnosed with T5 paraplegia is discharged from a rehabilitation hospital following 16 weeks of therapy. Assuming a normal recovery, which of the following most accurately describes the status of the patient's bathroom transfers?

   1. independent with the presence of an attendant
   2. independent with adaptive devices and a sliding board
   3. independent with bathroom adaptations
   4. independent

19. A physical therapist completes a manual muscle test on a patient that sustained a laceration to the anterior surface of the forearm. When performing the test on the flexor pollicis brevis, the therapist should direct the force:

   1. along the volar aspect of the proximal phalanx of the thumb
   2. along the volar aspect of the distal phalanx of the thumb
   3. along the dorsal aspect of the proximal phalanx of the thumb
   4. along the dorsal aspect of the distal phalanx of the thumb

20. A physical therapist from a home care agency examines a 50-year-old patient diagnosed with chronic bronchitis. The patient is overweight and presents with cyanosis at the fingertips and shallow breathing. The most immediate goal would be to:

   1. implement a low level exercise program
   2. implement breathing exercises and postural drainage techniques
   3. prescribe a wheelchair for mobility
   4. complete a manual muscle test of the upper and lower extremities

21. A physical therapist receives a referral for a two month old infant diagnosed with osteogenesis imperfecta. After completing the examination, the therapist discusses the physical therapy plan of care with the infant's parents. The primary goal of therapy should be:

   1. improve muscle strength and diminish tone
   2. facilitate protected weight bearing
   3. promote safe handling and positioning
   4. diminish pulmonary secretions

22. A patient with an I.V. in the antecubital region is treated in physical therapy. The physical therapist would like to instruct the patient in upper extremity active range of motion exercises, but is concerned about placing excessive pressure on the infusion site. Which of the following exercises would not be indicated?

   1. shoulder abduction and adduction
   2. shoulder flexion and extension
   3. elbow flexion and extension
   4. wrist flexion and extension

23. A physical therapist elects to utilize the six-minute walk test as a means of quantifying endurance for a patient rehabilitating from a lengthy illness. Which variable would be the most appropriate to measure when determining the patient's endurance level with this objective test?

   1. perceived exertion
   2. heart rate response
   3. elapsed time
   4. distance walked

24. Communication and perceptual problems are extremely common in patients with hemiplegia. Which clinical problem would be characteristic of a patient status post right CVA?

   1. inability to recognize symbols and perform basic math problems
   2. inability to plan and perform serial steps in activities
   3. distorted awareness of self image
   4. diminished functional speech

25. There are a variety of sizes of wheelchairs which can accommodate individuals of almost any size or build. Assuming a full grown adult of average size and build, which of the following wheelchair dimensions would be the most appropriate?

   1. seat width 14 inches, seat depth 12 inches
   2. seat width 16 inches, seat depth 14 inches
   3. seat width 18 inches, seat depth 16 inches
   4. seat width 20 inches, seat depth 18 inches

26. A physical therapist is concerned about the possibility of a patient developing a deep vein thrombosis following surgery. Which of the following special tests would be useful to identify the presence of this condition?

   1. Bunnel-Littler test
   2. Homans' sign
   3. Thompson test
   4. Froment's sign

27. A physical therapist completes an examination on a five-year-old boy diagnosed with Duchenne muscular dystrophy. The referral indicates that the boy was diagnosed with the disease less than one year ago. Assuming a normal progression, which of the following findings would be the first to occur?

   1. distal muscle weakness
   2. proximal muscle weakness
   3. impaired respiratory function
   4. inability to perform activities of daily living

28. A physical therapist attempts to document a patient's inability to achieve weekly goals with the following entry: "Patient may have performed poorly during the last week secondary to recent illness." Which section of a S.O.A.P. note would be the most appropriate for the entry?

   1. subjective
   2. objective
   3. assessment
   4. plan

29. A physical therapist completes a developmental assessment on a five month old infant. If the therapist elects to examine the infant's palmar grasp reflex, which of the following stimuli is the most appropriate?

   1. contact to the ball of the foot in upright standing
   2. maintained pressure to the palm of the hand
   3. noxious stimulus to the palm of the hand
   4. sudden change in the position of the hand

30. A physical therapist treats a 54-year-old male rehabilitating from a tibial plateau fracture. While completing a resistive exercise the patient indicates that lifting weights often causes him to void small amounts of urine. The most appropriate therapist action is:

   1. offer sympathy for the patient
   2. instruct the patient in pelvic floor muscle strengthening exercises
   3. discontinue resistive exercises as part of the established plan of care
   4. educate the patient about incontinence

31. A physical therapist completes an examination on a 14-year-old male with a genetic disorder caused by a chromosomal abnormality. The patient appears to be quite tall with a slender build and proportionately long arms. He is alert and oriented, however appears to possess below average intelligence. This type of clinical presentation is most consistent with:

   1. Down syndrome
   2. Edwards syndrome
   3. Klinefelter syndrome
   4. Turner syndrome

32. A physical therapist treats a nine-year-old child diagnosed with cystic fibrosis. As part of the treatment session the therapist attempts to improve the efficiency of the patient's breathing. The most appropriate technique to encourage full expansion at the base of the lungs is:

   1. manual percussion on the posterior portion of the ribs with the patient in prone
   2. manual contacts with pressure on the lateral borders of the ribs with the patient in supine
   3. manual vibration on the lateral portion of the ribs with the patient in sidelying
   4. manual cues on the epigastric area with the patient in supine

33. A physician discusses a patient's plan of care with a physical therapist. The patient is a 29-year-old male that sustained deep partial-thickness burns to the anterior surface of his upper legs. The physician discusses the possibility of discontinuing use of the topical antibiotic silver sulfadiazine after identifying an irregularity in the patient's laboratory results. Which finding could be most related to the use of silver sulfadiazine?

   1. leukopenia
   2. peripheral edema
   3. hypokalemia
   4. altered pH balance

34. A physical therapist reviews the medical chart of a patient with a history of recurrent dysrhythmias. The therapist is concerned about the patient's past medical history and would like to monitor the patient during all activities. Which of the following monitoring devices would be the most beneficial?

    1. pulmonary artery catheter
    2. electrocardiogram
    3. intracranial pressure monitor
    4. pulse oximeter

35. A patient with a lengthy history of substance abuse is referred to physical therapy after sustaining multiple injuries in a motor vehicle accident. Which of the following controlled substances does not foster physical dependence?

    1. depressants
    2. hallucinogens
    3. narcotics
    4. stimulants

36. A physical therapist employed in an acute care hospital conducts an initial interview with a patient referred to physical therapy. During the interview the therapist asks the patient if he feels dependent on coffee, tea or soft drinks. Which clinical scenario would most appropriately warrant this type of question?

    1. a 27-year-old female status post arthroscopic medial meniscectomy
    2. a 42-year-old male with premature ventricular contractions
    3. a 37-year-old female with restrictive pulmonary disease
    4. a 57-year-old male with respiratory alkalosis

37. A group of physical therapy students presents a research project entitled "Effects of Ultrasound on Blood Flow and Nerve Conduction Velocity." The dependent variables in the students' study is/are:

    1. ultrasound
    2. ultrasound and blood flow
    3. ultrasound and nerve conduction velocity
    4. blood flow and nerve conduction velocity

38. A physical therapist instructs a 65-year-old female in ambulation activities. The therapist instructs the patient to place the affected foot on the ground, but to avoid transmitting weight through the foot. The instructions best describe:

    1. non-weight bearing
    2. touch down weight bearing
    3. partial weight bearing
    4. full weight bearing

39. A physical therapist instructs a patient to close her eyes and hold out her hand. The therapist places a series of different weights in the patient's hand one at a time. The patient is then asked to identify the comparative weight of the objects. This method of sensory testing is used to examine:

    1. barognosis
    2. graphesthesia
    3. recognition of texture
    4. stereognosis

40. A nurse takes the temperature of a patient before a scheduled physical therapy session. Which of the following temperatures would be classified as normal?

    1. 35 degrees Celsius
    2. 36 degrees Celsius
    3. 37 degrees Celsius
    4. 38 degrees Celsius

41. Secretion removal techniques are an integral component of a pulmonary rehabilitation program. What is the simplest method to clear secretions from the upper airways?

    1. cough
    2. percussion
    3. shaking
    4. vibration

42. A patient with a lengthy medical history of cardiac pathology is referred to a phase II cardiac rehabilitation program. During the first session the physical therapist prepares to measure the patient's blood pressure by inflating the cuff 20 mm Hg above the patient's estimated systolic value. Which of the following values best describes the most appropriate rate to release the pressure when obtaining the blood pressure measurement?

    1. 2-3 mm Hg per second
    2. 3-5 mm Hg per second
    3. 5-7 mm Hg per second
    4. 8-10 mm Hg per second

43. A physical therapist performs goniometric measurements on a patient rehabilitating from injuries sustained in a motor vehicle accident. When measuring rotation of the cervical spine, which of the following landmarks would be the most appropriate for the axis of the goniometer?

   1. centered over the external auditory meatus
   2. centered over the center of the cranial aspect of the head
   3. centered over the C7 spinous process
   4. centered over the midline of the occiput

44. A physical therapist performs girth measurements on a patient rehabilitating from knee surgery. The therapist takes the measurements 5 cm and 10 cm above the superior pole of the patella with the patient in supine. The girth measurements are recorded as 32 cm and 37 cm on the right and 34 cm and 40 cm on the left. Which of the following conclusions can be made regarding the strength of the patient's quadriceps?

   1. The right quadriceps will be capable of producing a greater force than the left.
   2. The left quadriceps will be capable of producing a greater force than the right.
   3. The right and left quadriceps will be capable of producing equal force.
   4. Not enough information is given to form a conclusion.

45. A patient receiving physical therapy treatment complains that he is experiencing a great deal of pain around the I.V. site. The physical therapist's most appropriate response would be to:

   1. reposition the I.V.
   2. remove the I.V.
   3. turn off the I.V.
   4. contact nursing

46. A physical therapist instructs a woman with left unilateral lower extremity weakness to descend stairs. The most appropriate position for the therapist to guard the patient is:

   1. in front of the patient toward the left side
   2. in front of the patient toward the right side
   3. behind the patient toward the left side
   4. behind the patient toward the right side

47. A physical therapist monitors a patient's blood pressure using the brachial artery. What effect would you expect to see on the measured blood pressure value if the therapist selects a blood pressure cuff that is too narrow in relation to the circumference of the patient's arm?

   1. systolic values will be higher and diastolic values will be lower
   2. systolic values will be lower and diastolic values will be higher
   3. systolic and diastolic values will be higher
   4. systolic and diastolic values will be lower

48. A physical therapist is growing increasingly concerned about a patient that is demonstrating symptoms that are consistent with neoplastic activity. What is the most significant symptom of a rapidly growing neoplasm?

   1. fatigue
   2. swelling
   3. tenderness to palpation
   4. pain

49. A physical therapist instructs a patient to expire maximally after taking a maximal inspiration. The therapist can use these instructions to measure the patient's:

   1. expiratory reserve volume
   2. inspiratory reserve volume
   3. total lung capacity
   4. vital capacity

50. A patient diagnosed with an acute cervical strain is referred to physical therapy. During the examination the physical therapist asks the patient to bend his head to the right and then proceeds to apply a downward compressive force to the patient's head. Which of the following subjective findings would be considered indicative of a positive test?

   1. pain radiates into the right arm
   2. pain radiates into the left arm
   3. pain radiates into the arms bilaterally
   4. pain radiates into the arms and legs bilaterally

51. A physical therapist instructs a patient in diaphragmatic breathing exercises. Which of the following instructions would not be helpful in teaching diaphragmatic breathing?

   1. place your dominant hand over your midrectus area
   2. place your nondominant hand over your midsternal area
   3. inspire slowly through your nose
   4. as you expire watch your lower hand rise

52. A physical therapist volunteers to assist participants at the finish line in a 10K road race. The race takes place on a hot and humid day and some of the race organizers are concerned about the potential for heat related disorders. The most significant variables to differentiate between heat exhaustion and heat stroke are:

1. blood pressure and pulse rate
2. coordination and level of fatigue
3. mental status and skin temperature
4. pupil dilation and blood pressure

53. A physical therapist monitors a patient's vital signs while exercising in a phase I cardiac rehabilitation program. The patient is status post myocardial infarction and has progressed without difficulty while involved in the program. Which of the following vital sign recordings would exceed the typical limits of a phase I program?

1. heart rate elevated 18 beats per minute above resting level
2. respiration rate = 25 breaths per minute
3. systolic blood pressure decreases by 20 mm Hg from resting level
4. diastolic blood pressure less than 100 mm Hg

54. A physical therapist employed in a rehabilitation hospital performs an examination on a 52-year-old male diagnosed with amyotrophic lateral sclerosis. Which of the following signs and symptoms is not consistent with this disease?

1. mental deterioration
2. hyperactive deep tendon reflexes
3. weakness of the forearms and hands
4. impaired speech

55. A physical therapist examines a patient that recently sustained a cervical hyperextension injury. Results of the examination reveal a loss of proprioception and light touch with intact motor function. This type of incomplete spinal cord injury is most appropriately termed:

1. anterior cord syndrome
2. Brown-Sequard's syndrome
3. central cord syndrome
4. posterior cord syndrome

56. A physical therapist employed in a long-term care setting attempts to identify a screening tool that examines a patient's ability to perform a variety of activities of daily living independently. The therapist would like to readminister the tool to assess patient progress. The most appropriate screening tool is the:

1. Barthel Index
2. Berg Functional Balance Scale
3. Health Status Profile
4. Tinetti Performance Oriented Mobility Assessment

57. Health care facilities utilize a variety of employees including physical therapists, physical therapist assistants, and physical therapy aides. Which activity would be inappropriate for a physical therapy aide?

1. assist patients in preparation for treatment
2. make daily entries in the patient's medical record
3. assist patients with exercise activities
4. perform treatment procedures as determined by the physical therapist

58. A patient rehabilitating from a lower extremity injury is referred to physical therapy for hydrotherapy treatments. The physical therapist would like the patient to fully extend the involved lower extremity while in the hydrotherapy tank. Which type of whirlpool would not allow the patient to extend the involved lower extremity?

1. Hubbard tank
2. highboy tank
3. lowboy tank
4. walk tank

59. A patient recovering in the hospital from a total knee replacement is examined by a physical therapist. Assuming an uncomplicated recovery, how much knee range of motion is realistic prior to discharge?

1. 0-50 degrees
2. 0-90 degrees
3. 15-90 degrees
4. 15-105 degrees

60. A physical therapist orders a wheelchair for a patient with T9 paraplegia. Which wheelchair option would not be necessary for the patient?

1. detachable legrests
2. pneumatic tires
3. removable arms
4. wheel rim projections

61. A physical therapist instructs a patient ambulating with axillary crutches to move cautiously and deliberately on any potentially hazardous surface. Which gait pattern would allow the patient maximum security?

    1. swing-to
    2. swing-through
    3. three-point
    4. four-point

62. A physical therapist observes a patient's breathing as part of a respiratory assessment. Which muscle of respiration is most active during forced expiration?

    1. diaphragm
    2. external intercostals
    3. internal intercostals
    4. upper trapezius

63. A physical therapist performs a manual muscle test on a patient with unilateral upper extremity weakness. The patient is able to complete 75% of the available range of motion with gravity eliminated. The therapist should record the muscle grade as:

    1. poor plus
    2. poor
    3. poor minus
    4. trace plus

64. A physical therapist performs a manual muscle test on a patient's hip flexors. The therapist attempts to complete the test in supine, but the patient has difficulty holding the limb in the test position. What alternate test position would be appropriate to test the patient's hip flexors?

    1. prone
    2. sidelying
    3. sitting
    4. standing

65. A physical therapist measures a patient for a straight cane prior to beginning ambulation activities. Which gross measurement method would provide the best estimate of cane length?

    1. measuring from the head of the fibula straight to the floor and multiplying by two
    2. measuring from the iliac crest straight to the floor
    3. measuring from the greater trochanter straight to the floor
    4. dividing the patient's height by two and adding three inches

66. A physical therapist reviews the medical record of a patient with venous insufficiency. A recent entry in the medical record indicates that the physician ordered diagnostic testing in an attempt to rule out superficial or deep venous thrombosis. Which diagnostic test would be most beneficial to accomplish the physician's objective?

    1. Doppler ultrasonography
    2. hematocrit
    3. partial thromboplastin time
    4. pulmonary function tests

67. A physical therapist recommends a wheelchair for a patient rehabilitating from a CVA with the goal of independent mobility. The left upper and lower extremities are flaccid and present with edema. There is normal strength on the right, however the patient's trunk is hypotonic. The patient is cognitively intact. The most appropriate wheelchair for the patient is:

    1. solid seat, solid back, elevating legrests, and anti-tippers
    2. sling seat, sling back, arm board, and elevating legrests
    3. light weight, solid seat, solid back, arm board, and elevating legrests
    4. light weight, solid seat, solid back, arm board, and standard footrests

68. A physical therapist reviews the results of a pulmonary function test for a 58-year-old male patient recently admitted to the hospital. The therapist notes that the patient's total lung capacity is significantly increased when compared to established norms. Which medical condition would most likely produce this type of result?

    1. chronic bronchitis
    2. emphysema
    3. spinal cord injury
    4. pulmonary fibrosis

69. A physical therapist examines a patient status post traumatic brain injury. When examining neurologic tone the most appropriate method is:

    1. active range of motion of the involved extremities
    2. passive range of motion of the involved extremities
    3. passive range of motion of the involved and uninvolved extremities
    4. resisted motion of the involved extremities

70. A physical therapist treats a 47-year-old female with diminished lower extremity range of motion due to hamstrings tightness. As part of the treatment program, the therapist attempts to identify an appropriate active exercise technique to improve range of motion. Which objective finding would result in contract-relax being an undesirable treatment option?

1. the limitation of movement is accompanied by pain
2. the limitation of movement is greater than 50% of the normal available range
3. the limitation of movement involves multiple planes
4. the limitation of movement occurs in a noncapsular pattern

71. An elderly patient with a grade I right ankle inversion sprain is learning to use a straight cane. Which of the following instructions would be the most appropriate?

1. hold the cane in the right hand, step left, then step right
2. hold the cane in the left hand, step left, then step right
3. hold the cane in the right hand, step right, then step left
4. hold the cane in the left hand, step right, then step left

72. A 58-year-old female diagnosed with peripheral neuropathy returns from an appointment with an orthotist wearing a posterior leaf spring ankle-foot orthosis. Which of the following clinical descriptions would most warrant the use of this particular type of orthosis?

1. foot drop without medial or lateral instability
2. weak plantar flexors during swing phase
3. diminished knee stability
4. foot drop with multiplane instability

73. A physical therapist notices a small area of skin irritation under the chin of a patient wearing a cervical orthosis. The patient expresses that the area is not painful, but is becoming increasingly itchy. The most appropriate therapist action is:

1. instruct the patient to apply 1% hydrocortisone cream to the area twice daily
2. apply powder to the area and instruct the patient to avoid scratching
3. utilize an additional material for the liner of the orthosis
4. discontinue use of the orthosis until the skin has become less irritated

74. A physical therapist determines a patient's coronary artery disease risk factors as part of a health screening. The patient's heart rate is recorded as 78 beats per minute and blood pressure as 130/85 mm Hg. A recent laboratory report indicates a total cholesterol level of 170 mg/dL with high density lipoproteins reported as 20 mg/dL and low density lipoproteins as 150 mg/dL. Which of the following values would be considered atypical?

1. heart rate
2. blood pressure
3. high density lipoproteins
4. low density lipoproteins

75. A physical therapist assesses a one month old infant. During the treatment session the therapist strokes the cheek of the infant causing the infant to turn its mouth towards the stimulus. This action is utilized to assess the:

1. Moro reflex
2. rooting reflex
3. startle reflex
4. righting reflex

76. A physical therapist performs upper extremity passive range of motion exercises on a patient with an I.V. connected to the dorsum of his right hand. During the treatment session the therapist notices a small amount of blood which has backed up in the I.V. line. The therapist's most immediate response should be to:

1. turn off the I.V.
2. remove the I.V.
3. reposition the peripheral I.V. line
4. contact the primary physician

77. A physical therapist examines a patient referred to physical therapy diagnosed with peripheral vascular disease. Which of the following would be the most valid indicator that the patient is not a candidate for an active exercise program?

1. cool skin
2. resting claudication
3. decreased peripheral pulses
4. decreased vital capacity

78. A 17-year-old basketball player has completed six months of aggressive rehabilitation following a knee injury. The athlete was cleared for activity by his physician after completing a functional progression. Three days later the therapist identifies a small increase in effusion in the involved knee and a slightly antalgic gait pattern. What recommendation would be the most appropriate?

   1. "Continue to practice with the team, it's just your body's way of getting used to basketball again."
   2. "Avoid agility drills and scrimmaging at practice for a couple of days."
   3. "Make an appointment with your physician immediately."
   4. "It looks like your knee isn't ready for basketball. I think you should continue with rehabilitation and try again next year."

79. A physical therapist is growing more and more disenchanted with her job due to exceptionally high productivity expectations. The most appropriate therapist action is to:

   1. speak to the director of rehabilitation
   2. increase utilization of support staff
   3. communicate directly with the supervisor
   4. refrain from addressing the topic for fear of being labeled a troublemaker

80. While examining a patient diagnosed with Achilles tendonitis, a physical therapist notes that the foot and ankle appear to be pronated in standing. Which motions combine to create pronation?

   1. abduction, dorsiflexion, eversion
   2. adduction, dorsiflexion, inversion
   3. abduction, plantar flexion, eversion
   4. adduction, plantar flexion, inversion

81. A physical therapist measures a patient for a wheelchair. Which measurement is used to determine armrest height?

   1. seat to anterior superior iliac spine
   2. seat to olecranon distance
   3. femur to radial head distance
   4. elbow to acromion distance

82. A patient eight weeks status post right total hip replacement loses his balance and falls to the ground during a physical therapy session. The patient is visibly shaken by the fall, but insists that he is uninjured. The physical therapist examines the right hip and although active motion elicits pain, all other findings are inconclusive. The therapist should:

   1. continue with the current treatment so the patient does not focus on the incident
   2. notify the supervisor about the incident
   3. document the incident and contact a physician to examine the patient before resuming treatment
   4. document the incident and gradually resume prior treatment

83. A physical therapist administers a pulmonary function test to a patient with cardiopulmonary disease. When comparing the obtained value to a table of normal values, which variable would be the least relevant?

   1. age
   2. height
   3. gender
   4. weight

84. A work site examination is scheduled for a patient rehabilitating from a closed head injury eight weeks ago. The patient presents with mild dysarthria and right-sided hemiparesis with moderate upper extremity involvement. The patient's job duties are secretarial including: answering phones, filing, and organizing the office. The most appropriate clinician to participate in the work site examination is a/an:

   1. physical therapist
   2. occupational therapist
   3. speech therapist
   4. social worker

85. A physical therapist receives orders to design an exercise program for a 13-year-old boy recovering from thoracic surgery. The therapist explains the purpose and inherent risks of the exercise session as outlined on an informed consent form to the boy and his parents. After asking several additional questions the boy and his parents indicate that they would like to move forward with the session. The most appropriate therapist action is:

   1. ask the boy to sign the informed consent form
   2. ask one of the boy's parents to sign the informed consent form
   3. initiate the exercise program
   4. confirm the parameters of the exercise session with the referring physician

86. A squat pivot transfer is performed on a patient with a diagnosis of CVA, left hemiplegia. The physical therapist initiates the transfer to the patient's affected side. The benefits of transferring toward the affected side include all of the following except:

    1. retrains motor control through weight shift and weight bearing on the affected side
    2. decreases extensor synergy by weight bearing and maintaining minimal knee flexion
    3. directs attention and vision to the affected side
    4. allows affected upper extremity to remain unsupported which facilitates motion and decreases flexor synergy influence

87. A physical therapist works on range of motion of the lower extremities with a patient rehabilitating from a spinal cord injury. Independent range of motion of the lower extremities becomes a realistic goal at which spinal cord level?

    1. C2
    2. C4
    3. C5
    4. C7

88. A physical therapist measures body composition using skinfold measurements prior to initiating an exercise program. When measuring the abdominal skinfold the most appropriate method is:

    1. utilize a vertical fold approximately 2 cm to the right of the umbilicus
    2. utilize a horizontal fold approximately 2 cm to the right of the umbilicus
    3. utilize a vertical fold approximately 2 cm to the left of the umbilicus
    4. utilize a horizontal fold approximately 2 cm to the left of the umbilicus

89. A patient status post spinal fusion is referred for chest physical therapy. The physical therapist instructs the patient in diaphragmatic breathing exercises. Instructions are given to the patient to place his dominant hand over the midrectus abdominis area and his nondominant hand over the midsternal area. As the patient inhales slowly through the nose the therapist encourages the patient to:

    1. direct air so that the nondominant hand rises during inspiration
    2. direct air so that the dominant hand rises during inspiration
    3. direct air so that both hands rise equally during inspiration
    4. direct air so that both hands do not move during inspiration

90. A patient diagnosed with shoulder pain of unknown etiology is referred by his physician for magnetic resonance imaging. Results of the test reveal a partial tear of the infraspinatus muscle. Which muscle group would be the most seriously affected by the injury?

    1. shoulder lateral rotators
    2. shoulder medial rotators
    3. shoulder abductors
    4. shoulder adductors

91. The following description best describes a patient with a spinal cord injury at the _____ level? Biceps, deltoids, and rotator cuff musculature are intact. Independent transfers with a sliding board may be possible.

    1. C2
    2. C4
    3. C6
    4. C8

92. A physical therapist employed in an outpatient private practice notices that a patient has received the maximum number of physical therapy visits indicated on the physician referral form. The patient is scheduled for an appointment later in the week and has three additional appointments scheduled for the following week. The most appropriate therapist action is:

    1. contact the referring physician and request approval for the additional physical therapy visits
    2. ask the patient to contact the referring physician and seek approval for the additional physical therapy visits
    3. contact the insurance provider to authorize additional physical therapy visits
    4. discharge the patient from physical therapy

93. A physical therapist employed in an outpatient clinic provides physical therapy services for a patient rehabilitating from a tibial plateau fracture. Assuming the patient qualifies for Medicare, which description best explains the cost of therapy services to the patient?

    1. a maximum of $100 in a calendar year
    2. 10% of the cost of physical therapy services
    3. 20% of the cost of physical therapy services
    4. qualifying for Medicare eliminates out of pocket expenses

SAMPLE EXAMINATION: EXAM ONE

94. A physical therapist works as a team with a male physical therapist assistant in a fast paced orthopedic private practice. The therapist is unsure of the physical therapist assistant's orthopedic knowledge and therefore regularly delegates cleaning and filing responsibilities. What step would be the most appropriate to improve the quality of the team's performance?

   1. ask the physical therapist assistant how he feels about his present role in the clinic
   2. schedule a meeting with the physical therapist assistant to learn more about his education, career goals, and prior clinical experience
   3. encourage the physical therapist assistant to attend physical therapy school if he wants to become more involved in patient care
   4. continue to delegate various undesirable tasks to the physical therapist assistant

95. A patient status post motor vehicle accident is treated using skeletal traction. What bone when fractured is often associated with this type of traction?

   1. femur
   2. humerus
   3. tibia
   4. fibula

96. A physical therapist examines a patient with bicipital tendonitis. Which clinical finding would not be expected based on the patient's diagnosis?

   1. isometric resistance to the biceps brachii increases subjective pain levels
   2. referred pain in the C7-C8 dermatome
   3. a painful arc is noted with active range of motion of the involved shoulder
   4. tenderness to palpation over the bicipital tendon

97. A case manager reviews items that are reimbursed through Medicare Part B with a patient preparing for discharge from a rehabilitation hospital. Which of the following items would not be reimbursed through Medicare Part B?

   1. hospice care
   2. outpatient medical and surgical services
   3. clinical laboratory services
   4. vaccinations

98. Health maintenance organizations have been more successful than the majority of private health insurance companies in controlling escalating medical costs. The primary method used by health maintenance organizations to contain medical costs is:

   1. increasing premiums to discourage the unnecessary use of health care
   2. restricting the duration of physical therapy services
   3. limiting services to specific health care providers
   4. having the providers of care share in some aspect of the financial risk

99. A seven-year-old patient sustains a deep partial-thickness burn to his heel. When teaching the patient a stretching program the greatest emphasis should be placed in the direction of:

   1. plantar flexion
   2. dorsiflexion
   3. inversion with plantar flexion
   4. eversion

100. A physical therapist employed in an acute care hospital treats a patient who receives health care insurance through Medicaid. From a patient perspective, what is the primary problem with this type of insurance?

   1. large copayments and deductibles
   2. limited reimbursement for specific levels of care
   3. limited access to primary care providers
   4. no prescription drug benefit

101. A 25-year-old male is diagnosed with a first degree acromioclavicular sprain. The injury occurred two days ago after being checked into the boards while playing hockey. Which of the following would you not expect to observe during the initial examination?

   1. increased elevation of the clavicular end of the acromion
   2. inability to bring the arm completely across the chest
   3. inability to fully abduct the arm
   4. point tenderness on palpation of the injury site

102. A physical therapy department sponsors a program called "Healthy Heart" for individuals who have been identified as high risk candidates for developing coronary artery disease. One of the requirements of the program is that upon completion participants must be able to list three modifiable risk factors associated with coronary artery disease. Which domain of learning is emphasized with this particular requirement?

　1. affective
　2. basilic
　3. cognitive
　4. psychomotor

103. A physical therapist attempts to quantify a patient's endurance level by administering a maximal exercise test. What is the primary limitation of a maximal exercise test?

　1. Maximal exercise testing requires participants to exercise only to the point of volitional fatigue.
　2. Maximal exercise testing does not typically allow a steady state heart rate at each work rate.
　3. Maximal exercise testing is not useful in diagnosing coronary artery disease.
　4. Maximal exercise testing requires progressive stages of increasing work intensities without rest intervals.

104. A physical therapist administers a submaximal exercise test using the YMCA Cycle Ergometry Protocol. The test consists of a variable number of three minute stages of continuous exercise and requires the examiner to raise the patient's steady state heart rate to 110-150 beats per minute for two consecutive stages. Which of the following would be the most accurate guideline for terminating a submaximal exercise test?

　1. the subject reaches 75% of his/her age-predicted maximal heart rate
　2. the subject reaches 80% of his/her age-predicted maximal heart rate
　3. the subject reaches 85% of his/her age-predicted maximal heart rate
　4. the subject reaches 90% of his/her age-predicted maximal heart rate

105. A patient with neurological involvement is able to understand instructions and conversation, but cannot verbalize. The best term to describe this condition is:

　1. global aphasia
　2. receptive aphasia
　3. expressive aphasia
　4. agraphia

106. If a muscle crosses over more than one joint and it moves both of the joints at the same time, it will shorten to a point where it cannot move either of the joints through the full range of motion. This definition best describes:

　1. contracture
　2. substitution
　3. passive insufficiency
　4. active insufficiency

107. A physical therapist works on bed mobility exercises with a patient recently diagnosed with terminal cancer. The patient is extremely upset and tells the therapist, "I know I will never get better." The therapist's most appropriate response would be:

　1. Radiation treatments will make you feel much better.
　2. Many people have overcome larger obstacles.
　3. Having cancer must be very difficult for you to deal with.
　4. Physical therapy can improve your condition.

108. A physical therapist prepares to complete a formal sensory examination on a patient rehabilitating from a lower extremity burn. Which of the following would serve as the best predictor of altered sensation?

　1. presence of a skin graft
　2. depth of burn injury
　3. percentage of body surface affected
　4. extent of hypertrophic scarring

109. The treatment plan for a patient with hemiplegia includes reinforcing normal movement through key points of control and avoiding all reflex movement patterns and associated reactions. This approach most closely resembles:

　1. Bobath
　2. Kabat
　3. Trendelenburg
　4. Brunnstrom

110. Which statement concerning the APGAR newborn assessment is not true?

　1. the test is administered at 1 and 5 minutes after birth
　2. the maximum score is 5
　3. a score of less than 4 is indicative of respiratory distress
　4. the score for each assessed item ranges from 0-2

111. An 18-year-old male status post fractured right femur with open reduction and internal fixation is referred to physical therapy. After the initial session the patient states that therapy is a waste of time and he will not return for any additional appointments. The most immediate response would be to:

    1. inform the referring physician of the patient's decision
    2. instruct the patient to return for one additional treatment session
    3. discuss the importance of physical therapy with the patient
    4. discharge the patient from physical therapy

112. A physical therapist examines a patient with T1 paraplegia. As the therapist and patient perform balance activities in sitting, the patient begins to complain of a pounding headache. The patient exhibits profuse sweating above the T1 lesion, and blotching of the skin. The therapist should immediately identify this as:

    1. orthostatic hypotension
    2. autonomic dysreflexia
    3. Lowe's syndrome
    4. homonymous hemianopsia

113. A physical therapist instructs a physical therapist assistant to begin gait training with a patient one day status post noncemented total hip replacement. Assuming the patient has not had any significant problems postoperatively, the most likely weight bearing status would be:

    1. wheelchair use only
    2. toe touch weight bearing
    3. weight bearing as tolerated
    4. full weight bearing

114. A physical therapist completes a manual muscle test on the right lower trapezius muscle. In order to properly assess the muscle, the therapist should position the patient in:

    1. supine
    2. prone
    3. right sidelying
    4. left sidelying

115. A physical therapist attempts to have a patient with right hemiplegia brush his teeth while working on standing tolerance. The therapist notices that the patient attempts to put the toothpaste directly in his mouth and hair. The therapist would document this finding as:

    1. ideomotor apraxia
    2. ideational apraxia
    3. constructional apraxia
    4. conduction aphasia

116. A physical therapist examines a patient with shoulder subluxation secondary to a flaccid upper extremity. The therapist's short-term goal is to prevent further subluxation. The following techniques would be beneficial in treating the flaccid upper extremity except:

    1. distraction and stretching techniques
    2. approximation techniques
    3. neuromuscular electrical stimulation
    4. arm support when sitting and standing

117. A physical therapist monitors the vital signs of a 52-year-old male during a graded exercise test. The patient was prompted to seek medical assistance two weeks ago after becoming short of breath on two separate occasions. When interpreting the data collected during the exercise test, which finding would serve as the best indicator that the patient had exerted a maximal effort?

    1. failure of the heart rate to increase with further increases in intensity
    2. rise in systolic blood pressure of 50 mm Hg when compared to the resting value
    3. rating of 12 on a perceived exertion scale
    4. decrease in diastolic blood pressure of 20 mm Hg when compared to the resting value

118. A physical therapist suspects a patient may be under the influence of alcohol during a treatment session. The therapist has been treating the patient for over five weeks and during that time has failed to recognize any signs or symptoms of substance abuse. The therapist's most immediate action would be to:

    1. contact the referring physician and discuss the patient's problem
    2. ask the patient if he/she has been drinking
    3. discharge the patient from physical therapy
    4. refer the patient to a local Alcoholics Anonymous group

119. A physical therapist orders a wheelchair for a patient with C4 tetraplegia. Which power wheelchair option would be inappropriate for the patient?

   1. full length arm supports
   2. reclining frame
   3. hand controls
   4. elevating leg rests

120. A physical therapist instructs a patient to descend a flight of stairs with crutches. During the training session the patient loses his balance and falls to the ground. Although the patient denies being injured the therapist summons a physician to examine the patient. After completing an incident report the therapist should:

   1. document the daily treatment entry, however avoid describing any of the details associated with the incident
   2. document the daily treatment entry and include the details associated with the incident
   3. document the daily treatment entry and reference the completed incident report
   4. document the daily treatment entry after receiving an update on the patient's condition from the physician

121. Patella tracking dysfunction is a common problem encountered by physical therapists. Dynamic factors for patella tracking dysfunction include:

   1. increase in the angulation between the quadriceps muscle and the patella tendon
   2. a lateral femoral condyle that is not sufficiently prominent anteriorly
   3. vastus medialis obliquus muscle insufficiency
   4. shallow trochlear groove

122. A physical therapist instructs a patient in residual limb wrapping. Which bandage would be the most appropriate to utilize for a patient with a transfemoral amputation?

   1. two inch
   2. four inch
   3. six inch
   4. eight inch

123. A physical therapist instructs a female athlete to complete ten minutes of stretching before beginning her treadmill program. While observing the athlete the therapist notices repetitive bouncing and a failure to maintain the stretch for more than five seconds. Why is this type of stretching considered to be inadequate?

   1. The athlete should maintain each stretch for at least 30 seconds.
   2. The athlete should stretch only after running on the treadmill.
   3. The athlete is activating the stretch reflex.
   4. The athlete should remain activity specific and does not need to stretch the hamstrings if she is running on the treadmill.

124. A physical therapist initiates an exercise program with a patient diagnosed with chronic obstructive pulmonary disease. In order to assist the patient to improve the efficiency of respiration the therapist instructs the patient in pursed lip breathing. Which of the following instructions would be the most beneficial for the patient?

   1. breathe in through your mouth
   2. keep your lips tightly sealed during expiration
   3. breathe out twice as long as you breathe in
   4. use your abdominals to assist you during expiration

125. A physical therapist performs an examination on a patient with hip-knee-ankle-foot orthoses. The patient can ambulate independently with the orthoses and Lofstrand crutches, however due to the high energy expenditure often becomes fatigued very rapidly. Which disorder would be most consistent with this scenario?

   1. amyotrophic lateral sclerosis
   2. peripheral neuritis
   3. neurogenic arthropathy
   4. spina bifida

126. In what section of a S.O.A.P. note would the following entry belong? "Patient is not functional in activities of daily living due to lower extremity muscle weakness. Wife is unable to care for spouse at present level of functioning."

   1. subjective
   2. objective
   3. assessment
   4. plan

127. A therapist examines a patient's hamstrings length using a passive straight leg raise. While raising the tested lower extremity, the physical therapist attempts to stabilize the contralateral limb. If the patient has tight hip flexors which result in an excessive anterior pelvic tilt, what can the physical therapist conclude about the patient's measured hamstrings length?

   1. actual length is greater than measured length
   2. actual length is less than measured length
   3. shortened hip flexors do not influence apparent hamstrings length
   4. the apparent length measured is the actual length

128. A physical therapist attempts to secure a wheelchair for a patient with an incomplete spinal cord injury. The patient is a 28-year-old female that is very active and relies on a wheelchair as her primary mode of transportation. Which type of wheelchair design would be the most appropriate for the patient?

   1. standard chair with a rigid frame
   2. lightweight chair with a rigid frame
   3. standard chair with a folding frame
   4. lightweight chair with a folding frame

129. A physical therapist observes a patient walking at various speeds. Which of the following does not occur as the speed of ambulation increases?

   1. stride length increases
   2. angle of toe out increases
   3. width of the base of support decreases
   4. cadence increases

130. If a leg length measurement is 28.4 inches when taken in a supine position and 30.2 inches when taken in a standing position, the leg length difference is probably due to:

   1. poor standing posture
   2. pelvic asymmetry
   3. an actual leg length difference
   4. not enough information is given to form a conclusion

131. A physical therapist named in a lawsuit deliberately shreds several physical therapy records related to pending litigation. The legal term most consistent with this situation is:

   1. vicarious liability
   2. malpractice
   3. libel
   4. spoliation

132. A respiratory examination is performed on a patient with tetraplegia with the following results: the patient attains seventy percent of standard vital capacity, he is able to verbalize eight syllables per breath, and is able to mobilize and clear secretions from his lungs. Which level of injury does this best describe?

   1. C2-C3
   2. C4-C5
   3. C7-C8
   4. T2-T3

133. A patient with an amputation must be competent with residual limb care. The most objective long-term goal for bandaging would be:

   1. The patient will possess general knowledge regarding bandaging of the residual limb.
   2. The patient will attempt to bandage the residual limb twice a day.
   3. The patient will observe three styles of residual limb bandaging.
   4. The patient will perform proper bandaging of the residual limb 100% of the time.

134. A physical therapist attempts to select an assistive device for a patient rehabilitating from a traumatic brain injury. The patient is occasionally impulsive, however has fair standing balance and good upper and lower extremity strength. Which of the following would be the most appropriate assistive device?

   1. cane
   2. axillary crutches
   3. Lofstrand crutches
   4. walker

135. A physical therapist conducts a work site examination for a patient rehabilitating from a spinal cord injury. During the examination the therapist determines that the patient's desk height is inadequate for a wheelchair. The most cost efficient and acceptable accommodation would be to:

   1. secure a wheelchair with a smaller frame
   2. place bricks under the desk to increase desk height
   3. purchase a new desk
   4. eliminate job duties which require the use of a desk

136. A physical therapist prepares a presentation on preseason conditioning for a group of high school athletes. To maximize the effectiveness of the presentation the therapist should:

    1. develop specific learning objectives
    2. utilize a variety of audiovisual equipment
    3. assess the needs of the target audience
    4. provide an outline

137. A physical therapist determines that a patient rehabilitating from an anterior cruciate ligament reconstruction is not ready to return to athletic competition. Which of the following best supports the therapist's decision?

    1. a 20 percent quadriceps peak torque deficit at 60 degrees per second
    2. trace effusion in the knee after a therapy session
    3. a 5 degree limitation in knee flexion
    4. inability to complete a functional progression

138. A health care provider negotiates with an insurance company to provide health care services. As part of the agreement, the insurance company agrees to pay the health care provider a predetermined amount for each member in the plan on an annual basis. This type of arrangement is best termed:

    1. capitation
    2. fee for service
    3. case pricing
    4. negotiated compensation

139. A physical therapist attempts to have a patient quantify his pain using a subjective pain scale. The therapist explains to the patient that he should assign a numerical value between zero and ten to describe the pain. Which of the following would best describe a score of ten?

    1. no pain
    2. mild pain
    3. moderate pain
    4. most severe pain

140. A physical therapist prepares to initiate an exercise program for a patient with diabetes mellitus. Which objective measure would be the most appropriate to examine in order to avoid significant complications from exercise?

    1. systolic blood pressure
    2. respiratory rate
    3. blood glucose values
    4. oxygen saturation rate

141. A patient with cardiac disease rates the intensity of exercise as a 12 using Borg's Original Rate of Perceived Exertion Scale. What percentage of the patient's age-adjusted maximum heart rate best corresponds to a rating of 12 on the exertion scale?

    1. 50
    2. 60
    3. 75
    4. 85

142. A physical therapist observes that a patient has an exaggerated heel strike on the left during ambulation activities. Which term is most consistent with heel strike using Rancho Los Amigos nomenclature?

    1. pressuring
    2. loading response
    3. initial contact
    4. mid-stance

143. A patient rehabilitating from a stroke is referred to physical therapy. The medical record indicates the stroke primarily involved the right hemisphere of the brain. Which of the following objective findings would be least likely when examining the patient?

    1. diminished motor control of the left side of the body
    2. impaired awareness of the right side of the body
    3. impaired spatial ability
    4. diminished emotional depth

144. A physical therapist plans to administer ultraviolet radiation to the anterior trunk of a patient with psoriasis. Which form of protective equipment would be the most appropriate for the therapist to utilize?

    1. lead shield
    2. gloves, gown, mask
    3. eye goggles
    4. protective equipment is not necessary

145. A patient ambulating with crutches trips over an object on the floor and falls to the ground. The patient appears to be uninjured, however complains of diffuse pain in the involved knee. The most formal mechanism to describe the events associated with the fall is to:

    1. send a memo to the director of rehabilitation
    2. write a letter to the patient's insurance company
    3. complete an incident report
    4. dictate a letter to the referring physician

146. A physical therapist provides preoperative training for a patient scheduled for thoracic surgery. Which activity would be the most appropriate to prevent a deep vein thrombosis post surgery?

1. deep breathing
2. incentive spirometry
3. coughing
4. ankle pumps

147. A physical therapist attempts to gather information on the ligamentous integrity of a patient's knee. Which special test would be inappropriate based on the desired objective?

1. posterior sag sign
2. anterior drawer test
3. McMurray test
4. Lachman test

148. A physical therapist attempts to assess the dorsal pedal pulse of a patient diagnosed with peripheral vascular disease. To locate the dorsal pedal pulse the therapist should palpate:

1. between the extensor hallucis longus and the extensor digitorum longus tendons on the dorsum of the foot
2. between the flexor digitorum longus and the flexor hallucis longus tendons on the dorsum of the foot
3. immediately posterior to the medial malleolus
4. immediately posterior to the lateral malleolus

149. A physical therapist utilizes resistive testing as part of an initial examination. To assess the C5 myotome the therapist should resist:

1. wrist radial deviation
2. elbow extension
3. shoulder abduction
4. thumb extension

150. The parents of a patient with a C4 spinal cord injury request projected outcome information on their 18-year-old son. The most appropriate health care professional to answer the parents' question is the:

1. primary nurse
2. physiatrist
3. case manager
4. social worker

151. A patient positioned in kneeling works on weight shifting activities. Which stage of control is demonstrated with this activity?

1. mobility
2. stability
3. controlled mobility
4. skill

152. A patient with cerebellar dysfunction exhibits signs of dysmetria. Which of the following activities would be the most difficult for the patient?

1. alternate finger to nose
2. placing feet on floor markers while walking
3. walking at varying speeds
4. marching in place

153. A physical therapist employed by a home health agency treats a patient in a home that is dirty and unsanitary. When treating the patient in the home, the most appropriate location for the therapist's treatment and supply bag is:

1. in the car
2. on a countertop in the patient's house
3. on a piece of newspaper supplied by the physical therapist
4. on a chair in the treatment area

154. A physical therapist examines a patient with multiple sclerosis. The therapist documents that the patient presents with dysdiadochokinesia. Which objective finding is most representative of dysdiadochokinesia?

1. inability to perform rapid alternating movements
2. inability to discriminate selected tactile input
3. difficulty with speech articulation
4. presence of involuntary, rhythmic, and oscillatory movements at rest

155. Physical therapists are often faced with ethical issues in their daily clinical practice. Which of the following would be the most appropriate initial step when faced with an ethical dilemma?

1. determine an action plan
2. seek external support
3. gather relevant information
4. complete the action plan

156. A patient diagnosed with an acromioclavicular separation explains how the injury occurred. During the explanation the physical therapist identifies several inconsistencies and begins to question its authenticity. The most appropriate action is to:

1. document the patient's explanation
2. document the patient's explanation and identify each stated inconsistency
3. dismiss the patient's explanation
4. inform the patient that the explanation is difficult to believe

157. A physical therapist examines a 22-year-old baseball pitcher diagnosed with impingement syndrome. The athlete was prompted to see his physician after not being able to generate his usual velocity when throwing. Examination reveals positive impingement signs, mild anterior shoulder laxity, and limited flexibility in the posterior muscles and posterior capsule. The most appropriate treatment intervention is:

1. active abduction exercises using dumbbell weights in the frontal plane
2. medial and lateral rotation exercises with the arm at the side using elastic tubing
3. posterior capsule stretching
4. high voltage galvanic stimulation and ice

158. A physical therapist examines a patient referred to physical therapy diagnosed with a medial collateral ligament sprain. During the examination the patient appears to be relaxed and comfortable, however is extremely withdrawn. Which of the following questions would be the most appropriate to further engage the patient?

1. Is this the first time you have injured your knee?
2. Have you ever been to physical therapy before?
3. How long after your injury did you see a physician?
4. What do you hope to achieve in physical therapy?

159. A physical therapist working in a hospital notices that a particular patient recently diagnosed with pulmonary disease appears to be depressed. When treating the patient the therapist should:

1. provide additional information on the patient's medical condition
2. create an environment that promotes internal motivation
3. avoid activities that require prolonged verbal interaction
4. explain to the patient that his/her prognosis is good

160. A physical therapist reviews the results of a complete blood count taken on a 65-year-old male recently admitted to the hospital. Which of the following lab values may be considered a precaution for therapeutic exercise?

1. white blood cell count: 6.2×10^3 mm^3
2. hematocrit: 46 mL/dL
3. hemoglobin: 8 gm/dL
4. platelet count: 250×10^3 mm^3

161. A physical therapist completes a gait analysis on a patient diagnosed with Parkinson's disease. As part of the examination the therapist measures the distance between right heel strike and the next consecutive left heel strike. This measurement is used to measure:

1. left stride length
2. right stride length
3. left step length
4. right step length

162. A patient diagnosed with low back pain is referred to physical therapy. During the examination the physical therapist asks if the patient has had any formal diagnostic screening. The patient states that she had x-rays and a test where dye was injected into the spinal canal. This description most closely resembles:

1. arthrography
2. myelography
3. computed tomography
4. magnetic resonance imaging

163. A physical therapist participates in a study that examines knee range of motion at selected postoperative intervals. After collecting the necessary data, the therapist prepares to measure the spread or dispersion of the range of motion at each interval. Which statistical measure would be the most appropriate to meet the therapist's objective?

1. median
2. mode
3. mean
4. variance

164. A physical therapist attempts to identify an appropriate gait pattern for a patient with bilateral lower extremity involvement due to muscle weakness. The patient presents with balance and coordination deficits. The most appropriate gait pattern using axillary crutches is:

    1. swing-to
    2. swing-through
    3. four-point
    4. two-point

165. A physical therapist conducts a preoperative training session for a patient scheduled for surgery to repair a large rotator cuff tear. The patient is a 54-year-old male who is employed as an insurance agent. During the preoperative training session the patient inquires as to the amount of time before he is able to return to recreational activities such as tennis and golf. The most appropriate time frame is typically:

    1. 6–8 weeks
    2. 12-14 weeks
    3. 24-28 weeks
    4. 36-40 weeks

166. A physical therapist examines a patient referred to physical therapy with sacroiliac pain. As part of the examination, the therapist assesses the position of the sacrum by palpating the inferior lateral angles. Which spinal level is most consistent with the inferior lateral angles?

    1. S2
    2. S3
    3. S4
    4. S5

167. A physical therapist determines a patient's heart rate by counting the number of QRS complexes in a six second electrocardiogram strip. Assuming the therapist identifies eight QRS complexes in the strip, the patient's heart rate should be recorded as:

    1. 40 bpm
    2. 60 bpm
    3. 80 bpm
    4. 100 bpm

168. A patient with an irregular heart rate is monitored using a single lead electrocardiogram during exercise. Which of the following techniques would provide the physical therapist with the most accurate measurement of heart rate?

    1. count the number of QRS complexes that occur in sixty seconds
    2. count the number of R waves that occur in thirty seconds and multiply by two
    3. count the number of P waves that occur in fifteen seconds and multiply by four
    4. count the number of T waves that occur in six seconds and multiply by ten

169. A patient with superficial partial-thickness burns on the dorsal surface of the right foot refuses physical therapy services after being transported to the hydrotherapy area. The most immediate physical therapist action is to:

    1. continue with the treatment session
    2. discontinue the treatment session
    3. explain to the patient the expected consequences of refusing treatment
    4. notify the referring physician

170. A physical therapist receives a referral to instruct a patient in pelvic floor muscle strengthening exercises. Which of the following explanations would be the most effective to assist the patient to perform a pelvic floor contraction?

    1. tighten your muscles like you were trying to expel a large amount of urine in a very short amount of time
    2. pull your muscles up and in like when you have to go to the bathroom, but there is no toilet
    3. tighten your abdominal muscles and anteriorly rotate your pelvis
    4. gently push out as if you had to pass gas

171. A physical therapist and physical therapist assistant work as a team in an acute care medical facility. Which of the following responsibilities would be appropriate for the physical therapist to delegate to the physical therapist assistant?

    1. develop a patient treatment plan based on an initial examination
    2. revise an established patient care plan
    3. implement a therapeutic exercise program
    4. write a discharge summary

172. A physical therapist is responsible for supervising a physical therapist assistant at an off site location. Which guideline is most appropriate when determining the frequency of supervisory visits?

    1. supervisory visits should take place when convenient for the physical therapist and the physical therapist assistant
    2. supervisory visits should take place in accordance with patient need
    3. supervisory visits should take place on a weekly basis
    4. supervisory visits should take place at least once every third visit

173. A physical therapist orders a wheelchair with a reclining back for a patient in a rehabilitation hospital. Which type of legrests would be the most appropriate for the wheelchair?

    1. swing-away
    2. detachable
    3. elevating
    4. fixed

174. A physical therapy department attempts to establish a quality assurance program. The first step in developing the program should be to:

    1. identify important aspects of patient care provided by the department
    2. collect and analyze data for each established indicator
    3. identify quality indicators that will allow the department to monitor selected aspects of patient care
    4. determine a percentage of occurrence that will dictate a specified action

175. A patient rehabilitating from cardiac surgery is monitored using an arterial line. The primary purpose of an arterial line is to:

    1. measure right arterial pressure
    2. measure heart rate and oxygen saturation
    3. measure pulmonary artery pressure
    4. measure blood pressure

176. A physical therapist develops a chart detailing expected functional outcomes for a variety of spinal cord injuries. Which is the highest spinal level at which independent transfers with a sliding board would be feasible?

    1. C4
    2. C6
    3. T1
    4. T3

177. A physical therapist reviews the results of a patient's arterial blood gases. The report indicates the following: $PaO_2 = 45$ mm Hg, $PaCO_2 = 55$ mm Hg, $HCO_3 = 24$ mEq/L, pH = 7.20. These values are most indicative of:

    1. respiratory acidosis
    2. respiratory alkalosis
    3. metabolic acidosis
    4. metabolic alkalosis

178. A physical therapist alerts a nurse to skin breakdown on a patient's right heel. Which position would leave the patient most susceptible to additional tissue damage?

    1. right sidelying
    2. left sidelying
    3. prone
    4. supine

179. A patient with complete C5 tetraplegia works on a forward raise for pressure relief. The patient utilizes loops that are attached to the back of the wheelchair to assist with the forward raise. Which muscles need to be particularly strong in order for the patient to be successful with the forward raise?

    1. brachioradialis, brachialis
    2. rhomboids, levator scapulae
    3. biceps, deltoids
    4. triceps, flexor digitorum

180. A physical therapist treats a patient with complete C6 tetraplegia. Which of the following would not be an expected functional outcome for the patient?

    1. independent transfers with a sliding board
    2. independent bowel and bladder care
    3. independent manual wheelchair propulsion
    4. independent self feeding

181. A manual muscle test is conducted on the medial portion of the deltoid. The muscle is able to move through the full range of motion with gravity eliminated, but cannot function against gravity. The results of the manual muscle test should be recorded as:

1. trace
2. poor
3. fair
4. good

182. A physical therapist describes an exercise to a patient using terms such as flexion, extension, and abduction. The patient informs the therapist that she does not understand the instructions. The most appropriate action is to:

1. verbally define each term
2. provide a written definition of each term
3. define each term without using medical terminology
4. select a different exercise

183. A physical therapist uses rhythmic initiation to assist a patient in learning to roll from supine to prone. The therapist's initial command should be:

1. "Slowly roll over by yourself"
2. "Help me roll you over"
3. "Stop me from rolling you over"
4. "Relax and let me move you"

184. A physical therapist examines a 22-year-old soccer player who suffered an inversion ankle sprain 24 hours ago. The therapist notices the athlete's right ankle is moderately edematous. What valuable information has the therapist already acquired?

1. The athlete will probably be out of competitive soccer for at least two weeks because of the severity of the sprain.
2. The athlete should be non-weight bearing at all times due to the amount of edema.
3. The sprain is a third degree ligament sprain although no timetable for recovery is available.
4. The physical therapist still does not have an accurate indication as to the severity of the injury.

185. A physical therapist administers an isokinetic examination on a 24-year-old female status post anterior capsular shift. The patient is extremely excited about the testing since the surgeon expressed that a good performance on the isokinetic examination often signifies the completion of physical therapy and a return to athletic competition. After reviewing the results of the examination, the therapist concludes that the patient's strength deficit in the involved extremity is less than 5% when compared to the value obtained on the uninvolved extremity. The most appropriate therapist action is:

1. instruct the patient to gradually return to athletic competition
2. design a home exercise program for the patient
3. ask the patient to schedule an appointment with the physician
4. discharge the patient from physical therapy

186. A physical therapist employed in an outpatient orthopedic sports medicine clinic treats a 58-year-old female diagnosed with a traumatic anterior shoulder dislocation. The patient has no past history of shoulder instability, however has been treated for impingement syndrome. The patient is employed as a journalist and reports being an avid fisherman. Upon reading the physician referral the therapist is surprised that the period of shoulder immobilization was less than two weeks. Which of the following variables would have been the most significant when determining the length of immobilization?

1. age
2. sex
3. vocation
4. social history

187. A physical therapist obtains the past medical history of a patient recently referred to physical therapy after being diagnosed with adhesive capsulitis. Which medical condition is associated with an increased incidence of adhesive capsulitis?

1. diabetes mellitus
2. hemophilia
3. peripheral vascular disease
4. osteomalacia

188. A physical therapist uses proprioceptive neuromuscular facilitation to increase joint range of motion using the hold-relax technique. This technique utilizes an _____ contraction, which is used at the end point of the available range of motion?

   1. isotonic
   2. isometric
   3. isokinetic
   4. eccentric

189. Based on the "rule of nines", an adult who has burns on the anterior right arm, the anterior portion of the thorax, and the genital region would be classified as having burns over _____ percent of the body?

   1. 19
   2. 22.5
   3. 23.5
   4. 28

190. A physical therapist prepares to treat a patient with continuous ultrasound. Which general rule best determines the length of treatment when using ultrasound?

   1. 2 minutes for an area that is 2-3 times the size of the transducer face
   2. 5 minutes for an area that is 2-3 times the size of the transducer face
   3. 5 minutes is the maximum treatment time regardless of the treatment area
   4. 10 minutes is the maximum treatment time regardless of the treatment area

191. A patient is referred to physical therapy for range of motion and strengthening exercises after sustaining an anterior dislocation of the right shoulder. The patient was immobilized in a sling and swathe for four weeks and it has been five weeks since the injury date. Which activity would be the most appropriate for the patient to begin strengthening of the involved shoulder?

   1. medial and lateral rotation in sidelying with two pound weights within the available range of motion
   2. medial and lateral rotation using elastic tubing with the arm at the patient's side and elbow at 90 degrees
   3. isokinetic medial and lateral rotation at speeds less than 120 degrees per second
   4. isometric strengthening exercises with the arm positioned at the patient's side

192. A physical therapist monitors the vital signs of a patient completing a six stage exercise session on a treadmill. During the first two stages of the protocol the patient's heart rate does not increase enough to enter the calculated target heart rate range. The patient reports a subjective exercise intensity rating of 2 using Borg's 10 point rating of perceived exertion scale. The most appropriate therapist action is:

   1. increase the intensity of the exercise
   2. increase the length of the exercise session
   3. discontinue the exercise session
   4. consult with the referring physician

193. Which of the following factors is of least importance when selecting an assistive device?

   1. the patient's level of understanding
   2. the patient's height and weight
   3. the patient's upper and lower extremity strength
   4. the patient's level of coordination

194. A patient with a transfemoral amputation is referred to physical therapy for gait training. During the initial examination the physical therapist identifies lateral trunk bending towards the affected side during the stance phase of gait. A possible cause of this deviation is:

   1. the prosthesis is too long
   2. the prosthesis is too short
   3. the socket diameter is too small
   4. there is an increased amount of edema in the residual limb

195. A patient sustained a fracture of the acetabulum that was treated with open reduction and internal fixation. The injury occurred in a motor vehicle accident approximately seven weeks ago. Which objective measure would be the most influential variable when determining the patient's weight bearing status?

   1. visual analogue pain scale rating
   2. radiographic confirmation of bone healing
   3. lower extremity manual muscle testing
   4. balance and coordination assessment

196. A physical therapist treats a patient one day status post posterior hip dislocation. The injury was treated using closed reduction. As part of the treatment session the therapist educates the patient on hip precautions to avoid the recurrence of dislocation and implements an exercise program including gluteal sets, quadriceps sets, hamstrings sets, ankle pumps, upper extremity exercises, and bed mobility. Which activity would be the most essential for the physical therapy session the following day?

1. review the exercise program
2. initiate straight leg raises
3. begin ambulation activities
4. start active-assisted range of motion

197. A patient five days status post anterior cruciate ligament reconstruction using a patellar tendon autograft is referred to physical therapy. The patient uses a postsurgical rehabilitative brace that consists of a metal offset hinge with medial and lateral plastic supports. It is applied directly over the skin and is secured using a series of velcro straps. The brace has a flexion and extension setting and comes in six different sizes based on a series of circumferential measurements. The primary purpose of the brace is to:

1. reduce postoperative edema
2. increase anterior and posterior stability
3. enhance quadriceps activation time
4. limit knee flexion and extension

198. A physical therapist records grip strength measurements on a patient diagnosed with bilateral carpal tunnel syndrome. Which description does not accurately describe typical results when using a hand held dynamometer?

1. a bell curve is seen when charting multiple recordings from adjustable hand spacings in consecutive order
2. twenty to twenty five percent differences in grip strength may be observed between the dominant and nondominant hand
3. discrepancies of more than twenty five percent in a test-retest situation may indicate the patient is not exerting maximal force
4. an individual who does not exert maximal force for each test will not show the typical bell curve

199. A physical therapist designs an exercise program for a patient rehabilitating from anterior cruciate ligament reconstruction. Which of the following treatment options would place the least amount of stress on the reconstructed ligament?

1. walking with crutches
2. stationary cycling
3. walking
4. jogging at a slow speed on a level surface

200. A patient status post total hip replacement indicates to her physical therapist that she was instructed to avoid hip flexion greater than 90 degrees, adduction, and medial rotation. The most likely surgical approach utilized by the surgeon is:

1. anterolateral
2. anteromedial
3. posterolateral
4. posteromedial

Sample Exam: One – Answer Sheet

#		#		#	
1.	① ② ③ ④	36.	① ② ③ ④	71.	① ② ③ ④
2.	① ② ③ ④	37.	① ② ③ ④	72.	① ② ③ ④
3.	① ② ③ ④	38.	① ② ③ ④	73.	① ② ③ ④
4.	① ② ③ ④	39.	① ② ③ ④	74.	① ② ③ ④
5.	① ② ③ ④	40.	① ② ③ ④	75.	① ② ③ ④
6.	① ② ③ ④	41.	① ② ③ ④	76.	① ② ③ ④
7.	① ② ③ ④	42.	① ② ③ ④	77.	① ② ③ ④
8.	① ② ③ ④	43.	① ② ③ ④	78.	① ② ③ ④
9.	① ② ③ ④	44.	① ② ③ ④	79.	① ② ③ ④
10.	① ② ③ ④	45.	① ② ③ ④	80.	① ② ③ ④
11.	① ② ③ ④	46.	① ② ③ ④	81.	① ② ③ ④
12.	① ② ③ ④	47.	① ② ③ ④	82.	① ② ③ ④
13.	① ② ③ ④	48.	① ② ③ ④	83.	① ② ③ ④
14.	① ② ③ ④	49.	① ② ③ ④	84.	① ② ③ ④
15.	① ② ③ ④	50.	① ② ③ ④	85.	① ② ③ ④
16.	① ② ③ ④	51.	① ② ③ ④	86.	① ② ③ ④
17.	① ② ③ ④	52.	① ② ③ ④	87.	① ② ③ ④
18.	① ② ③ ④	53.	① ② ③ ④	88.	① ② ③ ④
19.	① ② ③ ④	54.	① ② ③ ④	89.	① ② ③ ④
20.	① ② ③ ④	55.	① ② ③ ④	90.	① ② ③ ④
21.	① ② ③ ④	56.	① ② ③ ④	91.	① ② ③ ④
22.	① ② ③ ④	57.	① ② ③ ④	92.	① ② ③ ④
23.	① ② ③ ④	58.	① ② ③ ④	93.	① ② ③ ④
24.	① ② ③ ④	59.	① ② ③ ④	94.	① ② ③ ④
25.	① ② ③ ④	60.	① ② ③ ④	95.	① ② ③ ④
26.	① ② ③ ④	61.	① ② ③ ④	96.	① ② ③ ④
27.	① ② ③ ④	62.	① ② ③ ④	97.	① ② ③ ④
28.	① ② ③ ④	63.	① ② ③ ④	98.	① ② ③ ④
29.	① ② ③ ④	64.	① ② ③ ④	99.	① ② ③ ④
30.	① ② ③ ④	65.	① ② ③ ④	100.	① ② ③ ④
31.	① ② ③ ④	66.	① ② ③ ④	101.	① ② ③ ④
32.	① ② ③ ④	67.	① ② ③ ④	102.	① ② ③ ④
33.	① ② ③ ④	68.	① ② ③ ④	103.	① ② ③ ④
34.	① ② ③ ④	69.	① ② ③ ④	104.	① ② ③ ④
35.	① ② ③ ④	70.	① ② ③ ④	105.	① ② ③ ④

SAMPLE EXAMINATION: EXAM ONE ANSWER SHEET

106.	①	②	③	④		138.	①	②	③	④		170.	①	②	③	④
107.	①	②	③	④		139.	①	②	③	④		171.	①	②	③	④
108.	①	②	③	④		140.	①	②	③	④		172.	①	②	③	④
109.	①	②	③	④		141.	①	②	③	④		173.	①	②	③	④
110.	①	②	③	④		142.	①	②	③	④		174.	①	②	③	④
111.	①	②	③	④		143.	①	②	③	④		175.	①	②	③	④
112.	①	②	③	④		144.	①	②	③	④		176.	①	②	③	④
113.	①	②	③	④		145.	①	②	③	④		177.	①	②	③	④
114.	①	②	③	④		146.	①	②	③	④		178.	①	②	③	④
115.	①	②	③	④		147.	①	②	③	④		179.	①	②	③	④
116.	①	②	③	④		148.	①	②	③	④		180.	①	②	③	④
117.	①	②	③	④		149.	①	②	③	④		181.	①	②	③	④
118.	①	②	③	④		150.	①	②	③	④		182.	①	②	③	④
119.	①	②	③	④		151.	①	②	③	④		183.	①	②	③	④
120.	①	②	③	④		152.	①	②	③	④		184.	①	②	③	④
121.	①	②	③	④		153.	①	②	③	④		185.	①	②	③	④
122.	①	②	③	④		154.	①	②	③	④		186.	①	②	③	④
123.	①	②	③	④		155.	①	②	③	④		187.	①	②	③	④
124.	①	②	③	④		156.	①	②	③	④		188.	①	②	③	④
125.	①	②	③	④		157.	①	②	③	④		189.	①	②	③	④
126.	①	②	③	④		158.	①	②	③	④		190.	①	②	③	④
127.	①	②	③	④		159.	①	②	③	④		191.	①	②	③	④
128.	①	②	③	④		160.	①	②	③	④		192.	①	②	③	④
129.	①	②	③	④		161.	①	②	③	④		193.	①	②	③	④
130.	①	②	③	④		162.	①	②	③	④		194.	①	②	③	④
131.	①	②	③	④		163.	①	②	③	④		195.	①	②	③	④
132.	①	②	③	④		164.	①	②	③	④		196.	①	②	③	④
133.	①	②	③	④		165.	①	②	③	④		197.	①	②	③	④
134.	①	②	③	④		166.	①	②	③	④		198.	①	②	③	④
135.	①	②	③	④		167.	①	②	③	④		199.	①	②	③	④
136.	①	②	③	④		168.	①	②	③	④		200.	①	②	③	④
137.	①	②	③	④		169.	①	②	③	④						

Sample Exam Answers: One

1. Answer: 2   Resource: Minor (p. 466)
The Americans with Disabilities Act is federal legislation designed to eliminate discrimination against individuals with disabilities. Physical therapists have an ethical obligation to make patients aware of their rights according to the ADA.

2. Answer: 1   Resource: Rothstein (p. 426)
The Glasgow Coma scale provides a quick and practical method for assessing the degree of conscious impairment in the critically ill patient. The scale utilizes eye opening, verbal responses, and motor responses to determine the level of consciousness and degree of dysfunction.

3. Answer: 3   Resource: Goodman (p. 6)
Physicians routinely specify the weight bearing status for their patients following surgical procedures such as a meniscus repair.

4. Answer: 2   Resource: Haggard (p. 71)
The physical therapist should answer questions asked by the family as long as they are within the therapist's scope of practice. A therapist should possess a basic understanding of expected functional outcomes of patients with spinal cord injuries.

5. Answer: 1   Resource: Adkins (p. 165)
A physical therapist should give the highest priority to educating the patient on appropriate skin care including pressure relief activities. A patient with C7 tetraplegia can perform lateral and forward weight shifting in the wheelchair to assist with pressure relief.

6. Answer: 1   Resource: Reese (p. 481)
A lesion involving the motor component of the facial nerve from damage to the nucleus is considered a lower motor neuron lesion. The most likely clinical presentation is facial muscle weakness ipsilateral to the lesion.

7. Answer: 4   Resource: Haggard (p. 39)
The cultural background of a patient without additional information offers little indication as to the patient's ability to comprehend a home exercise program.

8. Answer: 1   Resource: Guide to Physical Therapist Practice (p. S42)
Physical therapist assistants routinely perform physical therapy procedures such as fitting of an assistive device. The remaining options are activities that should only be performed by a physical therapist.

9. Answer: 3   Resource: Irwin (p. 357)
Diaphragmatic breathing is often used as a method to increase activity of the diaphragm during inspiration, while diminishing the reliance on accessory muscles.

10. Answer: 1   Resource: Long (p. 144)
Setting an ankle-foot orthosis in 5-10 degrees of dorsiflexion may serve to reduce genu recurvatum by inhibiting full extension of the knee during mid-stance.

11. Answer: 1   Resource: Currier (p. 284)
The degrees of freedom for two independent samples can be calculated using the formula $df = N + N - 2$. In the supplied example, the calculation is as follows: $df = 12 + 10 - 2 = 20$.

12. Answer: 3   Resource: Portney (p. 119)
Cluster sampling is defined as successive random sampling of a series of units in the population. Cluster sampling is often utilized when a researcher is unable to obtain a complete listing of an identified population. Since the technique requires two or more samples to be drawn, sampling error is increased.

13. Answer: 2   Resource: Best (p. 239)
A correlation coefficient of $r = .87$ is classified as high to very high. As a result, performance on the scholastic aptitude test and grade point average in a physical therapy academic program are strongly related.

14. Answer: 2   Resource: Magee (p. 460)
The hip is a ball and socket joint whose resting position is 30 degrees flexion, 30 degrees abduction, and slight lateral rotation. The close packed position is extension and medial rotation.

15. Answer: 4   Resource: Magee (p. 12)
Paresthesias of the long and ring fingers are commonly associated with the C7 nerve root, while the thumb and index finger are associated with C6.

16. Answer: 4   Resource: Magee (p. 129)
Lateral flexion, extension, and rotation are all components of the vertebral artery test. Extension is the most likely motion to assess the integrity of the intervertebral foramen, while lateral flexion and rotation have a greater effect on the vertebral artery.

17. Answer: 2   Resource: O'Sullivan - Physical Rehabilitation (p. 969)
Diplopia refers to double vision caused by defective function of the extraocular muscles. Often times a patient with diplopia is instructed to wear a patch alternately over one of his/her eyes. Specific strengthening exercises of the extraocular muscles can serve to improve the patient's vision.

18. Answer: 3   Resource: Sine (p. 25)
A patient with T5 paraplegia would have full innervation of the upper extremity muscles and limited trunk control. As a result the patient should be able to perform transfers independently, however would require bathroom adaptations such as grab bars and anti-slip mats to promote safety.

19. Answer: 1   Resource: Kendall (p. 241)
The flexor pollicis brevis inserts on the volar aspect of the base of the proximal phalanx of the thumb. The muscle flexes the metacarpophalangeal and carpometacarpal joints of the thumb and assists in opposition.

20. Answer: 2   Resource: Pauls (p. 601)
Chronic bronchitis is an obstructive disease characterized by increased mucus secretion of the tracheobronchial tree. Postural drainage techniques and breathing exercises can serve to clear secretions and improve ventilation.

21. Answer: 3   Resource: Ratliffe (p. 254)
Osteogenesis imperfecta is an autosomal disorder of collagen synthesis that affects bone metabolism. As a result, an infant with this condition is extremely susceptible to fractures during even basic activities such as being carried or bathing. The most common characteristic of osteogenesis imperfecta is bone fragility resulting in fractures.

22. Answer: 3   Resource: Pierson (p. 266)
The antecubital region refers to a triangular area immediately anterior to and below the elbow. Elbow flexion and extension place significant pressure on an infusion site in the antecubital region.

23. Answer: 4   Resource: Paz (p. 649)
The six-minute walk test provides an indirect measure of cardiovascular endurance by examining the distance a patient can walk in six minutes. Patients are instructed to walk as far and as fast as possible in six minutes.

24. Answer: 3   Resource: Rothstein (p. 445)
Patients with right CVA and left hemiplegia commonly have a distorted awareness of self image.

25. Answer: 3   Resource: Pierson (p. 149)
An average adult size wheelchair has the following dimensions: Seat depth = 16 inches, seat width = 18 inches, back height = 16-16.5 inches, arm rest length = 9 inches above the chair seat, seat height/leg length = 19.5-20.5 inches.

26. Answer: 2   Resource: Magee (p. 638)
Pain in the calf produced by passive dorsiflexion of the foot with an extended leg is typically referred to as Homans' sign. This objective finding can be indicative of thrombophlebitis or thrombosis.

27. Answer: 2   Resource: Ratliffe (p. 241)
A patient with Duchenne muscular dystrophy often exhibits significant proximal muscle weakness, particularly in the shoulders and pelvic girdle. As the condition advances, the muscular weakness encompasses the distal musculature and interferes with activities of daily living.

28. Answer: 3   Resource: Kettenbach (p. 110)
The assessment section of a S.O.A.P. note provides a physical therapist with the opportunity to discuss patient progress toward achieving established goals.

29. Answer: 2   Resource: Rothstein (p. 689)
The palmar grasp reflex is elicited through maintained pressure to the palm of the hand resulting in finger flexion. The reflex begins at birth and is integrated at approximately four to six months.

30. Answer: 4   Resource: Kisner (p. 616)
Incontinence refers to an inability to control the release of urine, feces, or gas. Education may include basic information related to incontinence as well as referral to the patient's primary care provider. Research demonstrates that a vast majority of patients with incontinence can be successfully treated with noninvasive techniques such as pelvic floor exercises, biofeedback, and electrical stimulation.

31. Answer: 3   Resource: Ratliffe (p. 230)
Klinefelter syndrome is characterized by the presence of an extra X chromosome. Individuals with this syndrome are characterized by small testes, abnormally long limbs, and below average intelligence. The syndrome is estimated to occur in one of 700 live male births.

32. Answer: 2   Resource: Frownfelter (p. 484)
Applying direct pressure with the hands on the lateral border of the ribs with the patient in supine can promote a more efficient breathing pattern. Physical therapy management for a child with cystic fibrosis may include bronchial drainage techniques, chest percussion, vibration, and suctioning.

33. **Answer: 1   Resource: Richard (p. 137)**
Silver sulfadiazine is a sulfa drug that can produce a decrease in the number of circulating white blood cells (leukopenia). The topical antibiotic works by interfering with bacterial nucleic acid production by disrupting folic acid synthesis in susceptible bacteria. Additional problems encountered with sulfa drugs include gastrointestinal distress and allergic reactions.

34. **Answer: 2   Resource: Pierson (p. 262)**
An electrocardiogram is a common monitoring device for patients with known or suspected cardiac abnormalities. The electrocardiogram measures the electrical activity of the heart as well as heart rate, blood pressure, and respiration rate.

35. **Answer: 2   Resource: Ciccone (p. 606)**
Hallucinogens may cause distortion of senses, altered perception, severe hallucinations, panic, and psychotic reactions. Physical dependence is not characteristic of hallucinogens.

36. **Answer: 2   Resource: Brannon (p. 206)**
Premature ventricular contractions are premature beats arising from ectopic foci in the ventricle. Premature ventricular contractions are the most common form of arrhythmia and may be precipitated by caffeine, anxiety, alcohol, and tobacco.

37. **Answer: 4   Resource: Best (p. 114)**
The dependent variable is defined as the conditions or characteristics that appear, disappear or change as the experimenter introduces, removes or changes the independent variable. In this particular study ultrasound is the independent variable, while blood flow and nerve conduction velocity are the dependent variables.

38. **Answer: 2   Resource: Pierson (p. 190)**
Touch down weight bearing allows the foot of an involved extremity to contact the ground for balance, but does not permit weight bearing.

39. **Answer: 1   Resource: O'Sullivan - Physical Rehabilitation (p. 147)**
Barognosis is a cortical sensation that is responsible for recognition of the weight of an object. It is responsible for the ability to differentiate weight between two or more objects.

40. **Answer: 3   Resource: Pierson (p. 45)**
98.6 degrees Fahrenheit or 37 degrees Celsius is considered normal body temperature.

41. **Answer: 1   Resource: Irwin (p. 380)**
Coughing is an efficient and effective method used to clear secretions from the airways. It is often a standard component of a chest physical therapy program.

42. **Answer: 1   Resource: Pierson (p. 54)**
A rate of 2-3 mm Hg per second will enable the physical therapist to identify normal Korotkoff's sounds and obtain a valid measure of the patient's blood pressure. Rates faster than 2-3 mm Hg will tend to increase the measurement error of the obtained readings.

43. **Answer: 2   Resource: Norkin (p. 196)**
The axis of the goniometer should be positioned over the center of the cranial aspect of the head. The stationary arm should be parallel to an imaginary line between the two acromial processes, while the moving arm should be aligned with the tip of the nose.

44. **Answer: 4   Resource: Guide to Physical Therapist Practice (p. S50)**
Anthropometric measurements can be used to quantify muscle atrophy and edema, however are not used to examine strength.

45. **Answer: 4   Resource: Pierson (p. 266)**
Patients should not experience significant pain around an I.V. site. A nurse may be able to modify or reposition the I.V. in order to reduce or eliminate the patient's pain.

46. **Answer: 1   Resource: Minor (p. 305)**
Guarding a patient in front and toward the affected side while descending stairs provides the physical therapist with the greatest opportunity to assist the patient in the event of a fall.

47. **Answer: 3   Resource: Pierson (p. 57)**
A blood pressure cuff that is too narrow in relation to a patient's arm will tend to artificially increase measured values. The width of the bladder should be 40% of the circumference of the midpoint of the limb. An average size adult requires a bladder that is 5-6 inches wide.

48. **Answer: 4   Resource: Goodman (p. 456)**
A rapidly growing neoplasm often results in pain due to direct pressure or displacement of specific nerves. Pain can also occur due to interference with blood supply or from blockage within an organ. Symptoms are magnified as the neoplasm continues to grow.

49. **Answer: 4   Resource: Irwin (p. 242)**
Vital capacity equals the sum of inspiratory reserve volume, tidal volume, and expiratory reserve volume.

50. **Answer: 1   Resource: Magee (p. 122)**
A foraminal compression test or Spurling's test is considered to be positive if pain radiates into the arm toward the side of head flexion during compression. The provocative test can be administered in progressive stages.

51. Answer: 4   Resource: Irwin (p. 357)
In diaphragmatic breathing exercises the patient should direct the air so that the dominant hand, placed over the midrectus abdominis area, rises during inspiration.

52. Answer: 3   Resource: National Safety Council (p. 145)
Altered mental status and elevated skin temperatures are classic signs associated with heat stroke. Heat stroke is a medical emergency that can result in death. Treatment should focus on attempting to rapidly cool the victim.

53. Answer: 3   Resource: Brannon (p. 3)
An increase in systolic blood pressure of greater than 20 mm Hg or a decrease of greater than 15 mm Hg both exceed the typical limits associated with a phase I cardiac rehabilitation program.

54. Answer: 1   Resource: Clinical Companion (p. 207)
Amyotrophic lateral sclerosis is a progressive syndrome marked by muscular weakness and atrophy with spasticity and hyperreflexia due to degeneration of the motor neurons of the spinal cord, medulla, and cortex. The disease is commonly referred to as Lou Gehrig's disease and is not associated with mental deterioration.

55. Answer: 4   Resource: Clinical Companion (p. 91)
Posterior cord syndrome is a relatively rare form of incomplete spinal cord injury that is characterized by a loss of proprioception, two-point discrimination, and stereognosis with preserved motor function. The injury is typically classified as a cervical hyperextension injury.

56. Answer: 1   Resource: Clinical Companion (p. 104)
The Barthel Index consists of 10 activities of daily living and is often used as a screening tool in rehabilitation, long-term care settings, and home care. Scoring on the assessment ranges from 0-100 in increments of 5. A score of 100 indicates that the patient is independent with mobility and self-care activities in the home. Observation and scoring should take approximately one hour.

57. Answer: 2   Resource: Guide to Physical Therapist Practice (p. S42)
Physical therapy aides are nonlicensed health care workers who perform routine tasks related to the operation of a physical therapy clinic. Aides are not typically allowed to make daily entries in the medical record.

58. Answer: 2   Resource: Michlovitz (p. 143)
The length of a highboy tank does not permit a patient to fully extend the lower extremities, however its depth permits immersion to the midthoracic region.

59. Answer: 2   Resource: Kisner (p. 431)
Range of motion activities are performed almost immediately following a total knee replacement. Failure to achieve 90 degrees of knee flexion range of motion prior to discharge from the hospital increases the incidence of additional medical intervention.

60. Answer: 4   Resource: Adkins (p. 184)
A patient with paraplegia does not require the use of projection wheel rims due to full innervation of the upper extremities. Patients with C5-C6 tetraplegia utilize projection hand rims in order to assist with manual wheelchair propulsion.

61. Answer: 4   Resource: Pierson (p. 202)
A four-point gait pattern offers maximum stability with low energy expenditure. The gait pattern requires bilateral ambulation aids and resembles a normal gait pattern, however is significantly slower.

62. Answer: 3   Resource: Kisner (p. 650)
The internal intercostals act to depress the ribs during forceful expiration.

63. Answer: 3   Resource: Kendall (p. 187)
The ability to move through partial range of motion in a gravity eliminated position is consistent with a muscle grade of poor minus.

64. Answer: 2   Resource: Kendall (p. 215)
Gravity eliminated testing positions are indicated when a patient cannot maintain the test position against the resistance of gravity. The gravity eliminated position for the hip flexors is sidelying.

65. Answer: 3   Resource: Pierson (p. 194)
The handgrip of a proper fitting cane should be at the level of the greater trochanter.

66. Answer: 1   Resource: Clinical Companion (p. 134)
Doppler ultrasonography is a diagnostic technique that uses ultrasound to produce an image or photograph of an organ or tissue. The noninvasive test is commonly used to evaluate blood flow in the major veins and arteries of the upper and lower extremities as well as in the extracranial cerebrovascular system.

67. Answer: 3   Resource: O'Sullivan - Physical Rehabilitation (p. 1061)
Independent propulsion is facilitated by the use of a lightweight wheelchair, while a solid seating system assists with posture and transfer activities. An arm board allows the flaccid upper extremity to be supported and elevating legrests assist to decrease dependent edema.

68. Answer: 2   Resource: Frownfelter (p. 516)
Emphysema is a chronic obstructive pulmonary disease characterized by an increase in the size of air spaces distal to the terminal bronchiole accompanied by destructive changes in their walls. As a result, the lungs become hyperinflated and the chest wall becomes fixed in a hyperinflated position. Total lung capacity and dead space in the lungs significantly increase.

69. Answer: 3   Resource: O'Sullivan - Physical Rehabilitation (p. 182)
Passive range of motion is utilized when assessing tone. The physical therapist should examine resistance to movement in all four extremities.

70. Answer: 1   Resource: Sullivan – Clinical Decision Making (p. 66)
In contract-relax the build up of tension is immediate and may therefore be problematic when the limitation in movement is accompanied by pain. In contrast, hold-relax requires a gradual buildup of tension over a period of several seconds and is therefore often the treatment of choice when pain is present.

71. Answer: 4   Resource: Minor (p. 420)
Using the cane with the left upper extremity allows the patient to increase his/her base of support and facilitates shifting the center of gravity away from the involved extremity. Advancing the involved leg with the assistive device allows the patient to transfer weight from the involved lower extremity.

72. Answer: 1   Resource: Clinical Companion (p. 313)
A posterior leaf spring ankle-foot orthosis is a plastic insert with a semirigid posterior upright that yields slightly at heel contact and recoils when the brace is unloaded during the swing phase. It is used to assist with dorsiflexion, however does not promote medial or lateral stability.

73. Answer: 3   Resource: Clinical Companion (p. 316)
Patients can experience itching or skin irritation as a result of a reaction to a liner of an orthosis. Since an orthosis is applied directly over the skin it is imperative to utilize a liner that maximizes patient comfort, promotes cleanliness, limits moisture, and reduces skin irritation. Failure to select an appropriate liner may result in skin breakdown or voluntary discontinuance of the orthosis.

74. Answer: 3   Resource: O'Toole (p. 1844)
Approximate normal ranges for cholesterol are as follows: cholesterol < 200 mg/dL, high density lipoproteins = 30-80 mg/dL, low density lipoproteins = 60-180 mg/dL.

75. Answer: 2   Resource: Ratliffe (p. 28)
The rooting reflex is a primitive reflex that is normally present from 28 weeks of gestation through three months of age. The reflex assists the mother when feeding an infant.

76. Answer: 3   Resource: Pierson (p. 266)
A small amount of blood backed up in an I.V. line is not an abnormal occurrence. By repositioning the peripheral I.V. line normal flow can often be reestablished.

77. Answer: 2   Resource: Irwin (p. 191)
Intermittent claudication is precipitated by exertion and relieved by rest. As a result, signs of resting claudication may be indicative of a more advanced vascular disorder, thus restricting the patient's ability to take part in an active exercise program.

78. Answer: 2   Resource: Booher (p. 243)
A small increase in effusion of an involved joint is a common objective finding following return to athletic competition, however an antalgic gait indicates the need to modify the athlete's level of participation. The patient should be required to complete another functional progression before being allowed to return to basketball without restriction.

79. Answer: 3   Resource: Walter (p. 5)
The physical therapist should discuss the situation with his/her immediate supervisor. It is important for a therapist to be aware of the established chain of commands within any health care organization.

80. Answer: 1   Resource: Booher (p. 404)
Pronation of the foot consists of eversion of the heel, abduction of the forefoot, and dorsiflexion of the subtalar and midtarsal joints.

81. Answer: 2   Resource: Pierson (p. 149)
Measuring the distance from the seat of the chair to the olecranon process with the elbow in 90 degrees of flexion, and then adding 1 inch determines armrest height in a wheelchair.

82. Answer: 3   Resource: Scott - Promoting Legal Awareness (p. 69)
Failure to have a patient examined by a physician after a fall can be considered a negligent act. In many facilities an incident report is required when a patient comes in contact with the floor.

83. Answer: 4   Resource: Mahler (p. 38)
Normal values for various spirometric tests are based on age, gender, and height. Physical therapists must be cautious when interpreting the results of pulmonary function tests since they rely on a high degree of subject cooperation.

84. Answer: 2   Resource: Neistadt (p. 315)
Occupational therapists focus on activities of daily living, work and leisure skills, and as a result may be best suited to address the obstacles that impact the patient's ability to return to work.

85. Answer: 2   Resource: Mahler (p. 41)
A legal guardian or parent must sign the informed consent form for a minor.

86. Answer: 4   Resource: Davies (p. 73)
A patient with left hemiplegia should be instructed to transfer toward the affected side. The patient's affected upper extremity should be supported in order to prevent injury, subluxation or increasing abnormal tonal patterns.

87. Answer: 4   Resource: Nixon (p. 174)
A patient with C7 tetraplegia has good shoulder and scapular strength. The latissimus dorsi and triceps are present as well as partial innervation of the finger flexors and extensors. These muscles are required for proper positioning during self range of motion activities.

88. Answer: 1   Resource: Mahler (p. 56)
All skinfold measurements should be taken on the right side of the body. Acceptable skinfold sites include the abdominal, biceps, chest/pectoral, medial calf, midaxillary, subscapular, suprailiac, and thigh. The abdominal skinfold site requires the therapist to utilize a vertical fold.

89. Answer: 2   Resource: Kisner (p. 665)
In diaphragmatic breathing, the patient's hand placed over the midrectus area should rise during inspiration and fall during expiration.

90. Answer: 1   Resource: Kendall (p. 281)
The infraspinatus functions as a lateral rotator of the shoulder and is innervated by the suprascapular nerve.

91. Answer: 3   Resource: Nixon (p. 119)
A patient with C6 tetraplegia can often perform independent sliding board transfers due to innervation of the deltoids, biceps, and rotator cuff muscles.

92. Answer: 1   Resource: Standards of Practice
The most appropriate physical therapist action is to contact the referring physician and request approval for the additional physical therapy visits. The patient has additional scheduled appointments and there is no information given that would indicate the patient has achieved the established therapy goals or exhausted his/her insurance benefits.

93. Answer: 3   Resource: Curtis (p. 35)
Patients with Medicare pay 20% for all outpatient physical therapy, occupational therapy, and speech therapy services.

94. Answer: 2   Resource: Guide to Physical Therapist Practice (p. S42)
The physical therapist is responsible for delegating tasks to the physical therapist assistant and as a result must be aware of the assistant's clinical competence. A meeting would enable the individuals to engage in dialogue addressing the working relationship.

95. Answer: 1   Resource: Miller (p. 1636)
Skeletal traction is often utilized to immobilize, position, or align a bone during a portion of the healing process. Force is applied to the bone through surgically inserted pins, wires or tongs. Although skeletal traction can be used on a number of bones, it is most commonly utilized on the femur.

96. Answer: 2   Resource: Kendall (p. 268)
The biceps brachii is innervated by the C5-C6 spinal level and therefore should not produce pain in the C7-C8 dermatome.

97. Answer: 1   Resource: Sultz (p. 221)
Medicare Part B covers outpatient medical and surgical services and supplies, diagnostic tests, ambulatory surgery center facility fees for approved procedures, preventive services, and durable medical equipment. Hospice care would be covered through Medicare Part A.

98. Answer: 4   Resource: Mathews (p. 114)
Health maintenance organizations pay participating physicians on a capitated or prospective basis and as a result provide incentives for physicians to utilize services in an effective and efficient manner.

99. Answer: 2   Resource: O'Sullivan - Physical Rehabilitation (p. 861)
A burn to the area surrounding the heel often results in a plantar flexion contracture. Special care must be taken to stretch the ankle into dorsiflexion to avoid a plantar flexion contracture.

100. Answer: 3   Resource: Sultz (p. 245)
Medicaid is a program that provides medical and health related services to qualifying individuals and families with low income and resources. Medicaid is a joint venture between the Federal and State government. Medicaid offers a broad range of services, however low product reimbursement rates makes it difficult for many Medicaid recipients to secure a primary care provider.

101. Answer: 1   Resource: Hertling (p. 564)
A third degree sprain of the acromioclavicular joint would be necessary to cause increased elevation of the clavicular end of the acromion (step deformity).

102. Answer: 3   Resource: Arends (p. 47)
The cognitive domain of learning is divided into six levels: knowledge, comprehension, application, analysis, synthesis, and evaluation.

103. Answer: 1   Resource: Mahler (p. 64)
Physical therapists gain information on a patient's response to exercise through various subjective and objective measures, however remain dependent on a patient's willingness to exert a maximal effort in order to collect meaningful data.

104. Answer: 3   Resource: Mahler (p. 70)
Termination guidelines for submaximal exercise testing indicate that a subject should not exceed 85% of his/her age-predicted maximal heart rate.

105. Answer: 3   Resource: Anderson (p. 114)
Expressive or motor aphasia is a condition that can occur due to a CVA. Patients with this condition can understand language, but cannot express themselves through language.

106. Answer: 4   Resource: Kendall (p. 179)
An example of active insufficiency of the hamstrings occurs when a patient attempts to achieve full hip extension with the knee already in a position of extreme flexion.

107. Answer: 3   Resource: Payton - Psychosocial Aspects (p. 8)
The statement "having cancer must be very difficult for you to deal with" acknowledges the patient's present condition without providing a false sense of hope. This type of approach is particularly important with patients who have recently diagnosed with a terminal disease.

108. Answer: 2   Resource: Richard (p. 44)
Patients with burns often experience a number of sensory changes. These changes can include impaired sensation or increased sensitivity. Although many factors contribute to sensory alteration, the depth of the burn appears to be the best predictor.

109. Answer: 1   Resource: Davies (p. 5)
The Bobath concept for neurological rehabilitation is often termed neurodevelopmental technique (NDT). This theory of rehabilitation emphasizes influencing normal movement through handling of the patient and does not utilize abnormal movement patterns or reflexes.

110. Answer: 2   Resource: Rothstein (p. 696)
The maximum score for the APGAR assessment is 10.

111. Answer: 3   Resource: Scott - Professional Ethics (p. 56)
The physical therapist must determine whether the patient understands the importance of physical therapy. If the patient continues to refuse treatment, the therapist should inform him of the expected consequences.

112. Answer: 2   Resource: Somers (p. 31)
Autonomic dysreflexia is a condition that occurs in patients with spinal cord injuries above the T6 level. The condition is triggered when a noxious stimuli is present followed by an increase in autonomic responses. Symptoms include headache, blotching of the skin, dilation of the pupils, nausea, and a dangerous increase in blood pressure.

113. Answer: 2   Resource: Brotzman (p. 287)
Total hip replacement using noncemented fixation requires toe touch weight bearing for a minimum of six weeks in order to allow adequate time for tissue and bone growth around the prosthesis.

114. Answer: 2   Resource: Kendall (p. 286)
To perform a manual muscle test of the lower trapezius, the patient should be positioned in prone with the shoulder abducted greater than 120 degrees. Pressure should be applied against the forearm in a direction towards the floor.

115. Answer: 2   Resource: Neistadt (p. 273)
Ideational apraxia is most commonly due to a lesion in the patient's dominant parietal lobe of the cerebrum. The condition deals with errors in concepts and sequencing of tasks.

116. Answer: 1   Resource: Umphred (p. 771)
Distraction and stretching techniques are used when there is a decrease in range of motion due to hypertonicity. The activity is not appropriate to prevent further subluxation in a patient with a flaccid upper extremity.

117. Answer: 1   Resource: Mahler (p. 126)
Failure of the heart rate to increase with further increases in intensity occurs when a patient is no longer able to meet the demands imposed by a given exercise intensity. This objective finding often signifies that the patient has produced a maximal effort.

118. Answer: 2   Resource: Goodman (p. 50)
A physical therapist should attempt to determine if a patient is under the influence of alcohol. Alcohol consumption can significantly influence a patient's ability to tolerate treatment. Asking the patient directly is an immediate step that can be used to gather additional information.

119. Answer: 3   Resource: Adkins (p. 182)
A patient with C4 tetraplegia does not have the upper extremity muscles innervated that are necessary to operate a hand control. Appropriate controls for a patient with C4 tetraplegia include sip and puff, chin or mouth control.

120. Answer: 2 Resource: Scott – Promoting Legal Awareness (p. 70)
An incident report does not relate to the patient examination or plan of care and as a result should not be referred to or included in the medical record. Physical therapists should include a concurrent treatment entry in the medical record that provides the necessary information related to the patient's injury and subsequent intervention.

121. Answer: 3 Resource: Hertling (p. 355)
Patellar tracking dysfunction can be influenced by each of the identified options, however the only dynamic factor involves the vastus medialis obliquus muscle.

122. Answer: 3 Resource: O'Sullivan - Physical Rehabilitation (p. 630)
A six inch ace wrap is the most appropriate bandage for wrapping the residual limb of a patient with a transfemoral amputation. The six inch wrap adequately covers the larger surface area of the residual limb.

123. Answer: 3 Resource: Kisner (p. 156)
Bouncing while attempting to stretch a muscle is synonymous with ballistic stretching. This specific stretching technique promotes tension in the muscle that is being stretched and therefore limits the effectiveness of the stretch.

124. Answer: 3 Resource: Mahler (p. 199)
Pursed lip breathing is a common breathing technique employed to assist patients with chronic obstructive pulmonary disease to deal with shortness of breath. Proper technique requires a patient to breathe in through the nose; breathe out twice as long as he/she breathes in; minimize the action of the abdominals; and keep the lips loosely pursed during expiration.

125. Answer: 4 Resource: Clinical Companion (p. 315)
Spina bifida is a neural tube defect characterized by a defective closure of the vertebral column. Although the exact clinical presentation of spina bifida can vary considerably, hip-knee-ankle-foot orthoses (HKAFO) are often employed to assist pediatric patients with ambulation activities. The high energy cost of ambulating with the orthoses often makes community ambulation difficult.

126. Answer: 3 Resource: Kettenbach (p. 110)
The assessment section of a S.O.A.P. note allows a physical therapist to express his/her professional judgment and discuss the patient's progress in physical therapy.

127. Answer: 1 Resource: Kendall (p. 42)
Tight hip flexors result in excessive anterior tilt of the pelvis, as a result actual hamstrings length will be greater than the measured length.

128. Answer: 2 Resource: Clinical Companion (p. 324)
A lightweight wheelchair will be significantly easier for the patient to propel and maneuver, while a rigid frame provides the necessary durability and strength required for an active individual.

129. Answer: 2 Resource: Norkin - Structure and Function (p. 458)
The normal degree of toe out during free speed walking is 7 degrees. Increased speed serves to diminish the degree of toe out.

130. Answer: 4 Resource: Magee (p. 478)
Not enough information is provided to determine if the variation in the measurements is due to a true leg length discrepancy or a functional leg length discrepancy.

131. Answer: 4 Resource: Scott – Health Care Malpractice (p. 142)
Spoliation refers to the loss or destruction of medical records.

132. Answer: 3 Resource: Nixon (p. 51)
A patient with C7-C8 tetraplegia should be able to attain between 60-80% of normal vital capacity, produce eight syllables per breath, and independently clear secretions. This goal can be attained through proper positioning, focus on breathing patterns, use of an abdominal binder, strengthening of the diaphragm, and assisted coughing techniques.

133. Answer: 4 Resource: Kettenbach (p. 83)
Long-term goals describe the functional abilities a patient will possess at the conclusion of therapy. A properly written long-term goal must include audience, behavior, condition, and degree.

134. Answer: 4 Resource: Pierson (p. 193)
A walker would be the most appropriate assistive device to use since the patient can stand without support, however has only fair standing balance and is impulsive at times. A walker does not require a great deal of coordination.

135. Answer: 2 Resource: Pierson (p. 340)
Placing bricks under a desk is a reasonable and cost efficient accommodation to increase desk height.

136. Answer: 3 Resource: Haggard (p. 27)
It is essential to assess the needs of the target audience prior to designing a formal or informal presentation.

137. Answer: 4 Resource: Booher (p. 243)
A functional progression is a series of progressive active movements designed to simulate a selected sport or activity. Failure to successfully complete a functional progression often indicates that a patient is not ready to return to competition.

138. Answer: 1   Resource: Mathews (p. 114)
Capitation is defined as a fixed payment to a provider per enrollee. Managed care organizations utilize capitation to shift some of the financial risk toward individual providers.

139. Answer: 4   Resource: Hertling (p. 66)
A score of ten on a subjective pain scale is best described as the most severe pain imaginable.

140. Answer: 3   Resource: Goodman (p. 310)
Decreased blood glucose levels result from inadequate food intake or excessive insulin levels. Symptoms include confusion, weakness, clammy skin, and increased pulse rate. Increased blood glucose levels indicate there is not enough insulin. Symptoms include polydipsia and polyuria.

141. Answer: 2   Resource: Brannon (p. 316)
Rating on a perceived exertion scale provides a subjective measure of exercise intensity. A rating of 12 on Borg's 20 - point scale corresponds to roughly 60 percent of the age-adjusted maximum heart rate.

142. Answer: 3   Resource: Levangie (p. 440)
Initial contact refers to the instant the foot of the leading extremity hits the ground.

143. Answer: 2   Resource: Bennett (p. 144)
A stroke involving the right hemisphere often affects the left side of the body. As a result it is common for a patient with a lesion in the right hemisphere to exhibit decreased awareness of the left side of the body. Neglect is often manifested as a disregard for the involved side of the body.

144. Answer: 3   Resource: Kahn (p. 30)
The physical therapist and the patient should wear ultraviolet opaque goggles during the treatment session.

145. Answer: 3   Resource: Scott - Promoting Legal Awareness (p. 69)
An incident report is a formal document that summarizes the facts associated with an adverse event.

146. Answer: 4   Resource: Irwin (p. 225)
Bedrest is the primary cause of acute postoperative thrombosis in the lower extremities. Ankle pumps can be an effective active exercise to facilitate venous return, and decrease the risk of deep vein thrombosis.

147. Answer: 3   Resource: Hertling (p. 339)
The McMurray test is designed to identify possible meniscal involvement.

148. Answer: 1   Resource: Hoppenfeld (p. 214)
The dorsal pedal artery is located between the tendons of the extensor hallucis longus and the extensor digitorum longus. The pulse can be absent in up to 15% of the population.

149. Answer: 3   Resource: Magee (p. 193)
Muscles responsible for abduction of the shoulder include the deltoid, supraspinatus, infraspinatus, subscapularis, and teres minor. Each of the muscles is innervated at the C5-C6 neurologic level.

150. Answer: 2   Resource: Neistadt (p. 792)
The physiatrist is the leader of the treatment team and therefore should address outcome potential with the family.

151. Answer: 3   Resource: Sullivan - An Integrated Approach (p. 86)
Lateral weight shifting, forward and backward shifting with or without upper extremity involvement are all forms of controlled mobility.

152. Answer: 2   Resource: Umphred (p. 722)
Dysmetria is an inability to modulate movement where patients will either overestimate or underestimate their targets. Dysmetria is a common clinical finding with cerebellar dysfunction.

153. Answer: 3   Resource: Pierson (p. 275)
The newspaper provides a barrier between the bag and any utilized surface within the patient's home. The newspaper limits the transmission of potentially infectious material.

154. Answer: 1   Resource: Umphred (p. 724)
Dysdiadochokinesia is the term used to describe the inability to perform rapid alternating movements. Dysdiadochokinesia is often observed in patients with multiple sclerosis due to demyelination in the cerebellum.

155. Answer: 3   Resource: Davis (p. 70)
Gathering relevant information is always the most immediate action when faced with an ethical dilemma. The step allows the physical therapist to be fully informed and may assist the therapist to resolve the dilemma.

156. Answer: 2   Resource: Goodman (p. 37)
Although stated inconsistencies should be documented, it is important to avoid making a definitive judgment until sufficient data has been gathered.

157. Answer: 3   Resource: Brotzman (p. 94)
A restriction in the posterior capsule may lead to anterior and superior translation of the humeral head. As a result, it is often advisable to incorporate posterior capsule stretching into the treatment program.

158. Answer: 4   Resource: Goodman (p. 38)
The question "What do you hope to achieve in physical therapy?" is an open-ended question that presents the patient with a myriad of possible responses.

SAMPLE EXAM ANSWERS: EXAM ONE   267

159. Answer: 2   Resource: Haggard (p. 49)
A physical therapist must attempt to engage the patient in his/her rehabilitation program by using a variety of motivational strategies. Possible strategies include emphasizing patient accomplishments, utilizing treatment activities that build confidence, and providing the patient with a sense of control over his/her current condition.

160. Answer: 3   Resource: Miller (p. 1843)
Hemoglobin refers to an iron based pigment that binds and transports oxygen in blood. The typical reference range for a male is 14-18 gm/dL, therefore a value of 8 gm/dL may result in decreased exercise tolerance, fatigue, and tachycardia.

161. Answer: 3   Resource: Levangie (p. 445)
Step length is defined as the distance between two successive points of contact of opposite extremities.

162. Answer: 2   Resource: Magee (p. 43)
Myelography can be used to detect disc herniation, nerve root entrapment, spinal stenosis, and tumors of the spinal cord.

163. Answer: 4   Resource: Best (p. 216)
The variance provides information on how scores in a distribution are dispersed about the mean. A small variance indicates that most of the scores are relatively close to the mean, while a large variance indicates that most of the scores are further away from the mean.

164. Answer: 3   Resource: Pierson (p. 202)
A four-point gait pattern is a deliberate, stable gait pattern using bilateral assistive devices. The gait pattern can be used as a transition to a two-point gait pattern.

165. Answer: 3   Resource: Brotzman (p. 100)
The majority of rotator cuff tears occur in individuals greater than 40 years of age with a history of recurrent shoulder symptoms. A large tear is typically considered to be between 3-5 cm in diameter and most often requires 24-28 weeks of rehabilitation before a patient is allowed to return to full activity without restrictions.

166. Answer: 4   Resource: Hertling (p. 709)
The inferior lateral angles of the sacrum are formed by the transverse processes of S5.

167. Answer: 3   Resource: Brannon (p. 193)
The QRS complex reflects the electrical activity of the ventricles during the cardiac cycle. If the physical therapist identifies eight QRS complexes in a six second interval, the therapist should multiply the number by ten to determine the patient's heart rate.

168. Answer: 1   Resource: Brannon (p. 190)
Measurement error decreases as the time associated with data collection increases.

169. Answer: 3   Resource: Scott - Professional Ethics (p. 56)
The physical therapist has a legal obligation to inform the patient of the expected consequences of refusing treatment.

170. Answer: 2   Resource: Hall (p. 365)
Correct technique includes pulling the muscles up and in. Placing a downward pressure on the pelvic floor serves to exacerbate the patient's condition. Research indicates that nearly 50% of patients who receive verbal instructions for pelvic floor contractions perform the exercises incorrectly.

171. Answer: 3   Resource: Guide to Physical Therapist Practice (p. S42)
Physical therapist assistants routinely implement therapeutic exercise programs based on an established plan of care.

172. Answer: 2   Resource: Guide to Physical Therapist Practice (p. S42)
State practice acts differ significantly in their rules and regulations associated with the supervision of support personnel at off site locations. In all cases, however the individual needs of the patient should be the most important priority.

173. Answer: 3   Resource: Pierson (p. 160)
Elevating legrests promote patient comfort and stability when the wheelchair is in a reclined position.

174. Answer: 1   Resource: Walter (p. 242)
Quality assurance programs are designed to assess the services provided and the outcomes achieved for the purpose of improving patient care. Prior to collecting, analyzing or interpreting specific data it is essential to identify the important aspects of patient care provided by the department.

175. Answer: 4   Resource: Pierson (p. 263)
An arterial line is inserted directly into an artery and is used to continuously monitor blood pressure or to obtain blood samples.

176. Answer: 2   Resource: Adkins (p. 140)
Key muscles that are partially or fully innervated at the C6 level include the brachialis, biceps, trapezius, deltoids, rhomboids, latissimus dorsi, rotator cuff, serratus anterior, and extensor carpi radialis.

177. Answer: 1   Resource: Rothstein (p. 529)
Respiratory acidosis is characterized by decreased pH, increased $PaCO_2$, and HCO_3 that is within normal limits.

178. Answer: 4   Resource: Pierson (p. 33)
Positioning in supine makes a patient susceptible to additional tissue damage on the posterior calcaneus.

179. Answer: 3   Resource: Adkins (p. 139)
A forward raise for pressure relief requires adequate strength of the biceps for elbow flexion and the deltoids for movement at the shoulder in the directions of flexion and extension.

180. Answer: 2   Resource: O'Sullivan - Physical Rehabilitation (p. 898)
Independence with bowel and bladder care would be extremely difficult for a patient with C6 tetraplegia. Triceps, flexor carpi radialis, finger extensors, and intrinsic hand muscles are often necessary in order to gain independence.

181. Answer: 2   Resource: Kendall (p. 187)
A grade of poor is assigned to a muscle that is capable of moving through the entire range of motion in a gravity eliminated position.

182. Answer: 3   Resource: Pierson (p. 13)
Physical therapists should attempt to limit the use of medical terminology when communicating with patients.

183. Answer: 4   Resource: Sullivan - An Integrated Approach (p. 135)
The rhythmic initiation technique should begin with passive movement of the patient by the physical therapist. Progression using this technique would include active-assistive movement, active movement, and finally resisted movement.

184. Answer: 4   Resource: Hertling (p. 421)
A complete examination of the ankle including ligamentous integrity testing is necessary before any prediction of severity can be made. Diagnostic testing such as x-rays may also be warranted to rule out the possibility of a fracture.

185. Answer: 3   Resource: Standards of Practice
Physical therapists do not have the authority to clear a patient to return to athletic competition. Although the results of the isokinetic examination appear to be excellent there is not enough information given to conclude that the patient should be discharged from physical therapy.

186. Answer: 1   Resource: Brotzman (p. 118)
Patients over 40 years old are more susceptible to shoulder stiffness with prolonged immobilization and as a result physicians tend to limit the length of the immobilization period. In addition, the recurrence rate for dislocation is relatively low in this age group.

187. Answer: 1   Resource: Brotzman (p. 130)
Adhesive capsulitis refers to an inflammation and adherence of the articular capsule resulting in limited joint play and restricted active and passive movement. The condition is more common in women than in men and tends to appear in the fourth, fifth, and sixth decades of life. Patients with diabetes mellitus are particularly susceptible to this condition and often experience a longer duration of symptoms and greater limitation of motion.

188. Answer: 2   Resource: Sullivan - An Integrated Approach (p. 138)
The hold-relax technique utilizes an isometric contraction at the end of available range of motion. The patient is then told to relax as the physical therapist moves the extremity into newly gained range.

189. Answer: 3   Resource: O'Sullivan - Physical Rehabilitation (p. 852)
The percentage of body surface burned in an adult can be calculated using the rule of nines: anterior arm (4.5%) + anterior thorax (18%) + genital area (1%) = 23.5%.

190. Answer: 2   Resource: Michlovitz (p. 200)
A gross estimate of treatment time can be estimated by allotting 5 minutes of time for each area that is 2-3 times the size of the transducer face.

191. Answer: 4   Resource: Kisner (p. 301)
Isometric exercise is the most appropriate form of exercise to promote strength following a prolonged period of immobilization. Isometric exercise allows the patient to utilize specific muscles without placing unnecessary stress on damaged structures.

192. Answer: 1   Resource: Mahler (p. 70)
A physical therapist should select an exercise intensity that is sufficient to elevate the patient's heart rate within the calculated target heart rate range. A rating of 2 on Borg's 10 point perceived exertion scale corresponds to "weak" which provides support for increasing the intensity of the exercise.

193. Answer: 2   Resource: Minor (p. 290)
Assistive devices can easily be adjusted to accommodate individuals of various height and weight.

194. Answer: 2   Resource: O'Sullivan - Physical Rehabilitation (p. 666)
Lateral trunk bending over the prosthetic limb during the stance phase of gait can be caused by a prosthesis with inadequate length.

195. Answer: 2   Resource: Brotzman (p. 147)
The status of bone healing as determined through a radiograph would provide the physician with the best information on the stability of the acetabulum. It is important to emphasize that the physician is the health care provider responsible for determining weight bearing status.

196. Answer: 1   Resource: Brotzman (p. 151)
It is often advisable to review an exercise program with a patient. It is particularly essential in the given scenario since failure to perform the exercises correctly could have a detrimental effect on the patient's condition. Although some of the other presented options may be appropriate, they would not offer the same degree of benefit for the patient.

197. Answer: 4   Resource: Brotzman (p. 191)
Rehabilitative braces with flexion and extension settings are designed to allow controlled motion within a specified range of motion. The braces function to protect the injured limb during the early phases of rehabilitation.

198. Answer: 2   Resource: Magee (p. 297)
Grip strength may vary by 5-10% when comparing the dominant and nondominant hand.

199. Answer: 1   Resource: Brotzman (p. 188)
A study performed by Henning et al. examined anterior cruciate stresses and elongation during functional and rehabilitative activities. The researchers concluded that the proper order of a rehabilitation program with regard to anterior cruciate ligament stress should be the following: crutch walking, stationary cycling, walking, slow running on level surface, faster running on level surface.

200. Answer: 3   Resource: Paz (p. 187)
Contraindications following total hip replacement using a posterolateral surgical approach include hip flexion greater than 90 degrees, adduction, and medial rotation.

Sample Examination: Two

1. A physical therapist supervising a physical therapy student observes the student performing an initial examination. During the examination the patient appears to be uncomfortable with the student and asks to be treated by the supervising therapist. The most appropriate physical therapist action is to:

   1. attempt to convince the patient to accept the student
   2. list the student's academic accomplishments
   3. inform the patient that the student is qualified to complete the examination
   4. complete the examination for the student

2. A patient in a rehabilitation hospital confides to her physical therapist that she has been physically abused by her husband in the past and is concerned about returning home following discharge. The most appropriate therapist action is to:

   1. contact the law enforcement agency
   2. contact the patient's case manager
   3. ask the patient to leave her husband
   4. question the patient's spouse

3. A physical therapist designs an exercise program for a patient rehabilitating from cardiac surgery. During the treatment session the therapist monitors the patient's oxygen saturation rate. Which of the following would be most representative of a normal oxygen saturation rate?

   1. 82%
   2. 87%
   3. 92%
   4. 97%

4. A physical therapist analyzes the gait of a patient rehabilitating from a motor vehicle accident. Which descriptive term is not associated with the stance phase of the gait cycle?

   1. heel strike
   2. deceleration
   3. loading response
   4. mid-stance

5. A patient rehabilitating from a total hip replacement receives home physical therapy services. The patient is currently full weight bearing and is able to ascend and descend stairs independently. The patient expresses that her goal following rehabilitation is to walk one mile each day. The most appropriate plan to accomplish the patient's goal is to:

   1. continue home physical therapy services until the patient's goal is attained
   2. refer the patient to an outpatient orthopedic physical therapy clinic
   3. design a home exercise program that emphasizes progressive ambulation
   4. admit the patient to a rehabilitation hospital

6. A physical therapist treats a 61-year-old male at home following thoracic surgery. As part of treatment, the therapist designs a general exercise program for the patient. The patient is extremely eager to begin the exercise program, however his spouse expresses serious doubt about the program's importance. The most appropriate therapist action is to:

   1. explain to the patient and spouse why the exercise program is an essential part of rehabilitation
   2. redesign the exercise program to address the spouse's concerns
   3. ask the spouse to leave the room during treatment sessions
   4. discharge the patient from physical therapy

7. A recent entry in the medical record indicates a patient exhibits dysdiadochokinesia. Based on the patient's documented deficit, which activity would be the most difficult for the patient?

   1. alternate supination/pronation of the forearm
   2. perform a standing squat
   3. march in place
   4. walk along a straight line

8. A physical therapist attempts to assess the integrity of the L4 spinal level. Which deep tendon reflex would provide the therapist with the most useful information?

   1. lateral hamstrings
   2. medial hamstrings
   3. patellar reflex
   4. Achilles reflex

9. A patient is scheduled to receive occupational and physical therapy services in his home. During the physical therapy examination the therapist determines that the patient requires assistance with tub transfers using a tub bench. The physical therapist is scheduled to treat the patient three times a week, however the occupational therapist cannot examine the patient for six days. The most appropriate physical therapist action is:

   1. practice tub transfers during physical therapy treatment sessions
   2. wait until an occupational therapist can examine the patient
   3. provide the patient with written information on tub transfers
   4. call another agency and request immediate occupational therapy services

10. An orthopedic surgeon instructs a patient to remain non-weight bearing for three weeks following a medial meniscus repair. During the examination it becomes obvious that the patient has not adhered to the prescribed weight bearing status. The most immediate physical therapist action is to:

    1. contact the orthopedic surgeon
    2. explain to the patient the potential consequences of ignoring the weight bearing restrictions
    3. draft a letter to the patient's third party payer
    4. complete an incident report

11. A physical therapist provides an inservice to the rehabilitation department on the Americans with Disabilities Act. Which of the following individuals would not be covered under the act?

    1. a 28-year-old with a documented learning disability
    2. a 46-year-old with severe mental retardation
    3. a 14-year-old that is blind
    4. a 36-year-old homosexual

12. While performing high level balance activities, a patient falls into a piece of equipment that causes a deep laceration to the calf. Immediate first aid includes direct pressure to the area and elevation, however the bleeding does not stop. The physical therapist should continue to administer first aid by providing:

    1. heat to the laceration site
    2. ice to the laceration site
    3. pressure to the dorsalis pedis artery pressure point
    4. pressure to the femoral artery pressure point

13. A physical therapist discusses how to perform pelvic floor muscle strengthening exercises with a 36-year-old female diagnosed with stress incontinence. The patient describes involuntary leakage of urine when she coughs, sneezes or exercises. The most appropriate ratio of rest to hold time when initiating pelvic floor muscle strengthening is:

    1. 1:2
    2. 1:5
    3. 2:1
    4. 5:1

14. A 45-year-old female involved in a phase II cardiac rehabilitation program refuses to take part in a group exercise session. The most appropriate physical therapist action is to:

    1. ask the patient why she is unwilling to participate
    2. inform the patient that she is only hurting herself
    3. notify the patient's insurance provider
    4. discharge the patient from therapy

15. A patient completes a D1 extension pattern for the upper extremity. The prime movers of the scapula during this pattern are the:

    1. trapezius and middle deltoid
    2. pectoralis minor and pectoralis major
    3. serratus anterior, pectoralis major, and anterior deltoid
    4. rhomboids, pectoralis minor, and levator scapulae

16. A physical therapist works with a 70-year-old patient diagnosed with general deconditioning. The patient is pleasant and cooperative, however has short-term memory deficits. The therapist initiates an exercise program that the patient is able to complete with verbal cueing. Which of the following home exercise programs would be the most beneficial for the patient?

    1. a program that allows for individual exercise selection
    2. a program that requires significant attention to detail
    3. a program that alternates exercises on consecutive days
    4. a program that varies based on the results of a subjective pain scale

17. A physical therapist treats a five-year-old with cerebral palsy. Initially the therapist was frustrated by the child's poor participation in therapy and as a result developed a reward system that enables the child to earn a sticker for good behavior. Since the therapist initiated the reward system the child has earned a sticker in each of the last five treatment sessions. This type of associated learning is termed:

    1. classical conditioning
    2. operant conditioning
    3. procedural learning
    4. declarative learning

18. A physical therapist working on an oncology unit reviews the medical chart of a patient prior to initiating an exercise program. The patient's cell counts are as follows: hematocrit 24 mL/dL, white blood cells 400 mm^3, platelet 4,000 mm^3, hemoglobin levels 7 gm/dL. Based on the patient's blood counts, which of the following would be the most accurate statement regarding the patient's allowable exercise level?

    1. no exercise is allowed
    2. light exercise is allowed
    3. active exercise is allowed
    4. resistive exercise is allowed

19. A physical therapist examines a patient diagnosed with rotator cuff tendonitis in physical therapy. The physician referral indicates the patient should be seen three times a week, however after examining the patient the therapist feels once a week is adequate. The most appropriate therapist action is to:

    1. schedule the patient once a week and notify the referring physician of your rationale
    2. schedule the patient as indicated on the physician referral
    3. ask the patient how often he/she would like to be seen in physical therapy
    4. attempt to determine if the patient's insurance will cover physical therapy visits three times a week

20. A physical therapist treats a patient using high voltage galvanic stimulation. During treatment the therapist observes smoke rising from the machine and smells an unusual odor. The most appropriate immediate response is to:

    1. unplug the machine and label it "Defective - Do Not Use"
    2. file an incident report
    3. contact the appropriate service group
    4. request an investigation by the biomedical instrumentation department

21. A physician refers a patient rehabilitating from an intertrochanteric fracture to physical therapy. On the referral form the physician specifies the use of continuous ultrasound at 2.4 W/cm^2 over the fracture site. The most appropriate physical therapist action is to:

    1. treat the patient as indicated on the referral form
    2. request that the patient obtain a new referral from the physician
    3. use another more acceptable modality
    4. contact the referring physician

22. A patient receiving physical therapy services in an outpatient clinic explains that he has felt nauseous since having his methotrexate medication level altered. The most appropriate physical therapist action is to:

    1. explain to the patient that nausea is very common when altering medication levels
    2. ask the patient to stop taking the prescribed medication
    3. request that the patient make an appointment with the physician
    4. request that the patient contact the physician's office to discuss the situation

23. A physical therapist prepares to instruct a patient in a three-point gait pattern using axillary crutches. The most appropriate initial step to facilitate patient learning is:

    1. distinguish a three-point gait pattern from other gait patterns
    2. demonstrate a three-point gait pattern
    3. provide the patient with direct feedback on his/her performance
    4. provide a written handout which illustrates the use of a three-point gait pattern

24. A physical therapist working in an acute care hospital attempts to determine the effectiveness of treating psoriatic lesions with ultraviolet. The most appropriate initial action is to:

    1. design a research study which examines the effectiveness of treating psoriatic lesions with ultraviolet
    2. determine if the current patient population would allow for an adequate sample size for a research study
    3. submit a research proposal to the hospital's institutional review board
    4. conduct a literary search for research related to treating psoriatic lesions with ultraviolet

25. As part of a total quality management program, a physical therapy department decides to collect patient satisfaction data. The most appropriate initial action is to:

    1. identify appropriate statistical techniques to analyze the data
    2. design a questionnaire for physical therapists
    3. design a patient satisfaction survey
    4. modify patient care standards based on the collected data

26. A physical therapist designs a research study that examines the effect of functional knee bracing on speed and agility. In this study speed and agility are the:

    1. dependent variables
    2. independent variables
    3. criterion variables
    4. extraneous variables

27. A physical therapist prepares to instruct a patient rehabilitating from a CVA in bed mobility activities. The most important initial step when designing an instructional program is to:

    1. assess the patient's cognitive status
    2. utilize a variety of teaching methods
    3. avoid using medical jargon
    4. speak loudly and directly to the patient

28. A physical therapist treats a 26-year-old male with complete C6 tetraplegia. During treatment the patient makes a culturally insensitive remark that the therapist feels is offensive. The most appropriate therapist action is to:

    1. document the incident in the medical record
    2. transfer the patient to another physical therapist's schedule
    3. discharge the patient from physical therapy
    4. inform the patient that the remark was offensive and continue with treatment

29. A physical therapist completes a fitness screening on a 34-year-old male prior to prescribing an aerobic exercise program. Which value is most representative of the patient's age predicted maximal heart rate?

    1. 168
    2. 174
    3. 186
    4. 196

30. An employee with a disclosed disability informs her employer that she is unable to perform an essential function of her job unless her work station is modified. Which of the following would provide the employer with a legitimate reason for not granting the employee's request?

    1. the accommodation would cost hundreds of dollars
    2. the accommodation would require an expansion of the employee's present workstation
    3. the accommodation would fundamentally alter the operation of the business
    4. the accommodation would not address the needs of other employees

31. A five-year-old patient is examined in physical therapy. The patient seems very uncomfortable during the examination and offers little useful information concerning her injury. The most appropriate physical therapist action is to:

    1. speak loudly and directly to the patient
    2. request that the patient's parents come into the treatment room
    3. explain to the patient the importance of physical therapy
    4. inform the patient that effective communication involves more than one individual

32. A patient rehabilitating from a grade I medial collateral ligament injury questions a physical therapist about his expected functional activity level following rehabilitation. The most accurate predictor of the patient's expected functional activity level is the:

    1. patient's age and past medical history
    2. patient's previous functional activity level
    3. duration of physical therapy services
    4. patient's compliance with the established home exercise program

33. A physical therapist reviews the results of a pulmonary function test for a patient with chronic obstructive pulmonary disease. Which of the following results is typical with chronic obstructive pulmonary disease?

    1. decreased functional residual capacity
    2. increased vital capacity
    3. increased residual volume
    4. increased forced expiratory volume in one second

34. A group of health care professionals participates in a family conference for a patient with a spinal cord injury. During the conference one of the participants summarizes the patient's progress with bathing and dressing activities. This type of information is typically conveyed by a/an:

    1. nurse
    2. physical therapist
    3. occupational therapist
    4. case manager

35. A physical therapist attempts to palpate the tibialis posterior tendon. To facilitate palpation of this structure the therapist should:

    1. ask the patient to invert and plantar flex the foot
    2. ask the patient to evert and dorsiflex the foot
    3. ask the patient to invert and dorsiflex the foot
    4. passively evert and plantar flex the foot

36. A patient diagnosed with spinal stenosis is referred to physical therapy three times a week for six weeks. During the examination the patient informs the physical therapist that the commute to therapy is over 90 miles. The most appropriate therapist action is to:

    1. schedule the patient once a week
    2. schedule the patient three times a week
    3. attempt to locate a physical therapy clinic closer to the patient's home
    4. discharge the patient with a home exercise program

37. A physical therapist participates in a discussion on health care reimbursement. During the session the group discusses various types of insurance. Which type of insurance provides reimbursement for the broadest array of services?

    1. Workers' compensation
    2. Medicaid
    3. Medicare Part A
    4. Medicare Part B

38. A patient status post total hip replacement surgery can reduce the risk of acquiring a deep vein thrombosis by performing all of the following except:

    1. repeated deep breathing exercises
    2. frequently turning from side to side in bed
    3. sitting with the legs in a dependent position
    4. active flexion and extension of the toes, ankles, knees, and hips

39. A physical therapist examines a 28-year-old male with burns covering 30 percent of his body. The patient sustained the burns approximately 24 hours earlier in a house fire. The medical record indicates an unremarkable medical history with the exception of a benign cardiac arrhythmia. Which of the following emergent conditions is the patient most susceptible to?

    1. aortic aneurysm
    2. autonomic dysreflexia
    3. diabetic coma
    4. shock

40. A physical therapist monitors a patient's vital signs during a submaximal exercise test. The exercise test protocol requires the patient to complete three stages of increasing intensity that are each three minutes in duration. Which of the following time parameters would be the most appropriate to assess heart rate during each of the three minute stages?

    1. 1 minute and 2 minutes
    2. 2 minutes and 3 minutes
    3. 1 minute and 3 minutes
    4. at the start and conclusion of exercise

41. During a balance assessment of a patient with left hemiplegia, it is noted that in sitting the patient requires minimal assistance to maintain the position and cannot accept any additional challenge. The physical therapist would appropriately document the patient's sitting balance as:

    1. normal
    2. good
    3. fair
    4. poor

42. A short-term goal for a patient with a neurological deficit is as follows: The patient will transfer from tall kneeling to half kneeling with supervision. This activity is an example of:

    1. mobility
    2. stability
    3. controlled mobility
    4. skill

43. A physical therapist administers a series of cranial nerve tests to a patient with a confirmed lower motor neuron disease. Assuming the patient has a lesion impacting the left hypoglossal nerve, which clinical presentation would be most likely?

    1. right sided tongue atrophy and deviation toward the left with tongue protrusion
    2. right sided tongue atrophy and deviation toward the right with tongue protrusion
    3. left sided tongue atrophy and deviation toward the left with tongue protrusion
    4. left sided tongue atrophy and deviation toward the right with tongue protrusion

44. A physical therapist is treating a patient with a head injury who begins to perseverate. In order to refocus the patient and achieve the desired therapeutic outcome, the therapist should:

    1. focus on the topic of perseveration for a short period of time in order to appease the patient
    2. guide the patient into an interesting new activity and reward successful completion of the task
    3. take the patient back to his room for quiet time and attempt to resume therapy once he has stopped perseverating
    4. continue with repetitive verbal cues to cease perseveration

45. A group of physical therapy students develops a physical activity survey as part of a community health screening. The survey consists of a series of questions in which subjects must respond by answering yes or no. What level of measurement does the survey utilize?

    1. nominal
    2. ordinal
    3. interval
    4. ratio

46. The goals for a patient status post total knee replacement include general conditioning and independent household mobility. Which component of the patient's treatment would be the most appropriate to delegate to a physical therapy aide?

    1. stair training
    2. progressive gait training with a straight cane
    3. patient education regarding the surgical procedure
    4. ambulation with a walker for endurance

47. A complete medical history should be conducted on all patients prior to initiating treatment. Questions asked during the patient history should not lead the patient. Which of the following questions would not be considered leading?

    1. Does this increase your pain?
    2. Does this alter your pain in any way?
    3. Does your pain increase at night?
    4. Does your pain decrease with activity?

48. A physical therapist examines the heart sounds of a 48-year-old female status post coronary artery bypass graft. When auscultating, the therapist identifies the heart sound associated with closing of the mitral and tricuspid valves. This heart sound best describes:

    1. S1
    2. S2
    3. S3
    4. S4

49. A 64-year-old male diagnosed with chronic bronchitis was admitted to the hospital three days ago after experiencing an acute exacerbation. While assessing the patient's vital signs the physical therapist determines the respiratory rate is 28 breaths per minute. Which breathing technique would be the most appropriate to decrease the patient's respiratory rate?

    1. glossopharyngeal breathing
    2. diaphragmatic breathing
    3. segmental breathing
    4. pursed lip breathing

50. A physical therapist measures a patient's respiration rate at rest. Which measurement time frame would provide the patient with the most accurate assessment of respiration rate?

    1. 10 seconds
    2. 15 seconds
    3. 30 seconds
    4. 60 seconds

51. A physical therapist commonly uses ice to decrease inflammation following arthroscopic surgery. Which type of pharmacological agent would have an antagonistic effect on joint inflammation?

    1. anti-inflammatory steroids
    2. nonsteroidal anti-inflammatory drugs
    3. peripheral vasodilators
    4. systemic vasoconstrictors

52. During an examination a physical therapist examines a patient's general willingness to use an affected body part. What objective information would provide the most useful information?

   1. bony palpation
   2. active movement
   3. passive movement
   4. sensory testing

53. A male physical therapist examines a female diagnosed with subacromial bursitis. After taking a thorough history, the therapist asks the patient to change into a gown. The patient seems very uneasy about this suggestion, but finally agrees to use the gown. The most appropriate course of action would be to:

   1. continue with treatment as planned
   2. attempt to treat the patient without using the gown
   3. bring a female staff member into the treatment room and continue with treatment
   4. offer to transfer the patient to a female physical therapist

54. A physical therapist examines a patient seated in a wheelchair. After completing the examination the therapist determines the wheelchair has inadequate seat width. Which of the following is the most likely consequence?

   1. excessive pressure under the distal thigh
   2. excessive pressure under the ischial tuberosities
   3. excessive pressure in the popliteal fossa
   4. excessive pressure on the greater trochanters

55. A physical therapist examines a patient diagnosed with an acute posterior cruciate sprain. The most common mechanism of injury for the posterior cruciate is:

   1. a forceful landing on the anterior tibia with the knee hyperflexed
   2. an anteriorly directed force applied to the tibia when the foot is fixed
   3. a valgus force applied to the knee when the foot is fixed
   4. hyperextension and medial rotation of the leg with lateral rotation of the body

56. A therapist attends an inservice on risk management. During the presentation the speaker describes guidelines to decrease the incidence of lawsuits. Which of the following would be considered the most essential action?

   1. conduct a thorough initial examination
   2. instruct patients carefully in all exercise activities
   3. keep the referring physician informed
   4. maintain accurate and timely documentation

57. A patient diagnosed with right shoulder adhesive capsulitis is limited to 25 degrees of lateral rotation. Which mobilization technique would be indicated based on the patient's limitation?

   1. lateral distraction and anterior glide
   2. medial distraction and posterior glide
   3. lateral distraction and posterior glide
   4. medial distraction and inferior glide

58. A former patient calls to ask for advice after injuring his lower back in a work related accident. The patient explains that he cannot bend down and touch his toes without severe pain and has muscle spasms throughout the entire lower back. The therapist works in a state without direct access, but would like to help the former patient. The most appropriate response would be:

   1. explain to the patient that you would be happy to treat him, however since you have not completed a formal examination it would be unfair to prescribe treatment over the phone
   2. arrange a time for the patient to come into your clinic for immediate treatment
   3. prescribe flexion exercises and ice every three hours
   4. refer the patient to a qualified physician

59. A therapist examines a patient diagnosed with patellar femoral syndrome. As part of the examination the therapist elects to measure the patient's Q angle. Which three bony landmarks are used to measure the Q angle?

   1. anterior superior iliac spine, superior border of the patella, tibial tubercle
   2. anterior superior iliac spine, midpoint of the patella, tibial tubercle
   3. anterior superior iliac spine, inferior border of the patella, midpoint of the patella tendon
   4. greater trochanter, midpoint of the patella, superior border of the patella tendon

60. A 55-year-old female diagnosed with a right hip intertrochanteric fracture is eight weeks status post open reduction and internal fixation with a plate and pinning. The patient has pain with active hip flexion and abduction. Acceptable modalities for the patient include all of the following except:

   1. hot packs
   2. whirlpool
   3. pulsed ultrasound
   4. shortwave diathermy

61. A physical therapist reviews the medical record of a 32-year-old male receiving intravenous fluid therapy. The medical record indicates that the patient's urine output for the last 24 hours is 300 ml. This amount of urine production is best termed:

   1. anuria
   2. hematuria
   3. oliguria
   4. polyuria

62. A patient sustains an injury to the dorsal scapular nerve. Which muscle not innervated by the nerve acts to elevate the scapula?

   1. latissimus dorsi
   2. levator scapulae
   3. rhomboid minor
   4. trapezius

63. A patient with an acute burn is referred to physical therapy. The patient's burns range from superficial partial-thickness to deep partial-thickness and encompass approximately 35 percent of the patient's body. Which of the following findings would be most predictable based on the patient's injury?

   1. increased oxygen consumption
   2. decreased minute ventilation
   3. increased intravascular fluid
   4. decreased core temperature

64. A patient rehabilitating from congestive heart failure is examined in physical therapy. During the examination the patient begins to complain of pain. The most immediate physical therapist action is to:

   1. notify the nursing staff to administer pain medication
   2. contact the referring physician
   3. discontinue the treatment session
   4. ask the patient to describe the location and severity of the pain

65. A 56-year-old female diagnosed with emphysema is referred to physical therapy. As part of the examination the physical therapist assesses tactile fremitus by asking the patient to repeat the term "ninety-nine" several times in succession. The most appropriate method when assessing tactile fremitus is:

   1. examine voice sounds through auscultation
   2. examine vibration using the ulnar border of the hand
   3. examine chest excursion with a tape measure
   4. examine the intensity and clarity of spoken words using a recording device

66. A physical therapist reviews the medical record of a patient diagnosed with chronic obstructive pulmonary disease. The medical record indicates that the patient's current condition is consistent with chronic respiratory acidosis. Which testing procedure was likely used to identify this condition?

   1. arterial blood gas analysis
   2. pulmonary function testing
   3. graded exercise testing
   4. pulse oximetry

67. A physical therapist examines a five-year-old child's gait. The therapist notes that the child is unsteady and uses a wide base of support. The child appears to lurch at times with minimal truncal bobbing in an anterior and posterior direction. The child cannot maintain a standing position with the feet placed together for more than five seconds. The area of the brain most likely affected is the:

   1. corticospinal tracts
   2. basal ganglia
   3. substantia nigra
   4. cerebellar hemisphere

68. A group of physical therapy students gather data on the public's perception of physical therapy. The students use a questionnaire of closed end questions which is randomly distributed to individuals throughout the country. All of the following are advantages of using closed end questions except:

   1. quicker and relatively inexpensive to analyze
   2. helps to ensure that answers are given in a frame of reference relevant to the research
   3. forces the respondent to choose an answer even if the choice that corresponds to that of the respondent is not listed
   4. makes the meaning of the question clearer

69. A group of senior physical therapy students attempts to determine if there is a relationship between intelligence and academic achievement. Which of the following correlation coefficients would indicate the strongest positive correlation?

   1. +.68
   2. +.81
   3. -.26
   4. -.91

70. A physical therapist designs an exercise program for a patient rehabilitating from a lower extremity injury. The single most important factor in an exercise program designed to increase muscular strength is:

   1. the recovery time between exercise sets
   2. the number of repetitions per set
   3. the duration of the exercise session
   4. the intensity of the exercise

71. A physical therapist treats a patient rehabilitating from a chemical burn sustained in a work-related injury. The patient has been in the hospital for 31 days and as a result the therapist is concerned about the patient's cardiovascular status. Which of the following would serve as the best indicator that the patient does not need to participate in a formal cardiovascular rehabilitation program?

   1. arterial blood gas analysis within normal limits
   2. functional capacity greater than 10 metabolic equivalents
   3. oxygen saturation rate greater than 90 percent
   4. resting heart rate of 58 beats per minute

72. A 45-year-old obese woman in a long leg cast attempts to transfer to a mat table using a sliding board. Which of the following instructions would be incorrect?

   1. lean away from the mat and place the sliding board under your buttocks
   2. perform a series of small pushups gradually moving closer to the mat
   3. grasp the edge of the sliding board with your fingers to secure additional support
   4. maintain a slight forward trunk position while transferring

73. A patient two months status post total knee replacement is referred to physical therapy for range of motion and strengthening exercises. Which treatment technique would be inappropriate for the patient?

   1. active stretching using the contract-relax technique
   2. joint mobilization to increase joint play
   3. exercise on a stationary bicycle against mild resistance
   4. performing straight leg raising, short arc extension, and knee flexion exercises using leg weights

74. A patient is given a prescription for a nonsteroidal anti-inflammatory medication that is to be taken three times a day with meals. What is the most common side effect of nonsteroidal anti-inflammatory medications?

   1. convulsions
   2. fever
   3. nausea and vomiting
   4. stomach discomfort

75. A physical therapist reviews the medical record of a patient with a peripheral nerve injury. The most common site for an ulnar nerve injury is at the:

   1. brachial plexus
   2. medial epicondyle of the humerus
   3. superficial surface of the flexor retinaculum
   4. distal wrist crease

76. A 12-year-old female that became anoxic in a near drowning performs dynamic activities in quadruped. The next posture to attain in the developmental sequence would be:

   1. half kneeling
   2. tall kneeling
   3. plantigrade
   4. standing

77. An 86-year-old female is partial weight bearing on the left lower extremity after a total hip replacement. Her upper extremity strength is 3+/5 and she resides alone. Which assistive device would be the most appropriate for the patient?

   1. Lofstrand crutches
   2. axillary crutches
   3. large base quad cane
   4. walker

78. A patient that sustained a lower extremity burn three months ago is treated in an outpatient physical therapy clinic. The patient's burns appear to be fully healed, however the patient exhibits decreased knee flexion due to scar tissue. As part of the treatment program the physical therapist performs passive stretching activities in an attempt to promote collagen extensibility. Which thermal agent would be the most beneficial to enhance the effectiveness of the treatment session?

    1. pulsed ultrasound
    2. continuous ultrasound
    3. hydrotherapy
    4. fluidotherapy

79. An order is received to perform chest physical therapy on a patient status post abdominal surgery. A chart review identifies right atelectasis. The most appropriate exercise to teach the patient is:

    1. reflex cough technique
    2. Codman's pendulum exercises
    3. segmental breathing
    4. quick paced shallow breathing

80. A physical therapist prepares to apply a topical antibiotic to a small portion of the upper arm of a patient with a deep partial-thickness burn. When applying the topical antibiotic the therapist should utilize which form of medical asepsis?

    1. gloves
    2. sterile gloves
    3. sterile gloves, gown
    4. sterile gloves, gown, mask

81. A physical therapist attempts to obtain information on a patient's endurance level by administering a low level exercise test on a treadmill. Which of the following measurement methods would provide the therapist with an objective measurement of endurance?

    1. facial color
    2. facial expression
    3. rating on a perceived exertion scale
    4. respiration rate

82. A physical therapist examines a patient status post stroke with a flaccid left side. In order to facilitate muscular activity, the treatment plan should include:

    1. weight bearing, tapping, elevation
    2. vibration, tapping, prolonged stretch
    3. weight bearing, tapping, approximation
    4. approximation, elevation, prolonged stretch

83. A physical therapist attempts to assess the Babinski reflex as part of an initial examination. To effectively elicit the Babinski reflex, the therapist should:

    1. stroke the lateral aspect of the foot beneath the lateral malleolus
    2. stroke the anteromedial tibial surface
    3. stroke the lateral aspect of the sole of the foot
    4. firmly squeeze the calf

84. A patient with a right radial head fracture is examined in physical therapy. The patient's involved elbow range of motion begins at 15 degrees of flexion and ends at 90 degrees of flexion. The physical therapist should record the patient's elbow range of motion as:

    1. 0 - 15 - 90
    2. 15 - 0 - 90
    3. 15 - 90
    4. 0 - 90

85. A physical therapist reviews the medical record of a patient with Broca's aphasia. This condition most often results from a CVA that affects the:

    1. anterior cerebral artery
    2. middle cerebral artery
    3. posterior cerebral artery
    4. basilar artery

86. A patient involved in a motor vehicle accident sustains a proximal fibula fracture. The fracture damages the motor component of the common peroneal nerve. Ankle dorsiflexion and eversion are tested as 2/5. The most appropriate intervention to assist the patient with activities of daily living would be:

    1. electrical stimulation
    2. orthosis
    3. exercise program
    4. aquatic program

87. A 72-year-old female involved in a motor vehicle accident fractures the middle third of her femoral shaft. The patient's physician is concerned about the effects of prolonged bed rest and would like the patient to begin walking as soon as possible. Which form of treatment would facilitate early weight bearing through the involved extremity?

    1. immobilization in a hip spica cast
    2. internal fixation with an intramedullary nail
    3. external mobilization
    4. skeletal traction

88. A 25-year-old female rehabilitating from a fractured tibia is cleared for 50 lbs. of weight bearing through the involved lower extremity. The patient has no other significant medical problems and is expected to progress to full weight bearing within two weeks. The most appropriate assistive device for the patient is:

    1. wooden axillary crutches
    2. walker
    3. cane
    4. aluminum Lofstrand crutches

89. A physical therapist examines a morbidly obese patient in physical therapy. The therapist would like to incorporate modalities into the patient's care plan, but is concerned about excessively elevating the patient's tissue temperature. Which modality would potentially be the most hazardous?

    1. shortwave diathermy
    2. hot packs
    3. paraffin
    4. pulsed ultrasound

90. A physical therapist implements an aquatic program for a patient rehabilitating from a total hip replacement. During the treatment session the patient indicates how much easier it is to walk in the water compared to on land. What factor is responsible for the patient's ability to walk in water?

    1. buoyancy
    2. pressure
    3. cohesion
    4. viscosity

91. A physical therapist instructs a patient with a pulmonary disease in energy conservation techniques. Which of the following techniques would be the most effective when assisting a patient to complete a selected activity without dyspnea?

    1. diaphragmatic breathing
    2. pacing
    3. pursed lip breathing
    4. ventilatory muscle training

92. A physical therapy practice attempts to demonstrate appropriate allocation of its resources. This process is best accomplished by:

    1. utilization review
    2. quality assurance program
    3. program examination
    4. peer assessment

93. A physical therapist prepares to perform volumetric measurements as a means of quantifying edema. Which patient would appear to be the most appropriate candidate for this type of objective measure?

    1. a 38-year-old female with a Colles' fracture
    2. a 27-year-old male with bicipital tendonitis
    3. a 48-year-old male with a rotator cuff tear
    4. a 57-year-old male with pulmonary edema

94. S.O.A.P. notes are a common form of documentation in a variety of health care settings. Which of the following would not be found in the objective section of a S.O.A.P. note?

    1. measurement of pertinent changes in mental status
    2. description of present treatment
    3. vital sign measurements
    4. short and long-term goals

95. A physical therapist performs a manual muscle test on a patient with unilateral lower extremity weakness. The therapist should test the patient's hip adductors with the patient positioned in:

    1. prone
    2. sidelying
    3. standing
    4. supine

96. A physical therapist attempts to assist a patient to clear secretions after performing postural drainage. What position would allow the patient to produce the most forceful cough?

    1. prone
    2. sidelying
    3. supine
    4. upright sitting

97. A physical therapist inquires about a child's activity level prior to beginning a treatment session. The child's mother indicates that the child frequently rides her tricycle in the driveway. Which age is most consistent with the onset of this activity?

    1. two
    2. three
    3. four
    4. five

98. A patient returns to an outpatient physical therapy clinic two hours after completing a treatment session complaining of increased back pain. The patient has been seen in physical therapy for three previous visits and has had little difficulty with a program consisting of palliative modalities and pelvic stabilization exercises. The patient was referred to physical therapy after straining his back two weeks ago while lifting his daughter out of a car seat. The most appropriate physical therapist action is:

   1. contact the referring physician to discuss the patient's care plan
   2. instruct the patient to discontinue the pelvic stabilization exercises and reexamine the patient at his next visit
   3. refer the patient to the emergency room of a local hospital
   4. instruct the patient to cancel existing physical therapy visits and schedule an appointment with the physician

99. A physical therapist employed in a nursing home routinely treats patients in excess of 70 years of age. Which of the following physical changes is not associated with aging?

   1. increased residual volume
   2. decreased vital capacity
   3. decreased cardiac output
   4. decreased total lung capacity

100. A physical therapist prepares to treat a patient in isolation. In what order should the protective clothing be applied?

   1. gloves, gown, mask
   2. gown, gloves, mask
   3. mask, gown, gloves
   4. gloves, mask, gown

101. A patient is referred to physical therapy 24 hours after total knee replacement. What exercise would be the most appropriate to begin treatment?

   1. quadriceps sets
   2. short arc quadriceps
   3. standing leg curls
   4. straight let raises

102. A physical therapist reviews a physician's examination of a patient scheduled for physical therapy. The examination identifies excessive medial displacement of the elbow during ligamentous testing. Which ligament is typically involved with medial instability of the elbow?

   1. annular
   2. radial collateral
   3. ulnar collateral
   4. volar radioulnar

103. A patient rehabilitating from a tibial plateau fracture is referred to physical therapy for instruction in gait training. The patient has been cleared by his physician for weight bearing up to 40 lbs. Assuming the patient has no significant balance or coordination deficits, which gait pattern would be the most appropriate?

   1. two-point
   2. four-point
   3. three-point
   4. swing-through

104. A patient reports to her physical therapist that she completely tore one of the ligaments in her ankle. If the patient's comment is accurate, the injury to the ligament should be classified as a:

   1. grade I sprain
   2. grade III sprain
   3. grade I strain
   4. grade III strain

105. A physical therapist treating a patient in a special care unit notices a marked increase in fluid on the dorsum of a patient's hand around an I.V. site. The therapist, recognizing the possibility that the I.V. has become dislodged, should immediately:

   1. continue with the present treatment
   2. contact the primary physician
   3. turn off the I.V.
   4. reposition the peripheral I.V. line

106. A patient rehabilitating from a radial head fracture performs progressive resistive exercises designed to strengthen the forearm supinators. Which muscle would be of particular importance to achieve the desired outcome?

   1. brachialis
   2. brachioradialis
   3. biceps brachii
   4. anconeus

107. A physical therapist examines the viscosity and color of a sputum sample after completing postural drainage activities. The sputum is a yellowish-greenish color and is very thick. The therapist can best describe the sputum as:

1. fetid
2. frothy
3. mucoid
4. purulent

108. The reliability of goniometric measurements taken by different physical therapists is measured by interrater reliability. Which joint motion would you expect to have the poorest interrater reliability?

1. ankle eversion
2. elbow flexion
3. knee flexion
4. shoulder lateral rotation

109. A physical therapist reviews the medical chart of a patient admitted to the hospital two days ago after being burned in a house fire. The chart specifies that the epidermal and dermal layers were completely destroyed and some of the subcutaneous tissue was damaged. Which type of burn does this best describe?

1. superficial partial-thickness
2. deep partial-thickness
3. full-thickness
4. subdermal

110. A patient using a standard wheelchair discusses the design of her home with a physical therapist in preparation for discharge. The patient informs the therapist that the home is 150 years old and has narrow doorways. If the patient is to safely propel the wheelchair through the doorway, the doorway width should be at least:

1. 20 inches
2. 26 inches
3. 32 inches
4. 38 inches

111. A patient is unable to take in an adequate supply of nutrients by mouth due to the side effects of radiation therapy. As a result the patient's physician orders the implementation of tube feeding. What type of tube is most commonly used for short-term feeding?

1. endobronchial
2. nasogastric
3. otopharyngeal
4. tracheostomy

112. A physical therapist employed in an acute care hospital prepares to work on standing balance with a patient rehabilitating from abdominal surgery. The patient has been on extended bed rest following the surgical procedure and has only been out of bed a few times with the assistance of the nursing staff. The most important objective measure to assess after assisting the patient from supine to sitting is:

1. systolic blood pressure
2. diastolic blood pressure
3. perceived exertion
4. oxygen saturation rate

113. A physical therapist treats a patient who sustained several orthopedic injures in a mountain climbing accident. Assuming the patient's upper extremity injuries include a partial tear of the ulnar collateral ligament, which of the following methods would most likely be used in the medical management of this injury?

1. short-arm thumb spica cast
2. long-arm thumb spica cast
3. short-arm thumb spica splint
4. long-arm thumb spica splint

114. A physical therapist treats a patient referred to physical therapy after sustaining a comminuted Colles' fracture. The fracture was stabilized with an external fixator device. Which postoperative time frame best represents the amount of time the external fixator device will be utilized?

1. 2-4 weeks
2. 6-8 weeks
3. 10-12 weeks
4. 14-16 weeks

115. A therapist attempts to quantify the amount of assistance a patient needs to complete a selected activity. Categories of assistance include maximal, moderate, minimal, stand-by or independent. This type of measurement scale is best classified as:

1. interval
2. nominal
3. ordinal
4. ratio

SAMPLE EXAMINATION: EXAM TWO

116. A physical therapist designs a treatment plan for an eight-year-old boy with cystic fibrosis. A major component of the treatment plan will include educating the patient's family in appropriate bronchial drainage techniques. Which of the following lung segments would be inappropriate for bronchial drainage?

   1. left middle lobe
   2. apical segments of the upper lobes
   3. anterior basal segments of the lower lobes
   4. anterior segments of the upper lobes

117. A physical therapist completes a developmental assessment on a seven month old infant. Assuming normal development, which of the following reflexes would not be integrated?

   1. asymmetrical tonic neck reflex
   2. Moro reflex
   3. Landau reflex
   4. symmetrical tonic neck reflex

118. A patient rehabilitating from a myocardial infarction prepares for a graded exercise test. Which of the following pharmacological agents would lower heart rate and blood pressure during the exercise test?

   1. antidepressants
   2. diuretics
   3. beta blockers
   4. bronchodilators

119. A physical therapist covering for a colleague on vacation examines a patient with a traumatic brain injury. The therapist has read the patient's medical chart, but remains anxious about the examination. The most important area for the therapist to assess immediately is:

   1. extent of orthopedic involvement
   2. level of communication
   3. muscle tone
   4. sensation

120. A physical therapist begins prosthetic training activities with a patient status post transtibial amputation. Which of the following would be the most appropriate initial activity?

   1. ascending and descending stairs
   2. marching in place
   3. walking on even ground
   4. weight shifting in standing

121. A patient is referred to physical therapy after being diagnosed with a partial tear of the ulnar collateral ligament of the thumb. Which objective finding would be most consistent with this type of injury?

   1. excessive angulation of the metacarpophalangeal joint of the thumb with valgus stress
   2. excessive angulation of the metacarpophalangeal joint of the thumb with varus stress
   3. excessive angulation of the carpometacarpal joint of the thumb with radially directed stress
   4. excessive angulation of the carpometacarpal joint of the thumb with ulnarly directed stress

122. A physical therapist measures the vertical leap of ten basketball players. The therapist then calculates the difference between the highest and lowest values in the distribution. What measure of variability has the therapist determined?

   1. mode
   2. range
   3. standard deviation
   4. variance

123. A physical therapist reviews the medical record of a patient recently admitted to the intensive care unit. A note from the patient's physician indicates an order for arterial blood gas analysis six times daily. Which type of indwelling line would be used to collect the necessary samples?

   1. intravenous line
   2. arterial line
   3. central venous line
   4. pulmonary artery line

124. A 42-year-old female is admitted to a rehabilitation hospital after sustaining a stroke. During the examination the physical therapist identifies significant sensory deficits in the anterolateral spinothalamic system. Which sensation would be most affected?

   1. barognosis
   2. kinesthesia
   3. graphesthesia
   4. temperature

125. A physical therapist discusses the importance of a proper diet with a patient diagnosed with congestive heart failure. Which of the following substances would most likely be restricted in the patient's diet?

   1. high density lipoproteins
   2. low density lipoproteins
   3. sodium
   4. triglycerides

126. A patient is instructed to lie supine with his knees bent to 90 degrees over the edge of a treatment table. The patient is then asked to bring his right knee to his chest. By examining the angle of the left knee, the physical therapist can obtain information on the length of the:

 1. biceps femoris muscle
 2. rectus femoris muscle
 3. sartorius muscle
 4. tensor fasciae latae muscle

127. A physical therapist examines a number of substances that influence circulation. Which of the following substances is stimulated by decreased arterial pressure and acts as a vasoconstrictor?

 1. angiotensin
 2. histamine
 3. epinephrine
 4. norepinephrine

128. A physical therapist identifies several inconsistencies between a patient's subjective complaints and the objective findings of an initial examination. When documenting the identified inconsistencies using a S.O.A.P. note, the most appropriate location for the entry is:

 1. subjective
 2. objective
 3. assessment
 4. plan

129. A physical therapy manager is responsible for enforcing employee compliance with departmental policies and procedures. Which of the following would be the most appropriate action for an employee who has violated the department dress code policy for the first time?

 1. private oral warning
 2. written warning
 3. probation
 4. suspension

130. A physical therapist records the vital signs of individuals at a health and wellness fair designed to promote physical therapy week. Which age group should the therapist expect to have the highest resting pulse rate?

 1. infants
 2. children
 3. teenagers
 4. adults

131. A 13-year-old girl discusses the possibility of anterior cruciate ligament reconstruction with an orthopedic surgeon. The girl injured her knee while playing soccer and is concerned about the future impact of the injury on her athletic career. Which of the following factors would have the greatest influence on her candidacy for surgery?

 1. anthropometric measurements
 2. hamstrings/quadriceps strength ratio
 3. skeletal maturity
 4. somatotype

132. A patient diagnosed with C5 quadriplegia receives physical therapy services in a rehabilitation hospital. The patient has made good progress in therapy and is scheduled for discharge in one week. During a treatment session the patient informs the physical therapist that one day in the future he will walk again. The most appropriate therapist response is:

 1. Your level of injury makes walking unrealistic.
 2. Future advances in spinal cord research may make your goal a reality.
 3. You can have a rewarding life even if confined to a wheelchair.
 4. Completing your exercises on a regular basis will help you to walk.

133. A patient rehabilitating from a lower extremity injury sustained in a motor vehicle accident ten days ago participates in a daily exercise session. The medical record indicates that the patient is currently taking beta blockers due to hypertension. When determining exercise intensity during the session the most appropriate variable to examine is:

 1. heart rate
 2. rate of perceived exertion
 3. respiratory rate
 4. blood pressure

134. A physical therapist employed in an acute care hospital treats a patient diagnosed with asthma. In order to assess the patient's activity tolerance the therapist elects to use oximetry. The most appropriate time periods to conduct a formal oximetry measurement is:

 1. during and after the exercise session
 2. before and during the exercise session
 3. before and after the exercise session
 4. before, during, and after the exercise session

135. A physical therapist conducts an initial examination on a patient with a traumatic brain injury. Which stimulus should the therapist utilize to test for clonus at the ankle?

   1. active-assistive dorsiflexion of the ankle
   2. active dorsiflexion of the ankle
   3. passive, rapid dorsiflexion of the ankle
   4. passive, slow dorsiflexion of the ankle

136. While working with a patient with a T6 spinal cord injury a physical therapist identifies a small reddened area over the patient's right ischial tuberosity. The therapist should immediately:

   1. notify nursing and remind the patient of his/her role in proper skin care
   2. order a water mattress for the patient
   3. alert the patient to the potential dangers of skin breakdown
   4. notify the primary physician

137. A physical therapist discusses the plan of care for a patient rehabilitating from total hip replacement surgery with the patient's surgeon. During the discussion the surgeon indicates that he would like the patient to continue to wear a knee immobilizer in order to help prevent hip dislocation. The primary rationale for this action is:

   1. The knee immobilizer serves as a constant reminder to the patient that the hip is susceptible to injury.
   2. The knee immobilizer reduces hip flexion by maintaining knee extension.
   3. The knee immobilizer facilitates quadriceps contraction during weight bearing activities.
   4. The knee immobilizer limits postoperative edema and as a result promotes lower extremity stability.

138. A physical therapist observes a video on the biomechanics of normal gait. The therapist notes that the subject's knee remains flexed during all of the components of stance phase except:

   1. foot flat
   2. heel strike
   3. mid-stance
   4. toe off

139. A physical therapist employed in an outpatient clinic discusses the daily treatment program with a patient three weeks status post medial meniscectomy. During the discussion the patient indicates that she is able to exercise, however did experience a low grade temperature three days ago. Assuming the therapist measures and records the patient's temperature as 98.9 degrees Fahrenheit, the most appropriate therapist action would be to:

   1. continue with treatment as planned
   2. continue with treatment, however avoid active exercise
   3. refer the patient to her primary care physician
   4. contact the patient's surgeon to discuss the situation

140. A physical therapist receives a referral for a 48-year-old female diagnosed with lung cancer. The patient reports smoking three packs of cigarettes a day for the last 25 years. Assuming the patient was diagnosed with cancer two years ago, which of the following pieces of data would provide the therapist with the most valuable information when establishing the plan of care and the associated goals?

   1. premorbid lifestyle
   2. staging of cancer
   3. past medical history
   4. motivation level

141. A physical therapist treats a patient that is on a waiting list for a heart transplant. The patient has a lengthy history of cardiac pathology and recently received a right ventricular assistive device due to persistent ventricular failure. Which two structures would house the tubes for this device?

   1. left atrium and aorta
   2. left atrium and pulmonary artery
   3. right atrium and aorta
   4. right atrium and pulmonary artery

142. A physical therapist uses repeated contractions to strengthen the quadriceps of a patient that fails to exhibit the desired muscular response throughout the entire range of motion. This proprioceptive neuromuscular facilitation technique should be applied:

   1. at the initiation of movement
   2. at the point where the desired muscular response begins to diminish
   3. at the end of the available range of motion
   4. only after a manual stretch to the hamstrings

143. A patient diagnosed with spastic hemiplegia wears an ankle-foot orthosis set in slight dorsiflexion. If the orthosis was set in excessive dorsiflexion, which of the following would you expect to observe during the stance phase of gait?

    1. increased knee stability
    2. decreased knee stability
    3. no effect on knee stability
    4. genu recurvatum

144. A patient is referred to physical therapy with a twenty degree restriction in wrist extension. Which mobilization technique would be the most appropriate based on the restriction?

    1. dorsal glide of the carpals
    2. stabilize lunate, volar glide radius
    3. stabilize capitate, volar glide lunate
    4. stabilize radius, volar glide scaphoid

145. A patient rehabilitating from extensive burns to the right upper extremity often complains of severe pain in the arm during physical therapy treatment sessions. The present plan of care emphasizes range of motion, stretching, and positioning. The most appropriate action to address the patient's complaint is to:

    1. reduce the frequency and duration of the treatment sessions
    2. schedule treatment sessions when the patient's pain medication is most effective
    3. avoid treatment activities that are uncomfortable for the patient
    4. request that the referring physician increases the dosage of the patient's pain medication

146. A physical therapist treats a patient diagnosed with chronic arteriosclerotic vascular disease. The patient exhibits cool skin, decreased sensitivity to temperature changes, and intermittent claudication with activity. The primary treatment goal is to increase the patient's ambulation distance. The most appropriate ambulation parameters to facilitate achievement of the goal are:

    1. short duration, frequent intervals
    2. short duration, infrequent intervals
    3. long duration, frequent intervals
    4. long duration, infrequent intervals

147. A patient rehabilitating from a bone marrow transplant is referred to physical therapy for instruction in an exercise program. The physical therapist plans to use oxygen saturation measurements to gain additional objective data related to the patient's exercise tolerance. Assuming the patient's oxygen saturation rate was measured as 95% at rest, which of the following guidelines would be the most appropriate?

    1. discontinue exercise if the patient's oxygen saturation rate is below 95%
    2. discontinue exercise if the patient's oxygen saturation rate is below 90%
    3. discontinue exercise if the patient's oxygen saturation rate is below 85%
    4. discontinue exercise if the patient's oxygen saturation rate is below 80%

148. A physical therapist reviews the medical record of a 46-year-old female diagnosed with myasthenia gravis. A recent physician entry indicates that the patient is currently taking immunosuppressive medication. Which laboratory test should be the most frequently monitored based on the patient's medication?

    1. hematocrit
    2. hemoglobin
    3. platelet count
    4. white blood cell count

149. A patient rehabilitating from a cerebrovascular accident uses an ankle-foot orthosis for ambulation activities. The patient is able to ambulate independently with the orthosis, however the physical therapist is concerned about the potential for skin breakdown since the patient has diminished sensation in the involved lower extremity. The most essential advice for the patient is:

    1. perform frequent skin checks
    2. limit wearing time to 30 minutes
    3. soak the foot and ankle in warm water after ambulation
    4. wear a minimum of two pairs of socks

150. A patient exhibits pain and sensory loss in the posterior thigh, lateral calf, and dorsal foot. Extension of the hallux is poor, however the Achilles reflex is normal. What spinal level would you expect to be involved?

    1. L4
    2. L5
    3. S1
    4. S2

151. An 18-year-old male six weeks status post open reduction of a Colles' fracture is referred to physical therapy. Examination reveals mild swelling on the dorsum of the hand and limited flexion of the metacarpophalangeal joints in all digits. The most appropriate heating agent for the patient is:

   1. paraffin
   2. hot packs
   3. vapocoolant sprays
   4. ultrasound

152. A female patient three weeks status post lateral ankle sprain reports for a treatment session wearing an oversized tank top that exposes a portion of her breasts and a pair of shorts. The physical therapist feels the tank top is inappropriate and is concerned that other patients in the clinic may be offended by the patient's dress. The patient's present treatment regimen includes lower extremity resistive exercises and various functional activities. The most appropriate therapist action is:

   1. drape the patient with a sheet
   2. provide the patient with a shirt
   3. treat the patient in a private treatment room
   4. discontinue the treatment session

153. A 26-year-old male involved in a motorcycle accident sustains a T10 vertebral fracture. The patient's physician attempts to restrict forward thoracic flexion by using an externally applied device. Which of the following would be the most appropriate selection?

   1. Minerva cervical-thoracic orthosis
   2. Philadelphia collar
   3. sternal-occipital-mandibular immobilizer
   4. thoraco-lumbar-sacral orthosis

154. A physical therapist employed in a rehabilitation hospital completes an examination on a patient diagnosed with Parkinson's disease. Results of the examination include 4/5 strength in the lower extremities, 10 degree flexion contractures at the hips, and exaggerated forward standing posture. The patient has significant difficulty initiating movement and requires manual assistance for gait on level surfaces. The most appropriate activity to incorporate into a home program is:

   1. prone lying
   2. progressive relaxation exercises
   3. lower extremity resistive exercises with ankle weights
   4. postural awareness exercises in standing

155. A physical therapist examines a patient's hip range of motion. Which pattern of limitation is typically considered to be a capsular pattern at the hip?

   1. limitation of flexion, abduction, and medial rotation
   2. limitation of flexion, adduction, and lateral rotation
   3. limitation of extension, abduction, and lateral rotation
   4. limitation of extension, adduction, and medial rotation

156. A patient diagnosed with an anterior cruciate ligament tear contemplates the option of surgery. The patient indicates that his insurance provider allows him to select an orthopedic surgeon and limits out of pocket expenses to a $250 deductible and 20% of the remaining fees. This type of arrangement best exemplifies:

   1. indemnity insurance plan
   2. preferred provider organization insurance plan
   3. point of service insurance plan
   4. health maintenance organization plan

157. A physical therapist performs a capillary refill test on a patient diagnosed with bronchitis by applying direct pressure to the nailbeds of the fingers. Which finding would be most indicative of a normal response after releasing the direct pressure?

   1. blanching should appear in less than two seconds
   2. blanching should appear in less than four seconds
   3. blanching should resolve in less than two seconds
   4. blanching should resolve in less than four seconds

158. A 62-year-old female is restricted from physical therapy for two days following surgical insertion of a urinary catheter. This type of procedure is most commonly performed with a:

   1. condom catheter
   2. Foley catheter
   3. suprapubic catheter
   4. Swan-Ganz catheter

159. A physical therapist instructs a patient to move her lower teeth forward in relation to the upper teeth. This motion is termed:

   1. protrusion
   2. retrusion
   3. lateral deviation
   4. occlusal position

160. A physical therapist examines a 27-year-old female with lower leg pain. The patient was referred to physical therapy after diagnostic imaging ruled out the possibility of a stress fracture. Which imaging technique would be the most appropriate when attempting to identify a stress fracture?

1. arthrography
2. bone densiometry
3. bone scan
4. x-ray

161. A patient in the intensive care unit rehabilitating from a serious infection is connected to a series of lines and tubes. Which lower extremity intravenous infusion site would be the most appropriate to administer an intravenous line?

1. antecubital vein
2. basilic vein
3. cephalic vein
4. saphenous vein

162. A patient four weeks status post arthroscopic medial meniscectomy is limited in knee flexion range of motion. Which mobilization technique would be the most beneficial to increase knee flexion?

1. anterior glide of the tibia
2. superior glide of the patella
3. posterior glide of the tibia
4. anterior glide of the fibula head

163. A 16-year-old high school track participant returns to physical therapy after a physician appointment. The patient indicates that after a series of diagnostic tests he was told that he had a tear in the medial meniscus of the left knee. Which of the following special tests would be the most appropriate to confirm the presence of the meniscal tear?

1. Lachman
2. pivot shift
3. McMurray
4. apprehension

164. After examining the respiratory status of a patient with a C6 spinal cord injury, which of the following clinical findings would you expect to be the most accurate?

1. partial innervation of the diaphragm
2. full epigastric rise in supine
3. a ventilator is required for assisted breathing
4. normal ventilatory reserve

165. A physical therapist instructs a patient with tight calf muscles to complete a closed kinematic chain standing wall stretch. Prior to beginning the stretch the therapist positions a folded towel under the medial arch of the patient's foot. The primary purpose of this action is to limit:

1. talocrural dorsiflexion
2. talocrural plantar flexion
3. subtalar supination
4. subtalar pronation

166. A physical therapist applies an electrical stimulation unit to a patient rehabilitating from an Achilles tendon rupture. Which of the following types of current has the lowest total average current?

1. low volt
2. high volt
3. Russian
4. interferential

167. A 50-year-old male rehabilitating from a recent stroke has good strength in the affected lower extremity with the exception of trace to poor strength in the right ankle joint. The patient's sensation is severely impaired for deep pressure, light touch, and sharp stimuli. The patient also has severe fluctuating edema at the ankle. The most appropriate orthosis for the patient is:

1. metal upright ankle-foot orthosis
2. polypropylene solid ankle-foot orthosis
3. prefabricated posterior leaf orthosis
4. metal upright knee-ankle-foot orthosis

168. A patient with a left transfemoral amputation ambulates in physical therapy. The physical therapist observes vaulting with left swing phase and occasional circumduction of the involved leg. The most likely cause of the gait deviation is:

1. the prosthesis is too short
2. the prosthesis is too long
3. weak plantar flexors on the right
4. there is decreased toe-out on the left

169. A patient is limited to 55 degrees in an active straight leg raise. When using the contract-relax technique to improve the patient's active range of motion, the therapist should emphasize contraction of the:

1. abductors and hip flexors
2. hamstrings and hip extensors
3. quadriceps and hip flexors
4. adductors and hip extensors

170. A developmental examination is completed on an eight month old infant. Findings from the examination include: the patient brings hands to mouth, requires assistance for ring sitting, presents with slight head lag, and does not reach across midline for objects. The child appears to be:

1. appropriate with normal development
2. developmentally delayed
3. developmentally accelerated
4. presents with cerebral palsy

171. A patient rehabilitating from a motor vehicle accident completes a series of closed kinetic chain exercises. One of the exercises requires the patient to perform a mini-squat in an erect position with the center of gravity placed directly over the knee joint. If the physical therapist modifies the activity by asking the patient to move the buttocks posteriorly in relation to the knees, what muscle is the therapist attempting to emphasize?

1. knee extensors
2. knee flexors
3. hip extensors
4. hip flexors

172. A physical therapist reviews a physician referral form that includes only the patient's name and the referring physician's signature. The therapist asks an administrative assistant to contact the physician's office to secure additional information while he begins the examination. During the examination the patient indicates that she had knee surgery two weeks ago, however is unable to provide more specific information. After completing the examination the therapist checks with the administrative assistant who indicates that she was unable to reach anyone at the physician's office. The most appropriate therapist action is:

1. initiate treatment based on the results of the examination
2. initiate treatment based on an established protocol following knee surgery
3. initiate treatment, however avoid resistive exercises and high level functional activities
4. delay treatment until orders are received from the referring physician

173. A physical therapist receives physical therapy orders for a patient that was recently injured in a motor vehicle accident. The patient's injuries include a Colles' fracture and a right tibial plateau fracture. The patient is mentally alert and does not exhibit any balance or coordination deficits. Assuming the patient is touchdown weight bearing, the most appropriate assistive device for the patient is:

1. Lofstrand crutches
2. rolling walker with platform attachments
3. axillary crutch and a straight crutch
4. walker with a platform attachment

174. A physical therapist employed in an acute care hospital reviews the results of recent laboratory testing for one of his patients. A note in the medical record indicates that the patient was dehydrated at the time the blood sample was taken. Which finding would be most likely based on the patient's hydration status?

1. increased coagulation time
2. decreased hematocrit level
3. increased blood urea nitrogen level
4. decreased hemoglobin level

175. A treatment program is designed to include late morning sessions involving aggressive stretching, moderate exercise, energy conservation, and stress management techniques. This program would be most appropriate for which diagnosis?

1. Guillain-Barre syndrome
2. myasthenia gravis
3. Osgood-Schlatter disease
4. multiple sclerosis

176. A patient with moderate chronic obstructive pulmonary disease performs an exercise test that will stress the patient to the point of limitation. During the test the physical therapist monitors the patient's physiologic response to exercise. Which of the following findings would not require cessation of the testing session?

1. a 20 mm Hg decrease in diastolic blood pressure with an increase in workload
2. systolic hypertension greater than 175 mm Hg
3. a PaO_2 of less than 55 mm Hg
4. maximal shortness of breath

177. A 28-year-old male referred to physical therapy by his primary physician complains of recurrent ankle pain. As part of the treatment program, the therapist uses ultrasound over the peroneus longus and brevis tendons. The most appropriate location for ultrasound application is:

1. inferior to the sustentaculum tali
2. over the sinus tarsi
3. posterior to the lateral malleolus
4. anterior to the lateral malleolus

178. A physical therapist positions a patient in supine prior to performing a manual muscle test of the supinator. To isolate the supinator and minimize the action of the biceps the therapist should position the patient's elbow in:

1. 30 degrees of elbow flexion
2. 60 degrees of elbow flexion
3. 90 degrees of elbow flexion
4. terminal elbow flexion

179. A patient involved in a cardiac rehabilitation program exercises on a treadmill. While exercising the patient reports his level of perceived exertion as a 7 on Borg's ten-point scale. Which option best describes the patient's rate of perceived exertion?

1. weak
2. moderate
3. strong
4. very strong

180. Laboratory testing reveals that a patient post chemotherapy has a platelet count of 60,000 mm^3. Which activity would be the most appropriate for the patient based on the platelet value?

1. strict bed rest
2. active range of motion
3. light activities of daily living
4. stationary cycling

181. A physical therapist reviews the surgical report of a patient that sustained extensive burns in a fire. The report indicates that at the time of primary excision cadaver skin was utilized to close the wound. This type of graft is termed a/an:

1. allograft
2. autograft
3. heterograft
4. xenograft

182. A physical therapist employed in a rehabilitation hospital treats a patient status post traumatic brain injury. During the treatment session the therapist notices that the patient's toes are discolored below a bivalved lower extremity cast. The cast was applied approximately five hours prior in an attempt to reduce a plantar flexion contracture. The most appropriate therapist action is to:

1. document the observation in the medical record and continue to monitor the patient's circulation
2. contact the staff nurse and request that the cast is removed
3. refer the patient to an orthotist
4. remove the cast

183. A physical therapist develops a problem list after completing an examination of a patient status post arthroscopic medial meniscectomy. The therapist identifies increased edema in the right knee as the first entry in the problem list. Which of the following short-term goals would be the most appropriate entry in the medical record?

1. decrease edema in the knee by one centimeter
2. decrease edema in the knee by one centimeter within two weeks
3. decrease right knee circumferential measurements by one centimeter at a level three centimeters and five centimeters above the knee
4. decrease right knee circumferential measurements by one centimeter at a level three centimeters and five centimeters above the superior pole of the patella within two weeks

184. A patient with a spinal cord injury positioned on a tilt table elevated to 60 degrees begins to complain of severe dizziness and nausea. The physical therapist's most immediate response should be to:

1. lower the tilt table 10 degrees and take off the patient's abdominal binder
2. leave the tilt table at 60 degrees and call for medical assistance
3. monitor the patient's vital signs with the tilt table at 60 degrees and continue to elevate the table as tolerated
4. lower the tilt table to horizontal and monitor the patient's vital signs

185. A group of senior physical therapy students utilizes ten patients from a local rehabilitation center with decubitus ulcers for a research project. This type of sampling most accurately describes:

1. cluster sampling
2. convenience sampling
3. stratified sampling
4. systematic sampling

186. A physical therapist examines a patient rehabilitating from a traumatic brain injury. The therapist makes the following entry in the medical record: The patient is able to respond to simple commands fairly consistently, however has difficulty with increasingly complex commands or lack of any external structure. Responses are nonpurposeful, random, and fragmented. According to the Rancho Los Amigos Cognitive Functioning Scale the patient is most representative of level:

1. III - localized responses
2. IV - confused-agitated
3. V - confused-inappropriate
4. VI - confused-appropriate

187. A physical therapist examines a 25-year-old male rehabilitating from a meniscus repair. The physician orders indicate the patient is non-weight bearing on the involved lower extremity. The most appropriate gait pattern for the patient is:

1. two-point
2. three-point
3. four-point
4. swing-to

188. A physical therapist examines a patient referred to physical therapy with olecranon bursitis. During the initial examination the therapist identifies diffuse swelling in the elbow joint. Which of the following joints would be affected with swelling in the elbow complex?

1. ulnohumeral joint
2. ulnohumeral and radiohumeral joints
3. radiohumeral and proximal radioulnar joints
4. ulnohumeral, radiohumeral, and proximal radioulnar joints

189. While treating a patient, a physical therapist notices a mixture of blood and urine in the patient's collection bag. The most immediate therapist response would be to:

1. temporarily disconnect the collection bag
2. continue with the patient's treatment program
3. contact a member of the nursing staff
4. document the observation in the physical therapy record

190. A patient with osteoarthritis in the right knee is referred to physical therapy. Examination reveals moderate inflammation in the involved knee and significant muscle weakness particularly in the quadriceps. The patient rates the intensity of pain in the knee as a 4 on a scale of 0 to 10. The most appropriate activity to address the muscle impairment is:

1. isometric quadriceps contraction
2. straight leg raises with ankle weights
3. limited range active knee extension in short sitting
4. avoid strengthening exercises until the patient is pain free

191. A 32-year-old female rehabilitating from a medial meniscus repair has been instructed by an orthopedic surgeon to remain non-weight bearing for three weeks following surgery. The patient has no significant past medical history and is expected to make a full recovery. Which of the following would be the most appropriate assistive device for the patient?

1. straight cane
2. axillary crutches
3. parapodium
4. walker

192. The practice of physical therapy in a given state is often defined according to the state physical therapy practice act. Which source of law is responsible for formalizing a practice act?

1. constitutional law
2. statutory law
3. common law
4. administrative law

193. A physical therapist treats a patient status post right cerebrovascular accident with resultant left hemiplegia for a colleague on vacation. A note left by the primary therapist indicates that the patient exhibits "pusher syndrome." When examining the patient's sitting posture, which of the following findings would be most likely?

1. increased lean to the left with increased weight bearing on the left buttock
2. increased lean to the right with increased weight bearing on the right buttock
3. increased forward lean with increased weight bearing on the right buttock
4. increased forward lean with increased weight bearing on the left buttock

194. A physical therapist performs goniometric measurements for elbow flexion with a patient in supine. In order to isolate elbow flexion the therapist should stabilize the:

1. distal end of the humerus
2. proximal end of the humerus
3. distal end of the ulna
4. proximal end of the radius

195. A physical therapist explains to a patient the benefits of using electrical stimulation for muscle reeducation. The patient appears to understand the therapist's explanation, however seems extremely frightened and asks the therapist not to use the electrical device. The most appropriate therapist action is to:

1. reassure the patient that the electrical stimulation will not be harmful
2. use only small amounts of current
3. select another appropriate treatment technique
4. discharge the patient from physical therapy

196. A physical therapist observes that a number of aides appear to be unfamiliar with appropriate guarding techniques. The most appropriate remedial strategy to improve their performance is to:

1. offer assistance to the aides when the inappropriate behavior is observed
2. refer the aides to text books that explain proper guarding technique
3. develop a mandatory inservice on guarding techniques for the aides
4. inform the director of rehabilitation that the aides are incompetent

197. A physical therapist prepares to treat a patient using ultraviolet light by determining the patient's minimal erythemal dose. The most common location for testing is:

1. on the posterior aspect of the upper arm
2. on the anterior aspect of the forearm
3. on the anterior aspect of the thigh
4. on the posterior aspect of the lower leg

198. A physical therapist examines a 24-year-old male recently admitted to the hospital with C3 tetraplegia. During the examination the therapist identifies several areas of reddened and mottled skin over selected bony prominences. The therapist is concerned that without proper care the patient's condition will worsen. The most immediate action is to:

1. discuss the situation directly with the nursing staff
2. ask the patient to perform pressure relief activities
3. contact the patient's family
4. contact the patient's referring physician

199. A physical therapist treating a patient overhears two of his colleagues discussing another patient's case in the charting area. The therapist is concerned that patients may overhear the same conversation. The most appropriate action is to:

1. discuss the situation with the director of rehabilitation
2. discuss confidentiality issues at the next department meeting
3. move the patient away from the charting area
4. inform the physical therapists that their conversation may be audible to patients

200. A physical therapist attempts to obtain information on the ability of noncontractile tissue to allow motion at a specific joint. Which selective tissue tension assessment would provide the therapist with the most valuable information?

1. active range of motion
2. active-assistive range of motion
3. passive range of motion
4. resisted isometrics

Sample Exam: Two – Answer Sheet

1.	① ② ③ ④	36.	① ② ③ ④	71. ① ② ③ ④
2.	① ② ③ ④	37.	① ② ③ ④	72. ① ② ③ ④
3.	① ② ③ ④	38.	① ② ③ ④	73. ① ② ③ ④
4.	① ② ③ ④	39.	① ② ③ ④	74. ① ② ③ ④
5.	① ② ③ ④	40.	① ② ③ ④	75. ① ② ③ ④
6.	① ② ③ ④	41.	① ② ③ ④	76. ① ② ③ ④
7.	① ② ③ ④	42.	① ② ③ ④	77. ① ② ③ ④
8.	① ② ③ ④	43.	① ② ③ ④	78. ① ② ③ ④
9.	① ② ③ ④	44.	① ② ③ ④	79. ① ② ③ ④
10.	① ② ③ ④	45.	① ② ③ ④	80. ① ② ③ ④
11.	① ② ③ ④	46.	① ② ③ ④	81. ① ② ③ ④
12.	① ② ③ ④	47.	① ② ③ ④	82. ① ② ③ ④
13.	① ② ③ ④	48.	① ② ③ ④	83. ① ② ③ ④
14.	① ② ③ ④	49.	① ② ③ ④	84. ① ② ③ ④
15.	① ② ③ ④	50.	① ② ③ ④	85. ① ② ③ ④
16.	① ② ③ ④	51.	① ② ③ ④	86. ① ② ③ ④
17.	① ② ③ ④	52.	① ② ③ ④	87. ① ② ③ ④
18.	① ② ③ ④	53.	① ② ③ ④	88. ① ② ③ ④
19.	① ② ③ ④	54.	① ② ③ ④	89. ① ② ③ ④
20.	① ② ③ ④	55.	① ② ③ ④	90. ① ② ③ ④
21.	① ② ③ ④	56.	① ② ③ ④	91. ① ② ③ ④
22.	① ② ③ ④	57.	① ② ③ ④	92. ① ② ③ ④
23.	① ② ③ ④	58.	① ② ③ ④	93. ① ② ③ ④
24.	① ② ③ ④	59.	① ② ③ ④	94. ① ② ③ ④
25.	① ② ③ ④	60.	① ② ③ ④	95. ① ② ③ ④
26.	① ② ③ ④	61.	① ② ③ ④	96. ① ② ③ ④
27.	① ② ③ ④	62.	① ② ③ ④	97. ① ② ③ ④
28.	① ② ③ ④	63.	① ② ③ ④	98. ① ② ③ ④
29.	① ② ③ ④	64.	① ② ③ ④	99. ① ② ③ ④
30.	① ② ③ ④	65.	① ② ③ ④	100. ① ② ③ ④
31.	① ② ③ ④	66.	① ② ③ ④	101. ① ② ③ ④
32.	① ② ③ ④	67.	① ② ③ ④	102. ① ② ③ ④
33.	① ② ③ ④	68.	① ② ③ ④	103. ① ② ③ ④
34.	① ② ③ ④	69.	① ② ③ ④	104. ① ② ③ ④
35.	① ② ③ ④	70.	① ② ③ ④	105. ① ② ③ ④

SAMPLE EXAMINATION: EXAM TWO ANSWER SHEET

106.	①	②	③	④	138.	①	②	③	④	170.	①	②	③	④
107.	①	②	③	④	139.	①	②	③	④	171.	①	②	③	④
108.	①	②	③	④	140.	①	②	③	④	172.	①	②	③	④
109.	①	②	③	④	141.	①	②	③	④	173.	①	②	③	④
110.	①	②	③	④	142.	①	②	③	④	174.	①	②	③	④
111.	①	②	③	④	143.	①	②	③	④	175.	①	②	③	④
112.	①	②	③	④	144.	①	②	③	④	176.	①	②	③	④
113.	①	②	③	④	145.	①	②	③	④	177.	①	②	③	④
114.	①	②	③	④	146.	①	②	③	④	178.	①	②	③	④
115.	①	②	③	④	147.	①	②	③	④	179.	①	②	③	④
116.	①	②	③	④	148.	①	②	③	④	180.	①	②	③	④
117.	①	②	③	④	149.	①	②	③	④	181.	①	②	③	④
118.	①	②	③	④	150.	①	②	③	④	182.	①	②	③	④
119.	①	②	③	④	151.	①	②	③	④	183.	①	②	③	④
120.	①	②	③	④	152.	①	②	③	④	184.	①	②	③	④
121.	①	②	③	④	153.	①	②	③	④	185.	①	②	③	④
122.	①	②	③	④	154.	①	②	③	④	186.	①	②	③	④
123.	①	②	③	④	155.	①	②	③	④	187.	①	②	③	④
124.	①	②	③	④	156.	①	②	③	④	188.	①	②	③	④
125.	①	②	③	④	157.	①	②	③	④	189.	①	②	③	④
126.	①	②	③	④	158.	①	②	③	④	190.	①	②	③	④
127.	①	②	③	④	159.	①	②	③	④	191.	①	②	③	④
128.	①	②	③	④	160.	①	②	③	④	192.	①	②	③	④
129.	①	②	③	④	161.	①	②	③	④	193.	①	②	③	④
130.	①	②	③	④	162.	①	②	③	④	194.	①	②	③	④
131.	①	②	③	④	163.	①	②	③	④	195.	①	②	③	④
132.	①	②	③	④	164.	①	②	③	④	196.	①	②	③	④
133.	①	②	③	④	165.	①	②	③	④	197.	①	②	③	④
134.	①	②	③	④	166.	①	②	③	④	198.	①	②	③	④
135.	①	②	③	④	167.	①	②	③	④	199.	①	②	③	④
136.	①	②	③	④	168.	①	②	③	④	200.	①	②	③	④
137.	①	②	③	④	169.	①	②	③	④					

Sample Exam Answers: Two

1. **Answer: 4**   Resource: Guide for Professional Conduct
   The physical therapist has an obligation to respect the patient's wishes despite the fact the student is qualified to complete the examination.

2. **Answer: 1**   Resource: Scott - Professional Ethics (p. 162)
   Physical therapists are required to report known or suspected abuse to enforcement agencies. These agencies include, but are not limited to, adult protective services and local or state law enforcement.

3. **Answer: 4**   Resource: Miller (p. 1845)
   Oxygen saturation rate refers to the percentage of oxygen bound to hemoglobin in the blood. Normal oxygen saturation rates range from 95-98%.

4. **Answer: 2**   Resource: Levangie (p. 443)
   Deceleration is a component of the swing phase. Deceleration occurs after mid-swing when the tibia passes beyond the perpendicular and the knee extends in preparation for heel strike.

5. **Answer: 3**   Resource: Guide for Professional Conduct
   The patient's goal of walking one mile each day does not warrant continued physical therapy services. Physical therapists should avoid overutilization of physical therapy services, however should assist patients to achieve individual goals through activities such as a home exercise program.

6. **Answer: 1**   Resource: Pierson (p. 13)
   A supportive spouse can be extremely helpful to a patient completing a home exercise program. In order for the spouse to be an asset, she must first recognize the value of the program.

7. **Answer: 1**   Resource: Thomas (p. 552)
   Dysdiadochokinesia is defined as the inability to perform rapidly alternating movements.

8. **Answer: 3**   Resource: Magee (p. 401)
   Lateral hamstrings reflex (S1-S2), medial hamstrings reflex (L5-S1), patellar reflex (L3-L4), Achilles reflex (S1-S2).

9. **Answer: 1**   Resource: Guide to Physical Therapist Practice (p. S34)
   A physical therapist is qualified to instruct and assist a patient with transfers to all surfaces. The therapist should perform tub transfers with the patient so that independence is attained as soon as possible.

10. **Answer: 2**   Resource: Haggard (p. 3)
    By addressing the issue directly with the patient, the physical therapist may improve compliance with the weight bearing restrictions and therefore promote a better environment for tissue healing.

11. **Answer: 4**   Resource: Pierson (p. 340)
    An individual who is a homosexual does not qualify under the Americans with Disabilities Act unless he/she has a physical or mental impairment that substantially limits one or more major activities or is regarded as having an impairment.

12. **Answer: 4**   Resource: Zydlo (p. 82)
    Pressure applied to an artery proximal to an injury site may be helpful to control bleeding.

13. **Answer: 3**   Resource: Hall (p. 363)
    Since the pelvic floor muscles are weak and the patient is "initiating" the strengthening exercises, it is desirable for periods of rest to exceed the periods of exercise. Weak pelvic floor muscles generally require twice as much rest time as hold time.

14. **Answer: 1**   Resource: Neistadt (p. 804)
    Requesting information provides the patient with the opportunity to express her feelings and may serve to promote dialogue.

15. **Answer: 4**   Resource: Sullivan - An Integrated Approach (p. 100)
    During a D1 extension pattern there is scapular depression, adduction, and downward rotation. The pectoralis minor assists with both depression and downward rotation. The rhomboids assist with adduction and downward rotation, while the levator scapulae assist with downward rotation.

16. **Answer: 1**   Resource: Haggard (p. 43)
    A patient with short-term memory deficits may have difficulty with an exercise program that is too complex. A program that allows for individual exercise selection offers the patient a limited number of options without compromising the integrity of the program.

17. Answer: 2   Resource: Wortman (p. 131)
Operant conditioning is a form of learning where a particular action or behavior is followed by the administration of a reward (positive reinforcement). B.F. Skinner first publicized this learning approach.

18. Answer: 1   Resource: Miller (p. 1843)
The patient's lab values for hematocrit, white blood cells, platelet, and hemoglobin are significantly below acceptable ranges. As a result exercise is not indicated.

19. Answer: 1   Resource: Guide for Professional Conduct
The frequency of physical therapy visits should be based on the results of the patient examination, and not solely on the physician referral.

20. Answer: 1   Resource: Robinson (p. 75)
By unplugging the machine and labeling it "defective- do not use", the physical therapist not only limits the danger to the current patient, but also ensures that other therapists will not place their patients in jeopardy.

21. Answer: 4   Resource: Michlovitz (p. 204)
Continuous ultrasound at 2.4 W/cm^2 over a fracture site is excessive and can be potentially dangerous to the patient.

22. Answer: 4   Resource: Ciccone (p. 222)
Methotrexate is used as a disease modifying agent in the treatment of rheumatoid arthritis. Adverse effects include nausea, gastrointestinal distress and/or hemorrhage, cough, shortness of breath, and lower extremity edema. Although nausea is not a medical emergency, it is appropriate for the patient to inform the physician of any persistent side effects as soon as possible.

23. Answer: 2   Resource: Minor (p. 289)
Demonstration promotes understanding and often limits the anxiety associated with learning a new task.

24. Answer: 4   Resource: Currier (p. 34)
It is essential to ascertain if research exists on the effectiveness of treating psoriatic lesions with ultraviolet prior to initiating a formal research project.

25. Answer: 3   Resource: Nosse (p. 155)
A patient satisfaction survey must be designed, disseminated, and analyzed prior to drawing specific conclusions or modifying existing patient care standards.

26. Answer: 1   Resource: Best (p. 114)
The dependent variable is defined as the conditions or characteristics that appear, disappear or change as the experimenter introduces, removes or changes the independent variable. In this particular study, functional knee bracing is the independent variable, while speed and agility are the dependent variables.

27. Answer: 1   Resource: O'Sullivan - Physical Rehabilitation (p. 540)
It is important to assess a patient's cognitive status in order to develop an appropriate plan of care. The examination should assess memory, attention span, ability to follow directions, and recall. This will allow the physical therapist to approach the patient at an appropriate level.

28. Answer: 4   Resource: Haggard (p. 40)
A physical therapist must make a patient aware of behavior that is unacceptable. Failure to address the issue directly with the patient may serve to reinforce the behavior.

29. Answer: 3   Resource: Minor (p. 39)
Age predicted maximal heart rate can be determined as follows: 220 – patient's age (34) = 186.

30. Answer: 3   Resource: Pierson (p. 340)
An accommodation that would fundamentally alter the operation of a business may not be considered reasonable. It is unlikely, however that a modification to a work station would fall into this category.

31. Answer: 2   Resource: Haggard (p. 136)
The presence of parents can often be reassuring to a young child when confronted with a new experience.

32. Answer: 2   Resource: Magee (p. 1)
The patient should return to his previous functional activity level in a matter of weeks following a grade I medial collateral ligament sprain.

33. Answer: 3   Resource: Brannon (p. 115)
Chronic obstructive pulmonary disease is characterized by a progressive reduction in expiratory flow rates. Hyperinflation of the lungs results in an increase in residual volume.

34. Answer: 3   Resource: Neistadt (p. 5)
Occupational therapy is described as the art and science of helping people perform day to day activities. Although professional boundaries differ from facility to facility, bathing and dressing activities are typically addressed by occupational therapists.

35. Answer: 1   Resource: Kendall (p. 202)
The tendon of the tibialis posterior is most prominent when the foot is inverted and plantar flexed. The tendon can be palpated posterior and inferior to the medial malleolus.

36. Answer: 3   Resource: Hertling (p. 530)
The distance to the clinic is excessive; particularly when sitting for prolonged periods of time may exacerbate the patient's condition. The patient should receive therapy services at a clinic closer to home.

37. Answer: 2   Resource: Sultz (p. 242)
Medicaid federal guidelines require states to offer a mandatory core of basic medical services including inpatient and outpatient hospital services, physician services, diagnostic services, nursing home care, home health care, preventive care, health screening services, and family planning services.

38. Answer: 3   Resource: Paz (p. 375)
Sitting with the legs in a dependent position promotes venous stasis and increases the incidence of a deep vein thrombosis.

39. Answer: 4   Resource: Richard (p. 36)
The primary cause of shock related to burns is hypovolemia or loss of circulating fluid. Symptoms of shock include a drop in blood pressure, increased pulse rate, and decreased urine output.

40. Answer: 2   Resource: Mahler (p. 70)
Measurements at 2 minutes and 3 minutes provide the therapist with the best opportunity to determine if a steady state heart rate has been achieved. Failure to reach a steady state heart rate at a given work load prohibits the work load from being increased.

41. Answer: 4   Resource: O'Sullivan - Physical Rehabilitation (p. 381)
Inability to sit unsupported without assistance is indicative of poor sitting balance.

42. Answer: 3   Resource: O'Sullivan - Laboratory Manual (p. 120)
Controlled mobility is the stage in motor control where a patient is able to have some mobility while maintaining postural stability. Tall kneeling represents static control, while the transfer to half kneeling requires the mobility to weight shift and change position.

43. Answer: 3   Resource: Reese (p. 493)
The hypoglossal nerve innervates the primary muscles of the tongue. As a result, a lower motor neuron disease affecting the left hypoglossal nerve will cause weakness and resultant deviation of the tongue to the left (toward the side of weakness). Muscle atrophy is a common finding in lower motor neuron lesions.

44. Answer: 2   Resource: O'Sullivan - Physical Rehabilitation (p. 375)
Perseveration is the continued repetition of a word, phrase, or movement. Initiating a new activity during therapy may allow the patient to redirect attention and subsequently receive positive reinforcement for attending to a selected task.

45. Answer: 1   Resource: Currier (p. 84)
A nominal scale describes differences by assigning them to a category or subset. The nominal scale is the weakest level of measurement.

46. Answer: 4   Resource: Guide to Physical Therapist Practice (p. S42)
A physical therapy aide is a nonlicensed worker trained under the direction of a physical therapist. A physical therapist may delegate ambulation activities to an aide if the physical therapist feels the aide's training is adequate to complete the activity. A physical therapy aide requires continuous on-site supervision.

47. Answer: 2   Resource: Goodman (p. 38)
Leading questions often bias a patient toward a specific response. The question "Does this alter your pain in any way?" provides the patient with the opportunity to provide additional insight into his/her present condition.

48. Answer: 1   Resource: Frownfelter (p. 220)
S1=closing of the mitral and tricuspid valves.
S2=closing of the aortic and pulmonic valves.
S3=early ventricular filling; noncompliant left vetricle
S4=rapid ventricular filling that occurs after atrial contraction.

49. Answer: 4   Resource: Kisner (p. 671)
Pursed lip breathing is a technique designed to improve ventilation and oxygenation. Studies indicate that pursed lip breathing decreases respiratory rate, increases tidal volume, and improves exercise tolerance.

50. Answer: 4   Resource: Pierson (p. 54)
The most accurate value for respiration rate is obtained using the longest measurement period.

51. Answer: 3   Resource: Ciccone (p. 299)
Vasodilators are drugs that directly inhibit smooth muscle contraction and decrease peripheral vascular resistance. A patient taking vasodilators may have difficulty with joint effusion due to subsequent fluid retention and the diminished contractility of the vascular system.

52. Answer: 2   Resource: Magee (p. 8)
Active movement requires direct patient participation.

53. Answer: 3   Resource: Scott - Promoting Legal Awareness (p. 104)
The physical therapist should utilize a female to serve as an observer. This type of action is a form of risk management in order to prevent allegations of alleged misconduct.

54. Answer: 4   Resource: Pierson (p. 152)
Inadequate seat width results in difficulty changing positions, pressure on the greater trochanters, and difficulty wearing bulky clothing or orthoses.

55. Answer: 1   Resource: Booher (p. 464)
The posterior cruciate ligament is responsible for preventing posterior displacement of the tibia on the femur. The ligament is most often injured by a direct force on the tibia, which displaces it in a posterior direction in relation to the femur.

56. Answer: 4   Resource: Scott - Promoting Legal Awareness (p. 65)
Although each of the presented options is important, maintaining accurate and timely documentation is the most important. Documentation often provides the primary evidence of what transpired during a given treatment session. The information is often utilized during litigation to determine if patient care standards were compromised.

57. Answer: 1   Resource: Kisner (p. 203)
Lateral distraction and anterior glide of the glenohumeral joint can be utilized to increase lateral rotation and extension.

58. Answer: 4   Resource: Guide for Professional Conduct
The most appropriate response is to refer the patient to a qualified physician. This action will allow the patient to receive a thorough examination and if indicated a referral to physical therapy.

59. Answer: 2   Resource: Hertling (p. 328)
The Q angle is defined as the angle between the quadriceps muscles and the patellar tendon. Normal Q angle values are 13 degrees for males and 18 degrees for females.

60. Answer: 4   Resource: Michlovitz (p. 233)
Internal or external metallic objects, including surgical metal implants, are contraindications for shortwave diathermy. Failure to recognize the presence of a surgical metal implant may result in excessive heat production and subsequent tissue damage.

61. Answer: 3   Resource: Richard (p. 43)
Oliguria refers to a decreased amount of urine output in relation to fluid intake. A typical healthy adult will excrete 1,000-1,500 ml in a 24 hour period.

62. Answer: 4   Resource: Kendall (p. 282)
The upper trapezius acts to elevate the scapula and is innervated by the spinal component of the accessory nerve. The dorsal scapular nerve innervates the levator scapulae and rhomboid minor.

63. Answer: 1   Resource: Richard (p. 39)
An acute burn produces hypermetabolism and therefore results in increased oxygen consumption, increased minute ventilation, and increased core temperature. Intravascular, interstitial, and intracellular fluids are all diminished.

64. Answer: 4   Resource: Magee (p. 2)
In order to adequately address the patient's subjective report of pain, it is essential to gather additional information.

65. Answer: 2   Resource: Frownfelter (p. 225)
Tactile fremitus is often examined by using a hand or portion of a hand to assess the vibration associated with spoken words. The examination technique can be used to provide information on the density of the lungs and thoracic cavity.

66. Answer: 1   Resource: Paz (p. 121)
Respiratory acidosis is characterized by elevated $PaCO_2$ and below normal pH due to hypoventilation.
An arterial blood gas analysis includes the following:
PaO_2 = partial pressure of oxygen in arterial blood
$PaCO_2$ = partial pressure of carbon dioxide in arterial blood
pH = the degree of acidity or alkalinity in arterial blood
HCO_3 = the level of bicarbonate in arterial blood

67. Answer: 4   Resource: Boissonnault (p. 211)
The cerebellum is the area of the brain responsible for modulation of movement. Lesions to the cerebellum may produce hypotonia, tremor, impaired reflexes, ataxic gait, and nystagmus.

68. Answer: 3   Resource: DePoy (p. 190)
Answers that do not correspond to the actual perception of a respondent may contribute to forming inaccurate conclusions.

69. Answer: 2   Resource: Best (p. 230)
The number that is closest to +1.00 represents the strongest positive correlation.

70. Answer: 4   Resource: Kisner (p. 57)
Gains in strength are greatest when a muscle is exercised against resistance at maximal intensity.

71. Answer: 2   Resource: Richard (p. 39)
Many patients on extended bed rest following a burn experience significant cardiovascular complications. A functional capacity of 10 or more metabolic equivalents is a good indication that a formal cardiovascular rehabilitation program is not necessary. An intensity of 10 METs corresponds to running at six miles per hour.

72. Answer: 3   Resource: Minor (p. 248)
The patient should not grasp the edge of a sliding board with her fingers since they may become pinched while completing the transfer.

73. Answer: 2   Resource: Kisner (p. 192)
Joint mobilization will not increase joint play in a prosthetic knee and therefore is not an appropriate intervention.

74. Answer: 4 Resource: Ciccone (p. 201)
The most common side effect of nonsteroidal anti-inflammatory medications is gastrointestinal discomfort. Discomfort occurs due to the direct irritation of the gastric mucosa and loss of protection in the mucosal lining of the stomach. Other side effects include vomiting, dizziness, headache, tinnitus, gastrointestinal hemorrhage, and rash.

75. Answer: 2 Resource: Hoppenfeld (p. 43)
The ulnar nerve is most susceptible to injury at its location between the medial epicondyle and the olecranon process.

76. Answer: 2 Resource: Sullivan - An Integrated Approach (p. 84)
Tall kneeling follows the quadruped position in the developmental sequence. Tall kneeling emphasizes hip extension in combination with knee flexion and serves to promote stability.

77. Answer: 4 Resource: Minor (p. 288)
A walker provides the patient with the necessary stability without relying on significant upper extremity strength. The walker allows for varying degrees of weight bearing on the involved lower extremity.

78. Answer: 2 Resource: Richard (p. 425)
Continuous ultrasound is commonly used to treat patients with healed burns due to its ability to increase the extensibility of collagen and decrease pain.

79. Answer: 3 Resource: Kisner (p. 708)
Atelectasis refers to a collapsed or airless condition of a lobe or segment of a lung. Segmental breathing is a technique that can be used to direct inspired air to a selected area.

80. Answer: 2 Resource: Richard (p. 138)
Topical antibiotics are often utilized in the treatment of burns. They serve to reduce bacterial count, provide a covering for the wound, reduce stiffness, and reduce evaporative loss. Since topical antibiotics are applied directly to the affected area sterile gloves should be worn. Due to the limited size of the wound additional medical asepsis would not be necessary.

81. Answer: 4 Resource: Pierson (p. 59)
Respiratory rate is an objective measure that is used to assess endurance. Respiratory rate typically increases as a patient becomes fatigued.

82. Answer: 3 Resource: Boissonnault (p. 220)
Normalization of tone is a priority in stroke rehabilitation. Facilitation techniques are utilized when hypotonia exists. Facilitation techniques include vibration, weight bearing, approximation, tapping, and quick stretch.

83. Answer: 3 Resource: Paz (p. 268)
A positive Babinski reflex is normal in infants up to six months of age. The reflex is elicited by stimulating the lateral aspect of the sole of the foot. If the great toe extends in a person older than six months of age, it may indicate the presence of an upper motor neuron lesion.

84. Answer: 3 Resource: Norkin (p. 26)
Since the patient's elbow range of motion begins at 15 degrees of flexion and ends at 90 degrees of flexion, the measurement should be recorded as 15-90 degrees of right elbow flexion. The amount of available range of motion is considered hypomobile.

85. Answer: 2 Resource: Umphred (p. 534)
Broca's area, located in the left hemisphere, receives its blood supply from the middle cerebral artery. Damage to Broca's area may result in expressive aphasia.

86. Answer: 2 Resource: O'Sullivan - Physical Rehabilitation (p. 1029)
The use of an orthosis would ensure adequate foot clearance and stability during activities of daily living.

87. Answer: 2 Resource: Kisner (p. 400)
Internal fixation provides the fracture site with the necessary stability to allow early protected weight bearing.

88. Answer: 1 Resource: Minor (p. 296)
Wooden axillary crutches provide the patient with an appropriate and cost effective assistive device to meet a short-term need.

89. Answer: 1 Resource: Michlovitz (p. 251)
Shortwave diathermy produces deep heating effects by introducing electromagnetic energy that is converted to heat.

90. Answer: 1 Resource: Michlovitz (p. 140)
Archimedes' principle of buoyancy states that a body immersed in a liquid experiences an upward force equal to the weight of the displaced liquid. In aquatic therapy, a patient may experience greater ease of movement due to the buoyant force of the water.

91. Answer: 2 Resource: Kisner (p. 672)
Pacing is a technique that can allow patients to complete functional activities without shortness of breath or dyspnea.

92. Answer: 1 Resource: Nosse (p. 161)
Utilization review is a process where a health care provider demonstrates appropriate allocation of resources through a formal review process. The primary purpose of utilization review is to ensure cost effective, quality patient care.

93. Answer: 1 Resource: Magee (p. 311)
Volumetric measurements are commonly used to measure edema in the distal extremities. The measurement is typically performed by examining the amount of water displaced from a cylinder following immersion of an affected body part.

94. Answer: 4 Resource: Kettenbach (p. 44)
The objective section of a S.O.A.P. note includes the physical therapist's objective observations and the results of examination and treatment procedures.

95. Answer: 2 Resource: Kendall (p. 228)
To test the right hip adductors, the patient should be positioned on his/her right side.

96. Answer: 4 Resource: Irwin (p. 369)
Upright sitting in a forward leaning posture with the neck flexed and arms supported is the optimal position to produce a forceful cough.

97. Answer: 1 Resource: Anemaet (p. 143)
A two-year-old child is typically able to perform the following gross motor skills: ride a tricycle, run on toes, walk downstairs alternating feet, and hop on one foot.

98. Answer: 2 Resource: Standards of Practice
It is not unusual for a patient to experience increased pain at various points during a rehabilitation program. As a result, it is not necessary to discontinue formal treatment or to refer the patient to another health care professional at this time.

99. Answer: 4 Resource: Irwin (p. 297)
Total lung capacity equals the sum of residual volume and vital capacity. Total lung capacity does not change significantly as a result of aging. Although residual volume increases with age, the net result on total lung capacity is negligible.

100. Answer: 3 Resource: Pierson (p. 282)
Although the order of application of the gown and mask may vary, gloves must be the last item to be applied.

101. Answer: 1 Resource: Kisner (p. 116)
Quadriceps setting exercises provide the opportunity for the muscle to contract without an appreciable change in length. The exercise places minimal stress on the knee and the surrounding tissues and as a result can be utilized during the initial stages of a rehabilitation program.

102. Answer: 3 Resource: Hertling (p. 220)
The medial collateral ligament, also termed the ulnar collateral ligament, is a fan shaped ligament that serves to restrict medial angulation of the ulna on the humerus. The ligament extends from the medial epicondyle to the medial margin of the ulna's trochlear notch and is assessed for potential instability by applying valgus force to the distal forearm.

103. Answer: 3 Resource: Pierson (p. 205)
The patient would likely utilize a three-point gait pattern using axillary crutches. A three-point gait pattern can accommodate different levels of weight bearing.

104. Answer: 2 Resource: Hertling (p. 349)
A third degree sprain involves a complete rupture or break in the continuity of a ligament. The injury usually results in significant joint play hypermobility.

105. Answer: 3 Resource: Pierson (p. 266)
When an intravenous line becomes dislodged from a vein it is appropriate to turn off the I.V. in order to prevent further accumulation of fluid.

106. Answer: 3 Resource: Kendall (p. 268)
In addition to flexing the elbow the biceps brachii acts to supinate the forearm. The musculocutaneous nerve innervates the biceps brachii.

107. Answer: 4 Resource: Rothstein (p. 533)
A sputum sample classified as purulent is described as a viscous fluid exudate that is often yellow or green and may be associated with acute or chronic infection.

108. Answer: 1 Resource: Rothstein (p. 122)
Ankle eversion has been shown to have an interclass correlation coefficient of 0.17. The value is significantly lower than the interclass correlation coefficients for the remaining options.

109. Answer: 3 Resource: Trofino (p. 22)
A full-thickness burn is characterized by complete destruction of the epidermal and dermal layers of the skin. In addition, some of the subcutaneous tissue is damaged. Grafts are required with full-thickness burns.

110. Answer: 3 Resource: Minor (p. 472)
Doorway width should be a minimum of 32 inches in order to accommodate a wheelchair.

111. Answer: 2 Resource: Pierson (p. 265)
Short-term tube feeding is often accomplished through the use of a nasogastric tube. A nasogastric tube is inserted through a nostril and terminates in the stomach.

112. Answer: 1 Resource: Pierson (p. 328)
Patients on extended bed rest may experience a significant decrease in systolic blood pressure with vertical positioning. A decrease in systolic blood pressure of 20 mm Hg or more is indicative of orthostatic hypotension.

113. Answer: 1 Resource: Brotzman (p. 57)
A partial tear of the ulnar collateral ligament is most often treated with a short-arm thumb spica cast. A long-arm thumb spica cast may be more appropriate for an injury such as a nondisplaced fracture of the scaphoid.

114. Answer: 2   Resource: Brotzman (p. 62)
The rate and amount of bone healing as determined through radiographs determines the actual amount of time an external fixation device is applied. A general estimate of the necessary time would be 6-8 weeks.

115. Answer: 3   Resource: Currier (p. 84)
An ordinal measurement scale allows for the ranking of items or individuals from highest to lowest. The amount of difference between rankings may not be equal.

116. Answer: 1   Resource: Irwin (p. 238)
The left lung does not have a middle lobe.

117. Answer: 3   Resource: Ratliffe (p. 30)
The Landau reflex is an equilibrium response that occurs when a child responds to prone suspension by aligning his/her head and extremities in line with the plane of the body. Although this response begins around three months of age, it is not fully integrated until the child's second year.

118. Answer: 3   Resource: Rothstein (p. 658)
Beta blockers' primary effect is to decrease heart rate and the force of myocardial contraction. As a result beta blockers act to decrease heart rate and blood pressure during exercise.

119. Answer: 2   Resource: Umphred (p. 426)
In order for a physical therapist to properly interact with a patient during an examination, it is essential to determine the patient's level of communication.

120. Answer: 4   Resource: O'Sullivan - Physical Rehabilitation (p. 667)
Weight shifting is a prerequisite activity for many higher level functional activities including gait.

121. Answer: 1   Resource: Brotzman (p. 57)
A complete tear of the ulnar collateral ligament of the thumb is often termed "gamekeeper's thumb" or "skier's thumb." The function of the ligament is to limit valgus stress at the metacarpophalangeal joint of the thumb.

122. Answer: 2   Resource: Payton - Research (p. 102)
Range is a common measure of dispersion that is expressed as the difference between the largest and smallest scores in a distribution.

123. Answer: 2   Resource: Paz (p. 616)
An arterial line consists of a catheter in an artery connected to pressure tubing, a transducer, and a monitor. The device can be used for continuous direct blood pressure readings and for access to the arterial blood supply. The radial and brachial arteries are the most common sites for an arterial line.

124. Answer: 4   Resource: O'Sullivan - Physical Rehabilitation (p. 139)
The anterolateral spinothalamic system is involved with the transmission of discriminative sensations such as pain and temperature. The system is activated by mechanoreceptors, thermoreceptors, and nociceptors.

125. Answer: 3   Resource: Paz (p. 39)
Patients with congestive heart failure tend to have excessive fluid retention in the pulmonary and systemic circulation. As a result a diet high in potassium is prescribed, while items high in sodium are restricted.

126. Answer: 2   Resource: Magee (p. 482)
The test knee remaining in 90 degrees of flexion over the edge of the table identifies adequate length of the rectus femoris. This is a common method of assessing the length of the two joint hip flexor.

127. Answer: 1   Resource: Paz (p. 9)
Angiotensin is a polypeptide in the blood that causes vasoconstriction, increased blood pressure, and the release of aldosterone from the adrenal cortex. Release of angiotensin is stimulated by decreased arterial pressure.

128. Answer: 3   Resource: Kettenbach (p. 110)
The assessment section of a S.O.A.P. note allows the physical therapist to express his/her professional judgment. The assessment section may include a statement about identified inconsistencies between subjective and objective data.

129. Answer: 1   Resource: Hickock (p. 45)
A manager should speak directly to an employee whenever an established policy is violated, however since it is the employee's first offense a private oral warning is the most appropriate option.

130. Answer: 1   Resource: Kisner (p. 137)
Infants have resting pulse rates of approximately 125-135 beats per minute.

131. Answer: 3   Resource: Magee (p. 40)
Due to the potential impact on future bone growth, lack of skeletal maturity can be a contraindication to anterior cruciate ligament reconstruction surgery.

132. Answer: 2   Resource: Umphred (p. 512)
The patient is making a general statement about his desire to walk again in the future. Although ambulation would not currently be realistic due to the level of injury, it would be inappropriate to dismiss the future chances of the patient being able to walk.

133. Answer: 2   Resource: Ciccone (p. 281)
Beta blockers decrease resting heart rate and the heart rate response to exercise. As a result, relying on heart rate as a means of monitoring exercise intensity can be problematic. A perceived exertion scale may be more appropriate since the patient is rehabilitating from a lower extremity injury and is participating in the exercise session on a daily basis.

134. Answer: 4   Resource: Paz (p. 124)
Oximetry is a noninvasive measure that examines oxygen saturation in a capillary bed. In order to determine the patient's activity tolerance it is necessary to examine the relative changes in oxyhemoglobin saturation during different periods including rest, activity, and recovery.

135. Answer: 3   Resource: Thomas (p. 400)
Clonus is an abnormal reflex that may occur with an upper motor neuron lesion. Clonus is defined as a spasmodic alternation of muscular contractions between antagonistic muscle groups and is commonly observed at the ankle joint with passive, rapid dorsiflexion.

136. Answer: 1   Resource: Adkins (p. 156)
A patient with T6 paraplegia should be able to perform independent pressure relief activities. It is essential that the patient understand his role in preventing skin breakdown. Nursing should also be alerted, however the most immediate action would be directed toward the patient.

137. Answer: 2   Resource: Paz (p. 185)
Hip flexion greater than 90 degrees is often considered a contraindication following total hip replacement surgery. The knee immobilizer limits hip flexion by maintaining the knee in an extended position.

138. Answer: 2   Resource: Levangie (p. 440)
Heel strike refers to the instant at which the heel of the leading extremity strikes the ground. The knee should be in a position of full extension at heel strike during normal gait.

139. Answer: 1   Resource: Pierson (p. 45)
A temperature of 98.9 degrees Fahrenheit represents a slightly elevated temperature when compared to the average temperature of 98.6 degrees Fahrenheit. Since the patient reports being able to exercise and the elevated temperature is within the accepted normal range (96.8°F – 99.5°F), the most appropriate action is to continue with treatment as planned.

140. Answer: 2   Resource: Paz (p. 312)
The TMN Classification System (T=tumor, M=metastasis, N=node) is a commonly used cancer classification system. This type of staging offers guidance to healthcare professionals when determining treatment options, life expectancy, and prognosis for complete resolution. The physical therapy plan of care may vary significantly based on the results of the staging.

141. Answer: 4   Resource: Paz (p. 612)
A right ventricular assistive device is designed to pump a percentage of the pulmonic blood flow around the right ventricle in order to decrease the workload on the myocardium. The right atrium would house one tube because it functions as a primer for the right ventricle and the other tube would be located in the pulmonary artery since its function is to deliver blood from the right ventricle to the lungs.

142. Answer: 2   Resource: Sullivan - An Integrated Approach (p. 132)
Repeated contractions should be applied at the point where the contraction begins to diminish. The technique utilizes an isometric contraction followed by subsequent manual stretching and resisted isotonic movement. Repeated contractions assist with enhancing motor neuron recruitment and strengthening of a muscle or group of muscles.

143. Answer: 2   Resource: Rothstein (p. 853)
An orthosis set in excessive dorsiflexion will promote knee flexion and instability.

144. Answer: 4   Resource: Kisner (p. 214)
To increase wrist extension, stabilize the radius and glide the scaphoid in a volar direction. The radius is considered to be the concave joint partner and the scaphoid is considered convex.

145. Answer: 2   Resource: Trofino (p. 156)
Rehabilitation following a burn can be extremely painful. Scheduling treatment sessions to coincide with the patient's pain medication schedule may reduce the patient's pain without compromising the established plan of care.

146. Answer: 1   Resource: Kisner (p. 631)
Intermittent claudication occurs as a result of insufficient blood supply and ischemia in active muscles. The condition occurs with activity and subsides during periods of rest and as a result can serve to limit the duration of exercise activities. Symptoms most commonly include pain and cramping distal to the occluded vessel.

147. Answer: 2   Resource: Paz (p. 332)
Oxygen saturation at rest is considered to be within normal limits between 95-98%. A rate of 90% or less is often used as a guideline to discontinue exercise activities. Supplemental oxygen may be indicated if oxygen saturation is 90% or less.

148. Answer: 4   Resource: Paz (p. 522)
Immunosuppressive pharmacological agents are desirable when the body loses its ability to differentiate between the body's own tissues and pathogenic tissues. White blood cell count provides valuable information related to the degree of immunosuppression.

149. Answer: 1   Resource: Umphred (p. 939)
Diminished sensation makes a patient particularly susceptible to skin breakdown when wearing an orthosis. Performing frequent skin checks allows the patient to closely monitor the status of the skin and avoid the development of a pressure ulcer.

150. Answer: 2   Resource: Magee (p. 12)
L5 nerve root:
    dermatome - buttock, posterior and lateral thigh, lateral aspect of leg, dorsum of foot, medial half of sole, first, second, and third toes
    myotome - extensor hallucis, peroneals, gluteus medius, dorsiflexors, hamstrings, soleus, plantaris
    reflexes - medial hamstrings, posterior tibial

151. Answer: 1   Resource: Michlovitz (p. 119)
Paraffin is a superficial heating agent that is commonly used to treat the distal extremities. Due to the number of joints involved, immersion in paraffin is an appropriate and practical selection.

152. Answer: 2   Resource: Code of Ethics
Providing the patient with a shirt allows the physical therapist to be sensitive to the needs of other patients and continue with the treatment session. In addition, the therapist should discuss the situation directly with the patient and offer examples of more acceptable attire.

153. Answer: 4   Resource: Clark (p. 339)
Thoraco-lumbar-sacral orthoses limit spinal motion of the lower thoracic and upper lumbar spine and are commonly used following surgery or as a result of an injury to the spine.

154. Answer: 1   Resource: Pauls (p. 343)
Prone lying is a commonly employed positional technique designed to stretch the hip flexors. Increased flexibility of the hip flexors will improve standing posture and enable the body's center of gravity to remain within the base of support. Although some of the other options are appropriate, they would not provide the same degree of benefit for the patient.

155. Answer: 1   Resource: Magee (p. 460)
The hip is a ball and socket joint whose capsular pattern is represented by a restriction in flexion, abduction, and medial rotation.

156. Answer: 1   Resource: Curtis (p. 26)
An indemnity insurance plan typically reimburses based on a fee for service model. This model reimburses each discrete element of service on a set fee schedule that is based on what is usual, customary, and reasonable. Patients have unlimited choices of health care providers and insurance companies have limited cost control measures.

157. Answer: 3   Resource: Magee (p. 734)
Blanching or whitening of the nailbeds occurs due to the interruption in circulation caused by the physical therapist's direct pressure. The capillary refill test is often used as a gross indicator of vascular perfusion.

158. Answer: 3   Resource: Pierson (p. 268)
A suprapubic catheter is an indwelling urinary catheter that is surgically inserted directly into the patient's bladder.

159. Answer: 1   Resource: Norkin (p. 215)
Protrusion refers to moving the lower teeth forward in relation to the upper teeth. Protrusion is measured by determining the distance between the lower central incisor teeth and the upper central incisor teeth. Normal protrusion is approximately 5 mm.

160. Answer: 3   Resource: Magee (p. 43)
A bone scan can identify bone disease or stress fractures with as little as 4-7% bone loss. Traditional radiographs are far less sensitive than bone scans, requiring 30-50% bone loss.

161. Answer: 4   Resource: Pierson (p. 266)
The saphenous vein is a superficial vein that extends from the foot to the saphenous opening. The antecubital, basilic, and cephalic vein are located in the upper extremity.

162. Answer: 3   Resource: Kisner (p. 222)
The tibiofemoral articulation consists of a concave tibial plateau articulating with the convex femoral condyles. A posterior glide of the tibia on the femur is indicated to increase knee flexion.

163. Answer: 3   Resource: Hertling (p. 339)
Common special tests to identify the presence of a meniscal lesion include the McMurray test, Apley's test, "bounce home" test, and Steinmann's test.

164. Answer: 2   Resource: Adkins (p. 79)
A patient with C6 tetraplegia should demonstrate full epigastric rise secondary to complete innervation of the diaphragm.

165. Answer: 4   Resource: Hall (p. 258)
Supporting the subtalar joint in a neutral or slightly supinated position limits subtalar pronation and promotes optimal stretching of the calf muscles.

166. Answer: 2   Resource: Robinson (p. 62)
High voltage current is characterized by a monophasic waveform usually delivered in spiked pulse pairs. High voltage current utilizes an extremely short pulse duration and voltage greater than 150 volts, as a result the total average current is quite low. High voltage current is most often used to provide sensory level stimulation.

167. Answer: 1   Resource: Umphred (p. 942)
Minimal contact with the skin allows a metal upright ankle-foot orthosis to accommodate for fluctuating edema while providing the appropriate support to the ankle joint.

168. Answer: 2   Resource: O'Sullivan - Physical Rehabilitation (p. 666)
A prosthesis that has excessive length may cause a patient to vault or circumduct in order to clear the floor during the swing phase of gait.

169. Answer: 2   Resource: Sullivan - Clinical Decision Making (p. 66)
Contract-relax is a therapeutic technique designed to increase range of motion to muscles on one side of a joint. Tightness of the hamstrings and hip extensors would serve to limit a straight leg raise.

170. Answer: 2   Resource: Long (p. 36)
The supplied description is characteristic of a child functioning at a four to five month old level. As a result, an eight month old child functioning at this level would be considered developmentally delayed.

171. Answer: 3   Resource: Hall (p. 257)
Moving the buttocks posteriorly in relation to the knees causes the patient's center of gravity to move behind the knees. As a result, the patient relies on eccentric contraction of the hip extensors to control the movement.

172. Answer: 4   Resource: Standards of Practice
Treating a patient following surgery without having specific information from the referring physician could be considered a negligent act. In this particular instance the physical therapist knows only that the patient had knee surgery two weeks ago.

173. Answer: 4   Resource: Pierson (p. 193)
A walker provides the necessary stability for a patient that is touchdown weight bearing. The platform attachment permits weight bearing through the involved arm without placing undue stress on the distal radius.

174. Answer: 3   Resource: Kee (p. 67)
Urea is the metabolic byproduct of the breakdown of amino acids used for energy production. The level of urea in the blood provides a gross estimate of kidney function. An increased blood urea nitrogen level can be indicative of dehydration, prerenal failure or renal failure. Normal blood urea nitrogen levels for adults are 5-25 mg/dL.

175. Answer: 4   Resource: Umphred (p. 607)
Multiple sclerosis is a progressive central nervous system disease marked by intermittent damage to the myelin sheath. Patients with multiple sclerosis tend to fatigue in the afternoon and as a result morning sessions are optimal. Stretching, exercise, energy conservation, and stress management are valuable components of a comprehensive plan of care for a patient with multiple sclerosis.

176. Answer: 2   Resource: Brannon (p. 260)
Systolic blood pressure of greater than 260 mm Hg or diastolic blood pressure greater than 115 mm Hg are indications to terminate an exercise test.

177. Answer: 3   Resource: Kendall (p. 203)
The peroneus longus and brevis tendons pass posterior to the lateral malleolus. The longus inserts on the lateral side of the base of the first metatarsal and first cuneiform, while the brevis inserts on the tuberosity of the fifth metatarsal.

178. Answer: 4   Resource: Kendall (p. 265)
Placing the biceps in a maximally shortened position significantly limits the muscle's ability to function as a supinator.

179. Answer: 4   Resource: Brannon (p. 319)
Selected levels of perceived exertion using Borg's ten point scale: 0 - nothing, 3 - moderate, 5 - strong, 7 - very strong, 10 - very, very strong.

180. Answer: 4   Resource: Goodman (p. 344)
Acceptable range for platelets is considered 150,000 - 400,000mm^3. Although a value of 60,000 mm^3 is significantly decreased, aerobic exercise is permitted with values greater than 50,000 mm^3.

181. Answer: 1   Resource: Anderson (p. 48)
An allograft refers to a graft or tissue between two genetically dissimilar individuals of the same species.

182. Answer: 4   Resource: O'Sullivan - Physical Rehabilitation (p. 379)
Discoloration of the patient's toes may be an indication that the cast is too tight and may be impeding the patient's circulation. Since the cast is bivalved, the cast can be easily removed by the physical therapist.

183. Answer: 4   Resource: Kettenbach (p. 96)
A properly written goal should provide adequate detail to allow the examiner to assess progress at a future date. All goals should include audience, behavior, condition, and degree.

184. Answer: 4   Resource: Somers (p. 93)
Lowering the table to a horizontal position will improve circulation and should significantly increase blood pressure. Vital signs should always be monitored when using a tilt table for vertical positioning.

185. Answer: 2   Resource: Currier (p. 108)
Convenience sampling utilizes available individuals willing to participate in a research study. This type of sampling is often utilized when other more formal types of sampling are not practical or unavailable.

186. Answer: 3   Resource: Rothstein (p. 450)
A patient at the confused-inappropriate level often exhibits inappropriate verbal output, poor memory, and difficulty performing new tasks. Physical therapy intervention may focus on following directions and goal oriented tasks.

187. Answer: 2   Resource: Pierson (p. 203)
A three-point gait pattern can be used when a patient is able to bear weight on one lower extremity, but is non-weight bearing on the other. The gait pattern requires good upper extremity strength and the use of crutches or a walker.

188. Answer: 4   Resource: Gross (p. 182)
The elbow complex consists of the ulnohumeral, radiohumeral, and proximal radioulnar joint. Each of the joints is affected by swelling in the elbow complex.

189. Answer: 3   Resource: Pierson (p. 267)
Blood in a patient's urine is a significant finding that should be reported to the nursing staff immediately.

190. Answer: 1   Resource: Hall (p. 192)
Isometric exercises are often the strengthening exercise of choice for patients with acute osteoarthritis. This form of exercise limits muscle atrophy while avoiding unnecessary stress on the joint. Avoiding strengthening exercises until the patient is pain free is unrealistic given the diagnosis of osteoarthritis.

191. Answer: 2   Resource: Pierson (p. 203)
A three-point gait pattern using axillary crutches would serve as the most efficient and cost effective gait pattern for the patient.

192. Answer: 2   Resource: Scott - Health Care Malpractice (p. 14)
Statutes are enacted by Congress or state legislatures and serve to define rights and obligations.

193. Answer: 1   Resource: O'Sullivan - Physical Rehabilitation (p. 535)
Pusher syndrome is characterized by a significant lateral deviation toward the hemiplegic side in all positions. A patient with left hemiplegia would exhibit a lateral lean to the left in sitting with increased weight bearing on the left buttock. Pusher syndrome is most common in patients with right cerebrovascular accidents and left hemiplegia.

194. Answer: 1   Resource: Norkin (p. 72)
The distal end of the humerus should be stabilized when measuring elbow flexion. Failure to adequately stabilize the humerus permits shoulder flexion.

195. Answer: 3   Resource: Scott - Health Care Malpractice (p. 59)
A physical therapist should not administer any form of treatment without patient consent.

196. Answer: 3   Resource: Purtillo - Health Professional (p. 91)
A mandatory inservice would enable the physical therapists to provide a formal educational session on guarding techniques for the aides.

197. Answer: 2   Resource: Michlovitz (p. 270)
The anterior aspect of the forearm is a common site utilized for determining the minimal erythemal dose since it is relatively easy to determine mild reddening of the skin in this area. It may at times, however be more appropriate to determine the minimal erythemal dose on the area to be treated.

198. Answer: 1   Resource: Adkins (p. 160)
A physical therapist should immediately notify the nursing staff when a reddened area is found on a patient with tetraplegia. Failure to adequately address the issue may result in the formation of a pressure ulcer and ultimately delay the rehabilitation process.

199. Answer: 4   Resource: Scott - Professional Ethics (p. 86)
The physical therapist must take immediate action to resolve the situation by speaking directly to the involved therapists. Patient information should not be discussed in or around a public area.

200. Answer: 3   Resource: Norkin (p. 8)
Passive range of motion provides a physical therapist with information on the integrity of the articular surfaces and the extensibility of the joint capsule and associated ligaments. Passive range of motion is independent of a patient's strength.

Sample Examination: Three

1. A physical therapist prepares a presentation on proper body mechanics for a group of 100 autoworkers. Which of the following media would be most effective to maximize learning during the presentation?

   1. lecture, handouts
   2. lecture, charts, statistics
   3. lecture, handouts, demonstration
   4. lecture, statistics

2. A physical therapist attempts to have a patient status post CVA reach for a cone by moving her trunk away from midline. The most appropriate type of manual contact to assist the patient with this movement is:

   1. firm, deep touch
   2. light, intermittent touch
   3. maintained touch
   4. no manual contact

3. A patient two weeks status post transtibial amputation is instructed by his physician to remain at rest for two days after contracting bronchitis. The most appropriate position for the patient in bed is:

   1. supine with a pillow under the patient's knees
   2. supine with a pillow under the patient's thighs and knees
   3. supine with the legs extended
   4. sidelying in the fetal position

4. A student physical therapist is treating a 65-year-old mildly obese patient. The patient is status post total hip replacement and is cleared for 25 pounds of weight bearing through the involved lower extremity. Appropriate assistive devices for gait training would include all of the following except:

   1. parallel bars
   2. walker
   3. axillary crutches
   4. straight cane

5. A physical therapist tests a small area of skin for hypersensitivity prior to using a cold immersion bath. The patient begins to demonstrate evidence of cold intolerance within 60 seconds after cold application. The most appropriate response is to:

   1. limit cold exposure to ten minutes or less
   2. select an alternative cryotherapeutic agent
   3. continue with the cold immersion bath
   4. discontinue cold application and document your findings

6. A physical therapist would not expect a seven month old infant to have completed which of the following developmental milestones?

   1. hold head erect when sitting
   2. crawl forward
   3. sit unsupported
   4. roll from supine to prone

7. A 21-year-old male suffers a primary dislocation of the right shoulder playing football. The athlete is referred to physical therapy after three weeks of immobilization. A physical therapist might elect to begin treatment with all of the following except:

   1. isometric shoulder exercises
   2. passive range of motion exercises
   3. active-assistive range of motion exercises
   4. high speed isokinetic exercises

8. A patient with a C3 spinal cord injury is positioned in supine. Which area is most susceptible to pressure in this position?

   1. greater trochanter
   2. anterior superior iliac spine
   3. medial malleolus
   4. sacrum

9. A 27-year-old female diagnosed with anterior compartment syndrome reports to an outpatient clinic for physical therapy services. While reviewing the physician referral supplied by the patient, the physical therapist identifies that the referral form is over 90 days old. The most appropriate therapist action is:

   1. continue with the session since the existing referral is acceptable
   2. attempt to contact the physician's office by telephone to receive verbal orders
   3. send the physician written correspondence requesting an updated referral
   4. discontinue the session until the patient secures an updated referral

10. A physical therapist assesses the deep tendon reflexes of a patient as part of a lower quarter screening examination. The therapist determines that the right and left patellar tendon reflex and the left Achilles tendon reflex is 2+, while the right Achilles tendon reflex is absent. The clinical condition that could best explain this finding is:

    1. cerebral palsy
    2. multiple sclerosis
    3. peripheral neuropathy
    4. vascular claudication

11. A physical therapist determines the maximum load a patient can squat ten times is 240 lbs. The patient's ten repetition maximum should be recorded as:

    1. 10 lbs
    2. 24 lbs
    3. 120 lbs
    4. 240 lbs

12. A patient demonstrates dizziness and nausea during vertebral artery testing. The physical therapist should pay particular attention when treating the patient to avoid positioning the neck in:

    1. extension and extremes of rotation
    2. flexion and extremes of rotation
    3. flexion and sidebending
    4. extension and sidebending

13. A patient lies supine with one knee over the edge of a treatment table and the other held against his chest. The physical therapist notes that the knee over the edge of the treatment table is flexed to 45 degrees. A probable cause of this position of the knee includes tightness of the:

    1. iliopsoas
    2. rectus femoris
    3. tensor fasciae latae
    4. vastus medialis

14. A 26-year-old male is referred to physical therapy after straining his lower back while playing softball. The patient is in obvious pain and reports being unable to perform even basic tasks such as putting on his socks or rising from a chair without tremendous difficulty. The patient is particularly concerned since he will be leaving on a two-week business trip to Europe in five days. Assuming the physician referral does not indicate the frequency of treatment, the most appropriate number of physical therapy visits prior to the patient's business trip is:

    1. one
    2. two
    3. three
    4. four

15. A physical therapist observes a patient with Parkinson's disease complete a series of functional activities. The therapist notes that the patient is slow to initiate movement and is slow to carry out a task once it has been initiated. This type of movement pattern is best termed:

    1. akinesia
    2. hypokinesia
    3. bradykinesia
    4. hyperkinesia

16. A therapist prepares to administer ultrasound to a patient with lateral epicondylitis. When applying ultrasound the amount of heat absorbed is least dependent upon:

    1. the intensity
    2. the duration of exposure
    3. the choice of coupling agent
    4. the size of the area sonated

17. A complete medical history can provide valuable information about a disorder, its prognosis, and the appropriate treatment. Which statement is not accurate when obtaining a medical history?

    1. The examiner should ask one question at a time and should receive an answer before proceeding with the next question.
    2. The questions should be easy for the patient to understand and should not be leading.
    3. The examiner should encourage the patient to discuss irrelevant information since it will foster the patient-therapist relationship.
    4. The history should be taken in an orderly sequence.

18. A physical therapist completes an examination on a patient diagnosed with facet impingement in the lumbar spine. The patient appears to be somewhat fixed in a position of side bending to the right and rotation to the left. When assessing lumbar range of motion, which motions would you expect to be most restricted?

    1. side bending to the right and rotation to the left
    2. side bending to the right and rotation to the right
    3. side bending to the left and rotation to the right
    4. side bending to the left and rotation to the left

19. A physical therapist observes a patient ambulating in the clinic. The therapist notes that the patient's pelvis drops on the left during left swing phase. This deviation is usually caused by weakness of the:

    1. left gluteus medius
    2. right gluteus medius
    3. left gluteus minimus
    4. right gluteus minimus

20. A physical therapist examines a patient diagnosed with cerebellar degeneration. Which of the following clinical findings is not typically associated with this condition?

    1. athetosis
    2. dysmetria
    3. nystagmus
    4. dysdiadochokinesia

21. A physical therapist examines the reflex status of a patient. The therapist should use which technique to assess the patient's superficial reflexes?

    1. brushing the skin with a light feathery object
    2. percussing a muscle over the musculotendinous junction
    3. stroking the skin with a noncutting, but pointed object
    4. tapping a tendon or bony prominence

22. Patients with cervical rib syndrome can experience tingling and numbness throughout the upper extremity when carrying heavy objects at their side. Which structures are commonly affected by the cervical rib?

    1. common carotid artery and inferior trunk of the brachial plexus
    2. common carotid artery and superior trunk of the brachial plexus
    3. subclavian artery and inferior trunk of the brachial plexus
    4. subclavian artery and superior trunk of the brachial plexus

23. A patient with a diagnosis of CVA presents with significant balance and coordination deficits. The patient has good upper and lower extremity strength, however ambulates with an ataxic gait pattern. Upon reviewing the patient's chart, you are not surprised to find that the area of the brain affected by the CVA is the:

    1. cerebellum
    2. cerebrum-left hemisphere
    3. frontal lobe
    4. Broca's area

24. A patient status post CVA exercises in supine. As the physical therapist resists adduction of the unaffected leg, the affected leg begins to adduct. This should be documented as:

    1. Souque's phenomenon
    2. overextension phenomenon
    3. Schunkel reflex
    4. Raimiste's phenomenon

25. A physical therapist is employed at a physician owned physical therapy clinic that charges for treatment by the modality. One of the physicians, who is an owner of the practice, requests that all of his patients receive a minimum of heat, ultrasound, and electrical stimulation during each treatment session. The therapist feels that the majority of patients receive little clinical benefit from the proposed treatment regime. The most appropriate immediate response would be to:

1. ignore the physician's request and treat each patient as you feel is indicated
2. discuss with the physician the rationale for requesting modalities on each patient
3. report the physician's conduct to the American Medical Association
4. inform the physician that he is abusing the health care system

26. A physical therapist completes a developmental assessment on an infant. At what age should an infant begin to sit with hand support for an extended period of time?

1. 6-7 months
2. 8-9 months
3. 10-11 months
4. 12 months

27. A physical therapist is required to train a 71-year-old patient to ascend and descend a flight of stairs. The patient presents with a fractured left tibia and is weight bearing as tolerated. There is moderate weakness in the involved lower extremity secondary to the fracture. The most appropriate instructions are:

1. "One step at a time, right foot first to ascend and to descend the stairs."
2. "One step at a time, right foot first to ascend the stairs and left foot first to descend the stairs."
3. "Step over step slowly."
4. "One step at a time, left foot first to ascend and to descend the stairs."

28. A physical therapist examines a 36-year-old female referred to physical therapy after experiencing back pain two weeks ago. The patient identifies the majority of pain in the buttock and lateral thigh and denies any referred pain down the posterior leg. Presently she rates the pain as a "3" on a 0-10 scale, however indicates that the pain is a "6" or a "7" during activity or at night. This description most closely resembles:

1. sacroilitis
2. iliolumbar syndrome
3. piriformis syndrome
4. trochanteric bursitis

29. A patient presents with orthostatic hypotension. The most appropriate treatment technique to assist the patient with standing is:

1. standing in parallel bars for increasing time intervals
2. using a standing table
3. standing in a pool
4. tilt table with progressive vertical positioning

30. A physical therapist can obtain valuable information during an examination by using special orthopedic tests. Which of the following tests is not performed with the patient in supine?

1. anterior drawer test
2. Apley's compression test
3. McMurray test
4. patella apprehension test

31. A physical therapist completes a sensory assessment on a 61-year-old female diagnosed with multiple sclerosis. As part of the assessment the therapist examines stereognosis, kinesthesia, and two-point discrimination. What type of receptor is primarily responsible for generating the necessary information?

1. deep sensory receptors
2. mechanoreceptors
3. nociceptors
4. thermoreceptors

32. A physical therapist records the blood pressure of a two-year-old child in the medical record. Assuming normal values, the most typical blood pressure reading is:

1. 80 systolic, 35 diastolic
2. 85 systolic, 60 diastolic
3. 105 systolic, 70 diastolic
4. 120 systolic, 80 diastolic

33. During an examination of a patient with a traumatic brain injury a physical therapist notes that the patient often mumbles phrases which are non-purposeful in nature. As the physical therapist initiates passive range of motion to the patient's lower extremities, the patient attempts to strike the therapist in the head. According to the Rancho Los Amigos levels of cognitive functioning, this patient would be best described at level:

1. II
2. III
3. IV
4. V

34. A physical therapist identifies excessive femoral neck anteversion during an examination of a patient diagnosed with trochanteric bursitis. This structural finding commonly results in:

    1. an increase in hip lateral rotation
    2. an increase in hip medial rotation
    3. an increase in hip extension
    4. an increase in hip flexion

35. A 63-year-old female referred to physical therapy for gait training suddenly loses her balance and falls to the floor. After rushing to the scene, it becomes obvious that the patient is unconscious. Which of the following would be the most appropriate immediate response?

    1. secure and maintain an airway
    2. file an incident report
    3. observe and record vital signs
    4. attempt to define the specific cause for the loss of consciousness

36. A physical therapist examines a patient placed in respiratory isolation. Which of the following diseases would require respiratory isolation?

    1. diphtheria
    2. pharyngitis
    3. pertussis
    4. hepatitis

37. A physical therapist working on a team with a physical therapist assistant would be incorrect in asking an assistant to perform which of the following tasks?

    1. modify treatment plan or goals
    2. apply and measure assistive or adaptive devices
    3. identify changes in treatment outcome
    4. administer therapeutic modalities

38. A therapist examines a patient with an acute grade II lateral ankle sprain. The most common mechanism for an anterior talofibular ligament sprain is:

    1. inversion and dorsiflexion
    2. inversion and plantar flexion
    3. inversion
    4. pronation, eversion, and dorsiflexion

39. A physical therapist employed in a work hardening program performs an examination on a patient diagnosed with fibromyalgia. During the examination the therapist identifies an inconsistency between the measured lumbar range of motion and the amount of lumbar range of motion observed while lifting a milk crate from the floor to a table. The most appropriate therapist action is:

    1. avoid discussing the identified inconsistency with the patient
    2. confront the patient with the identified inconsistency
    3. discuss the identified inconsistency with the referring physician
    4. discharge the patient from physical therapy

40. A patient is referred to physical therapy diagnosed with right hip trochanteric bursitis. Which clinical finding is usually not associated with trochanteric bursitis?

    1. resisted abduction reproduces symptoms
    2. full hip active range of motion
    3. positive Ober test
    4. joint play motions are limited in a capsular pattern

41. A patient is referred to physical therapy after surgery to repair a large rotator cuff tear. Which of the following motions would you initially expect to be the most restricted?

    1. extension
    2. abduction
    3. medial rotation
    4. lateral rotation

42. A patient is found to have limited knee extension. Which of the following mobilization techniques would be indicated?

    1. lateral glide of the patella
    2. caudal glide of the patella
    3. posterior glide of the tibia
    4. anterior glide of the tibia

43. If the axillary nerve was severed, what muscle could laterally rotate the humerus?

    1. teres major
    2. subscapularis
    3. infraspinatus
    4. teres minor

44. Exercise causes a significant increase in the body's cardiac output. During mild to moderate exercise what redistribution of the available cardiac output would you expect?

   1. an increase in cerebral and coronary blood flow
   2. a decrease in cerebral and active skeletal muscle blood flow
   3. an increase in coronary and active skeletal muscle blood flow
   4. a decrease in cerebral and coronary blood flow

45. A physical therapist performs passive range of motion on a patient with C7 tetraplegia. The patient's bilateral straight leg raise is measured passively to 90 degrees. What should the therapist conclude about the patient's ability to perform activities of daily living?

   1. The patient requires a straight leg raise of 110-120 degrees in order to perform long sit and activities of daily living.
   2. The patient is at a functional range to perform long sit and activities of daily living.
   3. The patient's range of motion is beyond the expected limit for long sit and activities of daily living.
   4. The patient requires a straight leg raise of 150 degrees in order to perform long sit and activities of daily living.

46. A note in a patient's medical record indicates a specific drug is taken through enteral administration. Which of the following is an example of enteral administration?

   1. inhalation
   2. injection
   3. topical
   4. oral

47. A physical therapist works with a patient status post stroke on a mat program. The therapist assists the patient in lateral weight shifting activities while positioned in prone on elbows. Which therapeutic exercise technique allows the patient to improve dynamic stability with this activity?

   1. alternating isometrics
   2. approximation
   3. rhythmic initiation
   4. timing for emphasis

48. A patient is positioned in supine with the hips flexed to 90 degrees and the knees extended. As the patient slowly lowers her extended legs toward the horizontal, there is an increase in lordosis of the low back. This finding is indicative of weakness of the:

   1. hip flexors
   2. back extensors
   3. hip extensors
   4. abdominals

49. A patient employed in a machine shop is referred to physical therapy with a diagnosis of carpal tunnel syndrome. The patient indicates that he is scheduled for a diagnostic test that may help to confirm the diagnosis. Which of the following electrodiagnostic tests would be the most appropriate?

   1. electroencephalography
   2. evoked potentials
   3. nerve conduction velocity
   4. electromyography

50. A patient with a transfemoral amputation ambulates with an abducted gait pattern on the prosthetic side. All of the following may cause this type of gait deviation except:

   1. high medial wall
   2. inadequate suspension
   3. abduction contracture
   4. prosthesis is too short

51. A patient with C4 tetraplegia requires a custom wheelchair upon discharge from the hospital. The patient's diaphragm is partially innervated. The most appropriate recommendation for proper seating is:

   1. light weight manual wheelchair, upright frame, seat and back cushions
   2. folding reclining wheelchair, power chin control, seat and back cushions
   3. nonfolding reclining wheelchair, power tongue control, underslung tray for ventilator
   4. upright power wheelchair, joystick hand control, seat cushion

52. A therapist examines a patient with a C6 spinal cord injury. Which muscle would not be innervated based on the patient's level of injury?

   1. biceps
   2. deltoids
   3. triceps
   4. diaphragm

53. A physical therapist attempts to assess the integrity of the vestibulocochlear nerve by administering the Rinne test on a patient with a suspected upper motor neuron lesion. After striking the tine of the tuning fork to begin vibration, which bony prominence should the therapist utilize to position the stem of the tuning fork?

   1. apex of the skull
   2. occipital protuberance
   3. inion
   4. mastoid process

54. Progress notes allow members of all health services to know what the patient is accomplishing in each given area. Which statement regarding physical therapy progress notes is not accurate?

   1. Observations and recordings should be the result of tangible tests and measurements.
   2. The progress note must contain patient identification, the date, and the signature of the physical therapist.
   3. Progress notes can include diagrams, graphs, and flow sheets.
   4. Progress notes should be written by physical therapists and not by other care providers such as physical therapist assistants.

55. A physical therapist reviews a laboratory report for a patient recently admitted to the hospital. The patient sustained burns over 25 percent of her body in a fire. Assuming the patient exhibits hypovolemia, which of the following laboratory values would be the most significantly affected?

   1. hematocrit
   2. hemoglobin
   3. oxygen saturation
   4. prothrombin time

56. A patient one week status post left total hip replacement is diagnosed with an acute deep vein thrombosis in the left calf. The physical therapist's role in the care of a deep vein thrombosis is:

   1. continued gait training with an assistive device and partial weight bearing
   2. progressive resistive exercises for bilateral lower extremities
   3. patient is on bedrest with no active therapy to the left leg
   4. postural drainage and diaphragmatic breathing

57. Health maintenance organizations differ from typical fee for service insurance providers in a variety of ways. Which of the following does not accurately describe health maintenance organizations?

   1. Members are limited to receiving services from specific providers.
   2. Payment to providers is often on a capitated or prospective basis.
   3. Health maintenance organizations provide services for a monthly fee which varies based on the amount of services utilized by each member.
   4. Health maintenance organizations are responsible for the provision and accessibility of care.

58. A patient with right hemiplegia is observed during gait training. The patient performs side stepping towards the hemiplegic side. The physical therapist may expect the patient to compensate for weakened abductors by:

   1. hip hiking of the unaffected side
   2. lateral trunk flexion towards the affected side
   3. lateral trunk flexion towards the unaffected side
   4. hip extension of the affected side

59. A patient in a pulmonary rehabilitation program is positioned in supine with a pillow under the knees. The physical therapist claps between the clavicle and nipple bilaterally. This technique is utilized for postural drainage of the:

   1. anterior segments of the upper lobes
   2. anterior basal segments of the lower lobes
   3. superior segments of the lower lobes
   4. posterior basal segments of the lower lobes

60. A 15-year-old male is referred to a local orthopedic surgeon after injuring his knee in a football game. The most appropriate initial step in the surgeon's care of the patient is to:

   1. complete a physical examination
   2. immobilize the injured knee
   3. aspirate the knee
   4. order x-rays

61. The open basketweave taping technique is commonly used as a form of treatment for an acute ankle sprain. Which of the following does not accurately describe the benefits of the open basketweave taping technique?

   1. allows freedom of movement in dorsiflexion
   2. allows freedom of movement in plantar flexion
   3. provides room for additional edema
   4. promotes proximal joint stability

62. A patient reports to a scheduled physical therapy session 25 minutes late. The patient has not been seen previously in physical therapy and was scheduled in a 45 minute block of time. The patient referral indicates the patient is 10 days status post arthroscopic medial meniscectomy. The most appropriate therapist action is:

1. begin the examination
2. design a home exercise program
3. consult with the patient's physician
4. ask the patient to reschedule

63. A patient with an ankle-foot orthosis demonstrates genu recurvatum during the stance phase of gait. Which action would be the most appropriate to decrease the recurvatum?

1. increase the plantar flexion stop
2. increase the dorsiflexion stop
3. allow full range of motion at the ankle
4. ankle joint position does not affect recurvatum

64. A physical therapist treats a patient with superficial partial-thickness burns to the anterior surface of his lower legs. In an attempt to assist the patient to control the pain associated with the burns, the therapist rewards the patient with a lengthy rest period after successfully completing an exercise sequence. This type of psychological approach is most representative of:

1. distraction
2. extinction
3. classical conditioning
4. operant conditioning

65. A physical therapist identifies that a child is unable to roll from prone to supine. Which reflex could interfere with the child's ability to roll?

1. asymmetrical tonic neck reflex
2. Moro reflex
3. Galant reflex
4. symmetrical tonic neck reflex

66. A physical therapist treats a patient with hemiplegia who has his right arm immobilized in a sling. What is the primary purpose of using a sling in the management of a subluxed shoulder?

1. correct the cause of the subluxation
2. decrease muscle spasticity
3. facilitate movement patterns
4. hold the upper extremity in proper alignment

67. A physical therapist reviews a laboratory report for a 41-year-old male diagnosed with chronic obstructive pulmonary disease. Which of the following would be considered a normal hemoglobin value?

1. 10 gm/dL
2. 15 gm/dL
3. 20 gm/dL
4. 25 gm/dL

68. A physical therapist instructs a patient with chronic obstructive pulmonary disease in diaphragmatic breathing exercises. Which patient position would be the most appropriate to initiate the training session?

1. sitting
2. standing
3. supine
4. walking

69. A patient with a history of rheumatoid arthritis is referred to physical therapy after being diagnosed with acute glenohumeral joint pain. Which treatment technique would be inappropriate for the patient?

1. passive range of motion in a pain free range
2. grade III and IV mobilization
3. periodic immobilization in a sling
4. gentle joint oscillation techniques

70. A patient diagnosed with an incomplete spinal cord lesion presents with muscle paralysis on the ipsilateral side of the lesion and a loss of pain, temperature, and sensitivity on the contralateral side of the lesion. This presentation best describes:

1. Steinert's disease
2. central cord syndrome
3. anterior spinal artery syndrome
4. Brown-Sequard's syndrome

71. A physical therapist applies a hot pack to the lumbar region of a patient rehabilitating from a laminectomy. Which mode of heat transmission is utilized when using the hot pack?

1. conduction
2. convection
3. evaporation
4. radiation

72. A physical therapist reviews the medical record of a patient rehabilitating from a stroke. The patient exhibits paralysis and numbness on the side of the body contralateral to the vascular accident. Which descending pathway is most likely damaged based on the patient's clinical presentation?

1. corticospinal tract
2. vestibulospinal tract
3. tectospinal tract
4. rubrospinal tract

73. A physical therapist performs a manual muscle test of the peroneus tertius on a patient diagnosed with anterior compartment syndrome. When providing resistance to the peroneus tertius, the physical therapist should direct pressure towards:

1. dorsiflexion and eversion
2. dorsiflexion and inversion
3. plantar flexion and eversion
4. plantar flexion and inversion

74. A patient diagnosed with emphysema is referred to physical therapy. Physical examination reveals increased accessory muscle use during normal breathing and a forward head posture. The primary goal for the patient is:

1. eliminate accessory muscle activity and decrease respiratory rate with pursed lip breathing
2. optimize accessory muscle strength to promote alveolar ventilation
3. utilize the accessory muscles to balance the activity of the upper and lower chest
4. diminish accessory muscle use and emphasize diaphragmatic breathing

75. Bed positioning is important for patients status post amputation. The prone position or prone lying is recommended for thirty minutes several times a day. This position is of particular importance for which type of amputation?

1. transfemoral amputation
2. transtibial amputation
3. Syme's amputation
4. hip disarticulation

76. A physical therapist observes excessive knee flexion from heel strike to mid-stance while observing a patient with a transtibial amputation during gait training. A possible cause for the deviation is:

1. the foot is set in neutral
2. the socket is set posterior in relation to the foot
3. the prosthesis is too short
4. the socket is aligned in excessive flexion

77. A physical therapist attempts to improve a patient's lower extremity strength. Which proprioceptive neuromuscular facilitation technique would be the most appropriate to achieve the therapist's goals?

1. contract-relax
2. repeated contractions
3. rhythmic stabilization
4. hold-relax

78. A physical therapist observes a patient with a transfemoral amputation during gait training. The therapist identifies marked lateral rotation of the prosthesis at heel strike. Which of the following would not be a contributing factor to the patient's gait deviation?

1. weak hip medial rotators
2. inadequate suspension
3. excessive toe-out built into the prosthesis
4. prosthesis is too short

79. A woman's pulmonary and cardiovascular systems are altered physiologically during pregnancy. Which of the following would a physical therapist expect to observe when treating a pregnant woman?

1. decreased oxygen reserve and decreased stroke volume
2. increased oxygen reserve and increased stroke volume
3. decreased oxygen reserve and increased cardiac output
4. decreased stroke volume and decreased cardiac output

80. A physical therapist instructs a patient diagnosed with rotator cuff tendonitis in transverse plane resistive exercises. Which motions would be appropriate based on the given information?

1. abduction and adduction
2. flexion and extension
3. medial and lateral rotation
4. pronation and supination

81. A physical therapist is concerned with a patient's lateral knee discomfort. The therapist attempts to determine if a contracture of the fasciae latae or iliotibial band could be contributing to the patient's symptoms. Which special test might help to identify a restriction in this area?

    1. Ober
    2. Thomas
    3. Apley's compression
    4. Thompson

82. A patient completing an exercise program starts to demonstrate signs of an insulin reaction including dizziness, vision difficulties, and a change in the level of consciousness. The most appropriate response for a conscious victim would include:

    1. give the patient sugar, candy or juice
    2. monitor airway, breathing, and circulation
    3. treat the patient for shock
    4. continue to supervise the patient, however do not intervene

83. A physical therapist performs a manual muscle test on a patient's shoulder medial rotators. Which muscle would not be involved in this test?

    1. pectoralis major
    2. subscapularis
    3. teres major
    4. teres minor

84. A physical therapist can use a variety of pulse sites to examine the general condition of the heart and the circulatory system. Which of the following pulse sites is not found on the lower extremity?

    1. brachial
    2. dorsalis pedis
    3. femoral
    4. popliteal

85. A physical therapist treats a patient status post surgical repair of the ulnar collateral ligament of the thumb. The patient injured the thumb approximately three weeks ago while skiing. Which of the following would be the most realistic postoperative time frame for the patient to resume unrestricted activity?

    1. 6 weeks
    2. 12 weeks
    3. 18 weeks
    4. 24 weeks

86. A physical therapist attempts to determine if a patient has muscular weakness in the gastrocnemius or soleus by observing the patient's gait. Which objective finding would not be consistent with weakness in this area?

    1. inability to dorsiflex the ankle during mid-swing phase
    2. inability to perform a calf raise against resistance
    3. inability to walk on toes
    4. decreased toe off

87. A physical therapist administers ultrasound to a patient rehabilitating from a burn in an attempt to increase range of motion and decrease joint stiffness in the foot. When applying ultrasound to the dorsum of the foot, the patient complaints of significant discomfort from the sound head contacting the skin. The most appropriate treatment modification is:

    1. decrease the intensity of the ultrasound beam
    2. reduce the size of the area being sonated
    3. utilize an underwater technique
    4. select another thermal agent

88. A patient is limited in passive ankle dorsiflexion when the knee is extended, but is not limited when the knee is flexed. The most logical explanation is:

    1. the gastrocnemius is responsible for the limitation
    2. the soleus is responsible for the limitation
    3. the popliteus is responsible for the limitation
    4. the gastrocnemius and soleus are both responsible for the limitation

89. A patient with chronic obstructive pulmonary disease receives two liters per minute of supplemental oxygen using a nasal cannula. The most relevant indicator for the use of supplemental oxygen for the patient would be:

    1. arterial saturation = 85%
    2. partial pressure of arterial oxygen = 70 mm Hg
    3. partial pressure of carbon dioxide = 40 mm Hg
    4. pH = 7.40

90. A patient with a C6 spinal cord injury relies on tenodesis to assist with functional activities. Which condition will reduce the benefits of tenodesis?

    1. lengthening of the long finger flexors
    2. excessive hamstrings length
    3. insufficient hamstrings length
    4. transferring with the fingers flexed

91. A physical therapist palpates the muscle bellies of the wrist extensors. The therapist follows the muscles proximally to their common origin. This bony landmark is termed the:

   1. lateral epicondyle
   2. medial epicondyle
   3. radial head
   4. olecranon

92. A patient sustains a deep laceration on the right anterior thigh after stumbling and falling into a modality cart. The physical therapist's most immediate response should be to:

   1. apply direct pressure over the wound
   2. apply heat
   3. apply ice
   4. fill out an incident report

93. When measuring hip abduction the stationary arm of the goniometer should be positioned:

   1. between the anterior superior iliac spines
   2. parallel to the anterior aspect of the femur
   3. along the midline of the tibia
   4. along a line from the crest of the ilium, femur, and greater trochanter

94. A patient is treated in physical therapy after injuring his hamstrings. The medical chart describes the injury as an avulsion fracture of the ischial tuberosity. This injury usually results from:

   1. forceful extension of the hip with an extended knee
   2. forceful extension of the hip with a flexed knee
   3. forceful flexion of the hip with an extended knee
   4. forceful flexion of the hip with a flexed knee

95. A physical therapist reviews the examination of a patient diagnosed with a cerebellar CVA. The therapist might expect the patient's primary impairment to be:

   1. visual field cuts
   2. gait disturbances
   3. impaired speech
   4. impaired comprehension skills

96. A physical therapist hypothesizes that a patient's persistent shoulder pain is caused by an injury to a specific upper extremity muscle. What selective tissue tension assessment would provide the therapist with the most useful information to test the hypothesis?

   1. active range of motion
   2. active-assistive range of motion
   3. passive range of motion
   4. resisted isometrics

97. A woman in her third trimester of pregnancy is referred to physical therapy with acute low back pain. During a postural examination the physical therapist identifies several significant findings. Which of the following postural findings is not commonly associated with pregnancy?

   1. decrease in cervical lordosis
   2. increase in lumbar lordosis
   3. hyperextension of the knees
   4. protraction of the shoulder girdle

98. A physical therapist completes an upper extremity goniometric examination. The therapist records right elbow range of motion as 15 - 0 - 150 degrees. The total available range of motion for this patient is:

   1. 135 degrees
   2. 150 degrees
   3. 165 degrees
   4. 180 degrees

99. A physical therapist classifies a patient's end-feel as soft after completing a specific passive movement. Which of the following joint motions would typically produce a soft end-feel?

   1. hip flexion with the knee extended
   2. knee flexion
   3. elbow extension
   4. forearm supination

100. A group of physical therapists conducts a research study which examines the effect of functional knee bracing on speed and agility. As part of the study the therapists determine measures of central tendency for each measured variable. Which of the following would not be considered a measure of central tendency?

   1. median
   2. mode
   3. mean
   4. range

101. A male physical therapist prepares to treat a female patient using a soft tissue massage technique. The therapist would like to ensure that the patient does not misinterpret the purpose of the treatment technique. The most appropriate action is to:

   1. transfer the patient to another physical therapist's schedule
   2. request a female staff member to be present during treatment
   3. select another less invasive technique
   4. discharge the patient from physical therapy

102. A physical therapist attempts to gain information on the ligamentous integrity of the knee. Which of the following special tests would not provide the therapist with the desired information?

   1. anterior drawer test
   2. apprehension test
   3. Lachman test
   4. pivot shift test

103. A physical therapist completes an examination on a young girl with spastic cerebral palsy. The therapist determines that the girl has involvement in all four extremities as well as the head, neck, and trunk. What type of cerebral palsy classification best describes the girl's condition?

   1. spastic diplegia
   2. spastic hemiplegia
   3. spastic tetraplegia
   4. spastic triplegia

104. A physical therapist employed in an acute care hospital treats a patient diagnosed with liver disease. The therapist notes that the patient's skin and eyes appear to have a yellow tint. Which condition is most consistent with this type of clinical presentation?

   1. human immunodeficiency virus
   2. hepatitis
   3. tuberculosis
   4. meningitis

105. A physical therapist positions a patient in the Trendelenburg position in preparation for postural drainage. Which of the following is not a relative precaution for the use of the Trendelenburg position?

   1. nausea
   2. obesity
   3. pulmonary edema
   4. secretion retention

106. Health care cost containment efforts have created incentives for inpatient care providers and hospitals to control the cost and utilization of inpatient services. Which of the following has not resulted as a product of cost containment efforts?

   1. a decrease in the average length of inpatient hospitalizations
   2. an increase in the utilization of home care and skilled long-term care
   3. a decrease in the use of diagnostic testing during inpatient hospitalization
   4. a decrease in the use of outpatient diagnostic testing and treatment

107. A physical therapist designs an exercise program to increase muscle strength and endurance in a patient rehabilitating from knee surgery. Which type of pharmacological agent would have an antagonistic effect on the desired objective?

   1. nonnarcotic analgesics
   2. nonsteroidal anti-inflammatory medications
   3. peripheral vasodilators
   4. skeletal muscle relaxants

108. A physical therapist reviews the medical record of a patient 24 hours status post total hip replacement. A recent entry in the medical record indicates that the patient was placed on anticoagulant medication. Which of the following laboratory values would be most affected based on the patient's current medication?

   1. hematocrit
   2. hemoglobin
   3. prothrombin time
   4. white blood cell count

109. A physical therapist participates in a community based screening program designed to identify individuals with osteoporosis. Which group would have the highest risk for developing osteoporosis?

   1. white females over the age of 60
   2. black females over the age of 60
   3. white females over the age of 40
   4. black females over the age of 40

110. A physical therapist instructs a 62-year-old female rehabilitating from an ankle sprain in the use of a straight cane. The patient is confused as to why it is necessary to use the cane in the left hand since it is her right ankle that is injured. The most appropriate explanation would be:

1. using the cane in the left hand will increase your base of support
2. using the cane in the left hand will improve your coordination and balance
3. using the cane in the left hand will reduce the pressure over your injured ankle
4. using the cane in the left hand will allow more weight bearing on your injured ankle and will therefore accelerate your rehabilitation time

111. A physical therapist discusses the plan of care for a 61-year-old male diagnosed with spinal stenosis with the referring physician. During the discussion the physician shows the therapist a picture of the patient's spine obtained through computed tomography. What color would vertebrae appear when using this imaging technique?

1. black
2. light gray
3. dark gray
4. white

112. A physical therapist completes a series of special tests designed to examine the ligamentous integrity of a patient's knee. After completing the tests, the therapist is unsure if the laxity is normal or if it is indicative of a ligamentous injury. The most appropriate step to gather more information is to:

1. attempt to quantify the millimeters of laxity and compare the values with established norms
2. contact the physician and suggest a referral for magnetic resonance imaging
3. directly compare the laxity in the involved knee to the laxity in the uninvolved knee
4. attempt to identify other special tests which can offer more information on the ligamentous integrity of the knee

113. A physical therapist performs the talar tilt test on a 22-year-old female rehabilitating from an inversion ankle sprain. Which ligament does the talar tilt test examine?

1. anterior tibiofibular
2. calcaneofibular
3. deltoid
4. posterior tibiofibular

114. A physical therapy department designs a study to examine rehabilitation outcomes in patients who have undergone anterior cruciate ligament reconstruction. The study will include a sample of patients from 25 orthopedic surgeons in the local region. If the physical therapists compile a list of all eligible patients and select every third patient to participate in the study, what type of sampling was used?

1. simple random sampling
2. stratified sampling
3. systematic sampling
4. cluster sampling

115. A physical therapist employed in an acute care hospital prepares to visit a former patient in strict isolation. The therapist was granted permission to visit the patient provided there is no body contact. What protective measures are necessary when entering the room?

1. mask
2. mask, gown
3. gloves, gown
4. mask, gown, gloves

116. A physical therapist attempts to palpate the lunate by moving his finger immediately distal to Lister's tubercle. Which wrist motion will allow the therapist to facilitate palpation of the lunate?

1. extension
2. flexion
3. radial deviation
4. ulnar deviation

117. A physician indicates that a patient rehabilitating from a cerebrovascular accident has significant perceptual deficits. Which anatomical region would most likely be affected by the stroke?

1. primary motor cortex
2. sensory cortex
3. basal ganglia
4. cerebellum

118. A patient with suspected cardiac dysfunction is placed on a continuous ambulatory ECG monitor. Which of the following is the name commonly used for this type of monitoring?

1. hemodynamic
2. Holter
3. phonocardiography
4. pulmonic

119. A physical therapist conducts a study which measures knee flexion range of motion two weeks following arthroscopic surgery. Assuming a normal distribution, what percentage of patients participating in the study would you expect to achieve a goniometric measurement value greater than one standard deviation below the mean?

    1. 49%
    2. 64%
    3. 68%
    4. 84%

120. A physical therapist positions a patient in prone with two pillows under the hips in preparation for bronchial drainage. If the therapist's goal is to perform bronchial drainage to the superior segments of the lower lobes, which area should the therapist's force be directed?

    1. between the clavicle and nipple on each side
    2. over the area between the clavicle and top of the scapula on each side
    3. over the lower ribs on each side
    4. over the middle of the back at the tip of the scapula on each side

121. Secretion removal techniques are often a necessary component of a pulmonary rehabilitation program. Which pulmonary disease is usually associated with a change in the composition of secretions?

    1. asthma
    2. bronchiectasis
    3. chronic bronchitis
    4. cystic fibrosis

122. A physical therapist treats a patient referred to physical therapy with incontinence. The patient describes her difficulty beginning after the birth of her son. After completing an examination the therapist concludes that the patient has extremely weak pelvic floor muscles. When instructing the patient in a pelvic floor muscle strengthening program, the most appropriate position to initiate treatment is:

    1. sidelying
    2. sitting
    3. standing
    4. supine

123. A physical therapist prepares to administer the Berg Functional Balance Scale to a patient rehabilitating from a cerebrovascular accident. Which of the following tools is considered a necessary piece of equipment when administering this outcome measure?

    1. reflex hammer
    2. goniometer
    3. stopwatch
    4. stethoscope

124. A physical therapist employed in a school setting observes a 10-year-old boy attempt to move from the floor to a standing position. During the activity, the boy has to push on his legs with his hands in order to attain an upright position. This type of finding is most commonly associated with:

    1. cystic fibrosis
    2. Down syndrome
    3. Duchenne muscular dystrophy
    4. spinal muscular atrophy

125. A physical therapist performs a respiratory assessment on a patient with restrictive lung disease. If the therapist records the respiration rate as 22 breaths per minute, which term is most appropriate to classify the patient's respiration rate?

    1. eupnea
    2. tachypnea
    3. bradypnea
    4. hyperpnea

126. Dysrhythmias can result in varying degrees of abnormal hemodynamics. Which of the following dysrhythmias would have the most significant effect on hemodynamics?

    1. sinus rhythm with first degree A-V block
    2. sinus rhythm with premature atrial contractions
    3. sinus rhythm with short episodes of paroxysmal supraventricular tachycardia
    4. ventricular tachycardia

127. After administration many drugs are stored at specific locations in the body. What is the primary site for drug storage in the body?

    1. adipose tissue
    2. bone
    3. muscle
    4. organs

128. A physical therapist uses ultrasound to elevate the tissue temperature at the insertion of the supraspinatus. What would be the most appropriate patient position for the ultrasound application?

 1. patient in supine with the arm abducted and laterally rotated
 2. patient in supine with the arm adducted and medially rotated
 3. patient in supine with the arm abducted and medially rotated
 4. patient in supine with the arm adducted and laterally rotated

129. A physical therapist treats a 15-year-old female of Spanish descent. The patient speaks only a few words of English and has significant difficulty understanding the therapist's instructions. The most appropriate therapist action is to:

 1. speak strongly and directly to the patient
 2. encourage frequent feedback from the patient
 3. utilize an interpreter
 4. emphasize nonverbal communication

130. A physical therapist uses a spirometer to administer a pulmonary function test to a patient with suspected pulmonary dysfunction. Which of the following measurements would the therapist be able to obtain directly without utilizing the results of other pulmonary function tests?

 1. expiratory reserve volume
 2. inspiratory reserve volume
 3. minute volume
 4. residual volume

131. A female diagnosed with a cervical spine injury reports to physical therapy for a scheduled treatment session. While walking with the patient to the treatment area the physical therapist notices that the patient's cervical orthosis is very loose. The most appropriate therapist action is:

 1. document the observation in the medical record
 2. reapply the orthosis correctly at the conclusion of the treatment session
 3. remind the patient of the donning instructions for the orthosis
 4. contact the referring physician

132. A physical therapist administers neuromuscular electrical stimulation to the quadriceps using a bipolar electrode configuration. After observing the muscle contraction, the therapist decides to modify the treatment set up in order to increase the depth of current penetration. The most appropriate action is to:

 1. utilize carbon-rubber electrodes
 2. increase the size of the electrodes
 3. utilize additional electrodes using a bifurcated lead
 4. increase the distance between the electrodes

133. A patient is able to actively hyperextend the right knee 5 degrees. Assuming the patient's total knee range of motion is 65 degrees, which of the following recordings would be the most representative of the patient's actual range of motion?

 1. 5 - 0 - 60
 2. 5 - 0 - 65
 3. 5 - 60
 4. 5 - 65

134. A physical therapist employed in an outpatient private practice informs a patient rehabilitating from an ankle sprain that she has exhausted her maximum allowable physical therapy visits from her health maintenance organization. The patient is presently independent with her home exercise program and has successfully achieved all of the established short and long-term goals. The most appropriate therapist action is:

 1. provide physical therapy services to the patient pro bono
 2. contact the referring physician and request approval for additional visits
 3. bill the patient directly for additional physical therapy sessions
 4. discharge the patient from physical therapy

135. A physical therapist develops a problem list after completing an examination on a patient diagnosed with rotator cuff tendonitis. Which section of the S.O.A.P. note would include the problem list?

 1. subjective
 2. objective
 3. assessment
 4. plan

136. A physical therapist palpates the bony structures of the wrist and hand. Which of the following structures would not be identified in the distal row of carpals?

    1. capitate
    2. hamate
    3. triquetrum
    4. trapezoid

137. A physical therapist examines the electrocardiogram of a patient during exercise. What change in the electrocardiogram would be indicative of myocardial ischemia?

    1. P wave changes
    2. PR interval changes
    3. QRS changes
    4. ST segment changes

138. A physical therapist treats a 72-year-old female who fractured her leg two weeks ago after losing her balance and falling to the floor in a nursing home. The patient's spouse died three years ago and left her with no appreciable assets or regular income. The patient has been a resident of the nursing home for eight years. Which form of insurance is the most likely to pay for the patient's daily care?

    1. private insurance
    2. health maintenance organization
    3. Medicaid
    4. Medicare

139. A physical therapist prepares a patient for ambulation. The patient has been in the hospital for six weeks with pneumonia and has only recently had enough strength to begin ambulation training. Which of the following treatment activities would be the last to occur?

    1. development of standing balance
    2. development of sitting balance
    3. training in a specific gait pattern
    4. training in weight shifting in a standing position

140. A physical therapist administers a submaximal exercise test to a patient in a cardiac rehabilitation program. The protocol requires the patient to ride a cycle ergometer for a predetermined amount of time using progressive workloads. In order to predict the patient's maximum oxygen uptake it is necessary to determine the relationship between:

    1. heart rate and perceived exertion
    2. heart rate and oxygen uptake
    3. perceived exertion and blood pressure
    4. blood pressure and oxygen uptake

141. A physical therapist examines a patient bedside when suddenly the patient's I.V. becomes disconnected. The therapist's most appropriate response would be to:

    1. reconnect the I.V.
    2. contact the primary physician
    3. contact the nurse
    4. continue with the present treatment

142. A physician orders the nursing staff to administer digitalis to a patient diagnosed with congestive heart failure. The physician's primary goal using this medication is to:

    1. increase cardiac pumping ability
    2. increase cellular metabolism
    3. regulate fluid and electrolyte levels
    4. regulate glucose metabolism

143. A physical therapist identifies a bluish discoloration of the skin and nailbeds of a 55-year-old male referred to physical therapy for pulmonary rehabilitation. What does this objective finding indicate?

    1. hyperoxemia
    2. hyperoxia
    3. hypokalemia
    4. hypoxemia

144. A physical therapist employed in a large medical center reviews the chart of a 63-year-old male referred to physical therapy for pulmonary rehabilitation. The chart indicates the patient has smoked 1-2 packs of cigarettes a day since the age of 25. The admitting physician documented that the patient's thorax was enlarged with flaring of the costal margins and widening of the costochondral angle. Which pulmonary disease does the chart most accurately describe?

    1. asthma
    2. bronchiectasis
    3. chronic bronchitis
    4. emphysema

145. A physical therapist performs a manual muscle test on a patient with bilateral upper extremity weakness. The therapist should test the patient's scapular adductors with the patient positioned in:

    1. prone
    2. sidelying
    3. standing
    4. supine

146. A physical therapist instructs a patient diagnosed with rotator cuff tendonitis in a home exercise program. The most important consideration when designing a home exercise program is to:

   1. focus the program on the individual needs of the patient
   2. limit the length of the program to 10 minutes
   3. provide written instructions that detail the frequency and duration of each exercise
   4. limit the amount of equipment required to complete the program

147. A physical therapist selects a wheelchair for a patient recently admitted to a skilled nursing facility. The patient is diagnosed with a right cerebrovascular accident with resultant left hemiplegia. After completing the examination the therapist concludes that the patient would benefit from a wheelchair with a one-arm drive. Which of the following variables would be the most critical to assess prior to prescribing this type of wheelchair?

   1. upper extremity strength and coordination
   2. sitting balance and upper extremity range of motion
   3. spatial orientation and kinesthesia
   4. sitting tolerance and skin integrity

148. A physical therapist reviews the results of pulmonary function testing on a 44-year-old female diagnosed with emphysema. Assuming the patient's testing was classified as unremarkable, which of the following lung volumes would most likely approximate 10% of the patient's total lung capacity?

   1. tidal volume
   2. inspiratory reserve volume
   3. residual volume
   4. functional residual capacity

149. A 26-year-old female is referred to physical therapy after being diagnosed with impingement syndrome. The patient is a competitive swimmer who complains of shoulder pain when performing strokes that require overhead motion. Which of the following results would be the most typical during the examination of the shoulder?

   1. excessive medial rotation
   2. diminished cutaneous sensation
   3. restricted posterior capsule
   4. weakness in the deltoid muscle

150. A patient rehabilitating from a spinal cord injury works on self range of motion activities in sitting. Suddenly, the patient begins to demonstrate signs and symptoms of autonomic dysreflexia. The most appropriate physical therapist action is to:

   1. keep the patient in sitting, monitor blood pressure, and check the bowel and bladder for impairment
   2. lie the patient flat, monitor blood pressure, and check the bowel and bladder for impairment
   3. lie the patient flat, monitor blood pressure, and give the patient fluids
   4. keep the patient sitting, monitor blood pressure, wait for medical assistance

151. A physical therapist administers the Body Mass Index Scale to a patient as a means of assessing total body composition. The therapist determines the body mass index by dividing the body weight in kilograms by height in meters squared. Which of the following values would be the most representative for a healthy male or female?

   1. 14 kg/m^2
   2. 22 kg/m^2
   3. 28 kg/m^2
   4. 35 kg/m^2

152. A patient diagnosed with patellofemoral syndrome discusses his past medical history with a physical therapist. The patient reports having anterior cruciate ligament reconstructive surgery in his right knee two years ago, however the therapist is not able to identify a scar over the anterior surface of the right knee. Assuming the surgeon utilized an autograft for the reconstruction, which of the following would be the most likely graft site?

   1. semitendinosus and semimembranosus
   2. semitendinosus and gracilis
   3. semimembranosus and gracilis
   4. semitendinosus and biceps femoris

153. A 36-year-old female distance runner diagnosed with Achilles tendonitis is referred to physical therapy. After completing an examination the physical therapist discusses selected elements of the patient's training program. Which recommendation would be the least beneficial based on the patient's diagnosis?

   1. decrease daily mileage
   2. introduce cross training in low impact activities
   3. implement interval training
   4. avoid running on hills

154. A physical therapist employed in a nursing home routinely treats patients in excess of 70 years of age. The therapist has noted several consistent postural changes in her patients. Which of the following does not accurately describe the postural changes associated with aging?

   1. forward head
   2. rounded shoulders
   3. increased hip extension
   4. increased knee flexion

155. A physical therapist orders a wheelchair for a patient with C5 tetraplegia. Which type of wheelchair would be the most appropriate for the patient?

   1. electric wheelchair
   2. manual wheelchair with handrim projections
   3. manual wheelchair with friction surface handrims
   4. manual wheelchair with standard handrims

156. A patient is instructed by the nursing staff to increase dietary consumption of food sources that are rich in vitamin A. Which of the following food groups would be the most appropriate to meet this goal?

   1. green leaves, nuts, seafood
   2. fish liver oils, butter, yellow vegetables
   3. milk, cheese, liver
   4. vegetable oil, wheat germ, dried yeast

157. A physical therapist reviews a medical chart to determine when a patient was last medicated. The chart indicates the patient received medication at 2300 hours. Assuming it is now 8:00 AM, how long ago did the patient receive the medication?

   1. 5 hours
   2. 9 hours
   3. 15 hours
   4. 18 hours

158. A 54-year-old male rehabilitating from a fractured ankle is referred to physical therapy for gait training. The patient is in a short leg cast and is not permitted to bear weight through the involved lower extremity. Which gait pattern is the most appropriate for the patient?

   1. three-point gait using axillary crutches
   2. three-point swing-through using a walker
   3. three-point swing-to using a walker
   4. four-point alternating gait using axillary crutches

159. A physical therapist attempts to auscultate over the aortic valve. Which of the following areas is the most appropriate to isolate the desired valve?

   1. second left intercostal space at the left sternal border
   2. second right intercostal space at the right sternal border
   3. fourth left intercostal space along the lower left sternal border
   4. fifth left intercostal space at the midclavicular line

160. A physical therapist presents the results of a research project entitled "Effects of an Aerobic Exercise Program on Heart Rate and Blood Pressure." The independent variable in the therapist's study is:

   1. exercise program
   2. exercise program and heart rate
   3. exercise program and blood pressure
   4. heart rate and blood pressure

161. A physical therapist completes a pulmonary function test on a male patient admitted to the hospital three days ago. What percentage of total lung capacity does residual volume represent?

   1. 10%
   2. 25%
   3. 35%
   4. 50%

162. A physical therapist positions a patient for bronchial drainage to the anterior segments of the upper lobes. The most appropriate patient position is:

   1. supine with a pillow under the knees
   2. supine with the head of the bed elevated 16 inches
   3. supine with the foot of the bed elevated 16 inches
   4. prone with the head of the bed elevated 12 inches

163. A physical therapist attempts to estimate the energy expenditure in calories for a patient performing a selected activity for 15 minutes. Assuming the therapist has a metabolic equivalent value for the activity, what other variables are necessary in order to obtain an estimate of the patient's energy expenditure?

   1. patient's height and weight
   2. patient's weight and oxygen consumption
   3. patient's stroke volume and heart rate
   4. patient's residual volume and heart rate

164. An acute myocardial infarction can often be diagnosed by analyzing the characteristic pattern and duration of selected enzymes in the blood. Which of the following enzymes is not commonly elevated following an acute myocardial infarction?

    1. aspartate aminotransferase
    2. creatine phosphokinase
    3. lactate dehydrogenase
    4. alkaline phosphatase

165. A physical therapist examines the cutaneous reflexes of a patient with suspected central nervous system involvement. Which of the following is the most appropriate to utilize when attempting to elicit the Babinski reflex?

    1. tuning fork
    2. index finger
    3. pointed end of a reflex hammer
    4. cotton ball

166. A physical therapist examines the foot of a 17-year-old female referred to physical therapy with lower leg pain. After placing the foot in subtalar neutral the therapist determines that the medial border of the foot along the first metatarsal is higher than the lateral border of the foot along the fifth metatarsal. This position would most appropriately be documented as:

    1. forefoot varus
    2. forefoot valgus
    3. rearfoot varus
    4. rearfoot valgus

167. A physical therapist prepares to administer a dressing change on a patient rehabilitating from a deep partial-thickness burn over the dorsal surface of the forearm and hand. The patient's current regimen consists of dressing changes twice daily and reapplication of a topical antibiotic. When sequencing the activities associated with the dressing change, which activity would occur second?

    1. gentle debridement in a hydrotherapy tank
    2. reapplication of the topical antibiotic
    3. application of gauze wraps in a distal to proximal pattern
    4. removal of current dressings

168. A patient is referred to physical therapy for gait training following an extended illness. The patient has poor balance, but is able to move her legs alternately. Which of the following gait patterns would be the most stable?

    1. two-point
    2. three-point
    3. four-point
    4. swing-through

169. A physical therapist reviews the medical record of a patient recently admitted to an inpatient rehabilitation hospital. The patient sustained a traumatic head injury in a motor vehicle accident five weeks ago. The medical record indicates that the patient is often disoriented and can frequently become agitated with little provocation. The most appropriate location for the therapist to make initial contact with the patient is:

    1. in the patient's room
    2. in the physical therapy gym
    3. in a private treatment room
    4. in the physical therapy waiting room

170. A physical therapist outlines a walking program for a patient rehabilitating from a prolonged illness. Which of the following recommendations would not be beneficial for the patient?

    1. wear comfortable, loose fitting clothing appropriate for the present temperature and weather
    2. walk at a rate designed to bring the heart to target levels
    3. walk continuously; frequent stops interfere with aerobic training
    4. when walking up steep hills lean backward slightly and lengthen your stride

171. A patient is referred to physical therapy after being diagnosed with cervical radiculopathy due to C7 nerve root impingement. When completing an upper quarter screening examination, which deep tendon reflex would you expect to be most affected?

    1. biceps
    2. brachioradialis
    3. triceps
    4. upper abdominal

172. Patients often progress through a predictable series of stages after being diagnosed with a terminal illness. According to Elizabeth Kubler Ross' Stages of Dying, what is the first stage a patient will experience?

   1. acceptance
   2. anger
   3. denial
   4. depression

173. A patient indicates that she is currently taking medication to control high blood pressure. Which of the following classifications of drugs would be helpful in the treatment of hypertension?

   1. diuretics
   2. narcotics
   3. nonsteroidal anti-inflammatories
   4. stimulants

174. A physical therapist monitors the blood pressure of a 28-year-old male during increasing levels of physical exertion. Assuming a normal physiologic response, which of the following best describes the patient's blood pressure response to exercise?

   1. systolic pressure decreases, diastolic pressure increases
   2. systolic pressure remains the same, diastolic pressure decreases
   3. systolic pressure and diastolic pressure remain the same
   4. systolic pressure increases, diastolic pressure remains the same

175. A physical therapist palpates the proximal row of carpals on a patient diagnosed with carpal tunnel syndrome. Which of the following bones does not articulate with the proximal row of carpals?

   1. hamate
   2. radius
   3. trapezium
   4. ulna

176. A physical therapist performs goniometric measurements at the carpometacarpal joint. If the therapist elects to measure carpometacarpal abduction, the stationary arm of the goniometer should be aligned with the:

   1. lateral midline of the second metacarpal
   2. lateral midline of the first metacarpal
   3. palmar midline of the radius
   4. palmar midline of the first metacarpal

177. A patient with degenerative joint disease is referred to physical therapy with right shoulder pain. During the initial examination the physical therapist identifies significant muscle guarding and spasm throughout the right shoulder. If the therapist elects to treat the patient using ultrasound, which patient position would be the most appropriate?

   1. supine with the upper extremity slightly flexed and adducted
   2. supine with the arm resting against the abdomen
   3. supine with the glenohumeral joint in the resting position
   4. a position where the patient is comfortable and relaxed

178. A physical therapist views a videotape that compares and contrasts the normal gait of toddlers and adults. Which of the following statements is not accurate when comparing the gait of these two groups?

   1. toddlers walk with a wider base of support
   2. toddlers walk with an increased single leg support time
   3. toddlers walk with a higher cadence
   4. toddlers walk with a shorter step length

179. A physician completes a physical examination on a 16-year-old male who injured his knee while playing in a soccer contest yesterday. The physician's preliminary diagnosis is a grade II anterior cruciate ligament injury with probable meniscal involvement. Which of the following diagnostic tools would be the most appropriate in the immediate medical management of the patient?

   1. bone scan
   2. computerized tomography
   3. magnetic resonance imaging
   4. x-rays

180. Performance appraisals are often conducted on a regular basis to assess an employee's performance in relation to the performance expectations. Which of the following statements describing a performance appraisal is not accurate?

   1. Employees should be aware of the performance standards after they are examined.
   2. A mechanism should be in place which employees can use to dispute or comment on appraisal outcomes.
   3. A manager's appraisal decisions should be audited by the organization.
   4. Performance discrepancies should be clearly documented on appraisal forms.

181. A physical therapist performs goniometric measurements on a 38-year-old female rehabilitating from an acromioplasty. The therapist attempts to stabilize the scapula while measuring glenohumeral abduction. Failure to stabilize the scapula will lead to:

    1. downward rotation and elevation of the scapula
    2. downward rotation and depression of the scapula
    3. upward rotation and elevation of the scapula
    4. upward rotation and depression of the scapula

182. A physical therapist measures a patient's shoulder medial rotation with the patient positioned in supine, glenohumeral joint in 90 degrees of abduction, and the elbow in 90 degrees of flexion. The therapist records the patient's shoulder medial rotation as 0 - 70 degrees and classifies the end-feel as firm. Which portion of the joint capsule is primarily responsible for the firm end-feel?

    1. anterior joint capsule
    2. posterior joint capsule
    3. inferior joint capsule
    4. superior joint capsule

183. A physical therapist treats a patient with limited right shoulder range of motion using a contract-relax technique. When completing a reexamination of the patient, which piece of objective information would most warrant discontinuing the selected treatment option?

    1. the patient does not experience pain with active muscle contraction
    2. the patient has full range of motion
    3. the patient can generate a maximal muscle contraction
    4. the patient has been treated for more than 10 sessions

184. A physician suspects a stress fracture in a 16-year-old distance runner after completing a physical examination. Assuming the physician's preliminary diagnosis is correct, which of the following diagnostic tests would be the most appropriate to identify the stress fracture?

    1. bone scan
    2. magnetic resonance imaging
    3. telethermography
    4. ultrasound scan

185. A physical therapist develops a problem list after completing an initial examination on a patient diagnosed with right shoulder impingement. Which of the following entries would not typically belong in the physical therapy problem list?

    1. decreased active right shoulder lateral rotation
    2. decreased strength of the right upper trapezius and middle deltoid
    3. increased pain with right shoulder active movement
    4. increased stress secondary to financial problems

186. A physical therapist performs an examination on a 46-year-old male patient diagnosed with piriformis syndrome. The patient indicates he has experienced pain in his lower back and buttock region for the last three weeks. Which motions would you expect to be weak and painful during muscle testing based on the patient's diagnosis?

    1. abduction and lateral rotation of the thigh
    2. abduction and medial rotation of the thigh
    3. adduction and lateral rotation of the thigh
    4. adduction and medial rotation of the thigh

187. Which type of joint receptor would a physical therapist expect to be most sensitive to high frequency vibration, deep pressure, and velocity changes in joint position?

    1. Free nerve endings
    2. Golgi-Mazzoni corpuscles
    3. Pacinian corpuscles
    4. Ruffini endings

188. A physical therapist examines a patient with a dorsal scapular nerve injury. Which muscles would you expect to be most affected by this condition?

    1. serratus anterior, pectoralis minor
    2. levator scapulae, rhomboids
    3. latissimus dorsi, teres major
    4. supraspinatus, infraspinatus

189. A physical therapist examines a patient with unilateral lower extremity weakness. As the patient performs hip flexion in supine, the therapist helps the patient complete the full range of motion. This would best be described as:

    1. active exercise
    2. passive exercise
    3. resistive exercise
    4. active-assistive exercise

190. A physical therapist positions a patient in prone to measure passive knee flexion. Range of motion may be limited in this position due to:

    1. active insufficiency of the knee extensors
    2. active insufficiency of the knee flexors
    3. passive insufficiency of the knee extensors
    4. passive insufficiency of the knee flexors

191. A patient injured in a work related accident is referred to physical therapy for work reconditioning. During the initial session the physical therapist identifies several selective behaviors that could be consistent with symptom magnification. The most appropriate therapist action is:

    1. avoid documenting the objective findings, however continue to monitor the situation
    2. document the objective findings
    3. document the objective findings and attempt to interpret the patient's behavior
    4. document the objective findings and list possible secondary gains

192. A physical therapist examines a four month old infant. During mat activities the infant suddenly becomes unconscious. The most appropriate location to check the infant's pulse is the:

    1. radial artery
    2. brachial artery
    3. popliteal artery
    4. carotid artery

193. A patient diagnosed with Parkinson's disease has difficulty initiating movement. What proprioceptive neuromuscular facilitation technique would be the most appropriate to treat this problem?

    1. contract-relax
    2. rhythmic initiation
    3. rhythmic stabilization
    4. slow reversal

194. A physical therapist instructs a patient to move from sitting through quadruped to tall kneeling. By moving through the developmental sequence a patient gains _____ control during movement and _____ during static positioning?

    1. isometric, isotonic
    2. isotonic, isometric
    3. isometric, isokinetic
    4. isokinetic, isotonic

195. A physical therapist examines the motor component of the trigeminal nerve by observing a patient open and close his mouth repeatedly. Which clinical finding would be most indicative of weakness of the right pterygoid muscles?

    1. right deviation of the jaw during opening of the mouth
    2. left deviation of the jaw during opening of the mouth
    3. difficulty depressing the mandible during opening of the mouth
    4. audible crepitation during opening of the mouth

196. A physical therapist observes a patient during gait training. The patient has normal strength and equal leg length. As the patient passes mid-stance he slightly vaults and has early toe off. The most likely cause of this deviation is:

    1. patient has excessive forefoot pronation
    2. patient has limited hamstrings length
    3. patient has limited plantar flexion
    4. patient has limited dorsiflexion

197. A physical therapist assesses kinesthesia in a 61-year-old male patient with Parkinson's disease. Which of the following patient responses would be the most appropriate during the testing?

    1. my arm is moving up toward the ceiling
    2. my arm is parallel with the floor
    3. my arm just started moving
    4. my arm is in approximately the same position as my other arm

198. Which clinical observation is not usually characteristic with a rotator cuff tear?

    1. the patient is less than 40 years old
    2. the patient is often unable to move the arm actively without pain
    3. scapulohumeral rhythm is altered
    4. night pain is a common patient complaint

199. A patient status post CVA with abnormal tone on the right side lies supine in bed. The patient's physical therapist discourages her from lying supine for long periods of time because:

    1. the position can cause shoulder-hand syndrome
    2. the position increases inferior subluxation
    3. the position encourages tonic neck and labyrinthine reflexes
    4. the position increases tone in the pectoralis

200. A physical therapist might select a metal upright ankle-foot orthosis instead of a plastic ankle-foot orthosis if the patient exhibits:

   1. mild sensory loss
   2. significant fluctuating edema
   3. cosmetic concerns
   4. mediolateral ankle instability

Sample Exam: Three – Answer Sheet

1. ① ② ③ ④	36. ① ② ③ ④	71. ① ② ③ ④
2. ① ② ③ ④	37. ① ② ③ ④	72. ① ② ③ ④
3. ① ② ③ ④	38. ① ② ③ ④	73. ① ② ③ ④
4. ① ② ③ ④	39. ① ② ③ ④	74. ① ② ③ ④
5. ① ② ③ ④	40. ① ② ③ ④	75. ① ② ③ ④
6. ① ② ③ ④	41. ① ② ③ ④	76. ① ② ③ ④
7. ① ② ③ ④	42. ① ② ③ ④	77. ① ② ③ ④
8. ① ② ③ ④	43. ① ② ③ ④	78. ① ② ③ ④
9. ① ② ③ ④	44. ① ② ③ ④	79. ① ② ③ ④
10. ① ② ③ ④	45. ① ② ③ ④	80. ① ② ③ ④
11. ① ② ③ ④	46. ① ② ③ ④	81. ① ② ③ ④
12. ① ② ③ ④	47. ① ② ③ ④	82. ① ② ③ ④
13. ① ② ③ ④	48. ① ② ③ ④	83. ① ② ③ ④
14. ① ② ③ ④	49. ① ② ③ ④	84. ① ② ③ ④
15. ① ② ③ ④	50. ① ② ③ ④	85. ① ② ③ ④
16. ① ② ③ ④	51. ① ② ③ ④	86. ① ② ③ ④
17. ① ② ③ ④	52. ① ② ③ ④	87. ① ② ③ ④
18. ① ② ③ ④	53. ① ② ③ ④	88. ① ② ③ ④
19. ① ② ③ ④	54. ① ② ③ ④	89. ① ② ③ ④
20. ① ② ③ ④	55. ① ② ③ ④	90. ① ② ③ ④
21. ① ② ③ ④	56. ① ② ③ ④	91. ① ② ③ ④
22. ① ② ③ ④	57. ① ② ③ ④	92. ① ② ③ ④
23. ① ② ③ ④	58. ① ② ③ ④	93. ① ② ③ ④
24. ① ② ③ ④	59. ① ② ③ ④	94. ① ② ③ ④
25. ① ② ③ ④	60. ① ② ③ ④	95. ① ② ③ ④
26. ① ② ③ ④	61. ① ② ③ ④	96. ① ② ③ ④
27. ① ② ③ ④	62. ① ② ③ ④	97. ① ② ③ ④
28. ① ② ③ ④	63. ① ② ③ ④	98. ① ② ③ ④
29. ① ② ③ ④	64. ① ② ③ ④	99. ① ② ③ ④
30. ① ② ③ ④	65. ① ② ③ ④	100. ① ② ③ ④
31. ① ② ③ ④	66. ① ② ③ ④	101. ① ② ③ ④
32. ① ② ③ ④	67. ① ② ③ ④	102. ① ② ③ ④
33. ① ② ③ ④	68. ① ② ③ ④	103. ① ② ③ ④
34. ① ② ③ ④	69. ① ② ③ ④	104. ① ② ③ ④
35. ① ② ③ ④	70. ① ② ③ ④	105. ① ② ③ ④

106.	①	②	③	④	138.	①	②	③	④	170.	①	②	③	④
107.	①	②	③	④	139.	①	②	③	④	171.	①	②	③	④
108.	①	②	③	④	140.	①	②	③	④	172.	①	②	③	④
109.	①	②	③	④	141.	①	②	③	④	173.	①	②	③	④
110.	①	②	③	④	142.	①	②	③	④	174.	①	②	③	④
111.	①	②	③	④	143.	①	②	③	④	175.	①	②	③	④
112.	①	②	③	④	144.	①	②	③	④	176.	①	②	③	④
113.	①	②	③	④	145.	①	②	③	④	177.	①	②	③	④
114.	①	②	③	④	146.	①	②	③	④	178.	①	②	③	④
115.	①	②	③	④	147.	①	②	③	④	179.	①	②	③	④
116.	①	②	③	④	148.	①	②	③	④	180.	①	②	③	④
117.	①	②	③	④	149.	①	②	③	④	181.	①	②	③	④
118.	①	②	③	④	150.	①	②	③	④	182.	①	②	③	④
119.	①	②	③	④	151.	①	②	③	④	183.	①	②	③	④
120.	①	②	③	④	152.	①	②	③	④	184.	①	②	③	④
121.	①	②	③	④	153.	①	②	③	④	185.	①	②	③	④
122.	①	②	③	④	154.	①	②	③	④	186.	①	②	③	④
123.	①	②	③	④	155.	①	②	③	④	187.	①	②	③	④
124.	①	②	③	④	156.	①	②	③	④	188.	①	②	③	④
125.	①	②	③	④	157.	①	②	③	④	189.	①	②	③	④
126.	①	②	③	④	158.	①	②	③	④	190.	①	②	③	④
127.	①	②	③	④	159.	①	②	③	④	191.	①	②	③	④
128.	①	②	③	④	160.	①	②	③	④	192.	①	②	③	④
129.	①	②	③	④	161.	①	②	③	④	193.	①	②	③	④
130.	①	②	③	④	162.	①	②	③	④	194.	①	②	③	④
131.	①	②	③	④	163.	①	②	③	④	195.	①	②	③	④
132.	①	②	③	④	164.	①	②	③	④	196.	①	②	③	④
133.	①	②	③	④	165.	①	②	③	④	197.	①	②	③	④
134.	①	②	③	④	166.	①	②	③	④	198.	①	②	③	④
135.	①	②	③	④	167.	①	②	③	④	199.	①	②	③	④
136.	①	②	③	④	168.	①	②	③	④	200.	①	②	③	④
137.	①	②	③	④	169.	①	②	③	④					

Sample Exam Answers: Three

1. Answer: 3   Resource: Haggard (p. 83)
   Lecture, handouts, and demonstration provide the broadest range of media for the presentation. A broad range of media allows for individuals with diverse learning styles to benefit from the presentation.

2. Answer: 2   Resource: Davies (p. 5)
   A physical therapist should attempt to facilitate movement of the patient's trunk and extremities using intermittent light touch. Intermittent light touch allows the patient to initiate movement and progress through the full range of movement with assistance as necessary.

3. Answer: 3   Resource: O'Sullivan - Physical Rehabilitation (p. 632)
   It is extremely important for a patient with a transtibial amputation to keep the knee in an extended position in order to avoid a knee flexion contracture.

4. Answer: 4   Resource: Pierson (p. 194)
   A straight cane can be used to compensate for balance deficits and to promote stability, however does not allow for various degrees of weight bearing.

5. Answer: 4   Resource: Michlovitz (p. 102)
   Signs of cold intolerance include pain, cyanosis, wheals, mottling, increased pulse rate, and a significant drop in blood pressure. A physical therapist should immediately stop the application of cold when any sign of cold intolerance is observed.

6. Answer: 2   Resource: Ratliffe (p. 37)
   A child that is seven months old is not usually able to crawl in a forward direction. Dissociation of the lower extremities occurs in the eighth or ninth month.

7. Answer: 4   Resource: Kisner (p. 301)
   High speed isokinetic exercises are considered extremely aggressive and would not be appropriate for a patient three weeks status post shoulder dislocation.

8. Answer: 4   Resource: Somers (p. 90)
   The area of the sacrum, which lies between the two innominate bones, is the most susceptible to skin breakdown with prolonged positioning in supine.

9. Answer: 2   Resource: Scott-Professional Ethics (p. 71)
   A physical therapist should attempt to secure an updated physician referral prior to administering formal treatment. Contacting the physicians office by telephone provides the fastest, most direct method to update the referral without further delaying treatment.

10. Answer: 3   Resource: Umphred (p. 879)
    Peripheral neuropathy is a broad term that describes a lesion to a peripheral nerve. The condition can be caused by a multitude of factors including diabetes, compression, trauma or nutritional deficiencies. Patients with peripheral neuropathy may exhibit motor, sensory, and autonomic changes including extreme sensitivity to touch, loss of sensation, muscle weakness, and loss of vasomotor tone. Deep tendon reflexes may be asymmetrical based on the location of the involved peripheral nerve and usually present as diminished or absent.

11. Answer: 4   Resource: Kisner (p. 89)
    The ten repetition maximum is equal to the maximum load a patient can lift ten times. The ten repetition maximum is used to determine the amount of weight used during each set of an exercise session using the DeLorme technique.

12. Answer: 1   Resource: Hertling (p. 535)
    Positioning the neck in extension and extremes of rotation places the vertebral artery in a compromised position. Extension, sidebending, and rotation are components of the vertebral artery test.

13. Answer: 2   Resource: Hertling (p. 722)
    The supplied description is the classic method for testing the length of the rectus femoris. Tightness of the rectus femoris is noted by failure to maintain a position of 90 degrees of knee flexion in the test leg.

14. Answer: 4   Resource: Kisner (p. 243)
    The patient's current functional level combined with his impending business trip makes daily physical therapy sessions the most appropriate option. Failure to make significant improvements in the patient's functional status will likely make the business trip unrealistic.

15. Answer: 3   Resource: Stokes (p. 61)
    Bradykinesia refers to an extreme slowness of movement. The finding is most common in patients with Parkinson's disease when initiating movement.

16. Answer: 3   Resource: Michlovitz (p. 198)
A number of factors play a significant role in determining the amount of heat absorbed using ultrasound, however the choice of coupling agent has a relatively small impact when compared to the other presented options.

17. Answer: 3   Resource: Goodman (p. 38)
Encouraging a patient to discuss irrelevant information typically results in inefficient use of available time.

18. Answer: 3   Resource: Saunders, D. (p. 93)
Facet impingement often results in a patient being locked in a selected position. In the thoracic and lumbar spine the position involves side bending and rotation occurring in opposite directions. The patient will experience the greatest discomfort and restriction of movement when moving away from the locked position.

19. Answer: 2   Resource: Hertling (p. 292)
A drop in the pelvis on the left during right stance phase is often indicative of right gluteus medius weakness. This type of deviation is termed a Trendelenburg gait pattern.

20. Answer: 1   Resource: O'Sullivan - Physical Rehabilitation (p. 162)
Athetosis is a term used to describe slow, writhing, and involuntary movements that may occur with damage to the basal ganglia.

21. Answer: 3   Resource: O'Sullivan - Physical Rehabilitation (p. 185)
Superficial reflexes are tested with some form of noxious stimuli. An example of this is the method of testing for the Babinski reflex.

22. Answer: 3   Resource: Tierney (p. 879)
A cervical rib that arises from the seventh cervical vertebra often compresses the inferior trunk of the brachial plexus and the subclavian artery. Adson's test may be useful in confirming the diagnosis of cervical rib syndrome. Additional findings include weakness and atrophy of intrinsic hand muscles and sensory alterations in the hand and forearm.

23. Answer: 1   Resource: Umphred (p. 745)
The cerebellum is the area of the brain that is associated with balance and coordination. Damage to the cerebellum often yields balance deficits and ataxia.

24. Answer: 4   Resource: O'Sullivan - Physical Rehabilitation (p. 532)
Raimiste's phenomenon is an associated reaction that is considered a form of overflow or irradiation.

25. Answer: 2   Resource: Guide for Professional Conduct
The Guide for Professional Conduct states that physical therapists seek remuneration for their services that is deserved and reasonable. Despite the fact the presented information indicates the physician may be inappropriate with his/her referrals, the most appropriate immediate response should be to discuss the situation directly with the physician.

26. Answer: 1   Resource: Ratliffe (p. 46)
Infants develop the stability necessary to sit with hand support for extended periods of time in the sixth or seventh month.

27. Answer: 2   Resource: Pierson (p. 233)
The uninvolved extremity leads when ascending stairs and the involved extremity leads when descending.

28. Answer: 4   Resource: Goodman (p. 438)
Trochanteric bursitis refers to inflammation of the trochanteric bursa, which is a pad-like sac that protects the soft tissue structures that cross the posterior portion of the greater trochanter. The condition can be differentiated from piriformis syndrome due to the lateral thigh pain and absence of radiating pain down the leg.

29. Answer: 4   Resource: Pierson (p. 328)
A patient with orthostatic hypotension would benefit from using the tilt table in order to slowly progress toward a standing position. Vital signs should be monitored during treatment.

30. Answer: 2   Resource: Magee (p. 560)
Apley's test is designed to detect the presence of a meniscal injury. The test is performed with the patient in a prone position with the knee flexed to 90 degrees.

31. Answer: 2   Resource: O'Sullivan - Physical Rehabilitation (p. 139)
Mechanoreceptors generate information related to discriminative sensations. The information is then mediated through the dorsal column-medial lemniscal system. Examples of mechanoreceptors include free nerve endings, Merkel's disks, Ruffini endings, and Pacinian corpuscles.

32. Answer: 2   Resource: Kozier (p. 487)
Normal blood pressure for a two-year-old ranges from 80-90 mm Hg systolic and 55-65 mm Hg diastolic.

33. Answer: 3   Resource: Rothstein (p. 450)
A patient classified as level IV, confused-agitated is likely to exhibit nonpurposeful speech, poor attention, diminished recall, and irritable behavior.

34. Answer: 2 Resource: Hertling (p. 287)
Patients with an anteverted hip typically present with excessive medial rotation and limited lateral rotation. The mean angle of anteversion in an adult is 8-15 degrees.

35. Answer: 1 Resource: National Safety Council (p. 25)
Securing and maintaining an airway is a necessary and immediate step when performing basic life support.

36. Answer: 3 Resource: Paz (p. 524)
Pertussis or whooping cough is an acute bacterial infection of the tracheobronchial tree. Pertussis often requires respiratory isolation since the disease is transmitted through airborne particles.

37. Answer: 1 Resource: Guide to Physical Therapist Practice (p. S42)
Modification of an established treatment plan or the associated goals is the responsibility of the physical therapist.

38. Answer: 2 Resource: Magee (p. 633)
The anterior talofibular ligament runs from the anterior portion of the lateral malleolus to the lateral aspect of the talar neck. The ligament is placed under stress with inversion and plantar flexion. The anterior talofibular, calcaneofibular, and posterior talofibular ligament make up the lateral collateral ligaments of the ankle complex.

39. Answer: 1 Resource: Saunders, R. (p. 34)
Symptom magnification is best identified by inconsistencies in the presentation of function. Although the physical therapist has identified a given inconsistency, it would be inappropriate to immediately confront the patient. The therapist would be better served by continuing the examination and gathering additional information during future treatment sessions.

40. Answer: 4 Resource: Hertling (p. 304)
Capsular patterns of restriction result from loss of mobility of the entire joint capsule. In trochanteric bursitis, passive and active range of motion are typically preserved, although there is often pain at end range with selected motions such as abduction.

41. Answer: 4 Resource: Kisner (p. 298)
Postoperative care of a rotator cuff repair often includes immobilization in abduction and medial rotation using an abduction splint. Lateral rotation is often restricted during the initial stages of rehabilitation since the position tends to place the repaired structures on stretch.

42. Answer: 4 Resource: Kisner (p. 225)
The tibiofemoral articulation consists of a concave tibial plateau articulating with the convex femoral condyles. An anterior glide of the tibia on the femur is indicated to increase knee extension.

43. Answer: 3 Resource: Magee (p. 193)
The infraspinatus is a lateral rotator of the shoulder and is innervated by the suprascapular nerve.

44. Answer: 3 Resource: Guyton (p. 336)
Mild-moderate exercise causes a significant increase in the blood flow to active muscles and the coronary system. Cardiac output can increase by up to five times the normal rate during strenuous exercise.

45. Answer: 1 Resource: Somers (p. 89)
A patient with C7 tetraplegia will not be able to independently perform activities of daily living secondary to inadequate hamstrings length. A patient requires between 110-120 degrees of straight leg raise in order to reach forward and don clothing.

46. Answer: 4 Resource: Ciccone (p. 15)
A drug that enters the body through the alimentary canal is defined as enteral administration. Taking medication orally is termed enteral administration.

47. Answer: 2 Resource: O'Sullivan - Physical Rehabilitation (p. 413)
Approximation is a therapeutic exercise technique designed to facilitate contraction and stability through joint compression.

48. Answer: 4 Resource: Kendall (p. 154)
The supplied description is a standard method to assess the strength of the lower abdominal muscles. Failure to maintain the low back flat on the treatment table as the legs are lowered is indicative of muscle weakness.

49. Answer: 3 Resource: Stokes (p. 41)
Nerve conduction velocity is often used to diagnose entrapment syndromes such as carpal tunnel syndrome. The diagnostic test measures conduction velocity along the sensory or motor component of a peripheral nerve. The conduction velocity is calculated by determining the amount of time for the action potential to move along a defined segment of the nerve.

50. Answer: 4 Resource: O'Sullivan - Physical Rehabilitation (p. 666)
A short prosthesis would have more than adequate clearance to advance the limb during swing phase without abducting.

51. Answer: 2 Resource: Adkins (p. 182)
A patient with C4 tetraplegia is appropriate for a reclining wheelchair with chin controls since the neck muscles are innervated. Back and seat cushions are necessary due to paralysis and inability to perform pressure relief.

52. Answer: 3 Resource: Somers (p. 82)
The triceps muscle is innervated by the radial nerve (C7-C8).

53. Answer: 4 Resource: Magee (p. 90)
The Rinne test is performed by placing the stem of the tuning fork on the mastoid process. The test is designed to compare bone conduction hearing with air conduction hearing.

54. Answer: 4 Resource: Guide to Physical Therapist Practice (p. S42)
Physical therapist assistants routinely complete progress notes in the medical record. Specific types of documentation such as an initial examination or a discharge summary are the responsibility of the physical therapist.

55. Answer: 1 Resource: Richard (p. 39)
Hematocrit is the volume percentage of red blood cells in whole blood. The hematocrit rises immediately after a severe burn and gradually decreases with fluid replacement.

56. Answer: 3 Resource: Paz (p. 375)
Pulmonary embolism is the primary complication of a deep vein thrombosis, as a result physical therapy intervention is not indicated.

57. Answer: 3 Resource: Knight (p. 2)
Health maintenance organizations offer health coverage to participants in exchange for a fixed, prepaid premium.

58. Answer: 3 Resource: O'Sullivan - Physical Rehabilitation (p. 559)
A patient with right hemiplegia can compensate for weak hip abductors while side stepping towards the right by leaning towards the left. This action unweights the right lower extremity and utilizes momentum along with the abductor muscles to perform sidestepping.

59. Answer: 1 Resource: Rothstein (p. 535)
The supplied description is the classic position for the anterior segments of the upper lobes.

60. Answer: 1 Resource: Magee (p. 1)
It is essential to complete a physical examination prior to initiating diagnostic imaging or any other form of direct intervention.

61. Answer: 4 Resource: Arnheim (p. 272)
An open basketweave taping technique provides room for edema while allowing ankle motion in the sagittal plane. The technique is often utilized immediately after an acute ankle sprain in combination with cryotherapy and elevation.

62. Answer: 1 Resource: Standards of Practice
The physical therapist should utilize the remaining time to begin the examination. Although the patient may benefit from a home exercise program, it would be inappropriate to design a home exercise program without first completing a thorough examination.

63. Answer: 1 Resource: O'Sullivan - Physical Rehabilitation (p. 1029)
A patient that presents with genu recurvatum while ambulating would benefit from increasing the plantar flexion stop of the ankle-foot orthosis. This would serve to prevent plantar flexion after heel strike and subsequently inhibit full extension of the knee during mid-stance.

64. Answer: 4 Resource: Richard (p. 486)
Operant conditioning is learning that takes place when the learner recognizes the connection between the behavior (completing an exercise progression) and its consequences (lengthy rest period).

65. Answer: 1 Resource: Ratliffe (p. 25)
Asymmetrical tonic neck reflex interferes with rolling due to the tonal influence of flexion to one side of the body and concurrent extension to the other.

66. Answer: 4 Resource: Umphred (p. 551)
The primary use of a sling in the treatment of hemiplegia is to hold the humerus and scapula in proper alignment during functional activities. Prolonged use of a sling can increase the incidence of contracture and flexor synergy in the upper extremity.

67. Answer: 2 Resource: Miller (p. 1843)
Normal hemoglobin values for a male range from 14-18 gm/dL.

68. Answer: 3 Resource: Frownfelter (p. 394)
The initial patient position should allow the patient to become familiar with his/her breathing pattern in a relaxed and comfortable position. Typically the most utilized teaching sequence is supine, sitting, standing, and walking.

69. Answer: 2 Resource: Kisner (p. 257)
Grade III and IV mobilization techniques are utilized primarily for stretching. Since patients with rheumatoid arthritis often present with inflammation, any joint mobilization technique must be utilized with great caution. Grade I and II mobilization techniques are often used to treat painful joints.

70. Answer: 4 Resource: Somers (p. 24)
Brown-Sequard's syndrome is a spinal cord injury due to a partial or full hemisection of the cord. The syndrome is frequently observed in stab wound victims.

71. Answer: 1   Resource: Michlovitz (p. 116)
Hot packs transfer heat to the body through conduction. Direct contact of the higher temperature hot packs result in heat being transferred to the cooler skin.

72. Answer: 1   Resource: Bennett (p. 20)
The corticospinal tract carries information from the cerebral cortex to the spinal nerves. The tract's projections are primarily contralateral and have a strong influence on spinal motor neurons which innervate distal muscles.

73. Answer: 4   Resource: Kendall (p. 198)
The peroneus tertius acts to dorsiflex the ankle joint and evert the foot. As a result, resistance should be applied against the lateral side of the dorsal surface of the foot in the direction of plantar flexion and inversion. The deep peroneal nerve innervates the peroneus tertius.

74. Answer: 4   Resource: Frownfelter (p. 517)
Emphysema is a disease of the alveoli with associated irreversible lung damage. Breathing exercises directed at increasing the activity of the diaphragm and decreasing the activity of the accessory muscles may influence the efficiency of the patient's breathing pattern.

75. Answer: 1   Resource: O'Sullivan - Physical Rehabilitation (p. 632)
Prone lying is an important positioning technique that stretches the hip flexors. Prone lying is essential to prevent hip flexion contractures in patients with transfemoral amputations.

76. Answer: 4   Resource: O'Sullivan - Physical Rehabilitation (p. 665)
When the socket of a transtibial prosthesis is aligned in excessive flexion it may cause exaggerated knee flexion during stance phase resulting in instability.

77. Answer: 2   Resource: Sullivan - An Integrated Approach (p. 130)
Repeated contractions is a technique that focuses on movement on one side of the joint. The technique is facilitated by quick stretch and utilizes an isotonic contraction. Providing resistance at the point of weakness can enhance repeated contractions.

78. Answer: 4   Resource: Rothstein (p. 838)
A prosthesis with insufficient length would not be responsible for excessive lateral rotation of the prosthesis upon heel strike. The deviation may be caused by weak hip medial rotators, poor suspension of the prosthesis or excessive toe-out of the prosthesis.

79. Answer: 3   Resource: Kisner (p. 600)
Cardiac output increases 30-60% and oxygen consumption increases 15-20% during pregnancy.

80. Answer: 3   Resource: Kendall (p. 15)
Shoulder medial and lateral rotation occur in a transverse plane around a longitudinal axis.

81. Answer: 1   Resource: Magee (p. 483)
A positive Ober test is indicative of a contracture of the iliotibial band or tensor fasciae latae.

82. Answer: 1   Resource: National Safety Council (p. 115)
An insulin reaction is often associated with hypoglycemia or low blood sugar. Treatment for hypoglycemia includes the administration of food or drink containing sugar.

83. Answer: 4   Resource: Kendall (p. 281)
The teres minor acts to laterally rotate the shoulder and stabilize the humeral head during shoulder movement. The axillary nerve innervates the teres minor.

84. Answer: 1   Resource: Pierson (p. 190)
The pulse of the brachial artery can be felt directly medial to the biceps tendon or along the medial aspect of the arm midway between the shoulder and elbow.

85. Answer: 2   Resource: Brotzman (p. 58)
Surgical repair of the ulnar collateral ligament of the thumb requires a pin to be inserted into the metacarpophalangeal joint of the thumb. The pin may remain in place for 3-6 weeks followed by the application of a wrist and thumb splint. Progressive strengthening typically commences at eight weeks and a return to unrestricted activity may occur at approximately 12 weeks.

86. Answer: 1   Resource: Kendall (p. 204)
The soleus acts to plantar flex the ankle joint, while the gastrocnemius plantar flexes the ankle and assists in flexing the knee. An inability to dorsiflex the ankle during mid-swing may be indicative of weakness of the tibialis anterior.

87. Answer: 3   Resource: Richard (p. 426)
Ultrasound using the underwater technique eliminates the need for contact between the sound head and the area being sonated.

88. Answer: 1   Resource: Kendall (p. 206)
By flexing the knee, the two joint gastrocnemius muscle is placed on slack. Since active ankle dorsiflexion is normal when the knee is flexed and is limited when the knee is extended, the gastrocnemius is likely responsible for the limitation.

89. Answer: 1   Resource: Paz (p. 597)
Supplemental oxygen is often warranted when the partial pressure of arterial oxygen is less than 60 mm Hg or when arterial saturation is below 90%. A partial pressure of arterial oxygen of 70 mm Hg corresponds to arterial saturation of 92-93%. Normal pH is 7.35-7.45.

90. Answer: 1   Resource: Somers (p. 88)
A patient with C6 tetraplegia relies on grasp through tenodesis. The grasp occurs through tension of the finger flexors when the wrist is extended. Tenodesis cannot occur if the finger flexors are stretched or lengthened.

91. Answer: 1   Resource: Hoppenfeld (p. 41)
The lateral epicondyle serves as the common origin for the wrist extensors. The wrist extensors include extensor carpi radialis longus, extensor carpi radialis brevis, and extensor digitorum.

92. Answer: 1   Resource: Pierson (p. 329)
Direct pressure is an appropriate first aid technique to control bleeding from a laceration.

93. Answer: 1   Resource: Norkin (p. 128)
The stationary arm of the goniometer should be positioned along a line extending from one anterior superior iliac spine to the other.

94. Answer: 3   Resource: Kendall (p. 208)
The medial and lateral hamstrings originate on the ischial tuberosity. Forceful hip flexion and knee extension places significant stress on the ischial tuberosity and can result in an avulsion fracture.

95. Answer: 2   Resource: Umphred (p. 724)
A patient status post cerebellar CVA often presents with an ataxic gait pattern.

96. Answer: 4   Resource: Magee (p. 12)
Resisted isometrics are strong, static isometric contractions that are performed in a neutral position. Resistive isometrics are designed to assess the integrity of a selected muscle or group of muscles.

97. Answer: 1   Resource: Kisner (p. 602)
Pregnancy does not have a significant effect on cervical lordosis.

98. Answer: 3   Resource: Norkin (p. 26)
Since the "15" is to the left of the "0", it is indicative of hyperextension. Therefore total available range of motion is determined as follows: 15 + 150 = 165.

99. Answer: 2   Resource: Norkin (p. 142)
The end-feel associated with knee flexion is typically described as soft due to contact between the posterior calf and thigh or between the heel and buttocks.

100. Answer: 4   Resource: Best (p. 215)
The range is considered a measure of spread or dispersion and not a measure of central tendency.

101. Answer: 2   Resource: Scott - Promoting Legal Awareness (p. 104)
The presence of another staff member often serves as a form of risk management. The physical therapist should not proceed with treatment until he has provided a thorough explanation of the technique and has obtained patient consent.

102. Answer: 2   Resource: Magee (p. 570)
Apprehension tests are provocative tests that attempt to simulate the mechanism of injury associated with a selected injury. The primary indication for an apprehension test is to assist with diagnosis. Common apprehension tests include anterior shoulder dislocation and patellar dislocation.

103. Answer: 3   Resource: Thomas (p. 1931)
Tetraplegia is defined as significant weakness of all four extremities. Tetraplegia is synonymous with quadriplegia.

104. Answer: 2   Resource: Paz (p. 470)
Hepatitis refers to an inflammation of the liver most commonly caused by one of five hepatitis viruses. The primary clinical signs of hepatitis include jaundice, fever, malaise, and nausea.

105. Answer: 4   Resource: Brannon (p. 424)
The Trendelenburg position is described as a position in which the patient's head is lowered and the body and legs are positioned on an inclined plane. The position is often utilized to assist with the elimination of secretions.

106. Answer: 4   Resource: Walter (p. 27)
As the length of stay steadily declines in hospitals, outpatient services continue to experience rapid growth.

107. Answer: 4   Resource: Ciccone (p. 170)
Sedation can be a significant side effect of skeletal muscle relaxants that can interfere with participation in a formal exercise regimen. Antispasticity drugs, which are a type of skeletal muscle relaxant, can result in decreased muscle tone and general muscle weakness.

108. Answer: 3   Resource: Clinical Companion (p. 145)
Anticoagulant drugs are often prescribed postoperatively for patients at risk of acquiring venous thrombosis. Prothrombin time is often used as a screening procedure to examine extrinsic coagulation factors and to determine the effectiveness of oral anticoagulant therapy.

109. Answer: 1   Resource: Thomas (p. 1368)
Osteoporosis is a metabolic bone disease characterized by increased bone resorption resulting in a reduction in bone mass. Osteoporosis is more prevalent in females than in males, in older more than younger individuals, and in whites more than in blacks.

110. Answer: 3 Resource: Minor (p. 420)
Using the cane in the left hand will allow the patient to shift her center of gravity away from the involved lower extremity and therefore reduce the pressure on the injured ankle.

111. Answer: 4 Resource: Magee (p. 43)
Computed tomography produces cross sectional images based on x-ray attenuation. Since vertebrae are made of bone and are extremely dense, they appear to be white. Soft tissue structures appear in various shades of gray, while cerebrospinal fluid is black.

112. Answer: 3 Resource: Magee (p. 539)
Performing ligamentous testing on an uninvolved joint provides a physical therapist with a valuable baseline that can then be compared to the involved joint.

113. Answer: 2 Resource: Magee (p. 635)
The talar tilt test can be used to identify the presence of a calcaneofibular ligament sprain.

114. Answer: 3 Resource: DePoy (p. 171)
A systematic sample is often used in place of a random sample when a population can be accurately listed or is finite. Members of the sample are automatically selected once the first subject has been chosen.

115. Answer: 4 Resource: Ignatavicius (p. 595)
Strict isolation always requires the use of a mask, gown, and gloves.

116. Answer: 2 Resource: Hoppenfeld (p. 68)
The lunate lies in the proximal row immediately distal to Lister's tubercle and proximal to the capitate. Wrist flexion acts to facilitate palpation of the lunate.

117. Answer: 2 Resource: Bennett (p. 33)
A lesion affecting the sensory cortex often results in numerous impairments including loss of sensation, perception, proprioception, and diminished motor control.

118. Answer: 2 Resource: Anderson (p. 769)
A Holter monitor is a portable unit that records electrocardiograph recordings during activities of daily living.

119. Answer: 4 Resource: Currier (p. 100)
In a normal distribution a known percentage of the population falls between specific standard deviation units. In the supplied example 50% of the population will fall above the mean and 34% of the population will fall between the mean and one standard deviation below the mean. Therefore, 50% + 34% = 84% of the population.

120. Answer: 4 Resource: Rothstein (p. 534)
The supplied description accurately describes the position and technique associated with bronchial drainage to the superior segments of the lower lobes.

121. Answer: 4 Resource: Pauls (p. 440)
Cystic fibrosis is an inherited disease affecting the exocrine glands. The disease is characterized by hypertrophy of goblet cells resulting in excessive airway secretions.

122. Answer: 4 Resource: Hall (p. 365)
Patients with very weak pelvic floor muscles should initiate strengthening exercises in a horizontal plane in order to avoid gravity exerting a downward force on the pelvic floor. Although sidelying would be an acceptable position, it is more awkward than the supine position for most patients. Patients should move to more challenging positions as their strength increases.

123. Answer: 3 Resource: Clinical Companion (p. 105)
The Berg Functional Balance Scale is used for assessing a patient's risk of falling. The Berg consists of 14 tasks of every day life that are scored according to a 0-4 scale. The maximum total score possible is 56, with a score of less than 45 indicating the patient is at risk for multiple falls. Necessary equipment to administer the Berg includes a stopwatch, two chairs, a ruler, and a step stool. Observation and scoring should take approximately 15-20 minutes.

124. Answer: 3 Resource: Ratliffe (p. 242)
Duchenne muscular dystrophy is a sex-linked disorder characterized by progressive muscular weakness beginning between the ages of two and five. Individuals typically lose the ability to ambulate and are dependent on a wheelchair by age 16. The majority of patients with Duchenne muscular dystrophy die by the end of their teenage years due to respiratory or cardiac failure. The described method of standing upright is termed Gowers' sign.

125. Answer: 2 Resource: Irwin (p. 336)
Tachypnea refers to a respiratory rate of greater than 20 breaths per minute.

126. Answer: 4 Resource: Brannon (p. 209)
Ventricular tachycardia is defined as three consecutive ventricular complexes with a rate of 150 –200 beats per minute. Sustained ventricular tachycardia can be life threatening due to inadequate cardiac output.

127. Answer: 1 Resource: Ciccone (p. 26)
The primary site for drug storage within the body is adipose tissue. Drugs that are fat soluble and are stored within adipose tissue can remain there for long periods of time due to diminished blood flow and reduced metabolic rate.

128. Answer: 3 Resource: Michlovitz (p. 204)
Shoulder abduction and medial rotation exposes the supraspinatus tendon from under the acromion process.

129. Answer: 3 Resource: Purtillo - Health Professional (p. 41)
The patient's inability to communicate using the English language necessitates the use of an interpreter.

130. Answer: 1 Resource: Clinical Companion (p. 147)
Expiratory reserve volume is defined as the maximal amount of air that can be expired after a normal exhalation. As a result, the measure can be obtained with relative ease using a spirometer.

131. Answer: 3 Resource: Clinical Companion (p. 315)
Reminding the patient of the donning instructions for the orthosis provides the patient with the best opportunity to learn the correct technique. Although reapplying the orthosis correctly at the conclusion of the treatment session is appropriate, the action does not provide any specific feedback to the patient.

132. Answer: 4 Resource: Cameron (p. 354)
The closer together electrodes are in a circuit the more superficial the flow of current and conversely the further apart electrodes are the deeper the flow of current.

133. Answer: 1 Resource: Norkin (p. 26)
If the total available knee range of motion is 65 degrees and the patient has 5 degrees of hyperextension, the patient must have 60 degrees of knee flexion. Therefore the patient's range of motion should be recorded as 5 - 0 - 60 degrees of right knee active range of motion.

134. Answer: 4 Resource: Standards of Practice
Physical therapists have an obligation to discharge patients from physical therapy services when the goals and projected outcomes have been attained.

135. Answer: 3 Resource: Kettenbach (p. 110)
The assessment section of a S.O.A.P. note includes the problem list, short-term goals, and long-term goals. The assessment section allows a physical therapist to express his/her professional judgment on a variety of issues related to patient care.

136. Answer: 3 Resource: Hoppenfeld (p. 65)
The distal row of carpal bones consists of the trapezium, trapezoid, capitate, and hamate.

137. Answer: 4 Resource: Brannon (p. 183)
ST segment depression of greater than 1 mm is indicative of ischemia and is often used to confirm the diagnosis of coronary artery disease.

138. Answer: 3 Resource: Sultz (p. 242)
Medicaid is the largest insurer of long-term care in the United States covering over two-thirds of nursing home residents.

139. Answer: 3 Resource: Pierson (p. 189)
Training the patient in a specific gait pattern is one of the final components of an ambulation program. Development of standing balance and weight shifting are prerequisite activities that should be addressed prior to ambulation.

140. Answer: 2 Resource: Mahler (p. 65)
The purpose of submaximal exercise testing is to determine the relationship between heart rate and oxygen uptake in order to predict maximum oxygen uptake. In order to do this it is necessary to determine the relationship between heart rate and oxygen uptake at two or more different submaximal exercise intensities.

141. Answer: 3 Resource: Pierson (p. 266)
A physical therapist should notify nursing immediately and avoid any attempt to reconnect the I.V.

142. Answer: 1 Resource: Boissonnault (p. 336)
Digitalis is utilized in the treatment of congestive heart failure. Digitalis works directly on electrolytes to improve the force and contractility of the heart.

143. Answer: 4 Resource: Anderson (p. 804)
Hypoxemia refers to a deficiency of oxygen in arterial blood.

144. Answer: 4 Resource: Thomas (p. 629)
Emphysema is an obstructive pulmonary disease characterized by overinflation and destructive changes in alveolar walls. Although closely related to other obstructive pulmonary diseases, the presence of a barrel chest is most characteristic of emphysema.

145. Answer: 1 Resource: Kendall (p. 282)
Scapular adductors including the rhomboids, middle trapezius, and the lower trapezius are tested with the patient in a prone position.

146. Answer: 1 Resource: Pierson (p. 13)
In order to provide maximum benefit a home exercise program must be designed to meet the individual needs of each patient.

147. Answer: 1   Resource: Clinical Companion (p. 324)
A one-arm drive wheelchair has two handrims attached to the same wheel. The far rear wheel is propelled by the outer handrim, while the near rear wheel is propelled by the inner handrim. Strength and coordination are required to grasp the handrims and simultaneously propel the wheelchair forward.

148. Answer: 1   Resource: Frownfelter (p. 150)
Tidal volume is defined as the amount of air inspired and expired per breath and is approximately 450-600 mL in an adult. This value represents approximately 10% of the total lung capacity.

149. Answer: 3   Resource: Brotzman (p. 94)
Athletes performing repetitive overhead activities are often subject to adaptive changes such as acquired anterior laxity, and a loss of flexibility in the posterior capsule and posterior muscles.

150. Answer: 1   Resource: Somers (p. 46)
The most immediate response in treating autonomic dysreflexia is to support the patient in a sitting position in an attempt to lower blood pressure. The patient's bowel and bladder should be assessed and vital signs should be monitored.

151. Answer: 2   Resource: Mahler (p. 59)
A desirable range for men and women according to the Body Mass Index scale is 20 – 24.9 kg/m^2.

152. Answer: 2   Resource: Brotzman (p. 185)
The semitendinosus and gracilis are acceptable grafts for anterior cruciate ligament reconstruction surgery. The grafts result in a decreased incidence of postoperative patellofemoral knee pain, however provide weaker initial fixation.

153. Answer: 3   Resource: Brotzman (p. 265)
Interval training requires participants to vary the rate and intensity of their training program. Since eccentric contraction of the gastrocnemius and soleus complex places the most stress on the Achilles tendon, this type of activity is not recommended during the early stages of a rehabilitation program.

154. Answer: 3   Resource: Lewis (p. 169)
Increased hip flexion is a postural change associated with aging.

155. Answer: 2   Resource: Adkins (p. 184)
The appropriate wheelchair for a patient with C5 tetraplegia is a manual chair with handrim projections. The projections should be angled at 30 degrees during the training period to assist with propulsion.

156. Answer: 2   Resource: Hamilton (p. 224)
Vitamin A is a fat soluble vitamin essential for functions such as bone growth, maintenance of body linings, and vision. Vitamin A is found in animal products such as butter, milk, liver, egg yolks, and in dark green, deep orange, and yellow vegetables.

157. Answer: 2   Resource: Anderson (p. 1666)
Military time operates on the premise that 2400 hours is equivalent to 12:00 AM and 1200 hours is equivalent to 12:00 PM. 8:00 AM or 0800 is nine hours after 11:00 PM or 2300 hours.

158. Answer: 1   Resource: Pierson (p. 203)
A three-point gait pattern with axillary crutches allows the patient to move in an efficient manner while maintaining the prescribed non-weight bearing status.

159. Answer: 2   Resource: Rothstein (p. 621)
The aortic valve is located at the junction of the left ventricle and the ascending aorta. The aortic valve prevents regurgitation at the entrance of the aorta to the heart.

160. Answer: 1   Resource: Payton - Research (p. 11)
Independent variables are the conditions or characteristics that are manipulated to determine the effect on the dependent variable. In the supplied example, the exercise program is the independent variable.

161. Answer: 2   Resource: Brannon (p. 48)
Residual volume is defined as the amount of gas in the lungs at the end of maximal expiration. Normal residual volume for a male is approximately 1500 ml, while total lung capacity is 6000 ml. Total lung capacity is equal to the sum of tidal volume, inspiratory reserve volume, expiratory reserve volume, and residual volume.

162. Answer: 1   Resource: Rothstein (p. 535)
To perform bronchial drainage to the anterior segments of the upper lobes the physical therapist should clap between the clavicle and nipple on each side with the patient positioned in supine.

163. Answer: 2   Resource: Rothstein (p. 664)
Energy expenditure expressed in the form of calories can be estimated using weight and oxygen consumption.

164. Answer: 4   Resource: Rothstein (p. 632)
Selected enzymes are released into the blood in a predictable fashion following myocardial infarction. These enzymes can be used to confirm the diagnosis of acute myocardial infarction. The most common enzymes analyzed after myocardial infarction include aspartate aminotransferase, creatine phosphokinase, and lactate dehydrogenase.

165. Answer: 3   Resource: O'Sullivan - Physical Rehabilitation (p. 183)
The Babinski reflex is tested by stroking the lateral sole of the foot from the heel to the ball of the foot with the pointed end of a reflex hammer. Although it is possible to elicit the reflex with the finger it is more appropriate to use a piece of equipment. A positive Babinski reflex is indicated by splaying of the toes and extension of the hallux. The reflex is normal in infants under the age of six months, however in an older population it may serve as an indication of a lesion in the corticospinal tract.

166. Answer: 1   Resource: Brotzman (p. 354)
Forefoot varus refers to an inverted position of the forefoot in relationship to the rearfoot with the subtalar joint in a neutral position.

167. Answer: 1   Resource: Richard (p. 138)
The correct sequence is as follows: removal of current dressings, gentle debridement in a hydrotherapy tank, reapplication of the topical antibiotic, application of gauze wraps in a distal to proximal pattern.

168. Answer: 3   Resource: Pierson (p. 202)
A four-point gait pattern is often prescribed for patients requiring significant stability. The gait pattern requires low energy expenditure, but is very slow.

169. Answer: 1   Resource: Campbell, M. (p. 210)
A patient with a traumatic brain injury that is disoriented will benefit from establishing contact with the physical therapist in familiar surroundings. Although the private treatment room would eliminate external stimuli, the patient is likely to be unfamiliar with the environment and therefore may become disoriented or agitated.

170. Answer: 4   Resource: White (p. 49)
When walking up hills it is advisable to shorten stride length and lean slightly forward to accommodate for the slope.

171. Answer: 3   Resource: Hoppenfeld (p. 122)
The triceps reflex (C7-C8) is best elicited with the patient sitting or standing with the arm supported by the physical therapist. The therapist passively moves the arm into a position of abduction and medial rotation with the elbow flexed to 90 degrees and strikes the triceps tendon with a reflex hammer where it crosses the olecranon fossa.

172. Answer: 3   Resource: Rothstein (p. 885)
Patients typically move through a predictable series of stages when experiencing dying. According to Elizabeth Kubler Ross theses stages include denial, anger, bargaining, depression, and acceptance.

173. Answer: 1   Resource: Boissonnault (p. 333)
Diuretics act to lower blood pressure by decreasing fluid levels in the vascular system, primarily through the excretion of urine.

174. Answer: 4   Resource: Pierson (p. 56)
Systolic pressure gradually increases as exercise intensity increases, however diastolic pressure remains relatively stable.

175. Answer: 4   Resource: Magee (p. 275)
The proximal row of carpals articulates with the radius at the radiocarpal joint and with the distal row of carpals at the midcarpal joints. The ulna does not form an articulation with the proximal row of carpals.

176. Answer: 1   Resource: Norkin (p. 108)
The stationary arm of the goniometer should be aligned with the lateral midline of the second metacarpal using the center of the second metacarpophalangeal joint for reference.

177. Answer: 4   Resource: Michlovitz (p. 204)
Failure to place a patient with muscle guarding and spasm in a comfortable position will only serve to exacerbate the patient's current condition.

178. Answer: 2   Resource: Levangie (p. 472)
When compared to the gait of an adult, toddlers tend to exhibit a wider base of support, decreased single leg support time, shorter step length, slower velocity, and higher cadence.

179. Answer: 4   Resource: Magee (p. 40)
Immediate medical management should focus on identifying potential complications such as a fracture. X-rays are a cost effective diagnostic tool commonly utilized with orthopedic injuries.

180. Answer: 1   Resource: Walter (p. 166)
Performance standards must be communicated openly to all employees on an ongoing basis. Introducing performance standards to an employee at a performance appraisal is unacceptable.

181. Answer: 3   Resource: Norkin (p. 58)
Failure to stabilize the scapula when measuring glenohumeral abduction will result in upward rotation and elevation of the scapula. When measuring shoulder complex abduction the thorax should be stabilized to prevent lateral flexion of the trunk.

182. Answer: 2   Resource: Norkin (p. 62)
The humeral head slides posteriorly on the glenoid fossa during shoulder complex medial rotation and as a result places pressure on the posterior capsule.

183. Answer: 2   Resource: Sullivan – Clinical Decision Making (p. 66)
Contract-relax is an active exercise technique designed to increase range of motion. As a result the presence of full range of motion would be an indication to discontinue treatment.

184. Answer: 1   Resource: Magee (p. 43)
A bone scan is a diagnostic test that utilizes radioactive isotopes to identify areas of bone that are hypervascular or have an increased rate of bone mineral turnover. Bone scans can demonstrate bone disease or stress fractures with as little as 4-7% bone loss.

185. Answer: 4   Resource: Kettenbach (p. 72)
The problem list typically provides a summary of the patient's physical therapy problems and forms the foundation for short and long-term goals. As a result the entry "increased stress secondary to financial problems" is not an appropriate entry in the problem list.

186. Answer: 1   Resource: Starkey (p. 229)
Piriformis syndrome is caused by hypertrophy or spasm of the piriformis muscle causing pressure on the sciatic nerve. Abduction and lateral rotation would likely be weak and painful since the motions serve as the prime function of the piriformis. The piriformis originates on the anterior surface of the sacrum and the sacrotuberous ligament and inserts on the greater trochanter of the femur. The muscle is innervated by sacral nerves I and II.

187. Answer: 3   Resource: Umphred (p. 90)
Pacinian corpuscles are encapsulated sensory nerve endings found in subcutaneous tissue. The receptors are stimulated by deep pressure, quick stretch to tissue, and vibration.

188. Answer: 2   Resource: Kendall (p. 282)
The dorsal scapular nerve innervates the levator scapulae and rhomboids. The levator scapulae function to elevate the scapula while the rhomboids adduct the scapula.

189. Answer: 4   Resource: Pierson (p. 71)
Active-assistive exercise is performed when the patient is able to produce some active movement, however relies on assistance from an external force.

190. Answer: 3   Resource: Kisner (p. 24)
Passive insufficiency occurs when a two joint muscle is stretched across two joints at the same time.

191. Answer: 2   Resource: Saunders, R. (p. 37)
Objective findings should not be withheld from documentation, however the physical therapist should avoid statements based purely on conjecture or speculation.

192. Answer: 2   Resource: Irwin (p. 535)
An infant's pulse is often assessed at the brachial artery, while the radial artery is utilized for an older child.

193. Answer: 2   Resource: Sullivan - An Integrated Approach (p. 135)
Rhythmic initiation is indicated when a patient has difficulty initiating movement. Rolling is usually one of the first tasks performed using this technique. Rhythmic initiation begins with passive range of motion and progresses to resisted movement as the patient acquires the skill.

194. Answer: 2   Resource: O'Sullivan - Laboratory Manual (p. 59)
Using the developmental sequence allows for treatment to focus on isometric control at each static position and isotonic control when moving from one position to the next.

195. Answer: 1   Resource: Reese (p. 476)
The trigeminal nerve innervates the primary muscles of mastication including the pterygoids. The pterygoids on one side function to open the jaw and cause the jaw to deviate to the opposite side. As a result, if the right pterygoids are weak the jaw will deviate to the right with opening.

196. Answer: 4   Resource: Magee (p. 694)
A patient with limited dorsiflexion may present with a vault or bounce through mid to late stance. Ten to twenty degrees of dorsiflexion is required for late stance through toe off.

197. Answer: 1   Resource: O'Sullivan - Physical Rehabilitation (p. 145)
Kinesthesia refers to the ability to perceive the extent or direction of movement. An appropriate patient response must include an indication of the direction of movement while the physical therapist actively moves the patient's extremity.

198. Answer: 1   Resource: Kisner (p. 292)
Rotator cuff tears typically occur in adults over the age of 40 as a result of repetitive microtears to the rotator cuff or long head of the biceps.

199. Answer: 3   Resource: Davies (p. 59)
A patient status post CVA should avoid prolonged supine positioning in bed. A supine position encourages abnormal reflexes including asymmetrical tonic neck reflex, symmetrical tonic neck reflex, and labyrinthine reflexes.

200. Answer: 2   Resource: O'Sullivan - Physical
                              Rehabilitation (p. 560)
A metal upright ankle-foot orthosis is able to accommodate fluctuating edema because the stirrups do not have total contact with the patient's lower extremity. The plastic ankle-foot orthosis is molded for total contact with the lower extremity.

Sample Examination: Four

1. A frequently administered treatment for cancer in which high doses of energy are administered to the body to stop cell replication is termed:

   1. immunotherapy
   2. radiation therapy
   3. chemotherapy
   4. surgical intervention

2. The intermittent use of tone reducing lower extremity bivalve casting for children with cerebral palsy hypothesizes that casting may:

   1. increase compensatory stabilizing efforts
   2. cause flexion of the toes which inhibits the plantar grasp response
   3. facilitate trunk stability by reducing contractures of the foot
   4. inhibit the use of extensor thrust by preventing plantar flexion

3. A physical therapist completes a manual muscle test where resistance is applied toward plantar flexion and eversion. This description best describes a manual muscle test of the:

   1. tibialis anterior
   2. tibialis posterior
   3. peroneus longus
   4. peroneus brevis

4. A physical therapist performs an examination on a 27-year-old male diagnosed with iliotibial band syndrome. The patient is an avid distance runner who routinely ran between 45-60 miles per week before experiencing pain in his knee. Standing posture reveals a varus position at the knee and a cavus foot. When palpating the lateral portion of the lower extremity, which area would you most likely identify marked tenderness?

   1. lateral femoral condyle
   2. lateral joint line
   3. lateral tibial condyle
   4. fibular head

5. A person with an anterior cruciate ligament insufficiency, who elects not to have surgical reconstruction, could probably expect to reach which minimal functional level?

   1. able to participate in all sports
   2. able to participate in light recreational sports
   3. cannot play any type of sport
   4. problems with normal walking

6. A 24-year-old soccer player is referred to physical therapy after being diagnosed with Achilles tendonitis. Which of the following actions would place the greatest stress on the Achilles tendon?

   1. concentric contraction of the gastrocnemius
   2. eccentric contraction of the gastrocnemius
   3. concentric contraction of the gastrocnemius and soleus complex
   4. eccentric contraction of the gastrocnemius and soleus complex

7. A physical therapist employed in a rehabilitation hospital discusses the merits of several different outcome assessment measures with a colleague. When discussing the Barthel Index, which of the following would be considered a valid limitation of the outcome measure?

   1. limited sensitivity for individuals with mild disabilities
   2. requires specialized equipment
   3. necessitates fasting for 12 hours
   4. may take 6-8 hours to administer

8. A physical therapist performs a manual muscle test on the primary hip abductor. The therapist should perform the test while palpating the:

   1. rectus femoris
   2. gluteus medius
   3. sartorius
   4. gluteus minimus

9. A physical therapist examines the forefoot position of a 36-year-old male referred to physical therapy with ankle pain of unknown etiology. After placing the foot in subtalar neutral the therapist determines that the patient has a forefoot varus. What compensatory finding is most likely at the rearfoot based on the alignment of the forefoot?

   1. subtalar eversion
   2. subtalar inversion
   3. talocrural dorsiflexion
   4. talocrural plantar flexion

10. A physical therapist designs an exercise program for a patient rehabilitating from a prolonged illness. Which of the following exercises is indicated for coordination training?

    1. Buerger-Allen exercises
    2. Codman's exercises
    3. DeLorme's exercises
    4. Frenkel's exercises

11. A 36-year-old female is limited to 30 degrees of lateral rotation at the right shoulder. Which shoulder mobilization technique would be the most appropriate to address the limitation?

    1. anterior glide of the humeral head
    2. posterior glide of the humeral head
    3. inferior glide of the humeral head
    4. superior glide of the humeral head

12. A physical therapist prepares a pair of orthoses for a patient referred to physical therapy with ankle pain. Results of a positional assessment of the foot reveal compensated forefoot varus. Which of the orthotic options would be the most appropriate to address this type of alignment?

    1. lateral forefoot posting
    2. medial forefoot posting
    3. lateral hindfoot posting
    4. medial hindfoot posting

13. Which progressive resistive exercise would function to strengthen the infraspinatus and teres minor?

    1. extension of the shoulder with dumbbell weights
    2. flexion of the shoulder with dumbbell weights
    3. lateral rotation of the shoulder with elastic tubing
    4. medial rotation of the shoulder with elastic tubing

14. A patient waiting for a scheduled therapy session in the gym suddenly begins to scream. The patient sustained a traumatic brain injury in a motor vehicle accident and is currently functioning at the confused-appropriate stage. The most appropriate therapist action is:

    1. ask the patient if he needs assistance
    2. seek assistance from other health care professionals
    3. request that the patient is transported back to his room
    4. contact a physician and request that the patient's medication dosage is increased

15. A physical therapist transfers a patient in a wheelchair down a curb with a forward approach. Which of the following actions would be the most appropriate?

    1. have the patient lean forward
    2. have the wheelchair brakes locked
    3. tilt the wheelchair backwards
    4. position yourself in front of the patient

16. A physical therapist positions a patient in supine in order to perform passive stretching of the rectus femoris on the right. In order to effectively stabilize the pelvis in a supine position, the therapist should:

    1. passively flex the right hip to the patient's chest
    2. passively flex the right hip and knee to the patient's chest
    3. passively flex the left hip to the patient's chest
    4. passively flex the left hip and knee to the patient's chest

17. A patient who is partial weight bearing on the left ambulates with a walker. The patient advances the walker followed by a step with the left and then a step with the right. This gait pattern is termed:

    1. two-point
    2. three-point
    3. four-point
    4. swing-to

18. A physical therapist observes the gait of a patient rehabilitating from a stroke. The patient was recently fitted with an ankle-foot orthosis that incorporates a posterior stop. The primary purpose of this type of device is to:

    1. limit dorsiflexion
    2. limit plantar flexion
    3. facilitate dorsiflexion
    4. facilitate plantar flexion

19. A physical therapist treats a patient with a fractured left hip. The patient is weight bearing as tolerated and uses a large base quad cane for gait activities. Correct use of the quad cane would include:

    1. using the quad cane on the left with the longer legs positioned away from the patient
    2. using the quad cane on the right with the longer legs positioned away from the patient
    3. using the quad cane on the left with the longer legs positioned toward the patient
    4. using the quad cane on the right with the longer legs positioned toward the patient

20. A therapist discusses postoperative instructions with a patient scheduled for total hip replacement surgery. Which of the following would be considered good advice to prevent subluxation or dislocation?

    1. use a raised toilet seat
    2. use an abduction pillow for one week postoperatively
    3. avoid sitting in high and hard chairs
    4. slowly bend forward when picking objects up from the floor

21. A 67-year-old patient is examined in physical therapy after having sutures removed following a transtibial amputation. The patient resides in a retirement community and describes herself as socially active. She is presently using a temporary prosthesis consisting of a plastic socket, a pylon, and a solid ankle cushion heel foot. When discussing a permanent prosthesis with the physical therapist the patient expresses concern that the device will look awful and will be obvious to everyone in her retirement community. Which type of prosthetic components would be the most appropriate for the patient?

    1. endoskeletal shank and single-axis articulated foot-ankle assembly
    2. endoskeletal shank and solid ankle cushion heel foot
    3. exoskeletal shank and single-axis articulated foot-ankle assembly
    4. exoskeletal shank and solid ankle cushion heel foot

22. A physical therapist treats a patient status post CVA. Which action would be most likely to facilitate elbow extension in a patient with hemiplegia?

    1. turn the head to the affected side
    2. turn the head to the unaffected side
    3. extend the lower extremities
    4. flex the lower extremities

23. Independent bed mobility is a realistic goal for a patient with C6 tetraplegia. In order to achieve this goal, a physical therapist should initiate strengthening to all of the following muscles except the:

    1. teres major
    2. flexor carpi ulnaris
    3. biceps brachii
    4. anterior deltoid

24. A physical therapist closely examines a small area of redness over the lateral portion of the lower leg of a patient diagnosed with peripheral neuropathy. The therapist is concerned that the skin irritation may have been caused by the leather calf band of the patient's metal upright ankle-foot orthosis. The most appropriate location for the calf band is:

    1. immediately inferior to the fibular head
    2. immediately superior to the fibular head
    3. immediately inferior to the tibial plateau
    4. immediately superior to the tibial plateau

25. A physical therapist examines a 16-year-old male diagnosed with left knee anterior cruciate ligament insufficiency. During the examination a Lachman test is performed. Ideally, the therapist should perform the test with the knee in:

    1. complete extension
    2. 20-30 degrees flexion
    3. 30-40 degrees flexion
    4. 40-50 degrees flexion

26. A physical therapist records a manual muscle test grade of poor for the right hip adductors. Which patient position would have been utilized to collect the data?

    1. supine
    2. prone
    3. right sidelying
    4. left sidelying

27. A physical therapist measures forearm supination range of motion on a patient rehabilitating from a radial head fracture. The patient is eager to show progress in therapy and as a result often attempts to substitute for his limited range of motion by manipulating his body. Which of the following motions would most often be used to substitute for a limitation in supination?

    1. shoulder abduction and lateral rotation
    2. shoulder abduction and medial rotation
    3. shoulder adduction and lateral rotation
    4. shoulder adduction and medial rotation

28. A patient with a full-thickness burn over the entire anterior aspect of the neck is examined in physical therapy. The physical therapist must plan a treatment program based on the anticipation of a possible contracture toward:

    1. flexion
    2. extension
    3. rotation with extension
    4. rotation with sidebending

29. A physical therapist examines a patient referred to physical therapy diagnosed with a lateral collateral ligament sprain. Which nerve can be palpated immediately inferior to the head of the fibula?

    1. common peroneal
    2. tibial
    3. sural
    4. lateral plantar

30. A physical therapist develops an aquatic therapy program for a patient diagnosed with a lower extremity injury. The therapist plans to monitor the patient's response to exercise using heart rate, however is concerned about the influence of the water on the patient's heart rate response. Which of the following best describes the effect of immersion in water on heart rate response when compared to traditional land activities?

    1. heart rate response is increased during low intensity exercise in water
    2. heart rate response is decreased during low intensity exercise in water
    3. heart rate response is increased during high intensity exercise in water
    4. heart rate response is decreased during high intensity exercise in water

31. A therapist recognizes that a child has great difficulty flexing the neck while in a supine position. Failure to integrate which reflex could explain the child's difficulty?

    1. tonic labyrinthine
    2. Moro
    3. asymmetrical tonic neck
    4. symmetrical tonic neck

32. A physical therapist completes a lower quarter screening examination on a 54-year-old male diagnosed with spinal stenosis. During the examination the therapist attempts to quantify hip flexion range of motion with the patient in supine and the knee in an extended position. What is the primary factor limiting range of motion in this position?

    1. active insufficiency of the hamstrings
    2. passive insufficiency of the hamstrings
    3. active insufficiency of the iliopsoas
    4. passive insufficiency of the iliopsoas

33. A patient with hemiplegia lying in supine demonstrates a synergistic pattern of movement when attempting to move his affected leg. The patient's hip is abducted and laterally rotated, knee flexed, ankle plantar flexed and inverted, toes flexed and adducted. This synergy pattern should be classified as:

    1. purely extension
    2. purely flexion
    3. a combination of flexion and extension synergy patterns
    4. isolated active movement

34. A physical therapist completes a postural examination on a patient with low back pain. Which structural deformity is often associated with weak abdominal muscles?

    1. increased lordosis
    2. decreased lordosis
    3. increased posterior pelvic tilt
    4. increased kyphosis

35. A 55-year-old patient, six months status post CVA and right hemiparesis, attends physical therapy on an outpatient basis. As the patient lies supine on the mat, the physical therapist applies resistance to right elbow flexion. The therapist notes mass flexion of the right lower extremity as the resistance is applied. The therapist should document this as:

    1. Raimiste's phenomenon
    2. Souque's phenomenon
    3. coordination synkinesis
    4. homolateral synkinesis

36. A patient with a grade II sprain of the acromioclavicular joint is referred to physical therapy. The patient sustained the injury after falling to the ground and landing on the shoulder in a lacrosse contest two weeks ago. When performing an examination on the patient, the first activity to occur would be:

    1. active movements
    2. passive movements
    3. resisted isometric movements
    4. special tests

37. A physical therapist completes a discharge summary on a patient following a six week hospital admission. A discharge summary is best described as:

    1. an explanation of the patient's condition at the time of discharge
    2. an overview of the patient's progress during therapy and his/her condition at discharge
    3. a document that indicates the reason for discharge and explains the patient's home program
    4. a record that indicates the frequency and number of appointments from the initial examination until discharge

38. An audit attempts to determine the quality of patient care through a review of patient records. All of the following are recommended to ensure that the results of an audit are accurate except:

    1. a comparison of the actual practice's level of care to the expected level of care
    2. specific objectives of the audit are defined prior to the collection of data
    3. an audit should not exceed a sample size of 15 to 20 charts
    4. the study should include records over a prolonged period to ensure a diverse sample

39. A physical therapist uses patient care gloves to prevent the transmission of infection. When is it appropriate to reuse patient care gloves?

    1. when the gloves are used to treat the same patient
    2. when the gloves are used by the same physical therapist
    3. when the gloves do not come in contact with any potentially infectious material
    4. gloves should not be reused

40. A patient with a transfemoral amputation begins gait training with a prosthesis. What effect will a hip flexion contracture have on the patient's gait?

    1. The patient will demonstrate increased stability in the prosthetic knee.
    2. The patient's step length on the prosthetic side will be increased.
    3. The hip flexion contracture will not affect the patient's gait pattern.
    4. The patient will not begin to ambulate until normal range of motion is restored.

41. A physical therapist examines a patient with a suspected acutely torn medial meniscus. Which symptom is not commonly associated with a medial meniscus tear?

    1. tenderness along the medial joint line
    2. moderate to severe pain
    3. joint locking
    4. hamstrings atrophy

42. A physical therapist uses infrared radiation as a form of superficial heat to treat a patient with arthritis. The therapist begins the treatment session with the infrared lamp 45 centimeters away from the target area. If the therapist later elects to move the lamp 90 centimeters away from the target area, what percentage of the original radiation intensity has been maintained?

    1. 25%
    2. 33%
    3. 50%
    4. 75%

43. A child with athetoid cerebral palsy is referred to physical therapy. Which of the following characteristics would a physical therapist typically identify when examining the child?

    1. continuous low tone and intermittent tonic spasms
    2. small range movements with full control within the range
    3. disorganized movement with fluctuating muscle tone
    4. little to no influence from tonic neck reflexes

44. A physical therapist treats a patient rehabilitating from a fracture at the distal end of the humerus. The therapist notes that the patient's elbow is grossly swollen. Which position of the elbow would best accommodate the increased fluid?

    1. full extension
    2. 15 degrees of flexion
    3. 70 degrees of flexion
    4. 120 degrees of flexion

45. A therapist discusses the importance of proper posture with a patient rehabilitating from back surgery. Which body position would place the most pressure on the lumbar spine?

    1. standing in the anatomical position
    2. standing with 45 degrees of hip flexion
    3. sitting in a chair
    4. sitting in a chair with reduced lumbar lordosis

46. A physical therapist reviews the medical record of a patient who sustained a brachial plexus injury. The record states that the medial cord of the brachial plexus was partially severed. Which nerve would you expect to be the most seriously affected by the injury?

    1. axillary
    2. median
    3. musculocutaneous
    4. medial pectoral

47. A patient begins to demonstrate signs and symptoms of a seizure including uncontrollable muscular movements, convulsions, and confused behavior. Appropriate intervention would include:

    1. attempt to check airway, breathing, and circulation
    2. place a soft object between the patient's teeth
    3. hold or restrain the patient
    4. protect the victim from injury, but do not restrain

48. A physical therapist works on transfer activities with a patient diagnosed with a complete C5 spinal cord injury. Which of the following muscles would the patient be able to utilize during the training session?

    1. brachioradialis
    2. pronator teres
    3. extensor carpi radialis brevis
    4. latissimus dorsi

49. Tenderness elicited through palpation on the floor of the anatomical snuffbox can often be indicative of a fracture. A fracture in this area would likely involve the:

    1. hamate
    2. lunate
    3. scaphoid
    4. pisiform

50. A physical therapist treats a patient using transcutaneous electrical nerve stimulation. Which condition would not be considered a contraindication for TENS?

    1. placement over the carotid sinus
    2. placement over a pregnant uterus
    3. use on a patient with a cardiac pacemaker
    4. use during labor and delivery

51. A physical therapist treats a 32-year-old female diagnosed with thoracic outlet syndrome. While exercising the patient begins to complain of feeling light headed and dizzy. The therapist immediately ushers the patient to a nearby chair and begins to monitor her vital signs. The therapist measures the patient's respiration rate as 10 breaths per minute, pulse rate of 45 beats per minute, and blood pressure of 115/85 mm Hg. Which of the following statements is most accurate?

    1. pulse rate and respiration rate are below normal levels
    2. pulse rate and blood pressure are above normal levels
    3. blood pressure and respiration rate are above normal levels
    4. the patient's vital signs are within normal limits

52. A physical therapist designs an exercise program for a patient rehabilitating from a myocardial infarction. During the exercise session the patient's blood pressure and pulse rate markedly exceed typical levels. The most appropriate course of action is to:

    1. consult with the referring physician
    2. ask the director of rehabilitation to examine the patient
    3. continue the exercise program when the patient indicates he/she is ready
    4. reexamine the patient prior to the beginning of the next treatment session

53. A physical therapist performs a test to measure the strength of a patient's lower abdominal muscles. The most appropriate technique to examine the strength of the abdominals is:

 1. partial sit-up
 2. full sit-up with rotation
 3. single leg lowering test
 4. double leg lowering test

54. A patient requires a walker for gait training. When fitting the walker for the patient the elbow should be placed in:

 1. 10-15 degrees of flexion
 2. 20-25 degrees of flexion
 3. 35-40 degrees of flexion
 4. complete extension

55. A physical therapist employed in a private practice observes the gait of a 68-year-old male as part of a fitness screening. Which of the following findings is most representative of the gait characteristics of an older adult compared to that of a young adult?

 1. increased stride length
 2. increased swing phase duration
 3. decreased stride width
 4. increased stance phase duration

56. Which statement best describes the realistic functional status of a patient with C4 tetraplegia after completing rehabilitation?

 1. able to ambulate independently
 2. independent in all activities of daily living
 3. able to propel a manual wheelchair independently
 4. able to operate a power wheelchair

57. A physical therapist examines a six month old infant with spina bifida. The infant suddenly begins to act strangely at the conclusion of treatment. A primary survey reveals the infant is not breathing, but does have a pulse. The most immediate response would be to:

 1. begin chest compressions
 2. begin mouth to mouth breathing
 3. begin mouth to nose breathing
 4. begin mouth to mouth and nose breathing

58. A physical therapy treatment plan for a patient rehabilitating from an anterior shoulder dislocation includes progressive resistive exercises. Which muscle groups should be emphasized during rehabilitation?

 1. abductors, lateral rotators
 2. adductors, lateral rotators
 3. abductors, medial rotators
 4. adductors, medial rotators

59. A physical therapist works with a patient diagnosed with anterior cruciate ligament insufficiency. The physician referral specifies closed kinematic chain rehabilitation. Which exercise would not be appropriate based on the physician order?

 1. exercise on a stair machine
 2. limited squats to 45 degrees
 3. walking backwards on a treadmill
 4. isokinetic knee extension and flexion

60. A physical therapist examines the gait of a 62-year-old male with peripheral neuropathy. The therapist observes that the patient's right foot has a tendency to slap the ground during the loading response. The observation can best be explained by weakness in the:

 1. iliopsoas
 2. tibialis anterior
 3. tibialis posterior
 4. gastrocnemius

61. A female distance runner complains of recurrent friction blisters whenever she increases the intensity of her training regimen. Appropriate physical therapy care of friction blisters includes all of the following except:

 1. pad the blister with a pressure pad
 2. use of skin tougheners with astringents
 3. soak regularly in ice water after activity
 4. make an incision along the periphery of the blister with a sterile instrument

62. A patient with patellar tracking dysfunction is examined in physical therapy. Physical examination reveals diminished vastus medialis obliquus activity. The most appropriate method to selectively train the vastus medialis obliquus is:

 1. quadriceps setting exercises and biofeedback
 2. short arc terminal extension with manual resistance
 3. straight leg raises with leg weights
 4. multiple angle isometric exercises

63. A physical therapist palpates along the lateral portion of the hamstrings musculature to the tendinous attachment on the fibular head. The hamstring muscle should be identified as the:

   1. biceps femoris
   2. gracilis
   3. sartorius
   4. semitendinosus

64. A physical therapist instructs a patient to reach behind her head and touch the superior medial angle of the opposite scapula. Which shoulder motions are necessary in order to follow this command?

   1. flexion and lateral rotation
   2. flexion and medial rotation
   3. abduction and lateral rotation
   4. abduction and medial rotation

65. A high school basketball player is treated in physical therapy after spraining her ankle. Palpation reveals an extremely painful area extending from the anterior portion of the lateral malleolus to the lateral aspect of the talar neck. The ligament most likely associated with the discomfort is the:

   1. deltoid
   2. calcaneofibular
   3. posterior talofibular
   4. anterior talofibular

66. In designing a wheelchair for a patient with bilateral transfemoral amputations, the axle should be moved in what direction?

   1. two inches laterally
   2. two inches backward
   3. two inches forward
   4. standard position is appropriate

67. A physical therapist examines a patient diagnosed with a wrist sprain. During the examination the therapist has difficulty identifying the scaphoid and attempts to use the tendinous radial and ulnar boundaries of the anatomical snuff box to assist him. Which of the following active motions would be the most helpful when locating the anatomical snuff box?

   1. abduction of the thumb
   2. adduction of the thumb
   3. extension of the thumb
   4. flexion of the thumb

68. A patient reports pain radiating down her posterior leg into the foot. She also exhibits weakness in plantar flexion and an absent Achilles reflex. Which spinal level would you expect to be involved?

   1. L2
   2. L3
   3. L5
   4. S2

69. A therapist performs an upper quarter screening examination on a patient prior to selecting an appropriate assistive device. Weakness in which muscle would make it particularly difficult to ambulate with crutches?

   1. medial deltoid
   2. erector spinae
   3. latissimus dorsi
   4. rhomboids

70. Transverse friction massage is a valuable treatment technique in a variety of common musculoskeletal disorders. Which of the following statements does not accurately describe the application technique of transverse friction massage?

   1. The physical therapist moves the skin back and forth in a direction perpendicular to the normal orientation of the fibers.
   2. A lubricant is used to prevent excessive skin friction.
   3. Fingers that are not involved directly in the massage are used to provide stabilization.
   4. The rate of movement is 2-3 cycles per second and rhythmical.

71. A physical therapist uses proprioceptive neuromuscular facilitation techniques to increase muscular strength. The therapist instructs the patient to actively perform a pattern of hip extension, abduction, and medial rotation. This pattern emphasizes strengthening of the:

   1. psoas major, psoas minor, iliacus
   2. tensor fasciae latae, biceps femoris
   3. gluteus maximus, gluteus medius, gluteus minimus
   4. gluteus maximus, piriformis, adductor magnus

72. A physical therapist employed in an ambulatory care center prepares to apply a hot pack to the lower back of a patient diagnosed with degenerative disk disease. When examining the patient the therapist identifies several blisters on the patient's right side. The patient indicates that the blisters were caused by heat from a hot pack applied during the previous treatment session. The patient blames himself for the incident because he was hesitant to tell the therapist that the heat was too intense. The most appropriate therapist action is to:

1. complete an incident report
2. contact the referring physician
3. modify the documentation from the previous treatment session
4. avoid documenting the event since it occurred during the previous treatment session

73. A physical therapist attempts to calculate the target heart rate range for a 32-year-old female with no significant past medical history. The patient's resting heart rate is recorded as 60 beats per minute and the maximal heart rate is 180 beats per minute. Using the heart rate reserve method (Karvonen formula) the patient's target heart rate range should be recorded as:

1. 96 – 120 beats per minute
2. 132 – 162 beats per minute
3. 144 – 174 beats per minute
4. 164 – 185 beats per minute

74. A patient in a work hardening program completes a training program consisting of ten different exercises requiring upper and lower extremity strength and endurance. The patient indicates that he is frustrated since he has been unable to increase the weight on a selected carrying activity in over two weeks. The most appropriate therapist action is:

1. provide the patient with verbal encouragement
2. attempt to substitute a different exercise for the carrying activity
3. vary the order of the exercises
4. decrease the number of repetitions

75. A physical therapist observes that a patient's medial longitudinal arch is extremely depressed. Which ligament helps to maintain the medial longitudinal arch?

1. talonavicular
2. anterior talofibular
3. calcaneonavicular
4. posterior talofibular

76. A 47-year-old patient with a diagnosis of CVA with left hemiplegia is referred for orthotic examination. Significant results of manual muscle testing include: hip flexion 3+/5, hip extension 3/5, knee flexion 3+/5, knee extension 3+/5, ankle dorsiflexion 2/5, and ankle inversion and eversion 1/5. Sensation is intact and no abnormal tone is noted. The most appropriate orthosis for this patient is a:

1. knee-ankle-foot orthosis with a locked knee
2. plastic articulating ankle-foot orthosis
3. metal upright ankle-foot orthosis locked in neutral
4. prefabricated posterior leaf orthosis

77. Tests for the length of the hamstrings typically involve stabilization of the uninvolved leg while raising the leg to be tested. It is important to stabilize the uninvolved leg because it:

1. prevents excessive posterior pelvic tilt and excessive flexion of the lumbar spine
2. prevents excessive posterior pelvic tilt and excessive extension of the lumbar spine
3. prevents excessive anterior pelvic tilt and excessive flexion of the lumbar spine
4. prevents excessive anterior pelvic tilt and excessive extension of the lumbar spine

78. A physical therapist conducts an examination on a patient diagnosed with Parkinson's disease. Which of the following clinical findings would you expect the therapist to identify?

1. aphasia
2. ballistic movements
3. severe muscle atrophy
4. cogwheel rigidity

79. What percentage of physical therapy students taking a standardized examination would you expect to score within plus one and minus one standard deviation of the mean?

1. 48%
2. 58%
3. 68%
4. 88%

80. A physical therapist employed in a rehabilitation hospital examines a patient prior to ordering a wheelchair. After completing the examination the therapist concludes that the patient would receive the greatest benefit from a tilt-in-space wheelchair. Which patient would be the best suited for this type of wheelchair?

   1. a 37-year-old male incapable of independent pressure relief
   2. a 42-year-old female with contractures at the hips and knees
   3. a 57-year-old male with poor upper extremity strength
   4. a 75-year-old female with significantly impaired sitting balance

81. A physical therapist prepares to treat a patient in isolation by donning a mask. Which of the following isolation categories would require only the use of a mask?

   1. strict isolation
   2. contact isolation
   3. respiratory isolation
   4. enteric precautions

82. A physical therapist examines a 15-year-old female distance runner diagnosed with foot pain of unknown etiology. As the therapist palpates along the medial aspect of the foot and ankle, she palpates the head of the first metatarsal bone and the metatarsophalangeal joint. Immediately proximal to the structures she identifies the first cuneiform. What large bony prominence would the therapist next identify if she continues to move in a proximal direction?

   1. talar head
   2. navicular
   3. medial malleolus
   4. cuboid

83. A patient rehabilitating from anterior cruciate ligament reconstruction surgery is examined in physical therapy. The physical therapist feels the patient has progressed as expected during the first three weeks of physical therapy, however is concerned about the excessive amount of effusion in the patient's knee. The primary effect of the effusion is:

   1. limited weight bearing status
   2. inability to engage in active exercise
   3. diminished knee extension range of motion
   4. impaired cutaneous sensation

84. A physical therapist receives a referral for lumbar traction on a 61-year-old female diagnosed with chronic lumbar pain. During the history the patient states that she sustained a compression fracture at the L4 level six weeks ago. The most appropriate action is:

   1. initiate lumbar traction in a prone position only
   2. initiate lumbar traction since the compression fracture was six weeks ago
   3. contact the physician and discuss your concerns
   4. inform the physician that the referral showed poor judgment

85. A therapist positions a patient in preparation for bronchial drainage. Which of the following lung segments would not require the foot of the bed to be elevated?

   1. anterior segments of the upper lobes
   2. lateral basal segments of the lower lobes
   3. posterior basal segments of the lower lobes
   4. right middle lobe

86. A physical therapist develops an exercise program for a young boy with insulin dependent diabetes. What effect does exercise have on the patient's insulin requirements?

   1. exercise may reduce a patient's insulin requirements
   2. exercise often increases a patient's insulin requirements
   3. exercise has no effect on a patient's insulin requirements
   4. exercise is contraindicated for patient's with insulin dependent diabetes

87. A patient with a traumatic brain injury and right hemiplegia receives an ankle-foot orthosis to assist with ambulation. After observing the patient the therapist notes that the patient's right knee occasionally buckles during stance phase. A modification to the ankle-foot orthosis that would enhance knee extension during loading and stance on the right is:

   1. position the ankle joint in 5 degrees of dorsiflexion
   2. shorten the toe plate
   3. extend the foot plate
   4. add a soft anterior shell

88. A patient ambulates outside a rehabilitation hospital as part of a therapy session. The physical therapist monitors the patient closely during the session due to extreme heat and humidity. What is the primary mode of heat loss during exercise?

1. conduction
2. convection
3. evaporation
4. radiation

89. A physical therapist develops a treatment program for a patient diagnosed with cystic fibrosis. Which of the following treatment activities would be the most essential to improve ventilation?

1. gait training
2. family education
3. postural drainage
4. home adaptations

90. A physical therapist debrides a decubitus ulcer after a whirlpool treatment. The therapist should take off sterile patient care gloves after:

1. completing debridement and transporting the patient to the patient waiting area
2. completing debridement
3. contact with the patient's decubitus ulcer
4. cleaning the whirlpool at the conclusion of patient treatment

91. A home visit is performed for a patient who resides alone and is three weeks status post total hip replacement. The patient is presently partial weight bearing on the affected side. The most appropriate recommendation to increase safety in the bathroom is:

1. raised toilet seat with rails, tub bench, hand held shower
2. grab bars in the shower and next to the toilet
3. handrails for the toilet, tub bench, hand held shower
4. the patient should not shower until her weight bearing status increases

92. A physical therapist attempts to strengthen the serratus anterior by utilizing proprioceptive neuromuscular facilitation techniques. Which pattern would be the most beneficial to strengthen the serratus anterior?

1. D1 flexion
2. D1 extension
3. D2 flexion
4. D2 extension

93. A physical therapist getting a cup of coffee in the staff room observes a physical therapist assistant reporting for work. The physical therapist notices that the physical therapist assistant smells like alcohol and appears to be slightly unsteady on his feet. The most appropriate physical therapist action is:

1. ask the physical therapist assistant if he is intoxicated
2. continue to monitor the physical therapist assistant at different points during the day
3. discuss the observation with the physical therapist assistant's immediate supervisor
4. report the incident to the state licensing agency

94. A laboratory report indicates that a patient's hematocrit and hemoglobin levels are decreased when compared to expected values. Which condition would not typically be associated with decreased hematocrit and hemoglobin levels?

1. anemia
2. hypoglycemia
3. trauma
4. iron deficiency

95. A physical therapist employed in a rehabilitation hospital works with a patient diagnosed with Parkinson's disease on preambulation activities. As part of the program the physical therapist focuses on improving the patient's lower trunk rotation. The most appropriate patient position to accomplish this goal is:

1. bridging
2. hooklying
3. prone on elbows
4. quadruped

96. A physical therapist treats a patient diagnosed with Parkinson's disease. When working on controlled mobility, which of the following would best describe the physical therapist's objective?

1. facilitate postural muscle control
2. promote weight shifting and rotational trunk control
3. emphasize reciprocal extremity movement
4. facilitate tone and rigidity

97. A physical therapist completes a sensory examination on a patient diagnosed with an incomplete spinal cord injury. To assess the C5 dermatome the therapist should utilize the:

1. neck
2. superior portion of the chest above the axilla
3. thumb and index finger
4. deltoid area of the lateral arm

98. A child is referred to physical therapy with physician orders to examine and treat the left knee. During the examination the patient describes diffuse pain throughout the area of the patella and proximal tibia/fibula. The mother states that the child has been extremely tired and has had a significant reduction in her appetite during the past two months. The medical record shows no evidence of any special testing and all other evaluative findings are inconclusive. The most appropriate physical therapist action is to:

1. utilize superficial modalities in an attempt to reduce the patient's pain
2. call the physician to discuss the patient's care
3. design an exercise program for the patient
4. inform the physician that the patient is not a candidate for physical therapy

99. A physical therapist examines a patient prior to ordering a wheelchair. The therapist measures from the patient's posterior buttock along the lateral thigh to the popliteal fold. The therapist then subtracts two inches from the measurement. This method can be used to measure:

1. seat height
2. seat depth
3. seat width
4. armrest length

100. A physical therapist instructs a patient diagnosed with multiple sclerosis to ambulate using two canes. Which gait pattern would be the most appropriate when using two canes?

1. swing-to
2. swing-through
3. three-point gait
4. four-point gait

101. A physical therapist monitors a patient's blood pressure during exercise. Which of the following responses would be considered normal?

1. diastolic pressure increases 10 mm Hg during exercise
2. systolic pressure does not decline as the intensity of exercise declines
3. systolic pressure does not increase during active exercise
4. systolic pressure declines during exercise before the intensity of the exercise declines

102. A physical therapist examines a patient three days following lumbar laminectomy. The most accurate predictor of the patient's functional status following rehabilitation is based on the patient's:

1. age
2. previous functional status
3. level of family/community support
4. past surgical history

103. Prior to performing a manual muscle test of the anterior deltoid, a patient is asked to perform active shoulder flexion. The patient is able to actively move the extremity from 0-160 degrees of shoulder flexion. Assuming the cause of the limitation is due to a capsular restriction, what is the most appropriate method when testing the anterior deltoid?

1. perform the manual muscle test in a horizontal plane
2. perform the manual muscle test in a gravity-eliminated position
3. perform the manual muscle test in an anti-gravity position
4. avoid performing the manual muscle test due to the limitation in range of motion

104. A physical therapist orders a wheelchair with anti-tip tubes for a patient in preparation for discharge from a rehabilitation hospital. Which patient would most significantly benefit from this option?

1. a patient with Guillain-Barre syndrome
2. a patient with C5 quadriplegia
3. a patient with hemiparesis
4. a patient with amyotrophic lateral sclerosis

105. A physical therapist working in a special care unit notices a tiny air bubble in a peripheral I.V. line. The therapist's most immediate response would be to:

    1. turn off the I.V.
    2. remove the I.V.
    3. reposition the peripheral I.V. line
    4. continue with the present treatment

106. A physical therapist selects an assistive device for a patient rehabilitating from an ankle injury. Which of the following would serve as the most significant obstacle to independent ambulation with axillary crutches?

    1. cognitive impairment
    2. weight bearing restrictions
    3. architectural barriers
    4. unilateral lower extremity weakness

107. A patient rehabilitating from a laminectomy informs a physical therapist that his work schedule has prohibited him from completing the prescribed home exercise program. The therapist is frustrated with the patient's admission, particularly since the home exercise program takes only 10 minutes to complete. The most appropriate therapist action is to:

    1. emphasize the importance of the home exercise program as part of the patient's rehabilitation program
    2. ask the patient to make a specific effort to complete the home exercise program
    3. inform the referring physician that the patient has been noncompliant
    4. discharge the patient from physical therapy

108. A physical therapist assistant completes daily documentation in the medical record. Which of the following documentation activities would be inappropriate for a physical therapist assistant?

    1. a reaction to treatment
    2. patient compliance
    3. discharge summary
    4. treatment or services provided

109. A physical therapist examines a 62-year-old female status post stroke with left hemiparesis. Which of the following perceptual deficits is not commonly associated with left hemiparesis?

    1. denial of disability
    2. rigidity of thought
    3. short attention span
    4. sequencing deficits

110. A physical therapist begins to suspect neurological involvement after completing an upper quarter screening examination. Which anatomic area would be most appropriate to gather information on the C8 dermatome?

    1. thumb and index finger
    2. radial border of the hand
    3. middle three fingers
    4. ulnar border of the hand

111. A physical therapist performs percussion over a selected area of the chest wall of a patient diagnosed with chronic obstructive pulmonary disease. The therapist documents the sound as dull. Which structure would not typically yield this type of sound?

    1. lung
    2. liver
    3. heart
    4. viscera

112. A patient with a lengthy cardiac history ambulates on a treadmill as part of a phase II cardiac rehabilitation program. Suddenly, the patient begins to experience signs and symptoms of an angina attack. The physical therapist's most immediate response should be to:

    1. contact emergency medical services
    2. stop the exercise session
    3. contact the patient's physician
    4. document the incident in the medical record

113. A physical therapist utilizes the results of a symptom-limited exercise treadmill test to determine the intensity of exercise for a patient who previously sustained a cardiac event. Which of the following guidelines would be the most appropriate when determining an appropriate exercise intensity for the patient?

    1. 20 percent of the maximal heart rate obtained on the treadmill test
    2. 40 percent of the maximal heart rate obtained on the treadmill test
    3. 60 percent of the maximal heart rate obtained on the treadmill test
    4. 80 percent of the maximal heart rate obtained on the treadmill test

114. A patient recently admitted to a hospital is examined in physical therapy after sustaining a cerebrovascular accident due to occlusion of the middle cerebral artery. During the examination the physical therapist identifies the presence of homonymous hemianopsia. The most immediate therapist action is:

    1. educate the patient about her condition
    2. ask the patient to turn her head toward the affected side
    3. rearrange the patient's room to ensure that necessary items are within the patient's available visual field
    4. provide frequent reminders to the patient about her limited visual field

115. A physical therapist reviews the medical record of a 54-year-old male prior to initiating treatment. A recent entry in the medical record by the patient's physician indicates an order for Doppler ultrasonography. Which scenario would most warrant the use of this diagnostic test?

    1. congestive heart failure
    2. coronary artery bypass graft surgery
    3. myocardial infarction
    4. artificial pacemaker insertion

116. A nurse on a cardiac unit describes a patient's pulse as thready. This description most accurately describes:

    1. slow and rhythmical pulse
    2. slow and forceful pulse
    3. weak and irregular pulse
    4. intermittent and pronounced pulse

117. A patient diagnosed with right bicipital tendonitis performs upper extremity resistance exercises using a piece of elastic tubing. What muscle is emphasized when laterally rotating the involved extremity against resistance?

    1. teres minor
    2. pectoralis major
    3. teres major
    4. subscapularis

118. A physical therapist attempts to take a history from a patient that is acutely ill. In an attempt to conserve the patient's energy, the therapist should ask questions that are:

    1. thought provoking and reflective
    2. easily answered with brief statements
    3. stimulating and invigorating
    4. sympathetic and endearing

119. A patient two days status post cardiac surgery complains of soreness in her right calf. Which of the following actions would be the most appropriate?

    1. gently massage the calf
    2. notify the patient's nurse of the symptoms
    3. assess the patient's dorsal pedal pulse
    4. have the patient ambulate and reassess the calf

120. A physical therapist examines a patient recently admitted to the hospital with uncontrolled diabetes mellitus. The physical therapy referral is for daily whirlpool treatments for a decubitus ulcer. Which of the following signs and symptoms would the therapist most expect based on the supplied information?

    1. fever and convulsions
    2. tremors and rigidity
    3. polydipsia and polyuria
    4. nausea and vomiting

121. A group of physical therapists utilize a statistical test to determine whether two means differ significantly from each other. Which parametric test of statistical significance is the most appropriate?

    1. t-test
    2. analysis of variance
    3. Chi-square test
    4. Mann-Whitney test

122. A physical therapist working in an acute care hospital reviews the results of laboratory testing prior to initiating treatment on a patient status post kidney transplant. Which of the following laboratory tests would be the most essential to monitor when looking for signs of transplant rejection?

    1. red blood cell count
    2. prothrombin time
    3. platelet count
    4. white blood cell count

123. A physical therapist examines the elbow of a patient rehabilitating from a radial head fracture. Which of the following most accurately describes the close packed position of the radiohumeral joint?

    1. 45 degrees flexion, 10 degrees supination
    2. 60 degrees flexion, 20 degrees supination
    3. 90 degrees flexion, 5 degrees supination
    4. 120 degrees flexion, 10 degrees supination

124. A patient rehabilitating from greater trochanteric bursitis completes active range of motion exercises. Which of the following best describes the arthrokinematics associated with hip flexion?

   1. superior glide of the femoral head
   2. anterior glide of the femoral head
   3. inferior glide of the femoral head in the acetabulum
   4. posterior and inferior glide of the femoral head in the acetabulum

125. A physical therapist examines a patient rehabilitating from an injury to the temporomandibular joint and concludes that the patient is restricted in a capsular pattern. Which of the following would be the most likely clinical presentation?

   1. protrusion is most restricted
   2. retrusion is most restricted
   3. mouth opening is most restricted
   4. mouth closing is most restricted

126. A patient is informed that her condition is terminal shortly before her scheduled therapy session. During the treatment session, the patient asks the physical therapist if she believes the physician's assessment is accurate. The most appropriate therapist response is:

   1. physicians are not infallible
   2. your present condition is serious
   3. channel your energy towards getting better
   4. focus on your therapy goals

127. A physical therapist orders a wheelchair for a patient in a rehabilitation hospital. Which of the following patients would be most in need of a wheelchair with handrim projections?

   1. a patient with a C3 spinal cord injury
   2. a patient with a C5 spinal cord injury
   3. a patient with hemiparesis
   4. a patient with a cauda equina lesion

128. A physical therapist reviews the results of ultraviolet testing. Which grade of erythemal dose best describes the time required for mild reddening of the skin?

   1. suberythemal dose
   2. minimal erythemal dose
   3. second degree erythema
   4. third degree erythema

129. A physical therapist assesses a patient's voice sounds as part of a respiratory examination. Which condition is typically associated with increased voice sounds?

   1. pneumothorax
   2. consolidation
   3. atelectasis
   4. pleural effusion

130. A patient rehabilitating from a myocardial infarction expresses to his physical therapist a desire to quit smoking. The most appropriate therapist action is to:

   1. supply the patient with the phone number of the American Heart Association
   2. refer the patient to a smoking cessation program
   3. provide the patient with general information on the dangers of smoking
   4. ask the patient to consider nicotine gum

131. A physical therapist examines a patient referred to physical therapy with bicipital tendonitis. Which of the following special tests would be the most useful to confirm the patient's diagnosis?

   1. Allen test
   2. apprehension test
   3. drop arm test
   4. Yergason's test

132. A physical therapist completes a selected resistive test as part of an examination. The patient reports feeling pain during the test, however strength is normal. Which of the following conclusions is most likely?

   1. capsular or ligamentous laxity
   2. a minor lesion of the muscle or tendon
   3. a complete rupture of the muscle or tendon
   4. intermittent claudication may be present

133. A note in a patient's medical chart indicates the presence of an acid-base disturbance of metabolic origin. Which condition is not typically associated with metabolic acidosis?

   1. vomiting
   2. secondary hyperventilation
   3. lethargy
   4. syncope

134. A therapist identifies signs and symptoms of neurovascular compression after examining a patient with an upper extremity injury. Which of the following special tests would not be helpful in identifying the presence of neurovascular compression?

    1. Tinel's sign
    2. Froment's sign
    3. Phalen's test
    4. Bunnel-Littler test

135. A physical therapist presents an inservice to the rehabilitation staff on the anatomy of the spine. As part of the presentation the therapist discusses the role of each of the ligaments of the spine. Which ligament acts to prevent hyperextension?

    1. ligamentum flavum
    2. interspinous ligaments
    3. anterior longitudinal ligament
    4. posterior longitudinal ligament

136. A physical therapist assigns a grade of good after completing a manual muscle test of the extensor digitorum. The most appropriate patient position to conduct the test would be:

    1. supine
    2. prone
    3. sidelying
    4. standing

137. A physical therapist completes a goniometric assessment of a patient's wrist. Assuming normal range of motion, which of the following motions would have the greatest available range?

    1. extension
    2. flexion
    3. radial deviation
    4. ulnar deviation

138. A physical therapist classifies a patient's posture as lordotic after completing a postural assessment. Which muscle group would you expect to be shortened based on the results of the postural assessment?

    1. intercostals
    2. hip flexors
    3. scapula retractors
    4. abdominals

139. A 63-year-old female status post stroke is screened for admission into a rehabilitation hospital. As part of the screen the physical therapist utilizes a standardized instrument to document the extent of the patient's impairments and disabilities. Which of the following standardized instruments would be most beneficial to provide an assessment of motor function?

    1. Barthel Index
    2. Functional Independence Measure
    3. Fugl-Meyer Assessment
    4. Rivermead Mobility Index

140. A physical therapist reviews an examination of a patient diagnosed with an upper motor neuron disease. The examination documents the existence of a positive Babinski reflex. A positive Babinski reflex is characterized by:

    1. extension of the great toe
    2. flexion of the great toe
    3. abduction of the great toe
    4. adduction of the great toe

141. A physical therapist measures passive forearm pronation and concludes that the results are within normal limits. Which measurement would be classified as within normal limits?

    1. 60 degrees
    2. 80 degrees
    3. 100 degrees
    4. 120 degrees

142. A physical therapist obtains a goniometric measurement with a patient in supine. The stationary arm of the goniometer is positioned at the midaxillary line of the trunk. The moveable arm is positioned along the lateral midline of the humerus using the lateral epicondyle as a reference. This positioning of the goniometer can be used to measure:

    1. shoulder flexion
    2. medial and lateral rotation of the shoulder
    3. shoulder extension
    4. elbow extension

143. A physical therapist examines a patient diagnosed with bicipital tendonitis. As part of the examination the therapist passively moves the upper extremity into a position that places maximum tension on the biceps tendon. Which motion would best accomplish this task?

1. elbow flexion and forearm pronation
2. elbow extension and forearm pronation
3. elbow flexion and forearm supination
4. elbow extension and forearm supination

144. A physical therapist examines a patient with lower extremity hypertonicity. All of the following can be used by the therapist to temporarily reduce tone except:

1. gentle rocking
2. cryotherapy
3. approximation
4. sustained stretch

145. A physical therapist transports a patient two days status post right total hip replacement to the parallel bars in preparation for ambulation activities. The patient has not placed any weight on the involved leg since surgery and appears to be extremely apprehensive. The most appropriate location for the therapist to stand when guarding the patient in the parallel bars is:

1. in front of the patient
2. behind the patient
3. on the right of the patient
4. on the left of the patient

146. A physical therapist reviews a physician's order prior to treating a patient with a deep partial-thickness burn over the volar surface of the forearm. Assuming a component of the treatment regimen includes use of a topical antibiotic, which of the following medications would be the most appropriate based on the depth and location of the burn?

1. Bacitracin
2. Furacin
3. Neosporin
4. silver sulfadiazine

147. What massage technique is commonly used at the beginning and conclusion of treatment and may be used during transitional periods prior to changing massage techniques?

1. effleurage
2. petrissage
3. tapotement
4. vibration

148. A physical therapist attempts to measure a patient's shoulder lateral rotation. Proper positioning of the upper extremity in supine would best be described by which of the following?

1. shoulder abducted to 90 degrees, elbow flexed to 90 degrees
2. shoulder abducted to 90 degrees, elbow fully extended
3. shoulder abducted to 90 degrees, elbow flexed to 45 degrees
4. shoulder in neutral, elbow flexed to 90 degrees

149. A physical therapist observes a patient performing active hip abduction in supine. The patient is limited by 10 degrees in abduction, but appears to be moving through the full range of motion. What compensatory measures might the patient use to seemingly increase hip abduction?

1. hip flexion and lateral rotation
2. hip flexion and medial rotation
3. hip hyperextension and lateral rotation
4. hip hyperextension and medial rotation

150. A physical therapist consistently falls behind with his documentation due to an excessive patient load. The most appropriate action is:

1. discuss the situation with other staff physical therapists
2. ignore the situation and attempt to complete the documentation in a timely fashion
3. discuss the situation with the immediate supervisor
4. discuss the situation with the director of rehabilitation

151. A physical therapist reviews a physician referral for a patient with incontinence. After completing an examination the therapist determines that the patient has weak pelvic floor muscles and as a result designs a home strengthening program. The therapist requests that the patient hold each contraction for three seconds and repeat each exercise five times. The most appropriate number of sets that the patient should perform in one day best corresponds to:

1. 1 set
2. 2 sets
3. 5 sets
4. 10 sets

152. A patient with a fractured right tibia who is partial weight bearing is referred to physical therapy for fitting and instruction with an assistive device. During the examination the physical therapist identifies poor lower extremity strength and coordination. Which assistive device would be most appropriate for the patient?

    1. axillary crutches
    2. cane
    3. Lofstrand crutches
    4. walker

153. Which of the following statements would probably not increase a patient's compliance with a home exercise program?

    1. The patient should receive both written and verbal instructions.
    2. The program should be goal oriented.
    3. The program should be individualized to the needs of the patient.
    4. The program should take in excess of 30 minutes to complete.

154. A physical therapist observes the gait of a patient status post right CVA with a metal upright ankle-foot orthosis. The therapist notes left knee instability with left stance. The ankle-foot orthosis most likely has:

    1. a long foot plate
    2. inadequate knee lock
    3. inadequate dorsiflexion stop
    4. inadequate plantar flexion stop

155. A physical therapist examines a patient with a limited straight leg raise of 40 degrees due to inadequate hamstrings length. Which proprioceptive neuromuscular technique would be most appropriate to increase the patient's hamstrings length?

    1. contract-relax
    2. rhythmic initiation
    3. rhythmic stabilization
    4. rhythmic rotation

156. A short-term goal for a patient status post CVA is to perform a stand pivot transfer from a bed to a wheelchair. Which section of a S.O.A.P. note would include the short-term goal?

    1. subjective
    2. objective
    3. assessment
    4. plan

157. A physical therapist practices assessing joint end-feel. The therapist would most accurately classify normal elbow extension end-feel as:

    1. firm
    2. hard
    3. soft
    4. empty

158. A physical therapist observes a patient dragging his toe during the swing phase of gait. All of the following are possible causes except:

    1. weakness of dorsiflexors
    2. spasticity of plantar flexors
    3. weakness of plantar flexors
    4. inadequate knee flexion

159. A physical therapist notices a student physical therapist using improper guarding technique on a patient that appears to be unstable. The most immediate physical therapist action should be:

    1. discuss the situation with the student's clinical instructor
    2. leave the student an anonymous note describing proper guarding technique
    3. offer suggestions to improve the student's guarding technique
    4. ignore the situation since you are not the clinical instructor

160. A physical therapist instructs a patient diagnosed with Parkinson's disease in ambulation activities. Which of the following would be helpful to improve the quality of the patient's gait?

    1. decrease stride length
    2. increase trunk rotation
    3. increase forward head posture
    4. decrease base of support

161. A physical therapist providing patient coverage for a colleague on vacation treats an 18-year-old male with lower back pain. After observing the patient in standing the therapist is convinced the patient has tight hip flexors, however a note from the initial examination indicates that the Thomas test was negative. Failure to limit which particular movements would best explain a false negative with the Thomas test?

    1. anterior pelvic tilt and increased lumbar lordosis
    2. anterior pelvic tilt and decreased lumbar lordosis
    3. posterior pelvic tilt and increased lumbar lordosis
    4. posterior pelvic tilt and decreased lumbar lordosis

162. A physical therapist positions a patient with hemiplegia in a plantigrade position to promote weight bearing through the affected upper extremity. The most appropriate hand position on the plinth is:

1. total palmar contact with the fingers fully extended
2. total palmar contact with fingers flexed
3. weight bearing on a closed fist
4. palmar contact with support of the palmar arches and weight through the heel of the hand

163. A physical therapist treats a 21-year-old male that sustained a fracture of the radial head six weeks ago. The physician referral specified aggressive joint mobilization to improve elbow range of motion. The patient has made progress in a limited number of visits, however continues to exhibit significant range of motion deficits. Assuming the patient is returning to school in one week and will not be able to return to the physical therapy clinic, which activity would be the most appropriate for the patient?

1. encourage the patient to make an appointment with a physician in the health center
2. encourage the patient to consult with an athletic trainer
3. encourage the patient to continue to receive physical therapy services
4. encourage the patient to limit activities until he has full elbow range of motion

164. A physical therapist treats a 32-year-old female rehabilitating from a closed head injury presently functioning at Rancho Los Amigos level IV. The therapist treats the patient in her home for 60 minute sessions, three times per week. Recently the therapist has noticed that the patient becomes increasingly combative as the session progresses and believes the deterioration in behavior is linked to the patient becoming fatigued. The most appropriate treatment modification is:

1. reduce the treatment sessions to 30 minutes, three times per week
2. reduce the frequency of the treatment sessions to two times per week
3. increase the rest periods during existing treatment sessions
4. increase the treatment sessions to 90 minutes, two times per week

165. A physical therapist assists a patient with C7 tetraplegia into a prone on elbows position on a mat. The therapist instructs the patient to push his elbows down, tuck his chin, and lift his trunk off of the mat while rounding out the shoulders. This exercise is helpful in strengthening the:

1. serratus anterior and scapular muscles
2. serratus anterior
3. latissimus dorsi and scapular muscles
4. sacrospinalis and semispinalis

166. A physical therapist performs a range of motion screening on a 14-year-old female. The therapist instructs the patient to stand on her tiptoes. The therapist uses this command to examine:

1. dorsiflexion and toe extension
2. dorsiflexion and toe flexion
3. plantar flexion and toe extension
4. plantar flexion and toe flexion

167. A forearm laceration causes damage to the median nerve. Which muscle not innervated by the median nerve can flex the wrist?

1. flexor carpi radialis
2. flexor carpi ulnaris
3. flexor digitorum superficialis
4. palmaris longus

168. A physical therapist examines a 37-year-old male referred to physical therapy with radicular pain in the lower extremity. A note from the referring physician indicates that magnetic resonance imaging confirmed the presence of a disc herniation with resultant L4 nerve root impingement. When completing muscle testing, which muscle would you expect to be the most affected by the patient's current condition?

1. iliopsoas
2. tibialis anterior
3. flexor hallucis longus
4. extensor digitorum brevis

169. A physical therapist performs a screening examination on a 43-year-old female diagnosed with carpal tunnel syndrome. The therapist attempts to pull the patient's fingers from a position of adduction to abduction. This action is used to test the strength of the:

1. finger extensors
2. opponens pollicis
3. dorsal interossei
4. palmar interossei

170. The middle score of a distribution which divides a group of scores into equal parts with half of the scores falling above and half of the scores falling below describes the:

   1. mean
   2. median
   3. mode
   4. range

171. A developmental examination is performed on an infant. The infant is able to play on extended arms and attempts to reach for objects. The infant can maintain good alignment of the head and trunk when pulled to a sitting position. The infant bears weight when placed in supportive standing. The physical therapist would expect the infant's age to be:

   1. 3 months
   2. 5 months
   3. 7 months
   4. 9 months

172. A physical therapist conducts an examination on a 27-year-old female rehabilitating from a tibial plateau fracture. During the examination the patient mentions that she is concerned about the muscle atrophy in her involved quadriceps. Assuming the therapist uses a S.O.A.P. note format for documentation, which section would be the most appropriate to record the information?

   1. subjective
   2. objective
   3. assessment
   4. plan

173. A physical therapist observes the standing posture of a patient from a lateral view. If the patient has normal anatomical alignment, a plumb line would fall:

   1. posterior to the lobe of the ear
   2. anterior to the greater trochanter of the femur
   3. slightly anterior to a midline through the knee
   4. slightly posterior to the lateral malleolus

174. A patient with latissimus dorsi and lower trapezius weakness would have the most difficulty performing which of the following activities?

   1. four-point gait with Lofstrand crutches
   2. two-point gait with a straight cane
   3. swing-through gait with axillary crutches
   4. wheelchair propulsion

175. A physical therapist instructs a 67-year-old female, four weeks status post total hip replacement in a home exercise program. Which exercise description would be inappropriate for the patient?

   1. Lie on your involved side and lift the involved leg towards the ceiling.
   2. Place a rolled up towel under your knee. Rest the weight of the thigh on the towel roll. Lift the heel off the table so that you straighten the knee.
   3. Lie on your back with the opposite knee bent. Tighten the thigh muscle, keeping the leg straight and lift the leg toward the ceiling.
   4. Lie on your back with knees bent. Raise your buttocks off the table.

176. A physical therapist performs a vertebral artery test on a patient prior to using traction and mobilization techniques in the upper cervical spine. During the test the patient begins to demonstrate nystagmus and blurred vision. The physical therapist should:

   1. repeat the vertebral artery test to confirm the original results
   2. proceed cautiously with traction and mobilization techniques in the upper cervical spine
   3. avoid traction or mobilization techniques in the upper cervical spine
   4. discharge the patient from physical therapy

177. A patient performs bridging in supine as part of an exercise program. The physical therapist increases the difficulty by applying agonistic reversals as the patient maintains the bridge position. The application of agonistic reversals promotes eccentric control of the:

   1. hip extensors, hamstrings
   2. hip flexors, quadriceps
   3. hip extensors, adductors
   4. adductors, hamstrings

178. A 16-year-old basketball player is anxious to return to athletic competition following rehabilitation from an Achilles tendon rupture. The athlete is objectively ready to return to competition, however continues to demonstrate a severe preoccupation with reinjury. The most appropriate response is to:

   1. allow the patient to return to basketball without restriction
   2. inform the patient that he should not participate in basketball this season
   3. design a functional progression for basketball that allows the patient to progress to higher level activities in a gradual fashion
   4. discuss other less demanding athletic activities with the patient

179. A physical therapist observes random changes in the intensity of an ultrasound generator during patient treatment. The most appropriate response is to:

1. ignore the changes in the intensity since they are normal when using ultrasound
2. continue to use the machine at intensity levels less than 1.0 W/cm^2
3. closely monitor the machine during use
4. discontinue use of the machine and contact a service technician

180. A physical therapist reviews literature which details the expected changes in endurance and physical work capacity as an individual progresses from middle age to an older adult. Which of the following measurements would not be affected by this transition?

1. resting heart rate
2. stroke volume
3. cardiac output
4. blood pressure

181. A physician requests that a physical therapist report to the orthopedic surgical center to instruct a patient in a preoperative training program. After completing the training program the therapist returns to the outpatient physical therapy area and finds a number of items that require her attention. Which of the following items should be given the highest priority?

1. an interim progress note for a patient scheduled to see a physician
2. unfinished documentation from a patient seen earlier in the day
3. a message from a patient that has been discharged from therapy
4. a scheduled patient that has been waiting for 15 minutes

182. A patient demonstrates unilateral neglect to the left. The physical therapist's short-term goals for the patient include reducing the patient's neglect. Which treatment technique would not be effective in improving the patient's condition?

1. have the patient participate in bilateral tasks to increase total body awareness
2. place the patient's food on the right side of the tray so the patient can eat by himself
3. have the patient observe himself massaging his left upper extremity
4. have the patient use a mirror while dressing

183. A physical therapist straps the ankle of a young athlete with a history of recurrent inversion ankle sprains. The therapist elects to use the closed basket weave strapping technique. Which of the following is not accurate when using this technique?

1. one and one half inch adhesive tape is traditionally used
2. stirrups should be applied pulling the foot into inversion
3. the foot should remain in dorsiflexion during strapping
4. to provide additional support use figure-eights with or without heel locks

184. A physical therapist attempts to obtain information on the integrity of the C7 dermatome. The most appropriate location to assess the dermatome is the:

1. little finger and ulnar border of the hand
2. lateral forearm and thumb
3. palmar distal phalanx of the middle finger
4. medial forearm

185. A physical therapist studies a normal resting electrocardiogram for one cardiac cycle. What wave or change in shape of the electrocardiogram results from atrial depolarization?

1. P wave
2. QRS complex
3. ST segment
4. T wave

186. A patient is referred to physical therapy after sustaining a Colles' fracture. A Colles' fracture refers to an injury of the:

1. ulna
2. radius
3. olecranon
4. scaphoid

187. A therapist prepares to measure forearm pronation range of motion on a patient rehabilitating from a Colles' fracture. When measuring forearm pronation the moving arm of the goniometer should be placed on the:

1. dorsal surface of the wrist
2. lateral surface of the wrist
3. medial surface of the wrist
4. volar surface of the wrist

188. When reviewing a medical record, a physical therapist identifies an entry which classifies the patient's pulse rate as bradycardic. This should be interpreted as:

    1. an increased pulse rate
    2. a decreased pulse rate
    3. an increase in the size of the heart
    4. an underdeveloped atria

189. A patient three weeks status post right total knee replacement complains of pain in the right calf. The patient's pain increases with ambulation and with quick passive range of motion into dorsiflexion. The patient's lower extremity is warm to touch. The most appropriate response would be to:

    1. disregard the findings as postoperative pain
    2. continue with ambulation to tolerance
    3. perform active calf stretching
    4. request a physician to rule out deep venous thrombosis

190. A 54-year-old male is referred to physical therapy four weeks status post acromioplasty. Examination reveals pain and limited motion in flexion, abduction, and lateral rotation. In order to increase the patient's shoulder range of motion, the physical therapist prepares to administer a hold-relax technique by assisting the patient's involved upper extremity to the point of limitation. Assuming the patient indicates that the position is painful, the most immediate therapist action is:

    1. administer the technique in a gravity-eliminated position
    2. reposition the upper extremity 5-10 degrees short of the point of limitation
    3. apply gradual pressure to the upper extremity in order to create an isometric contraction of the agonist
    4. apply gradual pressure to the upper extremity in order to create an isometric contraction of the antagonist

191. A physical therapist records the vital signs of a 45-year-old male prior to beginning treatment. The therapist palpates the patient's radial pulse for 15 seconds, but has difficulty computing the actual pulse rate since the rhythm is irregular. The most appropriate method to identify the actual pulse rate is to:

    1. recheck hand positioning and palpate the radial pulse for an additional 15 seconds
    2. select another pulse site and palpate for 15 seconds
    3. palpate the radial pulse for one minute
    4. record the original pulse rate and document the rhythm

192. When measuring ulnar deviation of the wrist, the moveable arm of the goniometer should be aligned with the:

    1. shaft of the second proximal phalanx
    2. shaft of the third proximal phalanx
    3. shaft of the second metacarpal
    4. shaft of the third metacarpal

193. A patient sustained a knife wound which severed the distal lateral cord of the brachial plexus. EMG testing reveals no damage to the median nerve. The injury will likely result in an impairment of:

    1. elbow flexion and forearm supination
    2. elbow extension and forearm pronation
    3. shoulder flexion and abduction
    4. shoulder lateral rotation

194. Kneading, wringing, and rolling are all specific variations of which basic massage technique?

    1. effleurage
    2. vibration
    3. petrissage
    4. tapotement

195. A patient in a rehabilitation hospital returns to physical therapy after meeting with a physiatrist. The patient indicates that during the meeting the physiatrist discussed the effect of his spinal cord injury on sexual function. Which of the following statements is typically not accurate for a male patient with complete T7 paraplegia?

    1. The patient will be able to sustain an erection.
    2. The patient will be able to ejaculate.
    3. The patient's fertility will be greatly diminished.
    4. The patient's medications may affect his sexual function.

196. A physical therapist attempts to identify subtalar neutral position as part of an orthotic assessment. The therapist positions the patient in prone and manipulates the foot by grasping the fourth and fifth metatarsal heads. Which anatomical landmark should be palpated when determining subtalar neutral?

    1. medial tubercle of the talus
    2. head of the talus
    3. sustentaculum tali
    4. sinus tarsi

197. A physical therapist treating a patient in supine elects to reinforce active movement of the lower extremity in a flexion, adduction, and lateral rotation pattern. This proprioceptive neuromuscular facilitation pattern is termed:

   1. D1 flexion
   2. D1 extension
   3. D2 flexion
   4. D2 extension

198. A physical therapist is hired as a consultant for a local business that has experienced a large increase in repetitive use injuries. The business employs over 50 workers who assemble plastic components while seated at small individual workstations. The workers are required to work eight-hour shifts with a 15 minute morning and afternoon break. Which recommendation would be the most beneficial?

   1. increase the size of the workstations
   2. institute group stretching activities at specified intervals
   3. expand the morning and afternoon breaks to 30 minutes
   4. decrease the length of all shifts to six hours or less

199. A physical therapist treats a patient with incomplete L4 paraplegia. The therapist uses proprioceptive neuromuscular facilitation techniques to strengthen the abdominals and improve trunk stability in sitting. The most appropriate technique to improve strength and control include:

   1. hold-relax alternating movement in sitting
   2. D1 flexion in quadruped
   3. D1 flexion in supine
   4. alternating isometrics and timing for emphasis in sitting

200. A patient is not able to whistle on command, but has been heard whistling while listening to music. The same patient is unable to walk in the gym after demonstration, but is observed walking across the room to get his dinner tray. This condition is termed:

   1. ideational apraxia
   2. ideomotor apraxia
   3. constructional apraxia
   4. dressing apraxia

Sample Exam: Four – Answer Sheet

1. ① ② ③ ④	36. ① ② ③ ④	71. ① ② ③ ④
2. ① ② ③ ④	37. ① ② ③ ④	72. ① ② ③ ④
3. ① ② ③ ④	38. ① ② ③ ④	73. ① ② ③ ④
4. ① ② ③ ④	39. ① ② ③ ④	74. ① ② ③ ④
5. ① ② ③ ④	40. ① ② ③ ④	75. ① ② ③ ④
6. ① ② ③ ④	41. ① ② ③ ④	76. ① ② ③ ④
7. ① ② ③ ④	42. ① ② ③ ④	77. ① ② ③ ④
8. ① ② ③ ④	43. ① ② ③ ④	78. ① ② ③ ④
9. ① ② ③ ④	44. ① ② ③ ④	79. ① ② ③ ④
10. ① ② ③ ④	45. ① ② ③ ④	80. ① ② ③ ④
11. ① ② ③ ④	46. ① ② ③ ④	81. ① ② ③ ④
12. ① ② ③ ④	47. ① ② ③ ④	82. ① ② ③ ④
13. ① ② ③ ④	48. ① ② ③ ④	83. ① ② ③ ④
14. ① ② ③ ④	49. ① ② ③ ④	84. ① ② ③ ④
15. ① ② ③ ④	50. ① ② ③ ④	85. ① ② ③ ④
16. ① ② ③ ④	51. ① ② ③ ④	86. ① ② ③ ④
17. ① ② ③ ④	52. ① ② ③ ④	87. ① ② ③ ④
18. ① ② ③ ④	53. ① ② ③ ④	88. ① ② ③ ④
19. ① ② ③ ④	54. ① ② ③ ④	89. ① ② ③ ④
20. ① ② ③ ④	55. ① ② ③ ④	90. ① ② ③ ④
21. ① ② ③ ④	56. ① ② ③ ④	91. ① ② ③ ④
22. ① ② ③ ④	57. ① ② ③ ④	92. ① ② ③ ④
23. ① ② ③ ④	58. ① ② ③ ④	93. ① ② ③ ④
24. ① ② ③ ④	59. ① ② ③ ④	94. ① ② ③ ④
25. ① ② ③ ④	60. ① ② ③ ④	95. ① ② ③ ④
26. ① ② ③ ④	61. ① ② ③ ④	96. ① ② ③ ④
27. ① ② ③ ④	62. ① ② ③ ④	97. ① ② ③ ④
28. ① ② ③ ④	63. ① ② ③ ④	98. ① ② ③ ④
29. ① ② ③ ④	64. ① ② ③ ④	99. ① ② ③ ④
30. ① ② ③ ④	65. ① ② ③ ④	100. ① ② ③ ④
31. ① ② ③ ④	66. ① ② ③ ④	101. ① ② ③ ④
32. ① ② ③ ④	67. ① ② ③ ④	102. ① ② ③ ④
33. ① ② ③ ④	68. ① ② ③ ④	103. ① ② ③ ④
34. ① ② ③ ④	69. ① ② ③ ④	104. ① ② ③ ④
35. ① ② ③ ④	70. ① ② ③ ④	105. ① ② ③ ④

SAMPLE EXAMINATION: EXAM FOUR ANSWER SHEET

106.	①	②	③	④	138.	①	②	③	④	170.	①	②	③	④
107.	①	②	③	④	139.	①	②	③	④	171.	①	②	③	④
108.	①	②	③	④	140.	①	②	③	④	172.	①	②	③	④
109.	①	②	③	④	141.	①	②	③	④	173.	①	②	③	④
110.	①	②	③	④	142.	①	②	③	④	174.	①	②	③	④
111.	①	②	③	④	143.	①	②	③	④	175.	①	②	③	④
112.	①	②	③	④	144.	①	②	③	④	176.	①	②	③	④
113.	①	②	③	④	145.	①	②	③	④	177.	①	②	③	④
114.	①	②	③	④	146.	①	②	③	④	178.	①	②	③	④
115.	①	②	③	④	147.	①	②	③	④	179.	①	②	③	④
116.	①	②	③	④	148.	①	②	③	④	180.	①	②	③	④
117.	①	②	③	④	149.	①	②	③	④	181.	①	②	③	④
118.	①	②	③	④	150.	①	②	③	④	182.	①	②	③	④
119.	①	②	③	④	151.	①	②	③	④	183.	①	②	③	④
120.	①	②	③	④	152.	①	②	③	④	184.	①	②	③	④
121.	①	②	③	④	153.	①	②	③	④	185.	①	②	③	④
122.	①	②	③	④	154.	①	②	③	④	186.	①	②	③	④
123.	①	②	③	④	155.	①	②	③	④	187.	①	②	③	④
124.	①	②	③	④	156.	①	②	③	④	188.	①	②	③	④
125.	①	②	③	④	157.	①	②	③	④	189.	①	②	③	④
126.	①	②	③	④	158.	①	②	③	④	190.	①	②	③	④
127.	①	②	③	④	159.	①	②	③	④	191.	①	②	③	④
128.	①	②	③	④	160.	①	②	③	④	192.	①	②	③	④
129.	①	②	③	④	161.	①	②	③	④	193.	①	②	③	④
130.	①	②	③	④	162.	①	②	③	④	194.	①	②	③	④
131.	①	②	③	④	163.	①	②	③	④	195.	①	②	③	④
132.	①	②	③	④	164.	①	②	③	④	196.	①	②	③	④
133.	①	②	③	④	165.	①	②	③	④	197.	①	②	③	④
134.	①	②	③	④	166.	①	②	③	④	198.	①	②	③	④
135.	①	②	③	④	167.	①	②	③	④	199.	①	②	③	④
136.	①	②	③	④	168.	①	②	③	④	200.	①	②	③	④
137.	①	②	③	④	169.	①	②	③	④					

Sample Exam Answers: Four

1. Answer: 2   Resource: Paz (p. 330)
   Radiation therapy has a number of useful clinical applications including reducing the size of tumors, relieving compression from tumors, and relieving pain. Radiation dosage is measured using Grays.

2. Answer: 4   Resource: Campbell, S. (p. 547)
   Lower extremity bivalve casting inhibits the extensor thrust reflex which is elicited through plantar flexion and pressure through the ball of the foot. The reflex interferes with mobility by stimulating a mass extension pattern.

3. Answer: 1   Resource: Kendall (p. 201)
   The tibialis anterior acts to dorsiflex the ankle joint and assists in inversion of the foot. During muscle testing, pressure should be applied against the medial side of the dorsal surface of the foot, in the direction of plantar flexion of the ankle joint and eversion of the foot.

4. Answer: 1   Resource: Brotzman (p. 225)
   The iliotibial band is a thickened strip of fascia that extends from the iliac crest to the lateral tibial tubercle. Activities requiring frequent flexion of the knee can produce an inflammatory reaction that occurs due to excessive contact between the iliotibial band and the lateral femoral condyle. Management of the condition often requires techniques for reducing inflammation and iliotibial band stretching.

5. Answer: 2   Resource: Kisner (p. 441)
   Although there is a wide range of outcomes with nonoperative anterior cruciate ligament injuries, most individuals are able to return to a minimum level of light recreational sports. Therapeutic management of an anterior cruciate ligament injury includes range of motion, progressive resistive exercises, functional activities, and bracing.

6. Answer: 4   Resource: Brotzman (p. 267)
   Eccentric contraction of the gastrocnemius and soleus complex places the greatest amount of stress on the Achilles tendon. Running on an incline or pushing off to accelerate while weight bearing are two examples of activities that produces this type of contraction. Although these activities place a significant amount of stress on the Achilles tendon, they are a necessary component of a rehabilitation program designed to return an individual to athletic competition.

7. Answer: 1   Resource: Clinical Companion (p. 104)
   The Barthel Index demonstrates limited sensitivity for individuals with mild disabilities since it does not record improvement in a patient's functional status until he/she reaches a specified level of independence.

8. Answer: 2   Resource: Kendall (p. 221)
   The gluteus medius functions as an abductor and medial rotator of the hip. The superior gluteal nerve innervates the muscle.

9. Answer: 1   Resource: Brotzman (p. 354)
   Subtalar eversion is a common compensatory finding in patients with forefoot varus. This position of the rearfoot allows the medial forefoot to come in contact with the ground, however can lead to hypermobility in the foot and a loss of the necessary rigid lever from mid-stance through toe off.

10. Answer: 4   Resource: O'Sullivan - Physical Rehabilitation (p. 730)
    Frenkel's exercises are designed to improve coordination by emphasizing the use of vision and hearing to compensate for altered or impaired proprioception.

11. Answer: 1   Resource: Kisner (p. 203)
    The glenohumeral joint consists of the concave glenoid fossa and the convex humeral head. An anterior glide of the humeral head is indicated to increase lateral rotation.

12. Answer: 2   Resource: Brontzman (p. 355)
    Forefoot varus refers to an inverted position of the forefoot in relation to the hindfoot with the subtalar joint in the neutral position. Compensatory forefoot varus allows the medial forefoot to come in contact with the ground due to eversion of the hindfoot. A medial forefoot posting limits compensatory pronation by allowing the foot to achieve a more stable position.

13. Answer: 3   Resource: Magee (p. 193)
    The infraspinatus and teres minor both serve as lateral rotators of the shoulder.

14. Answer: 1 Resource: O'Sullivan - Physical Rehabilitation (p. 802)
A patient with a traumatic brain injury functioning at Rancho Los Amigos level VI confused-appropriate typically demonstrates goal-directed behavior and is able to follow simple commands fairly consistently. Since the patient is no longer agitated, the verbal outburst would be considered an atypical event and therefore warrants direct contact with the physical therapist.

15. Answer: 3 Resource: Pierson (p. 170)
When descending a curb using a forward approach, the wheelchair must remain tipped backward until the rear wheels are in contact with the surface below the curb.

16. Answer: 4 Resource: Kisner (p. 175)
The rectus femoris is a two joint muscle that acts to flex the hip and extend the knee. Passively flexing the hip and knee of the contralateral lower extremity effectively serves to stabilize the pelvis.

17. Answer: 2 Resource: Pierson (p. 205)
The walker, uninvolved, and involved extremity are each considered one point. Since each of the points move independently, the gait pattern is considered to be three-point.

18. Answer: 2 Resource: Palmer (p. 83)
A posterior stop in the metal joint of an ankle-foot orthosis is often used to prevent foot drag during the swing phase of the gait cycle by limiting plantar flexion. An anterior stop is used to restrict dorsiflexion during the late stance phase.

19. Answer: 2 Resource: Minor (p. 405)
A quad cane should be utilized in the upper extremity that is opposite from the affected lower extremity. The device is designed so that the longer legs are positioned away from the patient.

20. Answer: 1 Resource: Kisner (p. 395)
A raised toilet seat helps to limit hip flexion. Hip flexion beyond 90 degrees is often considered a contraindication following total hip replacement surgery. Although a hip abduction pillow is employed postoperatively, it is used for more than one week.

21. Answer: 2 Resource: Palmer (p. 48)
An endoskeleton or modular shank is designed to incorporate a synthetic foam cover shaped like the opposite leg. As a result the device is more cosmetically attractive and would likely make the patient more comfortable in her social setting. A solid ankle cushion heel is the most frequently prescribed foot-ankle assembly. It is considered to be a nonarticulated foot since it does not incorporate a mechanical joint at the ankle.

22. Answer: 1 Resource: Sullivan - An Integrated Approach (p. 3)
The asymmetrical tonic neck reflex may produce extension of the affected upper extremity by turning the patient's head toward the affected side.

23. Answer: 2 Resource: Adkins (p. 54)
The flexor carpi ulnaris (C8-T1) would not be innervated in a patient with C6 tetraplegia.

24. Answer: 1 Resource: Palmer (p. 87)
The calf band of an ankle-foot orthosis should be placed immediately inferior to the fibular head. A calf band superior to the level of the fibular head may interfere with the normal function of the knee, while placement directly over the fibular head may result in impingement of the peroneal nerve.

25. Answer: 2 Resource: Magee (p. 543)
The Lachman test is perhaps the most common ligamentous instability test designed to assess the integrity of the anterior cruciate ligament. It is most commonly performed with the patient in a supine position and the knee flexed 20-30 degrees.

26. Answer: 1 Resource: Kendall (p. 228)
The gravity eliminated position for the hip adductors is supine.

27. Answer: 3 Resource: Clarkson (p. 172)
In order to secure valid measurements of available range of motion physical therapists should not permit any type of substitution. In addition to shoulder adduction and lateral rotation, patients can also attempt to substitute for limited supination by ipsilateral trunk sidebending.

28. Answer: 1 Resource: Garrison (p. 95)
A patient with burns over the anterior aspect of the neck will have a tendency to maintain the head in a flexed position and therefore is at risk for acquiring a flexion contracture.

29. Answer: 1 Resource: Hoppenfeld (p. 183)
The common peroneal nerve can be palpated immediately below the head of the fibula. An injury to the nerve may result in foot drop.

30. Answer: 4 Resource: Ruoti (p. 44)
Heart rate response when immersed in water appears to be similar to the response expected for land activities during periods of rest and during periods of low intensity exercise, however during periods of high intensity exercise the response is diminished.

31. Answer: 1 Resource: Ratliffe (p. 26)
The tonic labyrinthine reflex creates full extension of the body and extremities when positioned in supine. Extension serves to limit the child's ability to flex the neck.

32. Answer: 2   Resource: Clarkson (p. 14)
Hip flexion range of motion is most appropriately assessed with the knee in a flexed position. Flexion of the knee approximates the origin and insertion of the hamstrings and therefore avoids passive insufficiency.

33. Answer: 3   Resource: Davies (p. 27)
The described pattern is a combination of both flexor and extensor synergies. The hip and knee reflect flexor synergy, while the ankle and toes reflect the extensor synergy. A combination of the two patterns is common.

34. Answer: 1   Resource: Kisner (p. 534)
Increased lordosis refers to an abnormal anterior convexity of the lumbar spine. A lordotic posture is often associated with stretched or weakened abdominal muscles.

35. Answer: 4   Resource: Anderson (p. 772)
Homolateral synkinesis is an associated reaction that can occur after neurological damage. Resistance to flexion of the affected upper extremity will cause flexion in the lower extremity.

36. Answer: 1   Resource: Hertling (p. 77)
Active range of motion provides the examiner with cursory information related to a patient's willingness to move, ability to move, strength, and range of motion. If the patient can successfully complete active range of motion without difficulty or pain, further passive range of motion testing may not be necessary.

37. Answer: 2   Resource: Kettenbach (p. 170)
A discharge summary provides an overview of the treatment provided and the progress made toward achieving established goals. The note should include a description of the patient's status at the time of discharge.

38. Answer: 3   Resource: Hickock (p. 143)
Audit size should be based on available personnel, topic selected, and the monitoring system used. Audits often are composed of samples significantly greater than 20.

39. Answer: 4   Resource: Minor (p. 56)
Gloves worn during patient care activities should not be reused since they may contain contaminants.

40. Answer: 2   Resource: O'Sullivan - Physical Rehabilitation (p. 666)
Maintaining an angle of increased hip flexion during late swing through heel strike will create an increased step length.

41. Answer: 4   Resource: Hertling (p. 352)
An acute medial meniscus injury would not produce hamstrings atrophy.

42. Answer: 1   Resource: Kahn (p. 24)
The inverse square law indicates that radiation intensity is inversely proportional to the square of the distance from the source to the target. In the stated example, the source is moved from 45 centimeters from the target area to 90 centimeters from the target area, increasing by a factor of two. As a result the intensity of the radiation reaching the target will fall to one-fourth of its previous level.

43. Answer: 3   Resource: Long (p. 122)
A child with athetoid cerebral palsy typically demonstrates disorganized movements with tone that fluctuates between hypotonic and hypertonic. The child's cognitive ability usually remains age appropriate.

44. Answer: 3   Resource: Magee (p. 250)
A position of 70 degrees of flexion allows the elbow to reach its maximum volume and therefore accommodates the swelling with less discomfort.

45. Answer: 4   Resource: Saunders (p. 82)
According to a study performed by Nachemson, intradiskal pressure is greatest when sitting in a chair with reduced lumbar lordosis.

46. Answer: 4   Resource: Kendall (p. 385)
The medial pectoral nerve originates from the medial cord of the brachial plexus. The nerve innervates pectoralis major and minor.

47. Answer: 4   Resource: National Safety Council (p. 114)
A seizure occurs as a result of abnormal stimulation of brain cells. Intervention should be initially limited to protecting the patient from injury. A seizure typically lasts less than two minutes.

48. Answer: 1   Resource: Kendall (p. 266)
A patient with C5 quadriplegia would be able to utilize muscles innervated at or above the C5 spinal level. The patient should be able to utilize the brachioradialis to flex the elbow since the muscle is innervated at the C5-C6 spinal level.

49. Answer: 3   Resource: Hoppenfeld (p. 66)
The scaphoid, also known as the navicular bone, makes up the floor of the anatomical snuffbox. The bone is located in the proximal carpal row and is the most frequently fractured carpal bone.

50. Answer: 4   Resource: Robinson (p. 295)
Transcutaneous electrical nerve stimulators deliver controlled, low voltage electrical impulses that can be used for pain relief during labor and delivery.

51. Answer: 1   Resource: Pierson (p. 47)
Normal range for pulse rate is 60-100 beats per minute, while respiration rate is 12-18 breaths per minute.

52. Answer: 1   Resource: Brannon (p. 250)
Abnormal blood pressure and pulse rate in a patient rehabilitating from a myocardial infarction is a significant finding that warrants consultation with the referring physician. Serious complications associated with myocardial infarction include arrhythmias, heart failure, and thrombolytic complications.

53. Answer: 4   Resource: Kendall (p. 154)
The double leg lowering test assesses the strength of the lower abdominals. The test is performed by slowly lowering the legs from a vertical position with the knees extended.

54. Answer: 2   Resource: Pierson (p. 198)
A patient grasping a walker in standing should exhibit 20-25 degrees of elbow flexion.

55. Answer: 4   Resource: Anemaet (p. 331)
With aging, individuals tend to exhibit decreased stride length, decreased swing phase duration, increased stride width, and increased stance phase duration. In normal gait the stance phase represents 60% of the gait cycle.

56. Answer: 4   Resource: Adkins (p. 136)
A patient with complete C4 tetraplegia has innervation of the sternocleidomastoids and trapezius muscles. This allows the patient to operate a power wheelchair using a chin control.

57. Answer: 4   Resource: National Safety Council (p. 32)
Mouth to mouth and nose breathing is appropriate for an infant (less than one-year-old).

58. Answer: 4   Resource: Kisner (p. 301)
The shoulder medial rotators and adductors provide support for the anterior joint capsule and as a result strengthening of these muscles is an essential component of a rehabilitation program following anterior shoulder dislocation.

59. Answer: 4   Resource: Kisner (p. 88)
Isokinetic knee extension and flexion require the distal segment to move freely in space, as a result the exercise is considered to be an open kinematic chain exercise.

60. Answer: 2   Resource: Magee (p. 628)
The tibialis anterior dorsiflexes the ankle, inverts the foot, and is innervated at the L4, L5, S1 spinal level. Patients with significant weakness due to peripheral neuropathy often utilize an ankle-foot orthosis in order to avoid having the foot slap the ground.

61. Answer: 4   Resource: Guide for Professional Conduct
Making a large incision along the periphery of a blister with a sterile instrument may be considered outside the physical therapist's scope of practice.

62. Answer: 1   Resource: Kisner (p. 457)
Biofeedback and quadriceps setting exercises offer patients the ability to sense or feel activation of the vastus medialis obliquus in a comfortable and efficient position. The activity offers a tangible method to reinforce selective strengthening of the muscle during formal physical therapy sessions or as part of a home exercise program.

63. Answer: 1   Resource: Kendall (p. 209)
The biceps femoris muscle acts to flex and laterally rotate the knee joint and is innervated by the peroneal and tibial portions of the sciatic nerve.

64. Answer: 3   Resource: Hoppenfeld (p. 21)
The supplied instructions can be used to examine shoulder abduction and lateral rotation. This type of gross screening examination is a component of the Apley scratch test.

65. Answer: 4   Resource: Hoppenfeld (p. 216)
The anterior talofibular ligament runs from the anterior aspect of the lateral malleolus to the lateral aspect of the talar neck. The ligament is commonly injured with an inversion ankle sprain.

66. Answer: 2   Resource: Pierson (p. 148)
Bilateral amputations cause a patient's center of gravity to be moved posteriorly, as a result the wheels on a wheelchair must also be moved in a posterior direction in order to maintain an acceptable center of gravity.

67. Answer: 3   Resource: Hoppenfeld (p. 66)
Extension of the thumb causes the borders of the anatomical snuffbox to become more prominent and as a result can be used as a method to identify the exact location of the scaphoid. Extension of the thumb occurs in a frontal plane around an anterior-posterior axis. Passive ulnar deviation of the wrist can also be utilized to facilitate palpation since the action serves to move the scaphoid out from under the radial styloid process.

68. Answer: 4   Resource: Magee (p. 12)
S2 nerve root:
   dermatome - buttock, thigh, and posterior leg
   myotome - plantar flexors and hamstrings
   reflexes - Achilles

69. Answer: 3   Resource: Pierson (p. 189)
In addition to extending the shoulder, the latissimus dorsi acts to support the body's weight and assists to propel the body forward.

70. Answer: 2   Resource: De Domenico (p. 51)
Transverse friction massage requires firm contact with the skin and subcutaneous tissues. Using a lubricant would make this type of contact impossible.

71. Answer: 3   Resource: Moore (p. 444)
The gluteus maximus extends the hip. The medius and minimus are responsible for abduction and medial rotation of the hip.

72. Answer: 1   Resource: Scott – Promoting Legal Awareness (p. 69)
An incident report is a factual written summary of an adverse event designed to memorialize specific details of the event and to limit future liability of the organization. Information obtained from the incident report is often used to guide risk management initiatives. Since the physical therapist directly observed the blistered skin and heard the patient relate the cause of the burn to the hot pack it is essential to complete an incident report.

73. Answer: 2   Resource: Mahler (p. 160)
The American College of Sports Medicine recommends prescribing the intensity of exercise as 60 to 90% of maximum heart rate or 50-85% of $VO_{2\,max}$ or heart rate reserve. The heart rate reserve method (Karvonen formula) is determined as follows:
Target heart rate range = $[(HR_{max} - HR_{rest}) *0.60$ and $0.85] + HR_{rest}$

74. Answer: 3   Resource: Saunders, R. (p. 28)
Varying the order of an exercise program is a common technique to avoid stagnation. Other listed options may change the focus of the exercise program or fail to address the patient's frustration in an appropriate manner.

75. Answer: 3   Resource: Rothstein (p. 112)
The calcaneonavicular ligament helps to maintain the medial longitudinal arch by supporting the head of the talus between the navicular and the calcaneus.

76. Answer: 2   Resource: Umphred (p. 945)
Intact sensation along with the absence of tone allows for a plastic orthosis with an articulating ankle joint. This type of orthosis allows for a more normal gait pattern.

77. Answer: 1   Resource: Kendall (p. 40)
Stabilizing the opposite leg while assessing the hamstrings length serves to limit posterior pelvic tilt and flexion of the lumber spine. Failure to adequately stabilize results in exaggerated hamstrings length.

78. Answer: 4   Resource: Paz (p. 287)
Signs and symptoms of Parkinson's disease include cogwheel rigidity, resting tremor, poor initiation of movement, shuffling gait, and flat affect.

79. Answer: 3   Resource: Currier (p. 100)
In a normal distribution a known percentage of the population falls between specific standard deviation units. The area between +1 and –1 standard deviation units represents approximately 68% of the population.

80. Answer: 1   Resource: Clinical Companion (p.324)
A tilt-in-space wheelchair is designed to provide pressure relief without shearing forces. The wheelchair has a fixed seat to back angle even when reclined and as a result is often able to accommodate customized seating systems. The wheelchair is commonly prescribed for patients unable to perform independent pressure relief.

81. Answer: 3   Resource: Ignatavicius (p. 595)
Respiratory isolation requires the use of a mask, but does not require the use of gowns or gloves. Examples of diseases that may require respiratory isolation include measles, pneumonia, and pertussis.

82. Answer: 2   Resource: Hoppenfeld (p. 199)
The navicular is located along the medial aspect of the foot, proximal to the cuneiforms and distal to the talus.

83. Answer: 3   Resource: Starkey (p. 143)
Effusion refers to an increased volume of fluid within the joint capsule. Effusion in the knee may serve to decrease active and passive range of motion.

84. Answer: 3   Resource: Guide for Professional Conduct
The therapist must consult with the referring physician when the prescribed treatment procedure is contraindicated.

85. Answer: 1   Resource: Irwin (p. 364)
Bronchial drainage positioning for the anterior segments of the upper lobes is with the patient in supine with pillows under the knees.

86. Answer: 1   Resource: Tierney (p. 1018)
Insulin dependent diabetes mellitus usually has its onset before the age of 30. The disease is characterized by an absence of circulating insulin. Exercise has been shown to increase the effectiveness of insulin and as a result may slightly reduce a patient's insulin requirement.

87. Answer: 3   Resource: O'Sullivan - Physical Rehabilitation (p. 1048)
An extended toe plate on an ankle-foot orthosis creates an extension moment at the knee by diminishing toe extension during toe off and subsequently reducing the knee's ability to flex.

88. Answer: 3   Resource: Michlovitz (p. 142)
The primary mode of heat loss during exercise occurs through perspiration and exhaling. Both mechanisms are examples of evaporation.

89. Answer: 3   Resource: Campbell, S. (p. 749)
Postural drainage should be the highest priority in the care of a patient with cystic fibrosis. Postural drainage enhances gas exchange by removing mucus from the lungs and limits the incidence of infection.

90. Answer: 2   Resource: Minor (p. 56)
The therapist should remove the sterile gloves after completing debridement. Failure to remove the gloves may result in the spread of contaminants.

91. Answer: 1   Resource: O'Sullivan - Physical Rehabilitation (p. 340)
The most appropriate recommendation must adequately address safety and the patient's postoperative condition. A raised toilet seat is essential in order to avoid excessive flexion of the hip and a tub bench can significantly reduce the incidence of falls while bathing.

92. Answer: 1   Resource: Sullivan - An Integrated Approach (p. 99)
The serratus anterior is responsible for scapular upward rotation and abduction. D1 flexion produces scapular elevation, abduction, and upward rotation.

93. Answer: 3   Resource: Scott – Promoting Legal Awareness (p. 201)
The physical therapist's primary objective should be to ensure patient safety. By reporting the observation to the therapist's supervisor the physical therapist has effectively delegated responsibility to the appropriate party. Although the behavior could be reported to the state licensing agency this action would not address the immediate patient safety issue.

94. Answer: 2   Resource: Thomas (p. 946)
Hypoglycemia refers to decreased blood sugar levels. Signs and symptoms of hypoglycemia include fatigue, malaise, irritability, headache, and hunger. Causes of hypoglycemia include injection of an excessive quantity of insulin, hyperfunction of the islets of Langerhans or dietary deficiency. Hematocrit and hemoglobin levels are not significantly affected with hypoglycemia.

95. Answer: 2   Resource: O'Sullivan - Physical Rehabilitation (p. 415)
Hooklying is a term used to describe a position where a patient is in supine with the hips and knees flexed and the feet in contact with the floor. In this position the physical therapist can facilitate rotation by moving the lower extremities across the midline.

96. Answer: 2   Resource: O'Sullivan - Physical Rehabilitation (p. 164)
Controlled mobility activities should emphasize weight shifting and trunk control with rotation. This type of activity may serve to decrease rigidity and improve the fluidity of gait in a patient with Parkinson's disease.

97. Answer: 4   Resource: Magee (p. 12)
C5 nerve root:
   dermatome - deltoid area, anterior aspect of the entire arm to the base of the thumb
   myotome - supraspinatus, infraspinatus, deltoid, biceps
   reflexes - biceps, brachioradialis

98. Answer: 2   Resource: Guide for Professional Conduct
The patient exhibits several signs and symptoms that may be associated with a condition such as cancer. Since the examination findings are inconclusive, it is advisable to consult with the referring physician.

99. Answer: 2   Resource: Pierson (p. 149)
Seat depth in an average size adult chair is 16 inches.

100. Answer: 4   Resource: Pierson (p. 203)
Two canes do not offer an adequate platform to transmit the upper extremity force necessary to perform a swing-to, swing-through, or three-point gait pattern.

101. Answer: 1   Resource: Pierson (p. 56)
Systolic pressure gradually increases as exercise intensity increases, however diastolic pressure remains relatively stable.

102. Answer: 2   Resource: Saunders (p. 125)
A lumbar laminectomy refers to the excision of a vertebral posterior arch, usually for the purpose of removing a herniated disc or other lesion. After a comprehensive rehabilitation program, most patients are able to gradually return to an activity level similar to their previous functional status.

103. Answer: 3   Resource: Kendall (p. 184)
The patient can actively move through his/her full available range. As a result, the muscle should be tested in an anti-gravity (against gravity) position.

104. Answer: 2   Resource: Sine (p. 279)
Anti-tip tubes are mounted on the posterior frame of the wheelchair and serve to prohibit the wheelchair from falling over backwards. This wheelchair accessory would be most essential in a patient with high level quadriplegia due to the patient's limited ability to actively control the wheelchair.

105. Answer: 4   Resource: Pierson (p. 266)
Tiny air bubbles in a peripheral I.V. line are not typically indicative of a complication of intravenous therapy.

106. Answer: 1   Resource: Pierson (p. 189)
A significant cognitive impairment may result in a patient being unable to safely use axillary crutches.

107. Answer: 1   Resource: Pierson (p. 13)
The patient must develop an understanding of the importance of the home exercise program in order for it to be considered a priority.

108. Answer: 3   Resource: Guide to Physical Therapist Practice (p. S42)
The physical therapist is the health care professional responsible for establishing the discharge plan and documenting the discharge summary.

109. Answer: 4   Resource: Umphred (p. 755)
Sequencing and general language deficits are commonly identified with damage to the left hemisphere and therefore would be more commonly associated with right hemiparesis.

110. Answer: 4   Resource: Magee (p. 12)
C8 nerve root:
   dermatome - medial arm and forearm to long, ring, and little finger
   myotome – ulnar deviators, thumb extensors, thumb adductors
   reflexes - triceps

111. Answer: 1   Resource: Irwin (p. 345)
Percussion of the lungs should produce normal resonance. Liver, heart, and viscera typically yield a dull sound.

112. Answer: 2   Resource: Brannon (p. 251)
The most immediate response should be to stop the exercise session. This action allows the therapist to assist the patient in a safe and effective manner. Further intervention may include contacting emergency medical services or a referral to the patient's primary care physician.

113. Answer: 3   Resource: Garrison (p. 120)
Patients who have sustained a cardiac event often are prescribed an exercise intensity that corresponds to 60% of the maximal heart rate obtained on a symptom-limited treadmill test. Patients without a significant cardiac history should exercise at an exercise intensity of 70% of maximal heart rate at least three times per week. Exercise sessions should range from 30-60 minutes.

114. Answer: 1   Resource: O'Sullivan - Physical Rehabilitation (p. 969)
Homonymous hemianopsia is a loss of vision in the temporal half of the visual field of one eye and the nasal portion of the visual field in the other eye. A physical therapist should educate the patient regarding her condition before employing compensatory strategies.

115. Answer: 2   Resource: Clinical Companion (p. 134)
Doppler ultrasonography is a noninvasive test that is used to evaluate blood flow in major arteries and veins. The diagnostic test is commonly utilized to monitor patients who are status post bypass graft or arterial reconstruction.

116. Answer: 3   Resource: Pierson (p. 49)
Thready is a descriptive term used to characterize the quality of a pulse. A thready pulse indicates a weak force to each beat and an irregular pattern.

117. Answer: 1   Resource: Kendall (p. 281)
The teres minor laterally rotates the shoulder and stabilizes the head of the humerus in the glenoid. The muscle is innervated by the axillary nerve.

118. Answer: 2   Resource: Payton - Psychosocial Aspects (p. 5)
For a patient who is acutely ill answering questions that require detailed responses can be exhausting.

119. Answer: 2   Resource: Brannon (p. 103)
Patients on bedrest following cardiac surgery are susceptible to developing a deep vein thrombosis due to circulatory stasis. Any indication of a potential thrombosis including tenderness and pain in the calf should be reported immediately.

120. Answer: 3   Resource: Pauls (p. 102)
Diabetes mellitus is a disorder of carbohydrate metabolism that results from inadequate production or uptake of insulin. Signs and symptoms of diabetes mellitus include polyuria, polydipsia, rapid weight loss, polyphagia, and elevation of blood glucose levels.

121. Answer: 1   Resource: Payton - Research (p. 173)
A t-test is used to determine the significance of the difference between the means of two sets of data.

122. Answer: 4   Resource: Paz (p. 360)
White blood cell count can be used to identify the presence of infection, allergens or the degree of immunosuppression.

123. Answer: 3   Resource: Magee (p. 247)
The radiohumeral joint is composed of the radial head articulating with the capitulum of the humerus. The close packed position is 90 degrees of elbow flexion and 5 degrees of forearm supination.

124. Answer: 4   Resource: Levangie (p. 301)
The hip joint consists of a convex femoral head within a concave acetabulum. Hip flexion requires a posterior and inferior translation of the femoral head within the acetabulum.

125. Answer: 3   Resource: Magee (p. 152)
A patient with limited range of motion in a capsular pattern at the temporomandibular joint would have the most difficulty opening the mouth.

126. Answer: 2   Resource: Purtillo - Health Professional (p. 149)
The statement "your present condition is serious" acknowledges the patient's condition without providing false hope. Since the patient was just informed of her terminal condition prior to the scheduled therapy session, it is premature to remind the patient of the therapy goals.

127. Answer: 2 Resource: Nixon (p. 140)
A manual wheelchair with handrim projections is appropriate for a patient with C5 tetraplegia. The projection handrims are necessary due to distal weakness and diminished proprioception.

128. Answer: 2 Resource: Michlovitz (p. 271)
Minimal erythemal dose is defined as the time necessary for mild reddening of the skin which appears within eight hours of treatment and disappears within 24 hours.

129. Answer: 2 Resource: Irwin (p. 339)
A whispered sound will not typically be audible through a stethoscope with normal air-filled lung tissue, but may be distinctly audible with consolidation.

130. Answer: 2 Resource: Brannon (p. 391)
A smoking cessation program offers the patient the support and resources necessary to optimize his chances of quitting.

131. Answer: 4 Resource: Magee (p. 215)
Yergason's test and Speed's test are common special tests utilized to identify bicipital tendonitis.

132. Answer: 2 Resource: Magee (p. 18)
A minor lesion of a muscle or tendon will often yield mild to moderate pain with resistance, without a resultant decrease in strength.

133. Answer: 4 Resource: Rothstein (p. 529)
Syncope is often associated with respiratory alkalosis.

134. Answer: 4 Resource: Magee (p. 306)
The Bunnel-Littler test can be used to assess several structures acting on the metacarpophalangeal joint. A positive test is demonstrated by an inability to flex the proximal interphalangeal joint and is indicative of intrinsic muscle tightness or a contracture of the joint capsule.

135. Answer: 3 Resource: Hertling (p. 496)
The anterior longitudinal ligament extends from C2 to the sacrum and functions to limit extension of the vertebral column.

136. Answer: 1 Resource: Kendall (p. 255)
The most common patient position to utilize when testing the extensor digitorum is sitting, however a supine position is also acceptable.

137. Answer: 2 Resource: Norkin (p. 221)
According to the American Academy of Orthopedic Surgeons available range of motion for the wrist is as follows: extension 0-70 degrees, flexion 0-80 degrees, radial deviation 0-20 degrees, and ulnar deviation 0-30 degrees.

138. Answer: 2 Resource: Kendall (p. 106)
Lordosis refers to an abnormal anterior convexity of the lumbar spine. The postural condition is characterized by lumbar spine hyperextension and excessive anterior pelvic tilt resulting in shortening of the erector spinae and hip flexor muscles.

139. Answer: 3 Resource: Rothstein (p. 763)
The Fugl-Meyer is used to determine the level of recovery after a CVA. The assessment tool emphasizes the examination of motor function, range of motion, and balance.

140. Answer: 1 Resource: Thomas (p. 186)
The Babinski reflex occurs by stimulating the lateral sole of the foot with resultant extension of the great toe. The reflex normally occurs in infants up to six months of age.

141. Answer: 2 Resource: Norkin (p. 221)
According to the American Academy of Orthopedic Surgeons, normal pronation of the forearm is 80 degrees.

142. Answer: 1 Resource: Norkin (p. 54)
When measuring shoulder flexion, the axis of the goniometer should be aligned closely with the acromion process. Normal shoulder flexion range of motion is 0-180 degrees.

143. Answer: 2 Resource: Kendall (p. 268)
The action of the biceps is elbow flexion and forearm supination. As a result passive elbow extension and forearm pronation maximally lengthen the muscle and therefore place the greatest amount of tension on the biceps tendon.

144. Answer: 3 Resource: Rothstein (p. 467)
Approximation is a facilitation technique used to enhance muscle tone. Joint approximation attempts to facilitate cocontraction of muscles around a joint in order to increase joint stability.

145. Answer: 1 Resource: Pierson (p. 200)
The physical therapist should be positioned in front of the patient when beginning ambulation activities. The position enables the therapist to effectively guard the patient and at the same time monitor the patient's facial expressions for signs of distress. The width of the parallel bars would not permit the therapist to be positioned to the side of the patient and it would be inappropriate to guard the patient from outside of the parallel bars.

146. Answer: 4 Resource: Richard (p. 137)
All of the listed options are commonly utilized topical antibiotics, however Bacitracin, Furacin, and Neosporin are used on superficial burns, donor sites, and healing skin grafts. Silver sulfadiazine is more appropriate for use on deeper or infected wounds.

147. Answer: 1   Resource: De Domenico (p. 35)
Effleurage is defined as a slow, stroking movement performed over a large body area in the direction of the venous and lymphatic flow. The massage stroke is commonly incorporated into a treatment program to provide continuity between various massage strokes.

148. Answer: 1   Resource: Norkin (p. 64)
Abducting the arm to 90 degrees and flexing the elbow to 90 degrees allows for adequate exposure of the appropriate bony landmarks.

149. Answer: 1   Resource: Norkin (p. 128)
Hip abduction occurs in a frontal plane. Failure to stay within the frontal plane often yields compensatory motion such as flexion and lateral rotation.

150. Answer: 3   Resource: Hickock (p. 99)
Failure to complete documentation in a timely manner can have potentially serious ramifications. A function of the supervisor is to assist therapists with prioritizing patient needs and improving time management skills.

151. Answer: 3   Resource: Hall (p. 363)
Patient with weak pelvic floor muscles often experience rapid fatigue during strengthening exercises. As a result, exercise parameters typically include a relatively low number of repetitions and a high number of sets usually in the range of five or six per day.

152. Answer: 4   Resource: Minor (p. 292)
Poor lower extremity strength and coordination requires a stable assistive device such as a walker.

153. Answer: 4   Resource: Haggard (p. 43)
A home exercise program that is excessively lengthy will serve to decrease compliance.

154. Answer: 3   Resource: O'Sullivan - Physical Rehabilitation (p. 1031)
A metal upright ankle-foot orthosis with an inadequate dorsiflexion stop will allow the tibia to advance over the foot during the stance phase of gait. If there is inadequate quadriceps strength, the knee will remain flexed resulting in diminished stability.

155. Answer: 1   Resource: Sullivan - An Integrated Approach (p. 140)
Contract-relax is a proprioceptive neuromuscular facilitation technique utilized to increase range of motion on one side of a joint. The technique utilizes isometric as well as isotonic contractions.

156. Answer: 3   Resource: Kettenbach (p. 96)
Short-term goals are considered intermediate steps toward achieving established long-term goals. Both short-term and long-term goals are part of the assessment section of a S.O.A.P. note.

157. Answer: 2   Resource: Norkin (p. 74)
The end-feel associated with elbow extension is most often classified as hard due to contact between the ulna and the radius.

158. Answer: 3   Resource: Rothstein (p. 801)
Plantar flexor weakness would affect toe off during the late stance phase of gait.

159. Answer: 3   Resource: Guide for Professional Conduct
Failure to address the student's improper guarding technique may unnecessarily jeopardize patient safety.

160. Answer: 2   Resource: O'Sullivan - Physical Rehabilitation (p. 754)
A patient with Parkinson's disease would benefit from activities that emphasize rotation of the trunk and subsequent arm swing. Rotation allows for improvement in weight shifting, step length, and reciprocal arm swing.

161. Answer: 1   Resource: Konin (p. 185)
When completing the Thomas test the physical therapist stabilizes the pelvis in order to limit lumbar lordosis and anterior pelvic tilt. Failure to adequately stabilize the pelvis may allow the patient to lower the test leg to the table despite the presence of tight hip flexors.

162. Answer: 4   Resource: O'Sullivan - Physical Rehabilitation (p. 555)
A patient with hemiplegia should not bear weight through the palm in a flattened position. The position will eventually collapse the palmar arches and create more difficulty for motor return in the hand. Weight bearing should be directed through the heel of the hand.

163. Answer: 3   Resource: Standards of Practice
The patient has made progress in a limited number of physical therapy visits and as a result may significantly benefit from additional treatments. A physical therapist is the most appropriate health care professional to administer joint mobilization techniques.

164. Answer: 3   Resource: Campbell, M. (p. 157)
A patient functioning at Rancho Los Amigos level IV, confused-agitated, may be particularly susceptible to changes in behavior based on fatigue. Ideally the physical therapist should attempt to maintain the integrity of the current treatment regimen, however if increased rest periods do not produce an observable change in the patient's behavior it may be appropriate to modify other parameters such as the frequency or length of treatment.

165. Answer: 1   Resource: O'Sullivan - Physical Rehabilitation (p. 901)
A patient with C7 tetraplegia can strengthen the serratus anterior and scapular muscles in a prone on elbows position. This activity can be extremely useful to assist with bed mobility.

166. Answer: 3   Resource: Kendall (p. 205)
Standing on the tiptoes requires plantar flexion and toe extension. This activity provides a gross indicator of range of motion, but does not control for other variables.

167. Answer: 2   Resource: Kendall (p. 259)
The flexor carpi ulnaris acts to flex the wrist and is innervated by the ulnar nerve. The flexor carpi radialis, flexor digitorum superficialis, and palmaris longus are innervated by the median nerve.

168. Answer: 2   Resource: Reese (p. 305)
The tibialis anterior (p. L4, L5, S1) is innervated by the deep peroneal nerve. When testing the muscle the therapist offers resistance by pushing against the dorsal and medial aspect of the head of the first metatarsal bone in the direction of plantar flexion and eversion.

169. Answer: 4   Resource: Kendall (p. 249)
The palmar interossei act to adduct the thumb, index, ring, and little finger toward the axial line through the third digit. The muscles are innervated by the ulnar nerve.

170. Answer: 2   Resource: DePoy (p. 244)
The median is a measure of central tendency that lies at the midpoint of a distribution. Inspection rather than calculation can often determine the median.

171. Answer: 2   Resource: Ratliffe (p. 45)
A five month old infant is able to play on extended arms and grasp toys using an ulnar-palmar grasp. The infant is able to bear weight through the lower extremities when in supported standing and may be able to ring sit without support for short periods of time.

172. Answer: 1   Resource: Kettenbach (p. 31)
Since the patient verbalizes the concern about muscle atrophy, the information is best recorded in the subjective section of a S.O.A.P. note.

173. Answer: 3   Resource: Kendall (p. 75)
Assuming normal posture, a plumb line should fall through the lobe of the ear, midway through the trunk, through the greater trochanter, slightly anterior to a midline through the knee, and slightly anterior to the lateral malleolus.

174. Answer: 3   Resource: Pierson (p. 204)
A swing-through gait pattern relies on upper extremity strength to propel the body through the point where the assistive devices were advanced. Any significant upper extremity weakness would make this gait pattern extremely difficult to perform.

175. Answer: 1   Resource: Kisner (p. 397)
Hip adduction is contraindicated following total hip replacement surgery.

176. Answer: 3   Resource: Hertling (p. 535)
Nystagmus, slurring of speech, and loss of consciousness are contraindications to traction and mobilization in the upper cervical spine.

177. Answer: 1   Resource: Sullivan - Clinical Decision Making (p. 277)
The use of agonistic reversals in bridging promotes eccentric control of the hip extensors and hamstrings through applied resistance.

178. Answer: 3   Resource: Arnheim (p. 240)
A functional progression requires a patient to perform sport specific activities that demonstrate readiness to return to competition.

179. Answer: 4   Resource: Michlovitz (p. 71)
Random changes in the intensity of an ultrasound generator can be indicative of equipment malfunction. Failure to discontinue use of the machine is a potentially negligent act.

180. Answer: 1   Resource: Kisner (p. 139)
The resting heart rate of an adult is not influenced by age.

181. Answer: 4   Resource: Purtillo - Health Professional (p. 255)
A therapist should attempt to treat patients in a timely fashion. Since the remaining options do not require immediate action, the therapist's priority should be the patient who has been waiting.

182. Answer: 2   Resource: Umphred (p. 830)
A patient with unilateral left neglect must learn to compensate through scanning and conscious attention towards the left. Placing food on the right side of the tray will not improve the patient's ability to compensate for the neglect.

183. Answer: 2   Resource: Arnheim (p. 274)
Pulling the stirrups toward inversion will tend to place the ankle in a slightly inverted position and as a result will make the patient more susceptible to an inversion sprain.

184. Answer: 3　　Resource:　Magee (p. 12)
C7 nerve root:
　dermatome - lateral arm and forearm to index, long, and ring fingers
　myotome - triceps, wrist flexors
　reflexes - triceps

185. Answer: 1　　Resource:　Irwin (p. 51)
P wave - atrial depolarization, QRS complex - ventricular depolarization, T wave - ventricular repolarization.

186. Answer: 2　　Resource:　Hertling (p. 267)
A Colles' fracture is defined as a fracture of the radius within one inch of the wrist.

187. Answer: 1　　Resource:　Norkin (p. 76)
When measuring pronation of the forearm, the moving arm of the goniometer is aligned along the dorsal aspect of the wrist, immediately proximal to the styloid processes.

188. Answer: 2　　Resource:　Pierson (p. 49)
Bradycardic is an adjective that is used to describe the noun bradycardia. Bradycardia is a term used to describe a heart rate of less than 60 beats per minute.

189. Answer: 4　　Resource:　Paz (p. 375)
Signs and symptoms of a deep venous thrombosis include a positive Homans' sign, swelling, redness, and warmth in the calf. Physical therapy treatment should not continue until a physician clears the patient.

190. Answer: 2　　Resource:　Sullivan – Clinical Decision Making (p. 64)
Hold-relax is an active exercise technique designed to increase range of motion in situations where there is muscle tightness on one side of a joint. Failure to modify the technique to accommodate for pain will result in muscle splinting and increased pain during active contraction.

191. Answer: 3　　Resource:　Minor (p. 34)
Pulse rate should be measured for a full minute with any identified arrhythmia.

192. Answer: 4　　Resource:　Norkin (p. 90)
When measuring ulnar deviation of the wrist, the moveable arm of the goniometer is aligned with the dorsal midline of the third metacarpal.

193. Answer: 1　　Resource:　Kendall (p. 385)
An injury to the lateral cord of the brachial plexus would affect the musculocutaneous nerve. The musculocutaneous nerve innervates the coracobrachialis, biceps, and brachialis which are responsible for elbow flexion and supination of the forearm.

194. Answer: 3　　Resource:　De Domenico (p. 37)
Petrissage is characterized by firm pressure to a fold of skin and the underlying tissues. Massage strokes considered to be variations of petrissage include kneading, wringing, rolling, and pinching.

195. Answer: 2　　Resource:　O'Sullivan - Physical Rehabilitation (p. 882)
Sexual response in patients with spinal cord injuries is primarily based on the level of injury. Males with spinal cord lesions above the cauda equina will likely be able to achieve a reflexogenic erection, however will be unable to ejaculate.

196. Answer: 2　　Resource:　Brotzman (p. 345)
Palpating the head of the talus in a weight bearing or non-weight bearing position is the primary method for determining subtalar neutral. The head of the talus can be palpated using the thumb and forefinger of one hand while using the other hand to manipulate the foot or cue the patient. The subtalar neutral position is described as the position of the foot where the subtalar joint, talonavicular joint, and calcaneocuboid joint are all in a congruous relationship.

197. Answer: 1　　Resource:　Sullivan - An Integrated Approach (p. 12)
D1 flexion pattern of the lower extremity includes hip flexion, adduction, and lateral rotation. The knee can remain in extension or flexion, while the foot moves into dorsiflexion and inversion.

198. Answer: 2　　Resource:　Kisner (p. 253)
Performing stretching activities at specified intervals can be an effective means to limit repetitive use injuries. The activities provide workers with an opportunity to take an active role in managing their own health.

199. Answer: 4　　Resource:　Sullivan - Clinical Decision Making (p. 210)
Alternating isometrics and timing for emphasis are techniques that can be used in order to strengthen the abdominals and increase overall stability through the use of overflow.

200. Answer: 2　　Resource:　O'Sullivan - Physical Rehabilitation (p. 988)
Ideomotor apraxia occurs from an insult to the dominant hemisphere of the brain in the supramarginal gyrus. Ideomotor apraxia is a condition where a patient cannot perform functional movements or tasks upon command, but can perform tasks automatically.

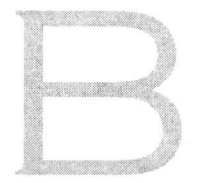

Bibliography

Adkins H: Spinal Cord Injury, Churchill Livingstone, 1985

American Heritage Dictionary, Dell Publishing Company, 1983

American Heart Association: BLS for Health Care Providers, American Heart Association, 2001

American Red Cross: Emergency Response, The American National Red Cross, 1997

Anemaet W, Moffa-Trotter M: Home Rehabilitation: Guide to Clinical Practice, Mosby, Inc., 2000

Anderson K, Anderson L: Mosby's Medical, Nursing & Allied Health Dictionary, Fifth Edition, Mosby, Inc., 1998

Arends R: Learning to Teach, Second Edition, McGraw-Hill Inc., 1991

Arnheim D: Essentials of Athletic Training, Third Edition, Mosby-Year Book, Inc., 1995

Bailey D: Research for the Health Professional: A Practical Guide, F.A. Davis, 1991

Bailey D, Robinson D: Therapeutic Approaches in Mental Health/Psychiatric Nursing, F.A. Davis Company, 1997

Basmajan J, Wolf S: Therapeutic Exercise, Williams and Wilkins, 1990

Bennett S, Karnes J: Neurological Disabilities: Assessment and Treatment, Lippincott-Raven Publishers, 1998

Berger K: The Developing Person Through the Lifespan, Worth, 1994

Berkow R: The Merck Manual, Merck Sharp & Dohme Research Laboratories, 1982

Best J, Kahn J: Research in Education, Fifth Edition, Prentice-Hall, 1986

Bickley L, Hoekelman R: Bates' Guide to Physical Examination and History Taking, Lippincott Williams and Wilkins, 1998

Bly L: Motor Skill Acquisition in the First Year, Therapy Skill Builders, 1994

Bobath B: Adult Hemiplegia: Evaluation and Treatment, Heinemann Medical Books Limited, 1978

Boissonnault W: Examination in Physical Therapy Practice: Screening for Medical Disease, Second Edition, Churchill Livingstone, 1995

Booher J, Thibodeau G: Athletic Injury Assessment, Mosby-Year Book, Inc., 1994

Bootzin R, Acoceila J: Abnormal Psychology, Random House, 1984

Brannon F, Foley M, Starr J, Saul L: Cardiopulmonary Rehabilitation: Basic Theory and Application, F.A. Davis, 1998

Brotzman S: Clinical Orthopedic Rehabilitation, Mosby-Year Book, Inc., 1996

Brunnstrom S: Movement Therapy in Hemiplegia, Harper and Row Publishers Inc., 1970

Buchanan L, Nawoczenski D: Spinal Cord Injury: Concepts and Management Approaches, Williams & Wilkins, 1987

Cameron M: Physical Agents in Rehabilitation: From Research to Practice, W.B. Saunders Company, 1998

Campbell M: Rehabilitation for Traumatic Brain Injury: Physical Therapy Practice in Context, Churchill Livingstone, 2000

Campbell S, Physical Therapy for Children, Second Edition, W.B. Saunders, 2000

Clarkson H: Musculoskeletal Assessment: Joint Range of Motion and Manual Muscle Strength, Second Edition, 1989

Carpenter M: Core Text of Neuroanatomy, Williams and Wilkins, 1985

Ciccone C: Pharmacology in Rehabilitation, Second Edition, F.A. Davis, 1996

Clark C, Bonfiglio M: Orthopaedics: Essentials of Diagnosis and Treatment, Churchill Livingstone, 1994

Code of Ethics, American Physical Therapy Association, 2001

Cohen H: Neuroscience for Rehabilitation, J.B. Lippincott Company, 1993

Cook A: Assistive Technologies: Principles and Practice, Mosby-Year Book, Inc., 1995

Currier D: Elements of Research in Physical Therapy, Second Edition, Williams & Wilkins, 1984

Curtis K: The Physical Therapist's Guide to Health Care, Slack Inc., 1999

Daniels K, Worthingham C: Muscle Testing Techniques of Manual Examination, W.B. Saunders, 1986

Davies P: Steps to Follow, Springer-Verlag, 1985

Davis C: Patient Practitioner Interaction, Third Edition, Slack Inc., 1998

De Domenico G, Wood E: Beard's Massage, W.B. Saunders Company, 1997

DePoy E, Gitlin L: Introduction to Research: Multiple Strategies for Health and Human Services, Mosby-Year Book, Inc., 1994

Domholdt E: Physical Therapy Research Principles and Application, Second Edition, W.B. Saunders Company, 2000

Edelman C, Mandle C: Health Promotion, Mosby, 1990

Edmond S: Manipulation and Mobilization: Extremity and Spinal Techniques, Mosby-Year Book, Inc., 1993

Educator's Guide to the Americans with Disabilities Act, American Vocational Association, 1993

Ellis D, Lamkowitz S, Maisey-Ireland M: Master Student, College Survival Inc., 1986

Fiorentino M: A Basis for Sensorimotor Development-Normal and Abnormal, Charles C. Thomas, 1981

Fox E, Mathews D: The Physiologic Basis of Physical Education and Athletics, Saunders College Publishing, 1981

Frownfelter D, Dean E: Principles and Practice of Cardiopulmonary Physical Therapy, Third Edition, Mosby-Year Book, Inc., 1996

Garrison S: Physical Medicine and Rehabilitation Basics, J.B. Lippincott Company, 1995

Giles S, Sanders R: Examination Preparation: A Complete Guide for the Physical Therapist, Mainely Physical Therapy, 1998

Giles S, Stuart J: Test Master: Physical Therapist Examination, Mainely Physical Therapy, 2001

Goldenson R: Disability and Rehabilitation Handbook, McGraw Hill, 1978

Goodman C, Snyder T: Differential Diagnosis in Physical Therapy, Third Edition, W.B. Saunders Company, 2000

Goold G: First Aid in the Workplace, Prentice Hall, 1995

Gross J, Fetto J, Rosen E: Musculoskeletal Examination, Blackwell Science Inc., 1996

Guide to Physical Therapist Practice, Second Edition, American Physical Therapy Association, 2001

Guide for Professional Conduct, American Physical Therapy Association, 2001

Guyton M: Textbook of Medical Physiology, W.B. Saunders Company, 1986

Haggard A: Handbook of Patient Education, Aspen Publishers, 1989

Hall C, Brody L: Therapeutic Exercise: Moving Toward Function, Lippincott Williams & Wilkins, 1999

Hamann B: Disease: Identification, Prevention, and Control, Mosby-Year Book, Inc., 1994

Hamill J, Knutzen K: Biomechanical Basis of Human Movement, Williams & Wilkins, 1995

Hamilton E, Whitney E, Sizer F: Nutrition Concepts and Controversies, Third Edition, West Publishing Company, 1982

Hermann N: The Creative Brain, Brain Books, 1990

Hertfelder S, Gwin C: Work in Progress: Occupational Therapy in Work Programs, American Occupational Therapy Association, 1989

Hertling D, Kessler R: Management of Common Musculoskeletal Disorders, Third Edition, Lippincott, 1996

Hickock R: Physical Therapy Administration and Management, Williams and Wilkins, 1982

Hill J: The Problem-Oriented Approach to Physical Therapy Care, American Physical Therapy Association, 1987

Hillegas E, Sadowsky H: Cardiopulmonary Physical Therapy, Second Edition, W.B. Saunders Company, 2001

Hilt N, Cogburn S: Manual of Orthopedics, 1980

Hoppenfeld S: Physical Examination of the Spine and Extremities, Appleton-Century-Crofts, 1976

Ignatavicius D, Workman L: Medical Surgical Nursing: A Nursing Process Approach, Volume I, Second Edition, W.B. Saunders Company, 1995

Irwin S, Tecklin J: Cardiopulmonary Physical Therapy, Third Edition, Mosby-Year Book, Inc., 1995

Kahn J: Principles and Practice of Electrotherapy, 2000

Kee J: Laboratory & Diagnostic Tests with Nursing Implications, Fourth Edition, Appleton & Lange, 1995

Kendall F, McCreary E, Provance P: Muscle Testing and Function, Williams and Wilkins, 1993

Kettenbach G: Writing S.O.A.P. Notes, Second Edition, F.A. Davis, 1995

Kisner C, Colby L: Therapeutic Exercise Foundations and Techniques, F.A. Davis, 1996

Knight W: Managed Care: What it is and How it Works, Aspen Publishers, 1998

Konin J, Wiksten D, Isear J: Special Tests for Orthopedic Examination, Slack Inc., 1997

Kozier B, Erb G: Techniques of Clinical Nursing, Addison-Wesley, 1989

Leek J, Gershwin ME, Fowler WM: Principles of Physical Medicine and Rehabilitation in the Musculoskeletal Diseases, Grune and Stratton Inc., 1986

Levangie P, Norkin C: Joint Structure and Function: A Comprehensive Analysis, Third Edition, F.A. Davis, 2001

Lewis B: Geriatric Physical Therapy: A Clinical Approach, Appleton & Lange, 1994

Long T, Cintas H: Handbook of Pediatric Physical Therapy, Williams & Wilkins, 1995

Magee D: Orthopedic Physical Assessment, W.B. Saunders Company, 1997

Mahler H: American College of Sports Medicine's Guidelines for Exercise Testing and Prescription, Fifth Edition, Lippincott Williams and Wilkins, 1995

Malone T, McPoil T, Nitz A: Orthopedic and Sports Physical Therapy, Third Edition, Mosby-Year Book, Inc., 1997

Mathews J: Practice Issues in Physical Therapy, Slack Inc., 1989

McConnell J: Understanding Human Behavior, CBS College Publishing, 1983

Meyer T: Review Books for Physical Therapy Licensing Exam, Volume I and II, Midwest Hi-Tech Publishers, 1989

Michlovitz S: Thermal Agents in Rehabilitation, Third Edition, F.A. Davis, 1996

Miller B: Miller-Keane: Encyclopedia & Dictionary of Medicine, Nursing & Allied Health, Sixth Edition, W.B. Saunders Company, 1997

Minor M, Minor S: Patient Care Skills, Fourth Edition, Appleton & Lange, 1999

Moore K: Clinically Oriented Anatomy, Williams and Wilkins, 1985

National Physical Therapy Examination Handbook, Federation of State Board, 2000

National Safety Council First Aid & CPR, Jones and Bartlett Publishers, 1997

Neistadt M, Crepeau E: Occupational Therapy, Ninth Edition, Lippincott, 1998

Nelson R, Hayes K, Currier DP: Clinical Electrotherapy, Third Edition, Appleton & Lange, 1999

Nixon V: Spinal Cord Injury-A Guide to Functional Outcomes in Physical Therapy Management, Aspen Publishers, 1985

Norkin C, White D: Measurement of Joint Motion: A Guide to Goniometry, Edition Two, F.A. Davis, 1995

Nosse L, Friberg D: Management Principles for Physical Therapists, Williams and Wilkins, 1992

O'Donoghue D: Treatment of Injuries to Athletes, W.B. Saunders Company, 1984

Ornstein, Thompson: The Amazing Brain, Houghton-Mifflin Company, 1984

O'Sullivan S, Schmitz T: Physical Rehabilitation: Assessment and Treatment, Fourth Edition, F.A. Davis, 2001

O'Sullivan S, Schmitz T: Physical Rehabilitation Laboratory Manual: Focus on Functional Training, F.A. Davis, 1999

Pagliarulo M: Introduction to Physical Therapy, Mosby-Year Book, 1996

Palmar L, Epler M: Clinical Assessment Procedures in Physical Therapy, J.B. Lippincott Company, 1990

Palmer M, Toms J: Manual for Functional Training, Third Edition, F.A. Davis, 1992

Paris S, Patla C: Extremity Dysfunction and Manipulation, Patris Inc., 1988

Pauls J, Reed K: Quick Reference to Physical Therapy, Aspen Publishers, 1996

Payton O: Psychosocial Aspects of Clinical Practice, Churchill Livingstone, 1986

Payton O: Research: The Validation of Clinical Practice, Edition Three, F.A. Davis, 1991

Paz J, Panik M: Acute Care Handbook for Physical Therapists, Butterworth-Heinemann, 1997

Physical Therapist's Clinical Companion, Springhouse Corporation, 2000

Pierson F: Principles and Techniques of Patient Care, Second Edition, W.B. Saunders Company, 1999

Portney L, Watkins M: Foundations of Clinical Research: Applications to Practice, Appleton & Lange, 1993

Post Stroke Rehabilitation, U. S. Department of Health and Human Services, 1995

Prentice W: Therapeutic Modalities for Allied Health Professionals, McGraw-Hill Companies, Inc., 1998

Purtilo R: Ethical Dimensions in the Health Professions, Second Edition, W.B. Saunders Company, 1993

Purtilo R: Health Professional and Patient Interaction, Fifth Edition, W.B. Saunders Company, 1996

Raffel M, Raffel N: The United States Health System, Delmar Publishers Inc., 1994

Ratliffe K: Clinical Pediatric Physical Therapy: A Guide for the Physical Therapy Team, Mosby Company, 1998

Reese N: Muscle and Sensory Testing, W.B. Saunders Company, 1999

Richard R, Staley M: Burn Care and Rehabilitation: Principles and Practice, F.A. Davis, 1994

Robinson A, Snyder-Mackler L: Clinical Electrophysiology, Williams & Wilkins, 1995

Rothstein J, Roy S, Wolf S: The Rehabilitation Specialist's Handbook, F.A. Davis, 1998

Roy S, Irvin R: Sports Medicine: Prevention, Evaluation, Management and Rehabilitation, Prentice-Hall, 1983

Ruoti R, Morris D, Cole A: Aquatic Rehabilitation, Lippincott Williams & Wilkins, 1997

Saidoff D: Critical Pathways in Therapeutic Intervention: Upper Extremities, Mosby-Year Book, 1997

Salter R: Textbook of Disorders and Injuries of the Musculoskeletal System, Third Edition, Williams & Wilkins, 1999

Saunders D: Evaluation, Treatment and Prevention of Musculoskeletal Disorders, Viking Press, 1985

Saunders J: Industrial Rehabilitation: Techniques for Success, Saunders Group, 1995

Scott R: Health Care Malpractice, Slack Inc., 1990

Scott R: Professional Ethics: A Guide for Rehabilitation Professionals, Mosby Inc., 1998

Scott R: Promoting Legal Awareness in Physical and Occupational Therapy, Mosby Inc., 1997

Shepard K, Jensen G: Handbook of Teaching for Physical Therapists, Butterworth-Heinemann 1997

Shumway-Cook A, Woollacott M: Motor Control: Theory and Applications, Williams & Wilkins, 1995

Sine R, Liss S: Basic Rehabilitation Techniques: A Self Instructional Guide, Fourth Edition, Aspen Publishers, 2000

Soderburg G: Kinesiology: Application to Pathological Motion, Williams and Wilkins, 1986

Somers M: Spinal Cord Injury: Functional Rehabilitation, Appleton & Lange, 1992

Standards of Practice for Physical Therapy and the Accompanying Criteria, American Physical Therapy Association, 2001

Starkey C, Ryan J: Evaluation of Orthopedic and Athletic Injuries, F.A. Davis, 1996

Stokes M: Neurological Physiotherapy, Mosby International Limited, 1998

Sullivan S, Markos P, Minor M: An Integrated Approach to Therapeutic Exercise, Reston Publishing Company, 1982

Sullivan P, Markos P: Clinical Decision Making in Therapeutic Exercise, Appleton & Lange, 1995

Sultz H: Health Care USA: Understanding its Organization and Delivery, Second Edition, Aspen Publishers, 1999

Thomas C: Taber's Cyclopedic Medical Dictionary, Edition 18, F.A. Davis, 1997

Tecklin J: Pediatric Physical Therapy, Edition Three, Lippincott Williams & Wilkins, 1999

Tierney L: Current Medical Diagnosis and Treatment, 34th Edition, Appleton & Lange, 1995

Trofino R: Nursing Care of the Burn Injured Patient, F.A. Davis, 1991

Umphred D: Neurological Rehabilitation, Fourth Edition, Mosby Inc., 2001

Van Deusen J: Assessment in Occupational and Physical Therapy, W.B. Saunders, 1997

Wade, Carole, Travis: Psychology, Harper Collins College Publishers, 1993

Wadsworth C: Manual Examination and Treatment of the Spine and Extremities, Williams and Wilkins, 1988

Walter J: Physical Therapy Management, Mosby, 1993

Waxman S, deGroot J: Correlative Neuroanatomy, Appleton & Lange, 1995

White T: The Wellness Guide to Lifelong Fitness, Health Letter Associates, 1993

Wortman C: Psychology, Third Edition, Alfred A. Knopf, Inc., 1988

Zadai C: Clinics in Physical Therapy - Pulmonary Management in Physical Therapy, Churchill Livingstone, 1992

Zydlo S, Hill J: The American Medical Association Handbook of First Aid & Emergency Care, Random House, 1990

Licensing Examination Resources

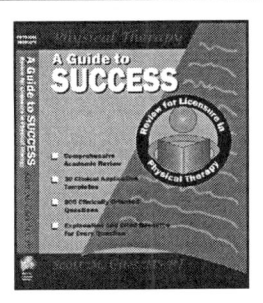

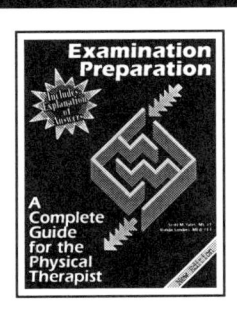

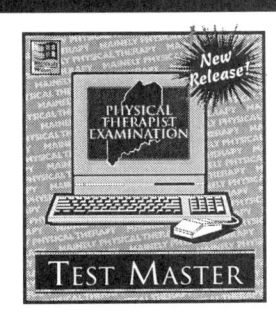

Acheive Your Goals... ORDER TODAY!

COMPREHENSIVE PACKAGE

TITLE	QTY	RETAIL PRICE	SUBTOTAL
Ultimate Review – PT		89.85	

INDIVIDUAL COMPONENTS

TITLE	QTY	RETAIL PRICE	SUBTOTAL
A Guide to Success – PT		39.95	
Examination Preparation – PT		33.95	
Test Master – PT (Diskettes)		35.95	

Shipping Charges $ 5.75

ORDER TOTAL

Method of Payment

☐ I've enclosed check # _____ payable to Mainely Physical Therapy

☐ Please charge to:

☐ Mastercard   ☐ Visa   Exp. Date __ __/__ __

☐ AMEX   ☐ Discover

☐ Card No. ____-____-____-____

☐ Signature _____
REQUIRED TO PROCESS ORDER

Ship to:

Name _____

Address _____

City _____

State _____ Zip _____

Phone (   ) _____

e-mail _____

Mainely Physical Therapy
P.O. Box 7242 ▪ Scarborough, ME 04070-7242
(207) 885-0304 ▪ Fax: (207) 883-8377 ▪ Web Site: www.ptexams.com
Toll Free: 866-PTEXAMS